FIFTH EDITION

KRAMER AND HINOJOSA'S FRAMES OF REFERENCE

for Pediatric Occupational Therapy

FIFTH EDITION

KRAMER AND HINOJOSA'S FRAMES OF REFERENCE

for Pediatric Occupational Therapy

PAULA KRAMER PhD, OTR, FAOTA
Professor Emeritus
University of the Sciences (now St. Joseph's University)
Philadelphia, Pennsylvania

TSU-HSIN HOWE PhD, OTR, FAOTA
Associate Professor and Chair
New York University
Department of Occupational Therapy
Steinhardt School of Culture, Education and Human Development
New York, New York

FRANCINE M. SERUYA PhD, MBA, OTR/L, FAOTA
Professor and Program Director, Masters in Occupational Therapy
Mercy University
Dobbs Ferry, New York

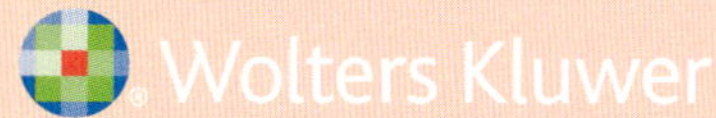

Wolters Kluwer

Philadelphia • Baltimore • New York • London
Buenos Aires • Hong Kong • Sydney • Tokyo

Senior Acquisitions Editor: Lindsey Porambo
Senior Development Editor: Amy Millholen
Editorial Coordinator: Vinodhini Varadharajalu
Editorial Assistant: Hillary Barry
Marketing Manager: Kirsten Watrud
Production Project Manager: Kirstin Johnson
Design Coordinator: Stephen Druding
Manufacturing Coordinator: Margie Orzech
Prepress Vendor: Aptara, Inc.

5th edition

9 8 7 6 5 4 3 2 1

Printed in Mexico

Library of Congress Cataloging-in-Publication Data

Names: Kramer, Paula, editor. | Howe, Tsu-Hsin, editor. | Seruya, Francine M., editor.
Title: Kramer and Hinojosa's frames of reference for pediatric occupational therapy / [edited by] Paula Kramer, Tsu-Hsin Howe, Francine M. Seruya.
Other titles: Frames of reference for pediatric occupational therapy
Description: Fifth edition. | Philadelphia, PA : Wolters Kluwer, [2026] | Preceded by Frames of reference for pediatric occupational therapy / [edited by] Paula Kramer, Jim Hinojosa, Tsu-Hsin Howe. Fourth edition. 2020. | Includes bibliographical references and index. | Summary: "Students in Occupational Therapy programs must learn how to evaluate pediatric patients, and effectively plan for intervention, programming, and support services-all based on theory-driven and evidence-based guidelines for practice. In Frames of Reference for Pediatric Occupational Therapy, students are introduced to several frameworks linking theory to practice through which they can evaluate child and adolescent clients and effectively plan for intervention"– Provided by publisher.
Identifiers: LCCN 2025004144 (print) | LCCN 2025004145 (ebook) | ISBN 9781975220204 (paperback) | ISBN 9781975220235 (epub)
Subjects: MESH: Occupational Therapy–methods | Children with Disabilities–rehabilitation | Developmental Disabilities–rehabilitation | Child Development | Infant | Child | Adolescent
Classification: LCC RM735.3 (print) | LCC RM735.3 (ebook) | NLM WS 370 | DDC 615.8/515–dc23/eng/20250317
LC record available at https://lccn.loc.gov/2025004144
LC ebook record available at https://lccn.loc.gov/2025004145

shop.lww.com

QUADM0725

We dedicate this book to our families who have continuously supported our growth and careers to make this book possible. To the families, children, and colleagues who have changed our lives and perspective and have helped to make this book possible.

Ultimately, this book is dedicated to the children whose lives may be changed by this book.

Contributors

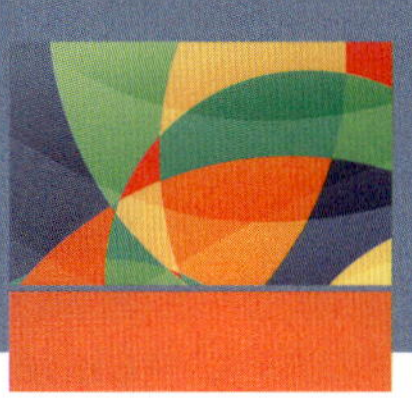

Joana Nana Serwaa Akrofi, OTD, OTR/L
PhD Candidate
Department of Occupational Therapy
Steinhardt School of Culture, Education and Human Development
New York, New York

Susan Cahill, PhD, OTR/L, FAOTA
Occupational Therapist
Chicago, Illinois

Cheryl Colangelo, MS, OTR
Retired Occupational Therapist
Instructor, Mercy College
Niantic, Connecticut

Katherine Dimitropoulou, PhD, OTR/L, MSPOR
Assistant Professor, Rehabilitation & Regenerative Medicine (Occupational Therapy Programs)
Director, Doctor of Education in Movement Sciences (Occupational Therapy)
Vagelos College of Physicians & Surgeons
Columbia University
New York, New York

Brad Egan, OTD, PhD, CADC, OTR/L, FAOTA
Associate Professor
Department of Occupational Therapy
DePaul University
Chicago, Illinois

Lauren Melissa Ellzey, MSLIS
Autistic Self Advocate
Consultant, Nest Support Project
New York University
Librarian & Media Specialist, Maria Regina High School
Hartsdale, New York

Margaret Folkes, OTR/L, TRBI Practitioner
OT Supervisor
Belmont Behavioral Health Hospital
Philadelphia, Pennsylvania

Mindy Garfinkel, OTD, OTR/L, ATP
Assistant Program Director
Associate Professor of Occupational Therapy
Katz School of Science and Health
Yeshiva University
New York, New York

Shawna Gigliotti, DrOT, OTR
Director of Training and Development/OT Services
Belmont Behavioral Health System
Philadelphia, Pennsylvania

Craig Greber, PhD, BOccThy, BHMS(Ed)
Allied Health Research Coordinator
Sunshine Coast Health
Queensland, Australia

Samuel J. Hendrickson, MA
Retired Public School Administrator
Parent of a Child with Special Needs
Plainsboro, New Jersey

Tsu-Hsin Howe, PhD, OTR, FAOTA
Associate Professor and Chair
New York University
Department of Occupational Therapy
Steinhardt School of Culture, Education and Human Development
New York, New York

Claire A. Sangster Jokić, PhD, MPhil Ed Res, BSc OT, BSc Psy
Department of Occupational Therapy
University of Applied Health Sciences
Zagreb, Croatia

Paula Kramer, PhD, OTR, FAOTA
Professor Emeritus
University of the Sciences (now St. Joseph's University)
Philadelphia, Pennsylvania

Rose Martini, PhD, OT Reg(Ont), OT(C), FCAOT
Professor, Director of the Occupational Therapy Program
School of Rehabilitation Sciences, Faculty of Health Sciences
University of Ottawa
Ottawa, Ontario

Annie Baltazar-Mori, OTD, OTR/L
CEO/owner
PlaySense Inc
Redondo Beach, California

Christine Rocchio Mueller, OTD, OTR/L, c/NDT, ATP
Clinical Director
Brave Wings Therapy
Fairfield, New Jersey

Kavitha Murthi, PhD, FHEA, OTR
Postdoctoral Candidate
University of Utah
Salt Lake City, Utah

Janet Njelesani, PhD, OTR/L, FAOTA
Associate Professor
Department of Occupational Therapy
New York University
Steinhardt School of Culture, Education and Human Development
New York, New York

Dora D. Onwumere, MS, OTR/L
PhD candidate
Department of Occupational Therapy
Steinhardt School of Culture, Education and Human Development
New York University
Supervisor of Occupational Therapy
New York City Public Schools
New York, New York

Meira L. Orentlicher, PhD, OTR/L, FAOTA, CRA
Professor & Associate Chairperson for Research and Scholarship
Director, Post Professional OTD Program
Occupational Therapy Department
School of Health Sciences
Touro University
New York, New York

Kristie K. Patten, PhD, OT/L, FAOTA
Counselor to the President
Professor
Department of Occupational Therapy
Steinhardt School of Culture, Education and Human Development
New York University
New York, New York

Mary "Betsey" Pohl, MEd, OT/L
School-Based Occupational Therapy Practitioner
Chicago Public School
Chicago, Illinois

Helene J. Polatajko, PhD, OT(C), FCAOT, FCAHS, LLD(h.c.), OC Occupationologist
Professor Emeritus
Department of Occupational Science and Occupational Therapy
Rehabilitation Sciences Institute
University of Toronto
Toronto, Ontario

Lisa M. Porter, PhD, OTD, OTR/L
Occupational Therapist/Assistant Professor
Occupational Therapy
Western Oregon University
Salem, Oregon

Susanne Smith Roley, OTD, OTR/L, FAOTA
Co-Founder
Collaborative for Leadership in Ayres Sensory Integration (CLASI)
Aliso Viejo, California

Roseann C. Schaaf, PhD, OTR/L, FAOTA
Director, Jefferson Autism Center of Excellence
Professor, Department of Occupational Therapy
Thomas Jefferson University
Director of Research, Collaborative in Ayres Sensory Integration
Philadelphia, Pennsylvania

Sarah A. Schoen, PhD, OTR/L
Former Director of Research, STAR Institute for Sensory Processing
Centennial, Colorado
Associate Professor
Rocky Mountain University of Health Professions
Provo, Utah

Francine M. Seruya, PhD, MBA, OTR/L, FAOTA
Professor and Program Director, Masters in Occupational Therapy
Mercy University
Dobbs Ferry, New York

Virginia Spielmann, PhD, OTR/L
Executive Director
STAR Institute for Sensory Processing
Centennial, Colorado

Tina Weisman, OTD, OTR/L
Adjunct Professor of Occupational Therapy
Mercy and Touro Universities
Clinical Supervisor
Cerebral Palsy of Westchester
Westchester, New York

Jenny Ziviani, AM, BAppSc(OT), MEd, PhD, FOTARA, AOTA
Emeritus Professor
School of Health and Rehabilitation Sciences
The University of Queensland
Brisbane, Australia

Foreword

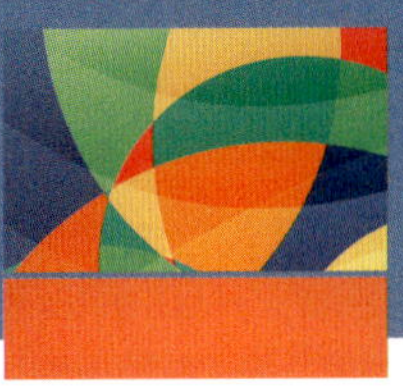

We have entered a period that expects professionals to have a rationale for the decisions they make in service to children, families, and service systems. Paired with this expectation is the fact that occupational therapy knowledge has expanded exponentially, creating a possible dilemma for those of us in practice. There is a lot of information available to consider, with little time for getting access to that knowledge.

Paula Kramer and Jim Hinojosa recognized this dilemma long ago and continue to provide a contemporary scaffolding for professional decision making. This is the 5th edition of their *Frames of Reference for Pediatric Occupational Therapy,* illustrating their foresight about needs for current information in practice. Their book provides an integrated resource that summarizes frames of reference relevant for colleagues serving children, families, and systems. Additionally, the fact that they continue to update their book demonstrates their commitment to supporting contemporary decision making. As editors, Kramer, Howe, and Seruya have solicited the best experts to provide updated information on frames of reference.

Colleagues in practice must rely on experts to sift through the wealth of information available to support their work; there is simply too much information available to honestly know what current practices are possible and are based on the best evidence. The authors provide a reliable summary of the available information along with strategies for systematic decision making in practice. The editors and authors are demonstrating their commitment to quality occupational therapy service through their translational approach to using frames of reference to support everyday practice.

Winnie Dunn, PhD, OTR, FAOTA
Distinguished Professor
Occupational Therapy, University of Missouri

Preface

"He who loves practice without theory is like the sailor who boards ship without a rudder and compass and never knows where he may cast."

Leonardo da Vinci

The quote above from da Vinci truly exemplifies our belief that theory must guide practice. We *continue to* strongly believe that practice needs to be based on and guided by theory, maybe even more now than before. Relying solely on habit or intuition is insufficient. The frame of reference provides an effective vehicle for translating theoretical information into practice. It serves as a blueprint for occupational therapy practitioners who work in pediatrics. As society evolves, a profession must adapt and develop to remain relevant. Theories are also continually changing, evolving, and adapting alongside the changing needs of clients and services. Subsequently, this ongoing transformation is supported and informed by published research. Therefore, to remain relevant, this book needs to evolve as well and include new knowledge that is being used in practice. We are very proud to be working on this fifth edition.

As before, we relied on feedback from users of the text and other expert reviewers to reorganize and update this new edition. All chapters have been updated to reflect latest changes in theory and practice, with new material added throughout. While some reviewers suggested other frames of reference, we only chose ones that are actively used with children and have been tested with research. The first section of the book holds critical background information for current pediatric practice. The structure of the frame of reference has been put up front as that remains the heart of the text. The second section contains the most commonly used frames of reference. The final section discusses the application of frames of reference, including how they can be used together and in sequence. This section covers frames of reference that are specific to particular areas of practice and how they are often used in conjunction with other frames of reference.

This fifth edition continues to focus on the importance of occupation, and all of the frames of reference have been revised to include examples that relate to the importance of occupation and active involvement in a meaningful life. We are proud that this edition includes the work of colleagues from Canada, Australia, and Croatia. This edition includes two new frames of reference: CO-OP, the Cognitive Orientation to daily Occupational Performance, and a frame of reference for secondary transition planning.

As with previous editions, this fifth edition is meant to be an effective tool for teaching pediatrics to entry-level students. However, it is equally beneficial for therapists looking to enhance their application of theory in practice or seeking new and updated approaches to interventions. The book continues to provide pediatric information organized through the structure of frames of reference.

For this edition, we continued to use the language of the World Health Organization's International Classification of Functioning, Disability, and Health (ICF), along with the updated *Occupational Therapy Practice Framework Domain and Process*, 4th ed. Incorporation of ICF language broadens the appeal of the book. This language resulted in an emphasis on the importance of the child's ability to participate in meaningful activities of life (occupations). It is our hope that both new and experienced therapists will use this text to bring new approaches into their practice and update their knowledge of their favorite frames of reference. We hope that practice never becomes habit and is continually updated through the use of current theory.

Paula Kramer, PhD, OTR, FAOTA
Tsu-Hsin Howe, PhD, OTR, FAOTA
Francine M. Seruya, PhD, MBA, OTR/L, FAOTA

Acknowledgments

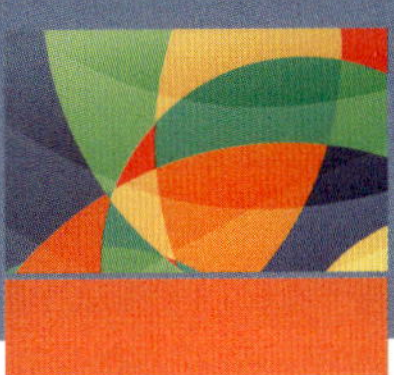

We are very pleased to be writing the fifth edition and are especially excited that all of the people at Wolters Kluwer supported the change in the title of the book to permanently include the names of Kramer and Hinojosa. Originally this book was a dream project for Paula and working with Jim helped to make it a reality. Working on this edition without Jim has been difficult. He was a very dear friend and colleague and is deeply missed. His thoughts and spirit live on through this book and he would be very proud to have his name in the title. We gratefully acknowledge how he influenced our development as educators and professionals.

While writing this book is a lot of work, in many ways, it is a labor of love because we strongly believe in the critical role that theory plays in practice. It is our goal that this edition contains updated knowledge and contemporary frames of reference that reflect current practices in pediatrics, thereby making a significant contribution to the field. We hope this fifth edition will meet the needs of those interested in pediatric occupational therapy practice, will strengthen the bridge between theory and practice, and enrich the current literature of our profession.

For this edition, Dr. Francine M. Seruya has joined us as a third editor. She brings an excellent understanding of theory and practice in pediatrics to this edition. She played a significant role in writing the first section of the book and in editing and revising many of the chapters throughout the text.

There are many people to thank who helped us, directly or indirectly, to make this edition possible. First and foremost, our families have always been there for us, providing love, support, and encouragement, even when writing took time away from them; notably, David and Andrew Hunt, Ching-Fan Sheu, Asher and Madelynn Seruya, and Young and Olivia Tran. As always, it is important for us to acknowledge the contribution that Dr. Anne Cronin Mosey has made in strongly influencing all of our thinking and professional development. We mourn her passing and gratefully recognize her contribution to us personally and to the body of knowledge of occupational therapy.

A special thanks to all the authors who contributed to this book, and to their spouses, significant others, families, and friends who were supportive to them and thus assisted them in producing such fine work. We are fortunate that they consider us to be their friends as well as their colleagues. We also extend our gratitude to our colleagues at the New York University and Mercy University for their unwavering support during the production of this new edition. We also thank our family at Wolters Kluwer for being wonderful supporters of this book, especially Matt Hauber, Lindsey Porambo, Amy Millholen, and Vinodhini Varadharajalu.

Our growth as educators and writers has always been stimulated by our students and colleagues. Their insights have greatly influenced this book, and we hope that they will continue to find it valuable to their practice.

The pictures in this book are critical to illustrating the text. We want to thank all the parents who have graciously allowed us to use the photos of their children to demonstrate concepts in this book. All the photographs make the text much richer.

Finally, we are indebted to our colleagues who continue to develop the art and science of pediatric occupational therapy.

Table of Contents

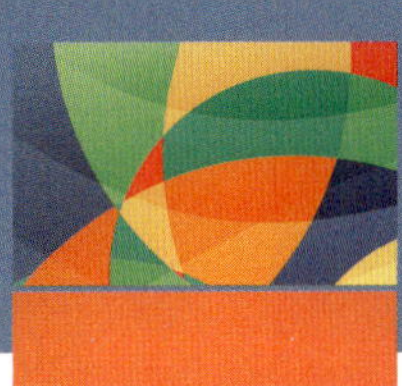

SECTION II • COMMONLY USED FRAMES OF REFERENCE 83

13 A Biomechanical Frame of Reference to Position Children for Function 353

Christine Rocchio Mueller, Cheryl Colangelo

Section I

Foundations of Pediatric Practice

Introduction to Section I

This section is meant to set the stage for this book. It contains essential information for readers, particularly students, to gain a comprehensive understanding of the frames of references discussed in Sections II and III. We firmly believe that one of the strengths of occupational therapy lies in conducting practice guided by theory. This section begins with the structure of the frame of reference, explaining each section and its purpose as part of the whole. Through an understanding of this format, readers will be able to grasp the specifics of each frame of reference that is presented later in the book.

It should be noted that we have changed some of the title headings of sections of the frame of reference to make it more reflective of current practice. We believe that the frame of reference as delineated by Dr. Anne Cronin Mosey (Mosey, 1970) is still very relevant to understanding the theories that are the basis of our practice; however, as society changes and our practice continues to evolve, we need to make some changes as well. In 1993, Kramer and Hinojosa added the "application to practice" section, which we consider essential for providing practitioners with a clear example of how the frame of reference is applied in the actual practice. In this edition, we have changed the title of Legitimate Tools to Contemporary Tools for intervention as we believe that is more reflective of our current practice.

The first chapter, Structure of the Frame of Reference: Transitioning From Theory to Practice, presents the format of the frame of reference and explains what information is included in each section. It is a road map describing how we move from a theory to practice. It begins with *the Theoretical Base*, which is the basis for understanding every aspect of a particular frame of reference, especially the essential knowledge required to develop an intervention. The next section, *the Function/Dysfunction Continua*, identifies those areas of function with which the frame of reference is concerned. This is followed by a section, *Guide for Evaluation*, describing what will be focused on in an evaluation. Some frames of reference suggest specific assessment tools, while others just present guidelines, as there may not be standardized assessments that are effective for the perspective. The next section, *Postulates Regarding Change*, describes how the practitioner promotes positive changes in client performance within the scope of the particular frame of reference, they allow the practitioner to theorize how and why changes would occur. The final section, *Application to Practice*, includes more specific examples of how to apply the frame of reference in intervention.

The second chapter, Developmental Perspective: Fundamentals of Developmental Theory, covers the various developmental theories that are reflected in contemporary occupational therapy education and practice. Understanding theories of development is critical for implementing the majority, if not all, of the frames of reference discussed in this text. We acknowledge that some of the references are dated; however, we maintain that it is important for readers to understand the historical context involved in these developmental theories. More recent writings about these theories have been included as well. We have also included newer theories of development that are relevant to occupational therapy practice, in particular the life theory of development that explores the importance of earlier experiences on the development of occupations.

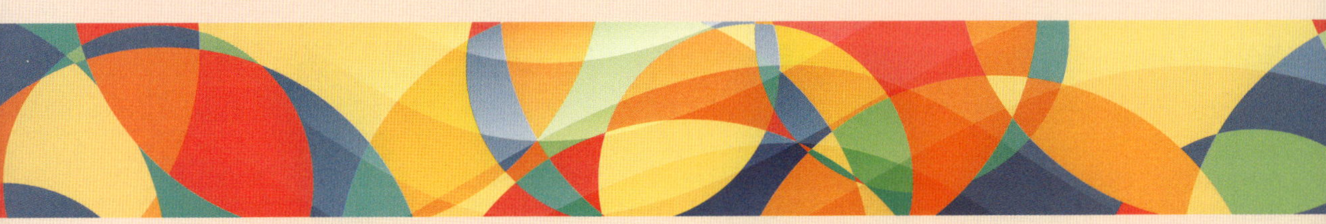

In the third chapter, titled "Domain of Concern of Occupational Therapy: Relevance to Pediatric Practice," we have incorporated updates to align with the current edition of the Occupational Therapy Practice Framework: Domain and Process (OTPF4) (AOTA, 2020). This revision involves a comprehensive comparison and contrast with the International Classification of Functioning, Disability and Health (ICF). By doing so, we contextualize American approaches and terminology within a global perspective on our domain of concern, highlighting the areas most important to pediatric occupational therapy practitioners. Further, this chapter identifies which frames of reference presented in the text relate to which specific areas in our domain of concern.

The next chapter, Pediatric Occupational Therapy's Contemporary Tools for Intervention, outlines the wide variety of tools for intervention used in pediatric practice. The focus is on occupations, activities, play, activity analysis and synthesis, and activity groups as they apply to pediatric practice. This chapter then discusses the important tools that practitioners must develop, including critical reasoning skills, conscious use of self, the teaching learning process, an understanding of physical modalities, sensory–response interaction, and the importance of the nonhuman environment. The nonhuman environment is an important aspect of child development and frequently used in treatment. It includes toys, animals, and technology. All or some of these tools will be used in the frames of reference presented in this book.

The last chapter in this section, Contextual Factors Shaping Pediatric Practice, covers the importance of considering context for those working with pediatric clients. It presents Bronfenbrenner's Ecological Systems Theory as an overarching framework for understanding context. It explores the various pediatric practice settings and how they influence interventions. Finally, it discusses the concept of cultural humility and underscores the importance of occupational therapy practitioners being mindful of their personal perspectives and interactions, recognizing their potential impact on interventions.

Summary

The chapters in this section provide an essential foundation for understanding the frames of reference presented in this book. This section emphasized the importance of the use of theory to provide a basis for our interventions, the mark of a true profession. Further, we hope these chapters will provide the readers with sufficient insight into the frame of reference to help them understand the next sections of the book, encouraging them to critically examine existing interventions or to create new ones based on the fundamental knowledge presented in this section.

REFERENCES

Kramer, P., & Hinojosa, J. (1993). *Frames of reference for pediatric occupational therapy* (1st ed.). Lippincott Williams & Wilkins.

Mosey, A. C. (1970). *Three frames of reference for mental health*. Slack.

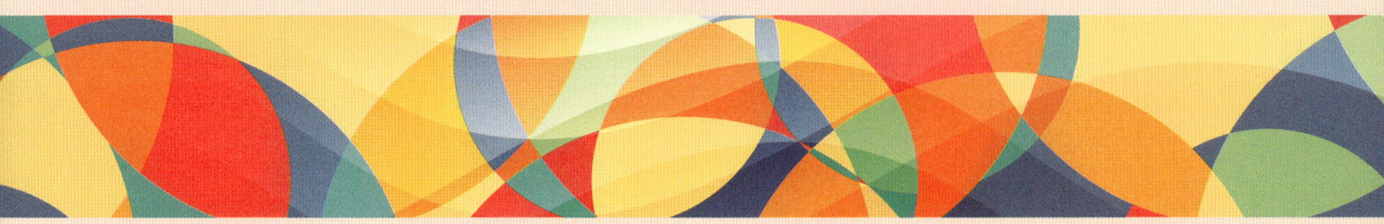

Structure of the Frame of Reference: Transitioning From Theory to Practice

Tsu-Hsin Howe ■ Paula Kramer ■ Francine M. Seruya

The premise of this textbook is that an intervention should be theoretically based, grounded in the specific needs of the child, rather than the diagnosis. Traditionally, occupational therapy textbooks focus on diagnostic categories (e.g., cerebral palsy, autism). Occupational therapy practitioners must learn about diagnostic categories, as they provide critical information needed to understand the child and their abilities and disabilities. When discussing treatment, diagnostic categories can also be linked with specific strategies for intervention. The inherent premise in these textbooks is that a therapist chooses an intervention based on the diagnosis of a client. Although a diagnosis may provide insight into a child's disabilities, occupational therapists are concerned primarily with functional performance. Occupational therapy practitioners are concerned with disabilities and impairments that may result from a diagnosis rather than the diagnosis itself. Material organized around diagnostic categories does not always address the essential focus of the occupational therapy process. In addition, a child may exhibit several other needs not described in the diagnostic category but still fundamental to intervention planning.

All occupational therapy interventions should be guided by theories. Before learning about frames of reference (Kramer & Hinojosa, 1993; Mosey, 1981, 1996), it is critical to have a basic understanding of theory. The purpose of a theory is to describe the theorist's intentions of explaining and predicting a certain aspects of physical world, and the use of theory refers to how professionals actually put the theory into practice and predict how the intervention with affect the functional outcome in their clients. In science, theories are based on the observation of phenomena. Scientists categorize what they have observed and then use that categorization to make predictions about the relationships between objects or events. When people hear the word "theory," they tend to think of something that is complex, esoteric, difficult to understand, and completely impractical. However, people develop simple theories all the time. When an individual observes something and believes that the observed occurrence is frequently repeated in the world, leading to the formation of a pattern, they are constructing a theory. For example, when we observe children playing on a slide in a playground, we might see that older children are more likely to go down the slide immediately and have fun. Younger children may get to the top of the steps of the slide and seem anxious and reluctant to come down without coaching or encouragement. Our "slide theory" might propose that young children are fearful of going down a slide until they have encountered enjoyment multiple times. Observing other children at various playgrounds can serve as a method to substantiate our theory about children's behavior on a slide. Repeated observations validate the credibility of our theory.

Theories are the formalized collection of concepts, definitions, and theoretical postulates, which predict relationships between behaviors and events in specified circumstances. Concepts, which provide the basis for categorization, are labels of a set of phenomena that have specific, definable characteristics. Definitions, which encompass specific and identifiable characteristics of concepts, play a vital role in theory formation. They identify the unique qualities of a concept, and enable individuals to differentiate which phenomena fall within the scope of the concept and which are excluded. Some of the concepts in the example mentioned earlier are older children, young children, height, slides, and anxiety. In this example, concepts have definitions based on our observations of the playground. Older children are physically larger, over 3 feet tall, and over 3 years of age. Younger children are smaller, shorter than 3 feet, and under 3 years of age. Height is the size of a child in inches and feet. Slides are structures in the playground that are often triangular in shape, with a means of going up on one side and a smooth sloping surface on the opposite side that allows a child to move down freely and smoothly. Anxiety within this context is defined as any behaviors displaying signs of fear including stopping at the top of the slide, crying, or whining. A theorist defines concepts in a way as they are observed or to explain a phenomenon, not necessarily using a dictionary definition or language that reflects common use. Once a theoretical concept is defined, the definition must be used consistently throughout the theory. If a new theory is developed or adapted, the theorist may modify the definition.

Theoretical postulates state the relationship between two or more concepts. Using the same example, one postulate maintains that younger children who hesitate at the top of a slide show anxiety (Figure 1.1). A second postulate holds that older children who go down the slide without stopping show no anxiety (Figure 1.2). A third postulate would be that the slide provokes anxiety in some children.

As explained earlier, a theory comprises concepts, definitions, and theoretical postulates. These concepts, definitions, and postulates define the parameters of the theory. A theory is formulated in

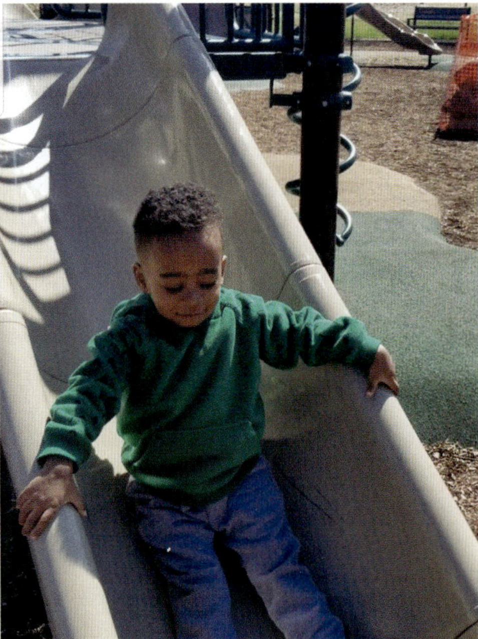

FIGURE 1.1 Child unsure about going down the slide.

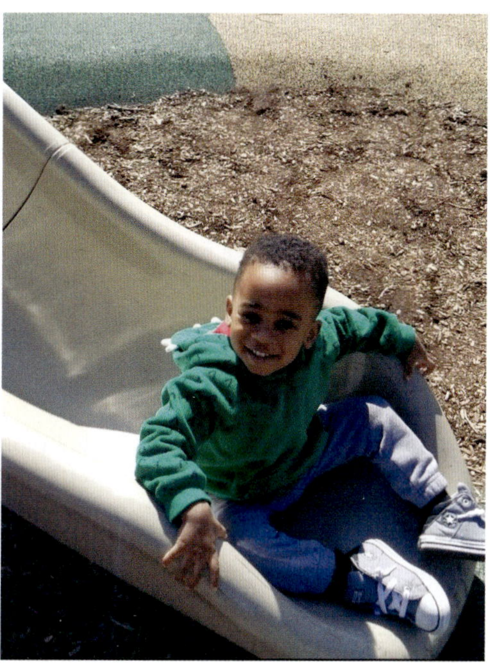

FIGURE 1.2 Child enjoying being successful going down the slide.

alignment with foundational assumptions that the theorists holds. An assumption is a belief that an individual accepts without ever subjecting it to questioning. All theories contain assumptions. In our example, we are assuming that children's behaviors are reflective of emotional state. Another assumption is that the age and size of the children is related to their ability and emotional state.

There are many ways of describing the application of theory into practice in occupational therapy. Theorists use many terms to describe this application of theory to practice, such as "perspectives," "model of practice," and "paradigms." Often these terms are used interchangeably; however, we strongly believe that these terms are not all equivalent. Some stress theories more, whereas others focus more on interventions. Most do not clearly describe the steps involved in moving from theory to intervention.

The frame of reference is one method of organizing theoretical material to provide a foundation to explain what we see and then postulate what we expect when applying intervention. It translates theoretical information into practice. It generally combines multiple theories or parts of theories in the theoretical base and then uses those theories in a clear, consistent manner to delineate function and dysfunction; to guide evaluations; to propose principles of change (postulates regarding change); and to facilitate the implementation of these theories (application to practice) (Kramer & Hinojosa, 1993). While various professions may share certain theories (e.g., developmental theories are used by psychologists, educators, and health care professionals), a frame of reference tailors theoretical information to suit the specific utilization of occupational therapy practitioners. It is our belief that the frame of reference is the clearest and most comprehensive approach to transitioning from the theoretical abstraction state to practical intervention. As a result, we have opted to adopt the structure of the frame of reference for this text.

The frame of reference is designed to first highlight traditionally used theories, then to relate that information to function, and, finally, to organize that information for the purpose of intervention that promotes function and engagement in meaningful occupation. Theories that serve as the basis for frames of reference address the strengths and limitations of the child and family. They do not focus solely on diagnosis, disability, or impairment. This book comprises articulated frames of reference that delineate the relationship between theory and practice to provide a blueprint for evaluation and intervention.

In the pediatric arena, the frame of reference offers an outline of fundamental theoretical concepts relative to particular areas of function. The frame of reference serves as a guiding principle for evaluating a child's functional capacities and provides a mechanism for formulating and executing intervention. Consequently, frames of reference empower the practitioners to apply theory in practice. The frame of reference provides a structure for identifying pertinent theories. Subsequently, it utilizes this information to establish directives that occupational therapy practitioners follow while evaluating and implementing intervention For credibility of the profession, interventions must be theory based.

This textbook comes from a perspective that all interventions begin with a thorough understanding of the child and family and their unique situation before choosing a frame of reference. In the following section, we will present a simulated frame of reference that illustrates the essential component parts. In this example, "Improving Constructive Block Play Skills of Kindergarten Children," we present each section of the frame of reference with a description of key components. This example is intended to clarify the structure of frame of reference while adding levity to this complex topic. It is not intended to be a completely developed frame of reference but, rather, a brief example that demonstrates the various parts needed to understand the structure of the frame of reference.

ESSENTIAL COMPONENT PARTS OF THE FRAME OF REFERENCE

The essential component parts of the frame of reference include the theoretical base, function/dysfunction continua, indicators of function and dysfunction, guide for evaluation, postulates regarding change, and application to practice. In each section, we discuss important aspects of the component parts and then provide a case example.

Theoretical Base

When therapists begin to use a new frame of reference, they should be certain to understand the theoretical base and its key components. The theoretical base sets the stage for the entire frame of reference. It is usually the most complex and abstract section in the frame of reference. Nonetheless, comprehending the theories used in the frame of reference is critical for practitioners as it facilitates the transition from theory to practical implementation of the frame of reference. The theoretical base includes both constant and dynamic theoretical information. Constant theoretical information describes phenomena as if they were static, and only describes the relationship between concepts. Dynamic theoretical information describes how change takes place; how the described concept may be initiated, inhibited, or maintained; and/or how the condition of homeostasis is sustained.

The theoretical base broadly delineates the areas of concern of the frame of reference within the context of occupational therapy. Specifically, the theoretical base identifies the various theories which the frame of reference uses to make predictions on how intervention will affect change and therefore, guide the intervention. It identifies all assumptions being made, names and defines the major concepts and describes the relationships between the major concepts.

Typically, the theoretical base incorporates a design that describes the interconnection of each of the individual parts to create a cohesive entirety. When learning a frame of reference, it is important to understand the theoretical base design or the way in which it is organized. The way that the theoretical base is organized should be reflected in all subsequent parts of the frame of reference. The key components of the theoretical base are assumptions, concepts, definitions, and theoretical postulates. For example, if the theoretical base presents concepts in a particular order, as if one flows from the next, then that order should be reflected in all other parts of the frame of reference. This format enables the practitioners to understand the design of the frame of reference and follow the same order in the application of the theoretical base to intervention. This again highlights the importance of the theoretical base.

Adequacy of Theory for Frames of Reference

When choosing a theory to support a guideline for intervention, practitioners must examine the suitability of the theory by examining the adequacy of concepts, definitions, and postulates of the theory. As for the concepts used in the theory, practitioners need to determine whether a theory's concepts are defined at an abstract level and need to examine how each individual concept is used throughout the theory. An important aspect of a theory is consistency of the concept label or how the theorist refers to the concept (set of phenomena) in each instance throughout the theory. Is the same label (concept) employed consistently by the theorist whenever referring to a particular set of phenomena? In order for a theory to have consistency in concept labeling, the response should be affirmative. In scientific writing, in contrast to creative writing, it is customary to use the same label for a specific set of phenomena throughout the theory. Thus, each concept has a label that captures a specific set of phenomena, and this label must be used consistently throughout the theory. To assess the definitions of concepts, the level at which a concept is defined needs to be evaluated. This evaluation is crucial because within a theory, the definition of a concept should ideally be stated at an abstract level, without referring to any particular object, instance, or circumstance. After examining the adequacy of the definitions within the theory, we consider the structure of the theory.

The other critical key component in the structure of the theory is its postulates. Postulates are statements that describe the relationship between two or more concepts. Postulates give meaning to theoretical information. To be an acceptable postulate, the relationship between concepts must be stated in a clear and concise manner, so it will easily be tested. Without postulates, concepts would contribute little to the description of a set of phenomena.

Theoretical Base: Improving Constructive Block Play Skills of Kindergarten Children

Play is the most common occupation of children. It is frequently used as an intervention tool in occupational therapy for children to improve a child's multifaceted skills, and to facilitate their overall development. Play is a subjective experience of joy and fun, that comes from engaging in freely chosen, intrinsically motivated, self-directed meaningful occupations (Lynch & Moore, 2016)

Constructive play is a type of play, and specifically refers to the manipulation of objects to build or to "create" something (Smilansky, 1968). Making a block structure, shaping an animal out of playdough, folding a sheet of paper into sculpture (origami), and putting a puzzle together are all examples of constructive play. This form of play actively engages motor skills in object manipulation, and the resulting creations may carry symbolic meaning. For instance, while simply stacking blocks constitutes a motor activity, stacking blocks to build a tower introduces the element of symbolism.

Guanella (1934) described five stages of block play. These stages are nonstructural or preorganized use of blocks in late infancy, stacks or rows of blocks, bidimensional construction (e.g., stacking blocks vertically to create a tower or horizontally to create a row), the tridimensional stage (e.g., use blocks to create a structure with an enclosed space), and representational play with blocks (e.g., The structure is named and symbolizes a real place or object). Tian et al. (2020) described the block playing further with specific required skills at specific ages. They are: exploring blocks and building in linear dimensions (6 months to 2 years), for example, piling blocks on one another; building in two dimensions and creating area structures (2 to 3 years), for example, adjoining stacks of blocks to form a vertical area arrangement; building in three dimensions, creating arches, bridges, and enclosures; adding symbolic representations to structures (3 to 4 years); producing multicomponent constructions and elaborations of symbolic representations (4 to 5 years); and Emerging integration (5 to 7 years).

Block play can be considered as a sequence of actions. Gagné (1977) states that for effective learning of a sequence of actions to occur, the individual must demonstrate interest in engaging with the materials. Additionally, they should be able to connect their existing knowledge or experiences related to the topic. Furthermore, they need to receive adequate learning guidance and support including cues, prompts or step-by step instructions, and feedback. Finally, it is essential for individuals to have opportunities to practice the newly acquired skills. Gagné's theory emphasizes the idea of a learning hierarchy, where skills are structured in a logical order of complexity. Learners progress from simpler prerequisite skills to more complex ones. Mastery of each skill is essential before moving to the next level. Using Gagné's proposed theory, examples of applying it in block play include creating an engaging environment that captures a child's attention, adjusting block sizes to match the child's developmental level, and designing block activities that align with their prior experiences and skill level. Utilizing Vygotsky's scaffolding approach in block play, providing support and guidance through means such as verbal instruction, modeling, encouragement, and feedback can further enhance a child's development and learning (Gregory et al., 2003).

Assumptions

Assumptions are ideas that are held to be true and are not questioned or tested in any way. In other words, they are basic beliefs. All theories have assumptions. If the theoretical base draws from several theories, then all the assumptions made must be accepted by all those theories and are not in conflict with each other. Assumptions in the theoretical base of *Improving Constructive Block Play Skills* of *Kindergarten Children* are as follows:

Assumption: Children's development follows in a predictable sequence
Assumption: Environment can shape learning experiences
Assumption: Play is inherently motivated, driven by a child's internal desire to engage in enjoyable and satisfying activities.

Concepts

Concepts are labels of sets of phenomena. They represent the concern and scope of the frame of reference. Because concepts describe sets of phenomena, they are abstract and do not refer to any single phenomenon (e.g., an object, a person, or an event). Because the concept is abstract, you can include other individual phenomenon into the concept if it shares the defining characteristics. Concepts selected from the theories must represent the concern and scope of the frame of reference. These concepts are used consistently with the same definitions across all sections of the frame of reference.

It is important to remember that the use of concept in everyday language is very different from its scientific use. In everyday language it is used to convey an idea or an impression, whereas in science it is formally defined to refer to an abstract description of characteristics that go together around a set of phenomena.

A concept can be categorized by its tangible characteristics, the manner in which it was defined, or its conceptual level. Furthermore, a concept may belong to more than one category. Categorization of the concepts is the first step to understanding how the theory is structured. Concepts can be categorized based on whether or not they have tangible or directly observable characteristics. *Simple concepts* are categories delineated by characteristics that are readily observable by visual, auditory, kinesthetic, or tactile sensation. For example, both "constructive play" and "block play" from the sample frame of reference "Improving constructive block play skills of kindergarten children" are simple concepts. These categories can be described verbally or represented pictorially.

Constructs, are categories of concepts delineated by characteristics that cannot be readily observable and are not based on directly observable phenomenon. They are defined by one's observations. In the occupational therapy, constructs concepts often refer to emotional states, such as anxiety or depression. Some theoretical bases may include a specific type of constructs labeled *"hypothetical constructs."* Hypothetical constructs differ from constructs in that hypothetical constructs are based on the originator's ideas or thoughts and are used to develop theories beyond the observable world. For example, Vygotsky's (1966) scaffolding is a hypothetical construct.

Concepts can also be categorized according to their relative order. A superordinate concept is at a higher conceptual level than another concept. A subordinate concept is at a lower conceptual level than another concept. When concepts are neither superordinate nor subordinate to each other, they are at the same conceptual level. Concepts in the theoretical base of *Improving Constructive Block Play Skills of Kindergarten Children* are as follows:

Concept: constructive play
Concept: block play

In this sample frame of reference, a conceptual hierarchy is play as superordinate concept (higher-level concept) followed by constructive play and block play. The "constructive play" is a subordinate concept (lower-level concept) to "play," and the "block play" is a subordinate concept to the "constructive play."

Definitions

Definitions explain the meaning of important concepts. Keep in mind that every concept in a theoretical base should be defined in terms of what it means to the particular frame of reference. Definitions describe the set of phenomena by its shared common characteristics that are unique to that set of phenomena.

Mosey (1996) proposes a taxonomy that classifies concepts according to their conceptual level (superordinate to subordinate). She identifies five levels of definition:

- *Abstract:* Abstract definitions do not refer to any specific object, circumstance, or incidence. They define the set of phenomena relative to its defining characteristics. All concepts in the theoretical information should be defined at this level.
- *Functional:* Functional definitions define the concept with consideration to application. The definition includes the kinds of actions or activity that one would do.

- *Operational:* Operational definitions are measurable and can be quantified or qualified in some particular manner.
- *Descriptive:* Descriptive definitions describe what the phenomena look like.
- *Example:* Example definitions are specific cases or illustrations of the set of phenomena (phenomenon).

In addition to these proper definitions, Mosey (1996) identifies another type of definition, a circular definition that is considered unacceptable. Circular definitions define the concept by using the concept within the definition. For example, defining musicality as "the quality or state of being musical" uses part of the term being defined (musical) in its definition.

As one goes from abstract to descriptive (superordinate to subordinate), the definitions become clearer and more understandable. However, when looking at definitions for a theory, being clearer and more understandable does not make definition "better." In a theory, it is the abstract definition that clearly captures the set of phenomena. Definitions in the theoretical base of *Improving Constructive Block Play Skills of Kindergarten Children* are as follows:

Definition: Constructive play is a type of play that involves manipulating objects to build or to "create" something.

Definition: Block play is a type of constructive play involves using blocks to build structures, patterns, and imaginative scenarios of varying complexity.

Postulates

Postulates are statements that describe the relationship between two or more concepts. Within the theoretical base, all concepts are related in some way; the relationship between important concepts is made clear by postulates. The postulate serves as the linking mechanism between concepts. Postulates give meaning to theoretical information. Without postulates, concepts would be isolated categories, contributing little to the description of theoretical information. There are eight types of theoretical postulates commonly used in theories: temporal, spatial, quantitative, qualitative, correlative, causal, hierarchical, and hypothesis. With the exception of hypothesis, postulates are categorized by the type of relationship they describe. Postulates often relate to more than one category. For example, the postulate "Students in Asia spend more time in school than students in the United States" is both quantitative and spatial.

Postulates in the frame of reference *Improving Constructive Block Play Skills of Kindergarten Children* are as follows:

Postulate: The block play progresses with the increased age and developmental skills

Postulate: Children can improve their performance with guided instruction.

Hypothesis

Hypothesis is a very specific type of postulate that is used to examine a theory; it is not used within the theory. Hypotheses are unique in that they predict expected behaviors. The hypothesis states the postulate in a way that it can be measured and tested. Typically, a hypothesis transforms a theoretical relationship into a statement about a real situation, allowing it to be observed and quantified. They are often not overtly written in the theoretical base but are implicit when the reader understands the meaning of the entire theoretical base. Hypotheses are based on concepts of the dynamic theory as they relate to the stated postulates. Within a frame of reference, hypotheses can be tested. Hypotheses in the frame of reference *Improving Constructive Block Play Skills of Kindergarten Children* are as follows:

Hypothesis: When guided instruction or modeling were provided during the block play, the child will use new skills to build blocks

When studying the theoretical base of a frame of reference, it may be helpful to keep the following questions in mind:

1. What are the assumptions? Are the assumptions compatible among various theories included in theoretical base section of the frame of reference?
2. What are the concepts? Are they at the same conceptual level and are they relatively mutually exclusive? Are the concepts explained in a way that ensures a clear understanding of their relationships?
3. What are the definitions of the concepts? Do you understand them? Is the superordinate/subordinate organization of concepts clear?
4. What are the postulates? Do you understand these relationships?
5. How is the theoretical base organized? What is the design of the theoretical base? Do you understand the design?

Function/Dysfunction Continua

The next section in a frame of reference is referred to as the function/dysfunction continua. This section clearly identifies those areas of function with which the frame of reference is concerned and is focused. As you read through the theoretical base, you should be able to identify the specific areas of performance important to the child's development of skills and abilities. These are the areas that the therapist evaluates to determine whether the child is functional or dysfunctional. Concepts and their definitions from the theoretical base identify what therapists who use this frame of reference consider to be functional. Likewise, concepts and definitions identify what represents dysfunction. Each function/dysfunction continuum covers one area of performance addressed by the particular frame of reference.

A frame of reference generally has several function/dysfunction continua, which are labeled as such because human performance rarely can be classified as good or bad and/or abled or disabled. The situation usually is not so clear-cut. Function is at one end of the spectrum and dysfunction is at the other end, and human performance may fall at any point along this scale:

Function______________________________________Dysfunction

The functional end of the continuum represents what the therapist expects the child to be able to do, whereas the dysfunctional end of the continuum represents disability:

Function______________________________________Dysfunction

Expected ability__________________________________Disability

Function/dysfunction continua derived directly from the theoretical bases of the frames of reference and, thus, are specific to those frames of reference. They cannot be taken out of context. The two function/dysfunction continua in frame of reference *Improving Constructive Block Play Skills of Kindergarten Children* are concerned with initiation and playing with blocks (see Tables 1.1 and 1.2).

Table 1.1 Indicators of Function: Initiate Block Play

Function	Dysfunction
Interacts with blocks when they are made available	Does not interact with blocks when they are made available
Indicators of Function	**Indicators of Dysfunction**
Show interests in blocks by exploring the blocks, i.e., touching them, and examining their shapes, colors, and textures.	Does not show interests or paying attentions in blocks
Spontaneously requests and/or retrieves blocks during free play	Do not spontaneously request and/or retrieve blocks during free play

Label—Initiate block play
Function—Ability to interacts with blocks when they are made available
Dysfunction—Does not interact with blocks when they are made available
Label—Block play
Function—Ability to manipulate blocks to create structures, patterns, and imaginative scenarios
Dysfunction—Inability to manipulate blocks to create structures, patterns, and imaginative scenarios

When examining function/dysfunction continua, you should consider the following:

- Are the continua compatible with the definition of the components of the problem as described in the theoretical base?
- Are the continua written in a manner that clarifies what is considered functional and what is not? They should not be written to address the specific behaviors and physical signs indicative of function and dysfunction that you have selected for each end of the continua.
- Are the labels for continua concise and impartial in relation to function and dysfunction?

Table 1.2 Indicators of Function: Block Play

Function	Dysfunction
Ability to manipulate blocks to create structures, patterns, and imaginative scenarios	Inability to manipulate blocks to create structures, patterns, and imaginative scenarios
Indicators of Function	**Indicators of Dysfunction**
Stacking and arranging blocks to create simple structure	Does not stack or arrange blocks to create simple structure
Creates complex structures with blocks that are representative of real objects or places	Does not create complex, representative structures

Indicators of Function and Dysfunction

Underneath each function/dysfunction continuum are lists of behaviors, physical signs, or some type of functional scale, such as a test score. These are called indicators of function and indicators of dysfunction. When the frame of reference uses lists of behaviors or physical signs, there is one list of expected abilities. This represents the functional end of the continuum. Another list identifies behaviors or physical signs that are considered areas of concern, which represent the dysfunctional end of the continuum. The function/dysfunction continua and the indicators of function and dysfunction are the guidelines for problem identification within a frame of reference. During the evaluation process, the therapist uses these lists of behavior and physical signs to identify strengths and areas of concern addressed by the particular frame of reference.

In some frames of reference, a functional scale is used to identify acceptable ranges of behaviors or performance rather than specified abilities. Alternatively, some areas of human performance that exhibit wide variations in acceptable performance can be listed as observable behaviors. For example, grasping an object involves many motoric steps. A child may have only partially acquired this and still be functional in relation to their age but may not have developed the whole sequence of grasping. This child, because they have not fully mastered grasping, still would not fall at the functional end of the continuum.

After therapists perform an evaluation, they can then look at the results and check them against these descriptive lists or functional scales. The more behaviors or physical signs that the child exhibits indicative of dysfunction, the closer the child will be to the dysfunctional end of the continuum, showing the need for intervention. Likewise, the fewer characteristics indicative of dysfunction that the child exhibits, the closer the child will be to the functional end of the scale.

The following are two function/dysfunction continua and the indicators of function and dysfunction from the sample frame of reference:

Initiating block play is the ability to interact with blocks when they are made available. The child may show interests in blocks by exploring the blocks, that is, touching them, and examining their shapes, colors, and textures, or they may spontaneously request and/or retrieve blocks during free play (Table 1.1, Figure 1.3).

Block play is the ability to manipulate blocks to create structures, patterns, and imaginative scenarios, and involves stacking and arranging blocks to create simple structure, or creates complex structures with blocks that are representative of real objects or places (Table 1.2, Figure 1.4).

When examining indicators of function/dysfunction, you should consider the following:

- Are the indicators of function and dysfunction compatible with the definition and description of each continuum?
- Are the indicators of function and dysfunction compatible with the behaviors/physical signs described in the theoretical base?
- Are the indicators unique to each continuum and not repeated across continua? The indicators must be specific and unique to the continuum.
- Are there a few indicators for each continuum for problem identification?
- Are the indicators written at the level of direct observation in settings typically used for problem identification?
- Are the indicators drawn from clinical observation or physical signs?

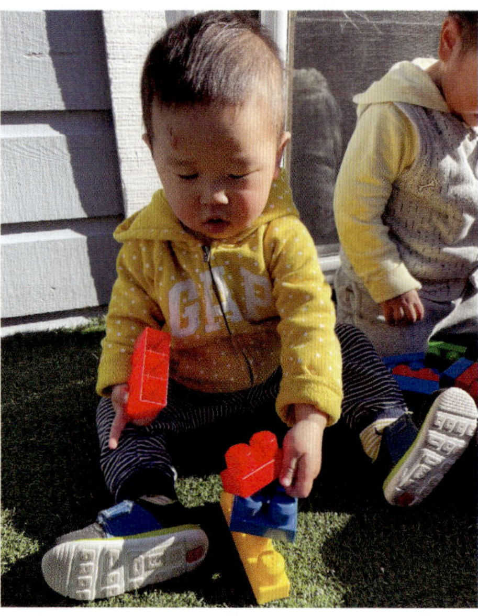

FIGURE 1.3 Child beginning to engage in constructional play.

Guide for Evaluation

This section identifies how therapists would approach the evaluation process within a particular frame of reference. It identifies potential assessments and methods and relates them to the indicators of function and dysfunction. This section may serve as a general guideline of evaluation in defining the areas of performance that therapists should assess. It is not, however, a specific assessment or

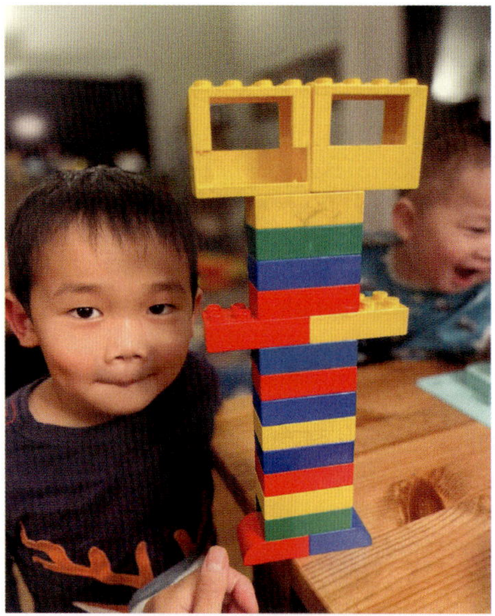

FIGURE 1.4 Child showing pleasure and proficiency in constructional play.

a specified evaluation protocol; it does not provide therapists with instructions on how to assess a child; instead, it highlights the aspects they should observe to determine whether the child requires intervention.

Through the evaluation process, therapists determine where the child falls on the function/dysfunction continuum. Is the child closer to function, or do they have so much difficulty with this area of performance that they are closer to dysfunction and therefore have to be considered in need of intervention?

Some frames of reference do not identify any specific assessments. In these situations, practitioners usually devise a set of tasks or observations that allow them to determine the child's therapists in the various function/dysfunction continua. This is perfectly acceptable as long as the tasks or observations chosen are directly related to the specified continuum. Although it is often difficult to choose or devise evaluative tasks, therapists should avoid falling back on "old favorites." Wherever possible, practitioners should attempt to choose standardized assessments that address the areas and skills that align with the scope of the frame of reference. If standardized assessments are not available, therapists need to choose tasks that demonstrate the specific behaviors outlined. Assessments or tasks should also not be chosen based on the therapists' comfort level but on whether assessments or tasks are designed to identify indicators of function and dysfunction listed under each of the continuum stated in the particular frame of reference.

Using the function/dysfunction continua as the guideline for the evaluation, therapists can determine whether the child can be considered functional or dysfunctional in terms of this specific frame of reference:

In this sample frame of reference, observation of the child's performance in block play could be used as an evaluation method. This observation would provide the practitioner with information about the child's behaviors and their development across various dimensions.

When examining the guide for evaluation, you should consider the following:

- Does the guide for evaluation identify any of the specific standardized and/or nonstandardized assessments that could be used in the particular frame of reference?
- If the occupational profile is used as a screening or assessment tool, does the profile guide you in describing information related to the stated continua and indicators?
- Is there an explanation within the evaluation description about modifying the specific assessment if needed for assessing the continuum?
- Do the suggested potential assessments address all the indicators of function/dysfunction?

Postulates Regarding Change

Postulates state the relationship between two or more concepts from the theoretical base of a frame of reference. Postulates regarding change states the relationships between concepts; however, these postulates describe the progression of problem remediation and the characteristics of and interactions between human and nonhuman environments that will facilitate problem remediation in the area addressed within the scope of the particular frame of reference. They are used as the guidelines for how the therapist should intervene with the child. Postulates regarding change, just like function/dysfunction continua, must relate back to the important concepts in the theoretical base. Postulates regarding change are derived from the dynamic theory stated in the theoretical base, as the thread of continuity must be present from one section to another.

Postulates regarding change are critical because they transition the frame of reference from a theoretical abstraction to the practical realm of tangible application. An essential feature of the postulates regarding change is the environment. In these postulates regarding change, the term "environment" encompasses both the physical surroundings, such as the space of the intervention setting, as well as the social, cultural, and psychological factors that shape a child's experiences and interactions, such as emotional climate, the social interaction with therapists and significant others, the various activities to which the child is exposed. It is important to note that therapists do not actually create the change in the child, but they do create an environment that allows the change to take place (Mosey, 1981, 1986). Practitioners may create an environment that enhances typical growth and development by providing the child with specific activities that they have not engaged in previously. Based on the theoretical postulates derived from dynamic theoretical information in the theoretical base, three categories of postulates regarding change are developed: general, directional, and specific.

General postulates regarding change explain the context in which intervention will take place. The general postulates regarding change are considered to be essential for remediation relative to all continua in the frame of reference. For example, a general postulate in the sample frame of reference is that intervention must be conducted in the social context with both males and females.

Some frames of reference have directional postulates regarding change that describe where to begin the process of problem remediation relative to the various continua and the recommended sequence of the change process. The sample frame of reference does not have a directional postulate regarding change, just the suggestions of one. An example of a directional postulate regarding change could be found in a frame of reference of reducing anxiety. The directional postulate regarding change would state that the process of dealing with anxiety is initiated at whatever point on the continuum that the individual appears to be within the process of dealing with anxiety. Because the process is often one of progression–regression–progression, therapists should be prepared to follow the individuals as they move between various points.

Specific postulates regarding change describe the interaction between the therapist, the environment, and specific techniques that the therapist will use to bring about change for each of the continua in the frame of reference. Specific postulates regarding change can be written as "if-then" statements. They state that if the therapist does something, then a resultant effect should occur. The statements are descriptive and guide the therapist's behavior and actions. As action-oriented statements, they convey to the therapist the type of environment that should be created to produce change or the type of technique needed to bring about change. The result can be a change in the child's behavior or an enhancement of typical growth and development that has been interfered with because of dysfunction.

In the statement of both general and directional postulates regarding change, only environmental elements are identified, not specific activities. While specific activities could be mentioned to provide examples, they should never serve as a substitute for clearly defined environmental elements. When a postulate regarding change relates to the use of a specific therapeutic technique, it states the type of action the therapist should take to bring about an explicit response in the child. For example, if the therapist lengthens the muscle fibers, then the muscle should relax. Because an environment that allows for change is important, it is rare that a frame of reference will have only postulates that describe the use of specific techniques. Most frames of reference include postulates regarding change that discuss the environment as well as the therapist's direct actions. In our example of lengthening the muscle fibers to promote muscle relaxation, the postulate regarding change must also address the therapists' conscious use of self and engagement in an activity.

Postulates regarding change serve as pivotal junctures within the frame of reference. They bridge the abstract concepts stated in the theoretical base and the practical actions that need to be taken by therapists to facilitate change in the child. The postulates regarding change give therapists a mechanism for using the frame of reference to plan the intervention.

Within the frame of reference of *Improving Constructive Block Play Skills of Kindergarten Children*, postulates regarding change might be the following:

General postulate regarding change: Block play is enhanced by providing children with opportunities to practice, receiving instructions and feedback.

Directional postulate regarding change: Intervention begins at a child's current level of block play, and progresses to performance of next level.

Specific postulate regarding change (for the continuum of "initiate block play"): If the child was provided with opportunities to explore blocks in different settings, the child will be more likely to initiate block play.

Specific postulate regarding change (for the continuum of "block play"): If a child was provided with opportunities to observe block play by others, receives verbal instructions or demonstrations from practitioners, and actively engages in practice, they are more likely to demonstrate improved block play skills.

When examining postulates regarding change, you should consider the following:

- Does a general postulate regarding change (1) identify environmental factors that apply to all continua and (2) state the characteristics, quality, quantity, and sequence of interaction with the human and nonhuman environment through which an individual is assisted in problem remediation?
- If appropriate, does the directional postulate regarding change address the order of continua to provide a sequence of delivering intervention?
- Is there a specific postulate regarding change for each continuum with consideration of the following: (1) each continuum is addressed by one specific postulate; (2) each specific postulate regarding change states the characteristics, quality, quantity, and sequence of interaction with the human and nonhuman environment through which an individual is assisted in problem remediation; and (3) each specific postulate regarding change is unique and only applies to the designated continuum?

Application to Practice

The postulates regarding change have stated the important guidelines that should be used by therapists to facilitate behavioral change in the child. Some frames of reference require a more in-depth explanation of the key strategies and techniques used to promote functional performance. Other frames of reference require additional descriptions of the actions to be taken by therapists or may require specific examples of the therapeutic process. Often it is difficult for even the most experienced therapists to make the transition from the abstract theoretical stage to practical application without additional explanation. This section eases that shift from theory to practice. In other words, the purpose of this section is to provide therapists with additional information to effectively implement this frame of reference in practical settings. Additionally, this section could suggest criteria for choosing appropriate activities and describe how these activities could be graded, enabling the child to transition from a state of dysfunction to one of function.

For example, within the sample frame of reference presented in this chapter, *Improving Constructive Block Play Skills of Kindergarten Children*, intervention would have to be done in an environment that allow individual or group free play.

The practioner should organize the room's physical layout, and allow ample time for children to engage in block play at their own pace. It is advantageous to store blocks on open, easily accessible shelves near the designated block-building area. Additionally, the practitioner should select and grade the activities to align with each child's abilities, ensuring that every activity is optimally effective. This may include modifying the sizes and types of blocks to match the child's motor skills and offering the right challenges that align with the child's skill level. The block play activities can be conducted individually or in a group setting.

This section is not meant to be a cookbook for application. Instead, it is meant to provide clarification, where necessary, by addressing the following questions:

- Does the application to practice section discuss practical and realistic implementation of the frame of reference clearly related to the theoretical base?
- Does the application to practice section discuss specific modalities or techniques that therapists use in this frame of reference such as therapeutic use of self (psychosocial or physical handling), activities, physical agents, teaching and learning, stimulus response and interaction, technologic products, and/or activity groups?
- Are the described interventions using specific modalities or techniques consistent with the postulates regarding change?
- Does the application to practice section discuss how the use of specific modalities or techniques facilitates engagement in occupation?

Evidence

We have emphasized throughout this chapter that all interventions are theoretically based. Because interventions are based on the hypotheses that are derived from theoretical postulates, therapists and researchers can examine the effectiveness of interventions by accepting or rejecting the working hypotheses via scientific methods. Examining interventions through the lens of frames of reference promotes best practice with supporting clinical evidence. For that reason, we have added a section to each chapter on evidence. Evidence is not a new section to the frame of reference, but it is an additional section to each chapter intended to show both students and therapists the current level of evidence regarding the frame of reference. It also indicates the work that still needs to be done, in terms of research, to determine the efficacy of the frame of reference.

Summary

As a scientific profession, interventions must be theoretically based. This text is based on frames of reference designed to meet the specific needs of children. Frames of reference assist therapists to organize theoretical guidelines for intervention. In addition, frames of reference provide a structure or a road map for therapists to identify, plan, and refine their interventions. This chapter describes the various sections of the frame of reference and gives examples for each section through a simulated frame of reference. It demonstrates the transition from the theoretical base through to application to practice, with clear statements about the consistency that is necessary throughout. This chapter provides a basis for understanding how to read and understand the frames of reference that are articulated in the following chapters.

REFERENCES

American Occupational Therapy Association. (2020). Occupational therapy practice framework: Domain and process (4th ed.), *The American Journal of Occupational Therapy*, *74*, Suppl. 2 7412410010p1

Gagné, R. M. (1977). *The conditions of learning* (3rd ed.). Holt, Rinehart and Winston.

Gregory, K. M., Kim, A. S., & Whiren, A. (2003). The effect of verbal scaffolding on the complexity of preschool children's block constructions. In D. E. Lytle (Ed.), *Play and educational theory and practice* (pp. 117–133). Praeger Publishers/Greenwood Publishing Group.

Guanella, F. M. (1934). Block building activities of young children. *Archives of Psychology*, *174*, 71–92.

Kramer, P., & Hinojosa, J. (1993). Structure of frames of reference. In P. Kramer & J. Hinojosa (Eds.), *Frames of reference for pediatric occupational therapy* (pp. 37–48). Williams & Wilkins.

Lynch, H., & Moore, A. (2016). Play as an occupation in occupational therapy. *British Journal of Occupational Therapy*, *79*(9), 519–520. https://doi.org/10.1177/0308022616664540

Mosey, A. C. (1981). *Occupational therapy: Configurations of a profession*. Raven Press.

Mosey, A. C. (1986). *The psychosocial components of occupational therapy*. Raven Press.

Mosey, A. C. (1996). *Applied scientific inquiry in the health professions: An epistemological orientation* (2nd ed.). American Occupational Therapy Association.

Smilansky, S. (1968). *The effects of sociodramatic play on disadvantaged children: preschool children*. Wiley.

Tian, M., Luo, T., & Cheung, H. (2020). The development and measurement of block construction in early childhood: A review. *Journal of Psychoeducational Assessment*, *38*(6), 767–782. https://doi.org/10.1177/0734282919865846

Vygotsky, L. (1966). Play and its role in the mental development of the child, *Voprosy Psikhologii*, *12*(6), 62–76.

2 Developmental Perspective: Fundamentals of Developmental Theory

Paula Kramer ■ Francine M. Seruya ■ Tsu-Hsin Howe

When working with children, an understanding and appreciation of human development is important. Typically, development is believed to be the sequential changes in functions that occur based on biologic maturation and environmental experience of children. Most developmental theories explain and describe the relationships between human biologic capacity (nature) and environmental experience (nurture). Developmental theorists emphasize nature or nurture to various degrees to form their personal perspectives and beliefs about development. Developmental theories used by occupational therapy practitioners as the foundation for interventions tend to fall into three general categories: stage-specific theories, ecological theories, and acquisitional learning theories.

TYPES OF DEVELOPMENTAL THEORIES

The stage-specific theories describe the developmental sequences and patterns in different domains including motor/physical, cognition, social/emotional, communication/language, and self-help. These theories also describe how the environment may enhance or inhibit development in some instances, but to a lesser degree.

The ecological theories focus more on how the environment and experiences within the environment can affect development in general and the developmental sequence overall. Information about these sequences and patterns provides practitioners with knowledge about biologic maturation and the potential influence of the environment. In a frame of reference, information from these theories provides a critical basis that become elements of important concepts in the theoretical base This information is then expanded in the function/dysfunction continua and indicators for functions and dysfunctions sections and application to practice guiding practitioners to conduct evaluation and intervention using specific context that described by these theories. Understanding the environment provides practitioners with the means to use it as an intervention tool.

More recently, there has been discussion in occupational therapy literature of the life course theory of development (Elder, 1998; Elder & Shanahan, 2006), particularly as it relates to the development of a child as an occupational being. Aspects of this theory are both developmental and environmental. This will also be discussed in this chapter.

On the other hand, acquisitional learning theories describe how children learn and what environmental factors facilitate or inhibit changes. In a frame of reference, these learning theories provide dynamic theoretical information that describes what practitioners can do to modify the environmental factors to promote changes in behaviors.

It is critical for occupational therapist practitioners to understand child development to adequately screen and assess children to determine the need for early intervention. Further, it is important for practitioners to be able to educate and explain to parents what is to be expected for their children and how to spot potential developmental delays.

Stage-Specific Theories

Theories that emphasize biologic determinants support the idea that development is genetically inherent, invariant among individuals, and with limited change by interaction with others or the environment (Bredekamp, 2019; Lerner, 2018). Many of these theories proposed development as distinct and separate stages, with all components of a process occurring before a skill is acquired or learned (e.g., Freud, 1966; Gesell & Armatruda, 1954; Kohlberg, 1969). Other theorists view progression as being more like building blocks in that there must be an underlying foundation from which skill development evolves (e.g., Ayres, 1972; Erikson, 1963; Maslow, 1970; Piaget, 1963).

Within the pediatric context, both perspectives on the developmental processes are used to describe progression, even though each differs significantly in its perspective of what development means. All of these viewpoints involve an attempt to understand the patterns of progression. Each of these theories describes a particular pattern of progression in children's development differently, yet each shares the accepted principles of stage specific human development.

Some view behaviors as representing a continual set of sequences, while others view the development of each level of functioning as important, but also as serving as the basis for higher level skills. Regardless of what aspect of stage specific theory one subscribes to, it is important to recognize that development is expected to occur within a prescribed sequence.

While these theories of how humans develop have evolved over the years, it should be noted that specific developmental milestones were updated in 2022 for the first time in 20 years by the Centers for Disease Control and Prevention (https://www.cdc.gov/ncbddd/actearly/milestones/index.html, retrieved July 2023) in conjunction with the American Academy of Pediatrics because of changes that have been documented in society (February 2022, https://publications.aap.org/pediatrics/article/149/3/e2021052138/184748/Evidence-Informed-Milestones-for-Developmental, retrieved May 2023). This was done through an extensive process, involving many professionals (though no occupational therapists) over a period of 3 years. It involved an extensive literature search, meetings of a broad panel of professionals, review of evaluative tools (some of which are used by occupational therapists), review by additional professionals, and then a final review to determine that the resulting document was "easy for families of different social, cultural and ethnic backgrounds to observe and review" (Zubler et al., 2022, p. 3).

Though there has been some criticism of these revised milestones, it was noted that in the previous document, the milestone was indicated when the 50th percentile of children were able to achieve the milestone. In the revised milestones, the indicator is set at the 75th percentile. The rationale for this was when the milestones were set at the 50th percentile, practitioners often took a "wait and see approach" rather than seeking intervention. With the revised milestones set at the 75th percentile, the panel felt that children will be more likely to get the needed intervention (Zubler et al., 2022).

Ecological Theories

Theorists who emphasized environmental experiences purport that based on systems theory, children are made up of subsystems and that the organism changes based on its interaction with the environment (Gibson, 1988; 2000; Humphrey, 2006; Von Bertalanffy, 1933). These theories put forth that children cannot learn about one part of an organism separate from the whole organism. This perspective views children as active and the source of their behaviors. Children are the center of development, and changes in children are self-directed based on the interaction children have with the environment.

The meta-theoretical stance emphasizes that both heredity and environment influence children's development. This perspective incorporates the perspective that the nervous system is plastic and that there is a strong influence on context to promote change and development of children (Lerner, 2018). These theories are consistent with the proposition of nurture as a way of promoting growth and change in children. Many practitioners prefer these theories. Occupational therapy practitioners are very cognizant that there are a myriad of factors that are now also believed to affect development.

Dynamic system theory can serve as an example of this perspective. Dynamic system theory views development as an open system, where genetic activity, neural activity, behavior, and environment (including physical, social, and cultural environment) interact in a specific way to promote children's development. There is a capacity for development throughout the life span. As these four systems interact, development occurs. These four systems are equally important in the developmental process; therefore, practitioners need to consider all aspects of these systems when evaluating and treating. There may be constraints on the interaction between these systems that influence development (Lerner, 2018). For example, while practitioners may think in terms of motor coordination, the younger child engaging in any sport may just think purely about the motor act of running (Figure 2.1). However, this may become more directed by internal genetic and neural activity, by the environmental response from parents and other children, or from the interaction with the sport itself.

Holistic Person–Context interaction theory (Magnusson & Stattin, 1998; 2006) is another theory grounded in the ecological perspective. It views children as active part of a complex, integrated, and dynamic person–environment system. Ecological theories assert that it is not possible to understand children's functioning and development without the knowledge of the environment. Processes of continuous reciprocal interaction among mental, behavior, and biologic aspects of children's functioning and social, cultural, and physical aspects of the environment guide children's development. Children and the environment function as an integrated dynamic totality, with both being equal in importance. Therefore, they must be studied together and not separately. Furthermore, these theories posit that an optimal environment supporting children's development is an environment that is patterned consistently. It would allow children to assign meaning to the world and to form valid conceptions about situation–outcome contingencies and behavior–outcome contingencies. Also, an optimal environment should be influenced by the children's action in a predictable way. That is, children must be able to exert active control of their environment. Family environment and peer networks are the two common contexts that practitioners should consider during evaluation and intervention planning.

The life course theory of development focuses on the importance of the environment in promoting the child as an occupational being. Elder (1998) states that "changing lives alters development" (p. 1). This is specifically related to the environmental factors of one's life. One example

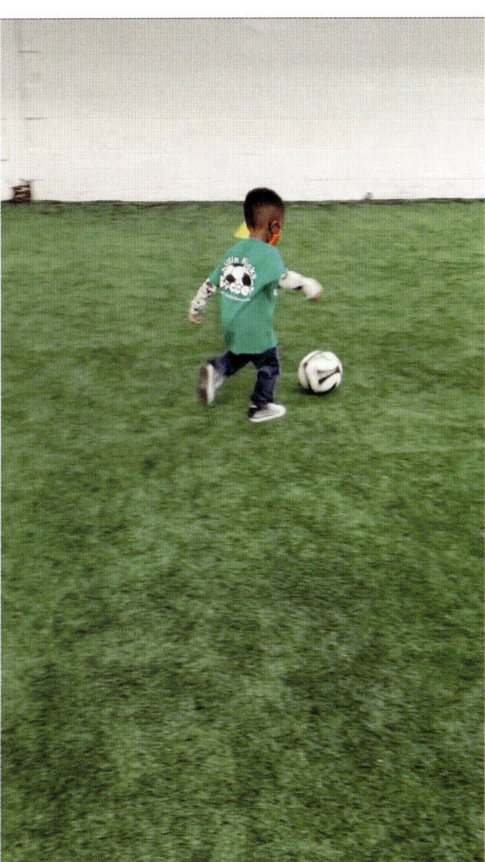

FIGURE 2.1 A child learning to play soccer and enjoying running. (Courtesy of B. DeVeaux.)

is when a child moves from one environment to a very different one, say an urban environment to a rural environment, the types of activities that they are exposed to may be very different which will influence their chosen occupations. Those experiences and occupations that the child sees and experiences in their personal environments are the skills and occupations that become meaningful to them. Additionally, those are the skills that they strive to develop because of the meaning of the occupations to those around them. A child who grows up with sports and views engagement in sporting activities as valuable to the adults in their environment is more likely to strive towards these types of skills. This perspective relates more to the person's actual experiences rather than the specific stages of life. Social history and geographic location play more of a role in this perspective than stage-specific development. This perspective provides a way for occupational therapy practitioners to see how ecological factors such as social situations can affect children's engagement in and choices of occupations rather than focusing on their developmental levels (Elder & Shanahan, 2006; Mayer, 2009). Lerner (2018) also presents a theory of relationship developmental systems where the human being is involved with others and the environment as a context, and that promotes changes and growth in the individual. He posits that humans by their interaction with others and the environment assist in constructing their own development. This is related to the life course theory of development and is based on earlier writings by Lerner and Spanier (1978).

Humphrey and Womack (2019) pointed out important principles relating to the life course theory to future occupations including that experiences transform over a lifetime and affect future occupations. In addition, past experiences, societal and historic events provide particular meaning to individuals and how they react.

Acquisitional Learning Theories

Development may occur through maturation, where subsequent skills are created based on pre-established foundations, or it may occur through learning and skill acquisition, or there can be a combination of learning and maturation. Acquisitional learning theories posit that behavior is a response to the environment, and that repeated interactions shapes children's behaviors. This is not the same as the ecological theories but based on the work of the early works of behavioral scientists of the early 20th century.

Behavioral scientists lay the groundwork for acquisitional learning theories based on the hypotheses and experimental research in areas of behaviorism, cognitive science, and neuroscience. Ivan Petrovich Pavlov (1941), Edward Lee Thorndike (1932), John B. Watson (1913), and Burrhus Frederic Skinner (commonly known as B.F. Skinner) (1953, 1971, 1974a, 1974b) were prominent behavioral theorists who believed that all behaviors, no matter how complex, can be reduced to simple stimulus–response association. Pavlov (1927), known for his experiments on classical conditioning, conducted the first systematic study of basic laws of learning through conditioning. Thorndike extended behaviorism's research from animal to human behaviors and introduced the concept of reinforcement (Donahoe, 1999). In his connectionism theory, Thorndike hypothesized that learning was the formation of a connection between stimulus and response. A neural bond would be established between the stimulus and response when the response was positive. A person learns when bonds form into patterns of behavior (Thorndike, 1932). Watson (1913) was among the first to use the term behaviorism, emphasizing the role of environmental factors in influencing behavior, to the near exclusion of innate or inherited factors.

B.F. Skinner's theory of operant conditioning (Skinner, 1953, 1971, 1974a, 1974b) with reinforcement (or reward) as a central focus has been widely applied to education and parenting. Albert Bandura (1965, 1977) expanded the role of observation and modeling in a learned behavior in his social learning theory. Carl Rogers' (Rogers, 1951, 1957; Rogers & Freiberg, 1994) "unconditional positive regard" forms the foundation of client-centered therapy. It places client at the center of the treatment setting, with partitioners continually offering support to promote client's positive behavioral changes. In their theory, the focus is on how the practitioner approaches intervention using principles of behaviorism.

Cognitive science, the second focus providing a basis for acquisitional learning theories, came from a blending of interdisciplinary researchers interested in attention, perception, communication, and information processing (Gardner, 1985). Cognitive theories emerged in response to limitations of behaviorism that tended to simplify behaviors and focus only on external influences, whereas cognitive scientists were more interested in complexity of inner working mental processes (Kandel, 2006).

In the 1970s and 1980s, behaviorists and cognitive scientists started collaborating with scientists studying higher brain function. The result of these collaborations resulted in the third focus of learning theories based on the neurosciences. Theorists based these theories on new knowledge that merged biologic science (concerned with brain processes) with behavioral and cognitive psychology (concerned with mental processes). Kandel's (2006) neuroscience research has shown that learning and memory are formed in stages and based on synaptic connections. Short-term memory, created by strengthening existing synapses, lasts minutes. His experiments propose that short-term memory grades naturally into long-term memory through repetition. According to Kandel (2006), "practice does make perfect" (p. 206). Acquisitional learning theories provide the dynamic theoretical information to promote change in some frames of reference.

USING DEVELOPMENTAL THEORIES IN FRAMES OF REFERENCE

Occupational therapy practitioners tend to accept developmental theories that have a broader perspective to explain children's learning and behavior. The acceptance by occupational therapy practitioners of diverse perspectives on development and interaction, rather than exclusively adhering to traditional developmental theories, has broadened their scope of practice and enhanced the effectiveness and flexibility of their interventions. These various perspectives are shown throughout the frames of reference in this text. Most practitioners accept that children interact with the environment, resulting in changes in children's behaviors, and that the children also have an impact on their surrounding environment, consequently changing the environment as well (Figure 2.2). As the environment changes and the child changes, there is a constant reciprocal interaction between the child and the environment, resulting in changes to both the child and environment (Davis & Polatajko, 2004). A limitation of all of these abovementioned developmental perspectives is the Western-based assumption that the environment is external to children. The Kawa model identifies that eastern philosophies view the person is interrelated with the environment rather than an independent self (Iwama, 2006).

The introduction of a wider variety of developmental theories presents an interesting conundrum for occupational therapy practitioners. The newer theories are very consistent with the views of practitioners regarding the importance of the environment, the plasticity of the neural system, the role of nurturing in development, and the criticality of involvement in meaningful activities to enhance growth. These same theories lessen the emphasis on the age-specific, stage-specific developmental theories that occupational therapy practitioners have used for many years, though we still look for specific milestones and view it as a "red flag" when they do not appear on time. The traditional developmental theories are mainstays in our educational programs. Additionally, they serve as the basis for a majority of our developmental evaluations.

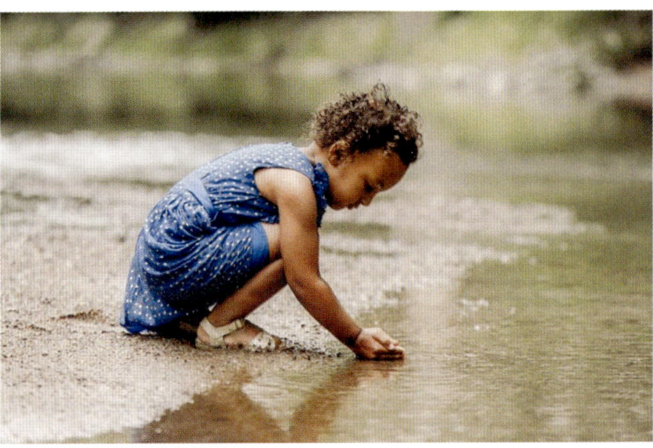

FIGURE 2.2 A child interacting with her environment. (Courtesy of J. Ngelesani.)

Philosophically, practitioners need to explore and understand all theories of development and determine how they can be used to support interventions. The unique advantage of frames of reference is that theoretical bases can be updated based on newer/updated versions of theories, thus leading to interventions with new directions. In addition, frames of reference provide clear structure so that research can be conducted to validate theories, accept/reject hypotheses, and thus to improve the effectiveness of intervention. Further, evaluations that are developed in the future or revised should consider the larger context of the child, rather than just on the developmental sequence.

At this point, occupational therapy practitioners are encouraged to embrace the knowledge from all these developmental perspectives to the extent possible, maintaining an understanding of age-specific and stage-specific development and incorporating an understanding of the vast additional perspectives on issues that can affect development. Although occupational therapy practitioners learn about all aspects of development, our primary concern is with the children's abilities to translate learned developmental skills into functional performance rather than the pure sequential nature of development. Our perspective of development focuses on understanding the ability of children to engage in meaningful occupations within the context of their environments. Regardless of which theories are used by the practitioner, the goal is to facilitate children learning different levels of functional skills.

Pediatric occupational therapy practitioners share a unique viewpoint in their concern for the development of performance skills. Occupational therapy practitioners are concerned with children being able to function within their environments to the best of their abilities. This viewpoint requires consideration of the many different factors that can influence children's overall development. We are inherently concerned with children's abilities and how human and nonhuman influences affect the development of these abilities. Practitioners can see children's abilities as a composite of various specific skills, and they focus on ascertaining the child's developmental level to address the development of these skills within their individual context.

Children do not develop in a vacuum. They are part of an ever-changing dynamic process because changes occur continuously in internal and external environments. Children's body and mind represent the internal environment, and yet their body and mind are greatly influenced by growth, maturation, and the external environment. Human and nonhuman objects are part of the external environment. Both human and nonhuman objects influence children's development separately and together. The importance of each environment varies with children's capabilities, the specific demands of a situation, the objects involved, and the performance required. Although children are considered to have many separate areas that develop independently, motor, psychological, cognitive, and social development are all interrelated and interdependent. In reality, although practitioners may discuss children's motor development in isolation, it cannot be considered independently of children's whole life. Children who are unable to walk may have limited access to interaction with their peers and, therefore, may have difficulty with age-appropriate social development. Other variables that may affect motor development include the neurophysiologic status, orthopedic conditions, early sensory and living experiences, and the family dynamics.

Rates of development vary among children, with no two children being exactly alike. There is a typical range, but not one normal, within progression and rates of development. Some children tend to walk earlier, while others move around in a variety of ways for a longer period of time before walking. Development does not always occur at a consistent rate but rather in spurts that alternate with rest periods, at which time consolidation of skills takes place, much influenced by external factors.

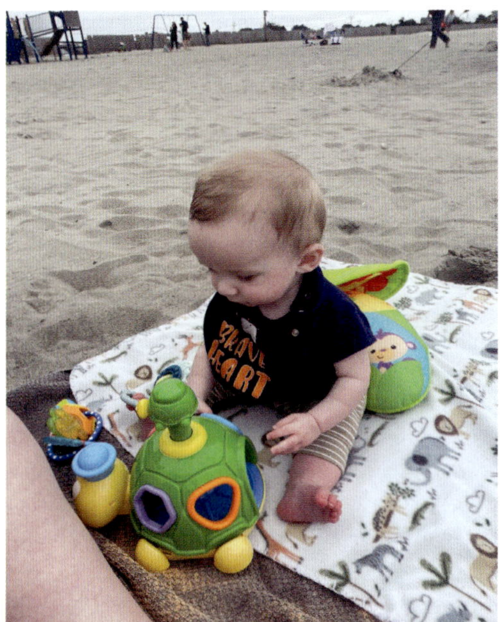

FIGURE 2.3 A young child enjoying sedentary play a toy. (Courtesy of the Barber family.)

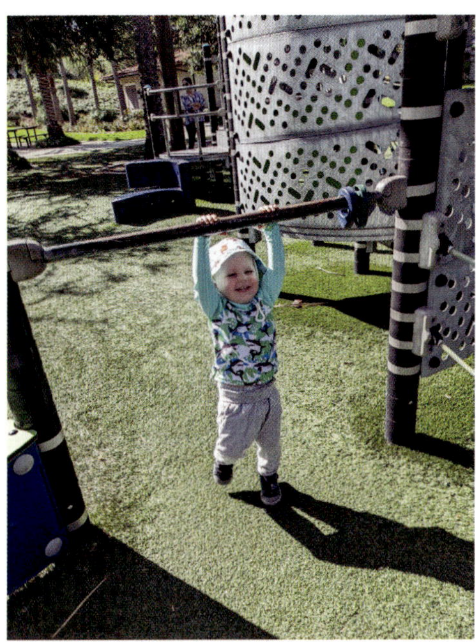

FIGURE 2.4 An older child exploring gross motor play. (Courtesy of J. Alfred.)

Environmental factors can enhance or inhibit skill progression. When practitioners view typical development, they describe it as orderly, predictable, and sequential. However, practitioners also need to explore the external factors of the environment, the interaction with care providers, the cultural climate, and physiologic changes in children. For example, as children begin to ambulate, they usually start to ignore previously favored toys that required them to be sedentary. Instead, they now want to explore the environment with their newfound freedom (Figures 2.3 and 2.4).

Traditionally, once children's patterns, sequences, and level of development are determined, occupational therapy practitioners can address children's needs in two ways. First, practitioners can determine the performance skills children have or can develop at their current level of function. Children who cannot walk or talk still may be able to participate actively in self-feeding. It is critical that practitioners focus on both the child's abilities as well as those skills that need to be attained. Second, based on a pattern or sequence of development, practitioners can determine children's deficits and the possible influencing factors. Based on some hypotheses, practitioners use knowledge about normal growth and development, anatomy, neurophysiology, and life tasks to develop an intervention plan that is sensitive to any sequela of disease or to any known data about the development of the particular systems in which children have deficits.

With the advent of new theories of development, occupational therapy practitioners can expand their focus to one that looks at functional skills and participation. They consider other factors that may also influence development. These include the environment, family life, cultural influences, nurturing, growth facilitating experiences, and other factors. Knowledge about the characteristic pattern of the development of particular performance skills must be balanced by the particular children's developmental direction, rate, and sequence, and the external factors of the environment and experiences that can influence the performance skill.

Perhaps the easiest area to understand is motor progression, which usually is presented in a format that identifies the sequence in which children acquire the ability to move. This progression, similar to those of other systems, inherently includes the acceptance of two basic assumptions: (1) development has a natural order and (2) development is sequential. Adding to this foundation is the perspective that factors such as environment, stimulation, interaction, and children's personal characteristics can affect and change the presumed natural progression of development. Therefore, that while there may be a general sequential order that children seem to follow, it is not necessarily the only order to achieve basic skills. This order may be modified and changed by the external factors that interact with children and the role of people who are nurturing the children. Development, therefore, becomes a much more multidimensional process, with influences from many more sources than just a set of age-specific and stage-specific skills and behaviors. Some children develop faster in one area, some slower, and children may not follow the same exact sequence as external forces may promote variations. Practitioners have to consider not only the chronologic age and developmental age but also the social and emotional age of the child. Experience tells us that children do not develop evenly across all of these areas, at any given time.

IS THERE A DEVELOPMENTAL FRAME OF REFERENCE?

Why do we raise this question? Many occupational therapy practitioners who work with children say that they use a developmental perspective or frame of reference for intervention. The developmental perspective, whether purely age and stage specific or influenced by a multitude of additional external forces, forms a foundational knowledge that is important to all pediatric occupational therapy practitioners. Most of the frames of reference presented in this textbook presume that practitioners have a firm knowledge of the developmental perspective and its impact on the skill acquisition of children. However, there is no one specific developmental frame of reference presented here, but rather a compendium of recent perspectives of development. We believe that there is no one specific developmental frame of reference that can be applied to intervene all issues occur in pediatric occupational therapy. We believe that what practitioners commonly refer to as the developmental frame of reference is truly a conventional approach where the practitioners use a variety of the accepted intervention tools of the profession to facilitate the traditionally accepted sequence of typical development. This involves practitioners' clinical reasoning, a manipulation of the environment, the use of teaching and learning theories, the provision of additional growth-enhancing experiences, and conscious use of self. In these situations, practitioners identify the critical skills needed by children within the accepted normal developmental sequence and use intervention tools to facilitate the development of those skills. The introduction and understanding of new perspectives on development that are consistent with the assumptions and values of occupational therapy can be effectively used to enhance our interventions with children.

CONCLUSION

The developmental perspective is not a single described view used in pediatric occupational therapy. Instead, there are multiple perspectives based on scientific, philosophical, or pragmatic views of a wide range of the theorists. Thus, occupational therapy practitioners need to be aware of the multiple perspectives and understand how they influence their interventions. In this book, the developmental perspectives are critical to the theoretical base of the many frames of reference. The specific theories in the theoretical base identify both constant and dynamic theoretical information. Specific theories provide constant theoretical information that describes how development is perceived and delineate the key elements that practitioners should address. On the other hand, dynamic theoretical information describes how to create environments that facilitate positive change of client's behaviors. Therefore, practitioners should possess a comprehensive understanding of diverse developmental theories and be comfortable to appreciate the interventions of other practitioners, even when these interventions are based on theoretical perspectives that differ from their own.

REFERENCES

Ayres, A. J. (1972). *Sensory integration and learning disorders.* Western Psychological Services.

Bandura, A. (1965). Influence of a model's reinforcement contingencies on the acquisition of imitative responses. *Journal of Personality and Social Psychology, 11*, 589–595.

Bandura, A. (1977). *Social learning theory*. Prentice-Hall.

Bredekamp, S. (2019). *Effective practices in early childhood education: Building a foundation*. Pearson Education.

Centers for Disease Control and Prevention. (2023). CDC's developmental milestones. Retrieved July 2023, from https://www.cdc.gov/ncbddd/actearly/milestones/index.html

Davis, J., & Polatajko, H. J. (2004). Occupational development. In C. H. Christiansen & E. S. Townsend (Eds.), *Introduction to occupation: The art and science of living* (pp. 91–119). Prentice Hall.

Donahoe, J. W. (1999). Edward L. Thorndike: The selectionist connectionist. *Journal of the Experimental Analysis of Behavior, 72*, 451–454.

Elder, G. H. (1998). The life course as developmental theory. *Child Development*, *69*(1), 1–12.

Elder, G. H., & Shanahan, M. J. (2006). The life course and human development. In R. M. Lerner (Ed.), *Handbook of personal psychology* (6th ed., Vol. 1, pp. 665–715). Wiley.

Erikson, E. H. (1963). *Childhood and society* (2nd ed.). Norton & Co.

Freud, S. (1966). *Standard edition of the complete psychological works of Sigmund Freud*. Hogarth Press.

Gardner, H. (1985). *The mind's new science: A history of the cognitive revolution.* Basic Book B.A.Bs.

Gesell, A., & Armatruda, C. S. (1954). *Developmental diagnosis* (2nd ed.). Harper & Brothers.

Gibson, E. J. (1988). Exploratory behavior in the development of perceiving, acting, and the acquiring of knowledge. *Annual review of Psychology, 39*, 1–41. https://doi.org/10.1146/annurev.ps.39.020188.000245

Gibson, E. J. (2000). Perceptual learning in development: Some basic concepts. *Ecological Psychology, 12*(4), 295–302. https://doi.org/10.1207/S15326969ECO1204_04

Humphrey, N. (2006). *Seeing red: A study in consciousness*. Belknap Press/Harvard University Press.

Humphrey, R., & Womack, J. (2019). Transformations of occupations: A life course perspective. In B. A. B. Schell & G. Gillen (Eds.) *Willards & Spackman's occupational therapy* (13th ed., pp. 100–112). Wolters Kluwer.

Iwama, M. K. (2006). *The Kawa model: Culturally relevant occupational therapy*. Churchill Livingstone, Elsevier.

Kandel, E. (2006). *In search of memory: The emergence of a new science of mind.* W.W. Norton & Co.

Kohlberg, L. (1969). Stage and sequence: The cognitive developmental approach to socialization. In D. Groslin (Ed.), *Handbook of socialization theory and research* (pp. 347–480). Rand McNally.

Lerner, R. M. (2018). *Concepts and theories of human development* (4th ed.). Routledge.

Lerner R. M., & Spanier, G. B. (Eds.). (1978). *Child influences on marital and family interaction: A life span perspective*. Academic Press.

Magnusson, D., & Stattin, H. (1998). Person-context interaction theories. In W. Damon & R. M. Lerner (Eds.), *Handbook of child psychology: Theoretical models of human* (5th ed., pp. 685–759). John Wiley.

Magnusson, D., & Stattin, H. (2006). The person in context: A holistic-interactionistic approach. In W. Damon, & R. M. Lerner (Eds.), *Handbook of child psychology: Theoretical models of human development* (6th ed., pp. 400–464). John Wiley.

Maslow, A. H. (1970). *Motivation and personality* (2nd ed.). Harper & Row.

Mayer, K. U. (2009). New directions in life course research. *Annual Review of Sociology, 35*, 413–443. https://doi.org/10.1146/annurev.soc.34.040507.134619

National Public Health Information Coalitions (2022). https://nphic.org/news/news-highlights/681-cdc-updates-child-developmental-milestones#:~:text=The%20CDC%20updated%20its%20developmental%20milestones%20f%20infants,adjusted%20by%20

Pavlov, I. P. (1927). *Conditioned reflexes* (G. V. Andrep, trans.). Oxford.

Pavlov, I. P. (1941). The conditioned reflex (pp. 166–185). In W. Horsley Gantt (Ed.), *Lectures on conditioned reflexes: Vol. 2. conditioned reflexes and psychiatry* (pp. 168–170). International Publishers.

Piaget, J. (1963). *Psychology of intelligence*. Littlefield, Adams & Co.

Rogers, C. R. (1951). *Client centered therapy*. Houghton Mifflin.

Rogers, C. R. (1957). The necessary and sufficient conditions of therapeutic personality change. *Journal of Consulting Psychology, 21*, 95–103.

Rogers, C. R., & Freiberg, H. J. (1994). *Freedom to learn* (3rd ed.). Merrill.

Skinner, B. F. (1953). The science of learning and the art of teaching. *Harvard Educational Review, 24*, 86–97.

Skinner, B. F. (1971). *Science and human behavior*. Macmillan.

Skinner, B. F. (1974a). *About behaviorism*. Vintage Books.

Skinner, B. F. (1974b). *Beyond freedom and dignity*. Knopf.

Thorndike, E. L. (1932). *Fundamentals of learning*. Teachers College, Columbia University.

Von Bertalanffy, L. (1933). *Modern theories of development: An introduction to theoretical biology*. Oxford University Press.

Watson, J. B. (1913). Psychology as the behaviorist views it. *Psychological Review, 20*, 158–177.

Zubler J. M., Wiggins L. D., Macias, M. M, Whitaker, T. M., Shaw, J. S., Squires, J. K., Pajek, J. A., Wolf, R. B., Slaughter, K. S., Broughton, A. S., Gerndt, K. L., Mlodoch, B. J., & Lipkin, P. H. (2022). Evidence-informed milestones for developmental surveillance tools. *Pediatrics, 149*(3), e2021052138. https://doi.org/10.1542/peds.2021-052138

Domain of Concern of Occupational Therapy: Relevance to Pediatric Practice

3

Francine M. Seruya ▪ Tsu-Hsin Howe ▪ Paula Kramer

Since a profession exists within the context of society, to be relevant it must identify how it meets the needs and concerns of society. Professions, therefore, identify their *domain of concern* to define the scope of professional practice, the breadth of the profession, and the expertise of practitioners. Unlike the overarching conceptualization of the professional domain, the *scope of practice* limits intervention based on federal and state legislation and institutional policy and defines what occupational therapy practitioners can do as part of their practice. As a means of further defining the scope of practice, professions use a *common language*. This common language provides the ability for smooth communication among professionals both internal and external to the profession. It also helps to define the scope of practice to stakeholders and the external world. Professions also use their common language to document services for reimbursement purposes and it is also used to show evidence that an intervention is effective. The scope of occupational therapy practice in the United States, is guided by the *Occupational Therapy Practice Framework: Domain and Process* (American Occupational Therapy Association, 2020). Other countries have published official documents (e.g., Canadian Association of Occupational Therapy, Occupational Therapy Australia) outlining their domain of concern and scope of practice as well.

CLASSIFICATION SYSTEMS

While health professions like occupational therapy have worked to define their domain of concern and scope of practice, these have been notably distinct to the specific needs and contexts of their own healthcare and educational systems. In 1980, the World Health Organization developed a classification system that was revised and subsequently published as the *International Classification of Functioning, Disability and Health (ICF)* with the intent to develop a single instrument that would be effective across different settings and cultures for communicating about health status and disability (World Health Organization, 2016b). The *ICF* is a framework for measuring health and disability at both individual and population levels (World Health Organization, 2001). It is a biopsychosocial framework of naming and measuring, based on a blending of medical and social models, designed to collect information about functioning, health, well-being, and other health-related domains. This classification was operationalized through the World Health Organization Disability Assessment Schedule, which was developed through a collaborative international approach.

Although initially designed for rehabilitation, this systematic standard framework for classification by functioning was designed to stand alone or work in conjunction with the *International Classification of Disease* to provide international statistics about health outcomes. After the World Health Organization published the *International Classification of Functioning, Disability and Health (ICF)*, occupational therapy scholars noted that it contains language very similar to the language used within occupational therapy, with its focus on activity and participation and some countries adopted similar language in their own documents related to scope of practice (AOTA, 2020). The *Occupational Therapy Practice Framework: Domain and Process*, 4th edition *(OTPF4)* document (American Occupational Therapy Association, 2020) has significant similarities in language and definitions to the *ICF*. While there are substantial commonalities shared by the two documents, the OTPF4's contextual underpinnings are American based, thus it does not necessarily hold universal applicability, however, it is extremely detailed in its definition of the domain and concern and process of occupational therapy services. It is beyond the scope of this book to provide an in-depth review of the entire *ICF* document or identify the whole domain of concern for the profession of occupational therapy. However, to provide common language for pediatric occupational therapy practitioners, this chapter provides an overview of the *ICF* to identify the domain of concern and scope of practice when working with children. In addition, this chapter, where appropriate, aligns more nuanced occupational therapy-based language utilizing the *OTPF4* document.

INTERNATIONAL CLASSIFICATION OF FUNCTIONING

This chapter uses the *International Classification of Functioning*, as it is a worldwide taxonomy that provides a uniform language while offering assessment capabilities to explore the scope of practice as it relates to occupational therapy in pediatrics. The classification system and definitions allow occupational therapy practitioners to provide consistent communication with other disciplines and reimbursement sources, using terminology such as activity, function, performance, functioning, and participation—words that have been part of the occupational therapy lexicon for decades. While the *OTPF4* is specific to occupational therapy in the United States, there is a distinct benefit to having occupational therapy practitioners use a language that is accepted internationally. Indeed, the viability of the profession may rest on the ability of occupational therapy to adapt the profession's language to the international standard naming and measuring system that allows coding, collection, storage, and analysis of statistics. For occupational therapy practitioners, using the *ICF* has an added benefit: This uniform language classification has an integrated coding system that allows measurement of baseline information for comparison with subsequent evaluation data. This universal classification and assessment tool provides a systematic method of building evidence to demonstrate the effectiveness of occupational therapy.

The *International Classification of Functioning (ICF)* has two parts—Part 1: Health Condition and Part 2: Contextual Factors. Each part has two subdivisions. Part 1: Health Condition is comprised by the subdivisions: (1) activities and participation and (2) body functions and structures. Part 2: Contextual Factors is comprised of the subdivisions: (1) environmental factors and (2) personal factors. Where appropriate, we will note the similarities to the *OTPF4* as a means of comparison and to increase applicability to occupational therapy specific terminology. See Table 3.1 for a comparison of the *OTPF4* and the *ICF* terminology.

Table 3.1 Comparison of the Occupational Therapy Practice Framework, 4th Edition (AOTA, 2020) and the International Classification of Function, Disability, and Health (WHO, 2001)

Occupational Therapy Practice Framework 4									**International Classification of Functioning (ICF)**								
Occupations									**Activities and Participation (Daily Life Area Domains)**								
Activities of Daily Living (ADLs)	Instrumental (ADLs)	Rest and Sleep	Education	Work	Play	Leisure	Social Participation	Health Management	Learning and Applying Knowledge	General tasks and Demands	Communication	Mobility	Self-care	Domestic life	Interpersonal interactions and relationships	Major Life Areas	Community, social and civic life
									Body Functions and Structures								
Client factors (values, beliefs and spirituality)		Performance skills (motor, process, and social interaction skills			Performance patterns (habits, routines, roles, and rituals)				Mental	Sensory	Voice and speech	Cardiovascular, hematologic, immunologic, and respiratory	Digestive, metabolic, and endocrine	Genito-urinary and reproductive	Neuro-muscular and movement related	Skin and related structure	
Context									**Contextual Factors**								
Environmental		**Personal**							**Environmental**					**Personal**			
Same environmental factors as noted in the ICF		Age Gender Sexual identity Race and ethnicity Cultural identification and cultural attitudes Social background, social status, socioeconomic status Upbringing and life experiences Habits and past and current behavioral patterns Individual psychological assets Education Profession and professional identity Lifestyle Other health conditions and fitness							Products and Technology	Natural environment and Human Made changes to environment	Support and relationships	Attitudes	Services, systems, and policies	Age and gender Coping style Social background Education Profession Past experience Character style and habits			

Health Conditions: Activities and Participation

In the *International Classification of Functioning*, the activities and participation subdivision (of Part 1. Functioning and Disability) has nine daily life area domains: learning and applying knowledge, general tasks and demands, communication, mobility, self-care, domestic life, interpersonal interactions and relationships, major life areas, and community and social and civic life.

To an occupational therapy practitioner, items within the nine *International Classification of Function* daily life domains are considered occupations, a core concept of the profession of occupational therapy. "Occupation, a collection of activities that people use to fill their time and give life meaning, is organized around roles or in terms of activities of daily living, work and productive activities or play/leisure" (Hinojosa & Kramer, 1997, p. 865). Occupations serve a multitude of purposes; people become involved in them for survival, necessity, pleasure, and personal meaning. Each individual's occupations comprise a unique combination of activities that are meaningful to that person. "Occupations are the ordinary and familiar things that people do every day" (Christiansen et al., 1995, p. 1015). People engage in occupations throughout their everyday lives to fulfill their time and give their lives meaning. An individual's unique occupations define that person. Depending on life situation and circumstances, the occupations that are important to the individual may change over time (Hinojosa & Kramer, 1997). Although the occupational therapy profession uses the term "occupation," the *ICF* uses the term "activities and participation" in nine daily life areas, also called "domains." This chapter works to integrate and unite occupational therapy terminology with *ICF* language. Therefore, the term "occupation-based life areas" is used in this chapter interchangeably with *International Classification of Function* activities and participation, *International Classification of Function* life areas, or *International Classification of Function* domains.

The flexibility of the *International Classification of Functioning* allows items within the activities and participation domains to be reclassified as an activity, defined as "the execution of task or action by an individual," or as participation, "involvement in a life situation" (World Health Organization, 2001, p. 10). A simplified way of looking at activity versus participation is from a role standpoint. If a person does something in their "self" role, then that action is likely to be categorized as an activity. Keep in mind that the root word of activity is active, so the person has to be engaged in doing something. A person involved in a role beyond the self (e.g., functioning as a son, brother, student, or pet owner) is operating in participation mode, is the person part of something. In other words, from an occupational therapy standpoint, occupations (tasks or actions) a person completes in the self-role would be classified as *ICF* activities and occupations (tasks and actions) an individual completes in other role are termed participation.

In addition to determining whether a part of a daily life domain is categorized as an activity or participation, qualifiers can be added to each. When qualifiers are used during the assessment process, the list of nine daily life area domains becomes a classification that allows quantitative measurement of baseline information to be compared with subsequent reevaluation data. For activities and participation, the two qualifiers are *performance* and *capacity*. In the *ICF*, performance is used in the same way occupational therapy practitioners have used the term for years. Performance is what an individual can do in their current context (e.g., home, school) within society. For an individual, assessment of performance includes all equipment typically used in that environment. For example, if a person used eyeglasses (considered a "technical aid" under the *ICF* category of environmental factors) to correct visual disabilities, the person would be assessed using their glasses. Capacity, as identified by the *ICF*, determines the person's ability within the standard environment, alone and without aids. To assess capacity, the individual would be evaluated in a standard environment (e.g., a rehabilitation unit bathroom that is part of a simulated apartment). The person is evaluated without any equipment (not even eyeglasses) in such an evaluation. Capacity assesses a person's true ability in a standard environment.

Many of the *ICF* domains can be likened to the main areas of occupations (Activities of Daily Living [ADL], Instrumental Activities of Daily Living [IADLs], Health Management, Rest and Sleep, Education, Work, Play, Leisure, and Social Participation) identified by the *OTPF4* (AOTA, 2022) and components of these occupations can be observed in of all nine daily life area domains of the *ICF.* Practitioners apply information from the *learning and applying knowledge domain* when they work on specific school functioning of students, such as focusing attention, solving problems, and making decisions. Activities identified in this domain of the *ICF* when considering pediatric intervention aligns with the *OTPF4 occupation of Education*. Practitioners use aspects of the *general tasks and demands domain* when working with a child on carrying out a daily routine, handling stress and other responsibilities, and operating alone or in a group. Here we can see similarities to the tasks identified in the *OTPF4* as part of *occupations of ADL and IADL*. Although speech and language pathologists are responsible for many of the items in the *communication domain*, occupational therapy practitioners work with children on various communication domain aspects such as comprehending body gestures or using a tablet computer to access alternative communication apps. Communication is interwoven throughout all of the familiar occupations in which we engage and does not align with any one specific occupation. Similarly, mobility is a major ICF-identified domain for occupational therapy practitioners working with children but not specific to any of the noted areas occupations. While physical therapists frequently address many of the areas noted in the mobility domain, there is significant overlap with occupational therapy in this area. The *mobility domain* includes changing and maintaining body positions, transferring from one surface to another, lifting and carrying objects, walking and moving, driving (e.g., bikes, four-wheelers, boats, cars), and riding animals. The self-care domain is also a primary area for pediatric occupational therapy and aligns with several occupations including *ADL, IADL,* and *Rest and Sleep*. These occupations are of primary concern to the pediatric practitioners and are often a primary focus for intervention.

The *domestic life domain* is akin to the *occupation of IADL* and includes acquiring goods and services, preparing meals, doing housework, and taking care of domestic animals. Pediatric practitioners address this domain when they work with children on tasks involving making a bed, doing household chores, shopping, or taking responsibility for a pet. The *interpersonal interactions and relationships domain* is another area within the occupational therapy scope of practice that is analogous to components of the *occupation of social participation*. The focus is on this domain when practitioners work with children on completing actions needed for basic and complex interactions with others (e.g., tolerance in relationships, interacting according to rules, and family relationships). Pediatric occupational therapy practitioners frequently address these areas while addressing *occupations of play and leisure*.

Another primary area for pediatric occupational therapy practitioners is the *International Classification of Functioning* domain *major life areas*, which includes education (informal, daycare, preschool, school), vocational training, and higher education. This domain also aligns with the *occupations of education* and *work in OTPF4*. Many pediatric practitioners practice in natural settings such as school systems that include aspects of major life areas. Practitioners may also address work and employment activities when they are working with older children or youth who are involved in transitioning to employment or have remunerative employment, such as mowing lawns or shoveling snow. Within all domains, practitioners will evaluate for supports for participation, which may include human supports such as parents or teachers and environmental support such as the integration of assistive technology.

In the *International Classification of Functioning*, the *community, social, and civic life domain* includes community life, recreation and leisure, religion and spirituality, human rights, and political life and citizenship. This domain has an aspect that is a primary focus of pediatric occupational therapy—*play* and *leisure*—which includes sports, arts and culture, crafts, hobbies, and socializing.

As main areas of focus for pediatric occupational therapy practitioners tends to be in the occupation-based life areas of self-care and play, this section provides further review of self-care as a whole domain and on the recreation and leisure section of the community, social, and civic life domain.

Self-Care

The self-care domain includes washing oneself, caring for body parts, toileting, dressing, eating, drinking, and looking after one's health (Figure 3.1). Depending on the individual situation of the child, the practitioner may intervene with the child, the care provider, or both to address aspects of the self-care domain. The ability to perform self-care activities independently is crucial to an individual's dignity and the preparation for transitions in roles and routines. Therefore, this is a primary area of concern for the pediatric occupational therapy practitioner and should not be overlooked in intervention.

Although it may be difficult for therapy practitioners to work with some self-care domain activities, it is critical that they do so because this may enable the child to become as independent as possible and to develop a positive sense of self. Although some frames of reference in this text do not address the self-care domain directly, such as the *Ayres Sensory Integration Frame of Reference* (Chapter 6) and the *Frame of Reference for Neurodevelopmental Treatment* (Chapter 8), it is understood that they are laying the foundation that allows the child to become independent in

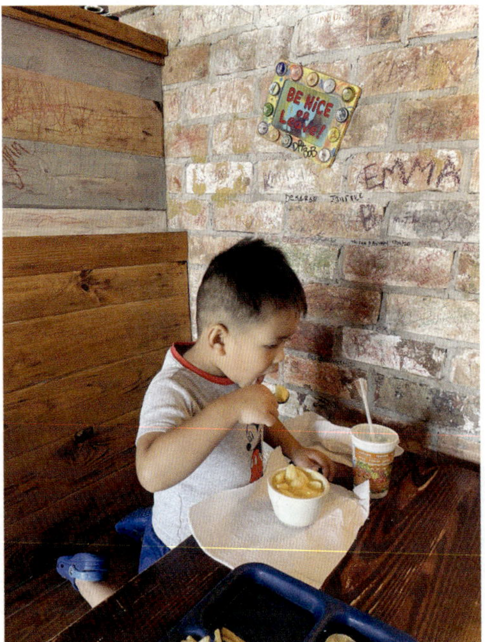

FIGURE 3.1 Child eating soup. (Courtesy of L. Mai.)

self-care. Other frames of reference, such as the *Frame of Reference for Teaching and Learning: The Four Quadrant Model of Facilitated Learning* (Chapter 10) and the *Frame of Reference for Motor Skill Acquisition* (Chapter 11), lend themselves to address self-care more directly.

Play, Recreation, and Leisure

The community, social, and civic life domain includes sections dealing with community life, recreation and leisure, religion and spirituality, human rights, and political life and citizenship. The recreation and leisure section encompasses play (ranging from spontaneous, informal play as seen with younger children to rule-based games such as cards or video games, more frequently seen in older children), sports (e.g., soccer or bowling), arts and culture (e.g., reading for enjoyment, playing musical instruments, or going to the movie theater, art museum, art gallery), crafts (e.g., painting, sewing, scrapbooking), hobbies (e.g., collecting action figures, bugs, shells), and socializing (e.g., informal or casual gatherings, structured play dates, accessing social networking Web sites).

For occupational therapy practitioners, play is a primary intervention when working with the pediatric population. Play activities are those things chosen by children because they are amusing, enjoyable, relaxing, or self-expressive. Play often promotes skill development and interaction with others. The occupational therapy practitioner uses play in two separate ways. First, the practitioner tries to facilitate play exploration so that children can try out diverse types of play and decide which ones they find enjoyable. Second, the practitioner uses play as a therapeutic modality to facilitate the functioning and development of children. The importance of play and its use in intervention is discussed in many frames of reference in this text.

Play, recreation, and leisure include those inherently gratifying activities in which children choose to engage. When used in therapy, play activities are selected for a child's amusement, enjoyment, or self-expression (Figure 3.2). Intrinsically, play, recreational, and leisure activities should be pleasurable, promoting children's enjoyment or relaxation. Involvement in play,

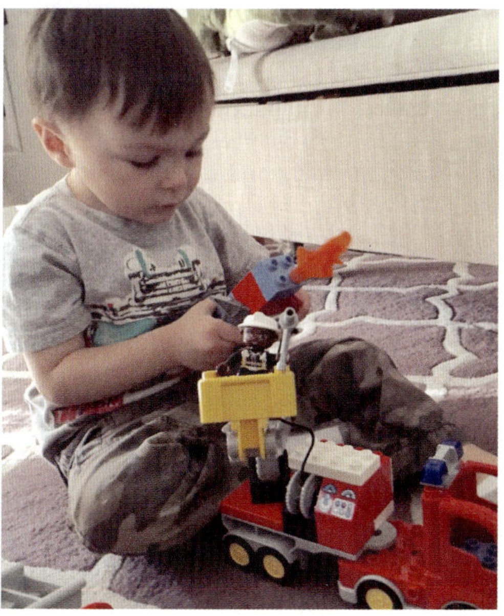

FIGURE 3.2 Young boy enjoying constructional and fantasy play.

recreation, and leisure activities hopefully should encourage skill development through involvement with objects and interaction with others.

Play, recreation, and leisure activities are a natural part of children's life, and children without disabilities have many opportunities to engage in these activities. However, children with disabilities may not have as many occasions to become involved. The primary exposure that children have to play, recreation, and leisure activities may be in the context of a therapeutic experience. The expertise of the occupational therapy practitioner can be used to assist children in playing as a means of self-expression and fun and as a means of assisting parents to strengthen their interaction with their children to provide a typical childhood experience (Hinojosa & Kramer, 1997), using adaptations, accommodations, and equipment as needed. Furthermore, it is incumbent on the practitioner to work with the parent or caregiver to encourage the involvement of children in situations that can increase play opportunities.

Health Conditions: Body Functions and Structures

The second subdivision of Part 1: Health Conditions in the *ICF* is the Body Structures and Functions section. The body structures section is related to the anatomical parts of the body (e.g., organs, limbs, and components). The body structures include structures of the nervous system; the eye, ear, and related structures; structures involved in voice and speech; structures of the cardiovascular, immunologic, and respiratory systems; structures related to the digestive, metabolic, and endocrine systems; structures related to the genitourinary and reproductive systems; structures related to movement; and skin and related structures. The body functions represent the physiologic functions of the body systems and include mental functions; sensory functions and pain; voice and speech functions; functions of the cardiovascular, hematologic, immunologic, and respiratory systems; functions of the digestive, metabolic, and endocrine systems; genitourinary and reproductive functions; neuromusculoskeletal and movement-related functions; and functions of the skin and related structures. *The Client Factors: Body Structures and Functions* of the *OTPF4,* are specifically aligned with these *ICF* categories (AOTA, 2020). Body functions and body structures can be further coded as either positive or negative. The positive aspect is known as "functioning" (having functional integrity and having structural integrity for body functions and body structures, respectively). The negative aspect is called an "impairment," which has three qualifiers: extent (how much), nature (e.g., total absence, qualitative changes), and location (where).

Foundational body-level components—body functions and structures—are closely interrelated, and each aspect embodies an area of the child's development. Understanding body-level functions and structures and their interrelation provides basic information about the child. From this point, the occupational therapy practitioner can develop appropriate interventions after considering the child's biologic potential and developmental status. Separating body function and structure into foundational components allows the occupational therapy practitioner to understand the individual sections that make up the whole. By looking at the small sections, a practitioner gains a better understanding of how children process information in these discrete areas. Through this specific examination of each discrete part, a more comprehensive understanding of children's skills and challenges can be gained. A practitioner's knowledge and understanding of the complex human organism increases by examining and understanding the foundational components of the human at the body level. This is analogous to an activity analysis—instead of analyzing the activity, the practitioner is analyzing the relationship of the physical components to the skill development. This is an essential distinction in pediatric intervention as children often have not learned or acquired skills and interventions are typically geared to facilitate growth rather than seek to rehabilitate lost or declining skills.

Occupational therapy practitioners have expertise in three primary systems at the body function and structure level: (1) sensory functions and pain, (2) neuromusculoskeletal and movement-related functions, and (3) mental functions that are particularly germane when working with children. Each of these areas will be discussed as they are related to pediatric occupational therapy.

Sensory Functions and Pain

In the *International Classification of Function*, the sensory functions and pain subcomponent comprise seeing functions (visual acuity, visual field functions, quality of vision, functions of the structures adjoining the eye such as nystagmus, and sensations associated with the eye and adjoining structures), hearing functions, vestibular functions, sensations associated with hearing and vestibular functions, additional sensory functions (taste, smell, proprioception, touch, temperature, vibration, pressure, and noxious stimuli), and pain. In this conceptualization, the critical concepts are the ability to take in sensory information and process this information.

Sensory functions are also based on the status of the central nervous system and the child's neurophysiologic responses. Sensory function responses are thought to develop from a generalized response to a more sophisticated discrete response to specific stimuli. The tactile system, for example, develops the ability to recognize internal as opposed to external sensation, such as interpreting light touch and pressure. The visual system likewise develops more sophisticated responses through recognition of pattern and color.

Understanding the sensory functions and pain subcomponent is critical to comprehending the *Ayres Sensory Integration Frame of Reference* (Chapter 6), the *Frame of Reference for Sensory Processing Difficulties: Sensory Therapies and Research* (Chapter 7), and the *Frame of Reference for Neurodevelopmental Treatment* (Chapter 8). The occupational therapy student should be aware when reading each of these frames of reference that the theoretical bases of each may conceptualize these subcomponents somewhat differently.

Neuromusculoskeletal and Movement-Related Functions

Neuromusculoskeletal and movement-related functions involve areas of development that underlie the motor aspects of behavior. Function depends on the maturity of the central nervous system and the neurophysiologic system. The neuromusculoskeletal and movement-related functions subcomponent includes functions of the joints and bones (mobility and stability of bones and joints), muscle functions (strength, tone, and endurance), and movement functions (reflexes, involuntary movements, control and coordination of voluntary movements, involuntary movement functions such as tremors, gait patterns, and sensations related to muscles and movement functions such as muscle stiffness or spasm).

When pediatric occupational therapy practitioners consider these neuromusculoskeletal and movement-related functions, each is considered relative to the typical development of the child. It is not simply a case of whether the child has reflexes, for example, but at what level are the reflexes relative to the child's chronologic and developmental age and, even more importantly, how they influence functioning. Most often these subcomponents are viewed relative to other motor behaviors and skills such as standing and climbing (Figure 3.3). These subcomponents are an important element of the *Frame of Reference for Neurodevelopmental Treatment* (Chapter 8),

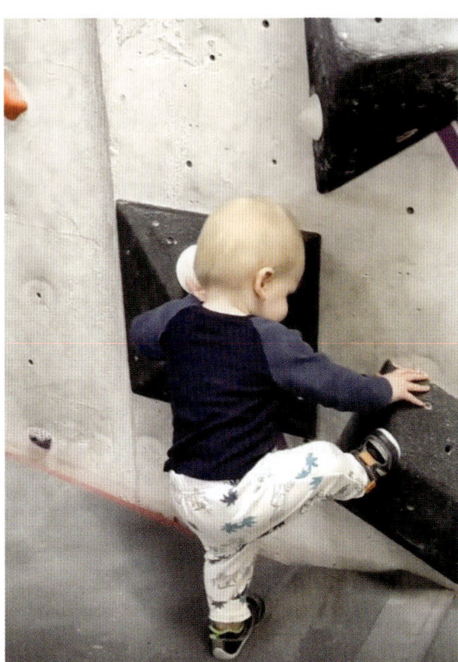

FIGURE 3.3 Child learning how to climb. (Courtesy of J. Alfred.)

the *Frame of Reference for Motor Skill Acquisition* (Chapter 11), and the *Biomechanical Frame of Reference for Seating and Positioning in Children* (Chapter 13).

Mental Functions

In the *International Classification of Function*, mental functions encompass two broad areas: global mental functions and specific mental functions. These broad areas allow the child to develop the cognitive and psychosocial abilities to handle life situations. Global mental functions include consciousness (state, continuity, and quality), orientation (time, place, person), intellectual (general cognitive functions and development across a life), global psychosocial (development of interpersonal skills needed to establish reciprocal meaningful social interactions), temperament and personality functions (extraversion, agreeableness, conscientiousness, psychic stability, openness to experience, optimism, confidence, trustworthiness), energy and drive (energy level, motivation, appetite, craving, impulse control), and sleep (amount, onset, maintenance, quality, functions involving the sleep cycle). An example of addressing global mental functions is an occupational therapy practitioner who is working with a child on the ability to focus on a task, working with others in a group, and exploring a variety of toys and environments (Figure 3.4).

Specific mental functions include attention functions (sustaining, shifting, dividing, and sharing attention), memory (short term, long term, and retrieval), psychomotor functions such as control (regulation of speed or response time such as moving and speaking slowly or excessive behavioral and cognitive activity), and quality (e.g., hand–eye coordination). Other specific mental functions are emotional functions (appropriateness, regulation, and range of emotion), perceptual functions (auditory, visual, olfactory, gustatory, tactile, and visuospatial perception), and thought functions (pace, form, content, and control of thought). A practitioner who is working

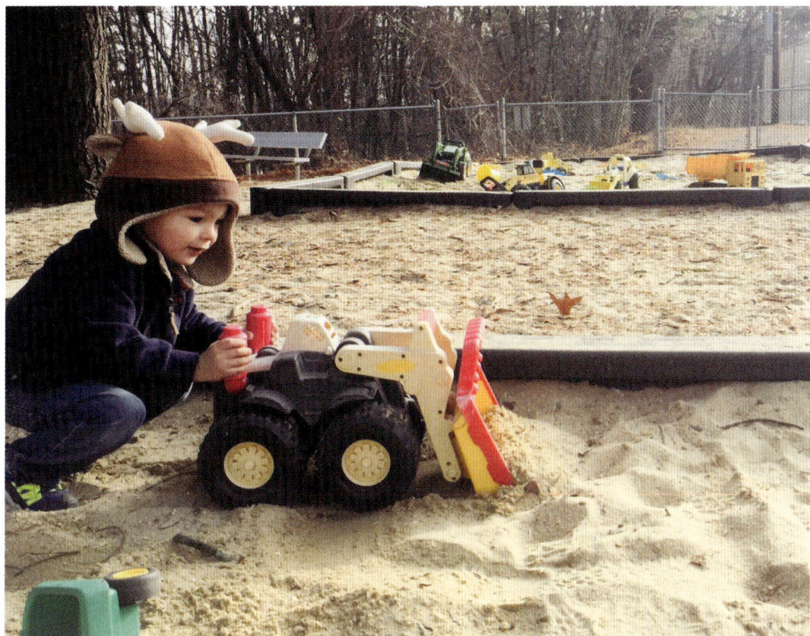

FIGURE 3.4 Young boy concentrating on playing with a new toy in a different environment.

with a child to improve perceptual skills in the area of form constancy or figure-ground or to regulate emotions is addressing these foundational body-level subcomponents.

In addition, specific mental functions also involve higher-level cognitive functions of abstraction, organization and planning, time management, cognitive flexibility, insight, judgment, problem solving; mental functions of language (reception and expression of spoken, written, and sign language); integrative language functions (organization of semantic and symbolic meaning, grammatical structure and ideas for the production of spoken and written language); calculative functions (simple and complex calculation); mental function of sequencing complex movements (commonly called "praxis" in the occupational therapy profession); and experience of self and time functions (experience of self, body image, experience to time). A practitioner who addresses a child's organizational and time management skills or sequencing of movements (motor planning or praxis) is working on specific mental functions, a foundational body-level subcomponent.

These foundational body-level components appear to be directly related to the *Frame of Reference for Teaching and Learning: The Four Quadrant Model of Facilitated Learning* (Chapter 10) and the *Frame of Reference for Developing Handwriting Sills* (Chapter 12). However, the importance of foundational body-level components is much broader because it affects every area of the child's life. There is a complex interplay between and among the foundational body-level components, occupation-based life areas, and contextual factors.

Contextual Factors

Contextual factors are situations or factors that influence an individual's engagement in desired and required occupation-based life areas. The *International Classification of Function* Part 2:

Contextual Factors has two subdivisions: (1) environmental factors and (2) personal factors. Here again, we see the similarities between the language of the *ICF* and the *OTPF4*. The *ICF* environmental factors include the following categories: products and technology; natural environment and human-made changes to the environment; support and relationships; attitudes; and services, systems, and policies. While occupation-based life areas and foundational body-level components are internal to the child, environmental factors are external to the child. These external factors have an impact on the child's ability to engage in life areas. These factors may have a positive or negative effect. Positive environmental factors are "facilitators," whereas negative factors are known as either "barriers" or "hindrances."

One category, products and technology, comprises both general products and technology as well as assistive products and technology. Products and technology include those for personal consumption (e.g., food, drugs); personal use in daily living; personal indoor and outdoor mobility; communication; education; employment; culture, recreation, and sport; and practice of religion and spirituality. Examples of products are prescription medications, an adapted saddle for hippotherapy, a walker, pullover shirts for someone who cannot manipulate fasteners, and reachers. Technology may include computer devices, screen reader programs on a computer, communication boards, lighted pointers, and computer tablets.

This category also includes design, construction, and building products and technology of buildings for public use and private use, land development, and assets. Providing reasonable accommodations in the form of a ramp that allows a student who uses a wheelchair to enter a school and has an equal opportunity to engage in learning is one example of these types of products and technology. Another example is a community that develops an area of land for an accessible playground.

Another category is the natural environment and human-made changes to the environment, which includes physical geography, population, flora and fauna, climate, natural events, human-caused events, light, time-related changes, sound, vibration, and air quality. Children with disabilities who live in rural areas may have a different level of access to occupational therapy services compared with those who live in a city with a therapy clinic down the street, and may benefit from telehealth services. A second example is an occupational therapy practitioner who may help children find fun activities for engagement inside buildings on days with a high pollen count.

Support and relationships are the third category of environmental factors. Included in support and relationships are immediate family; extended family; friends; acquaintances, peers, colleagues, neighbors, and community members; people in positions of authority; people in subordinate positions; personal care providers and personal assistants; strangers; domesticated animals, health professionals; and other professionals. The support and relationships category refers to all people and other living things with which the child interacts. This includes family members, peers, significant others, and pets (Figure 3.5).

The primary function of the family is to provide a supportive and nurturing environment for the child's development. The family shapes the child's ideologic system and provides opportunities to develop interpersonal relationships (Seligman & Darling, 2017; Turnbull et al., 1986). Family configurations have evolved to address the changing dynamics of society. There are a variety of ways to define the family unit, however, defining family via kinship has been the primary means of understanding family configurations (Sharma, 2013). Although there are variations to family configurations, the nomenclature regarding family configurations has largely utilized the concepts of the immediate, extended, expanded, and single-parent households. The immediate (also called "nuclear") family consists of a couple who shares the responsibility of raising a child.

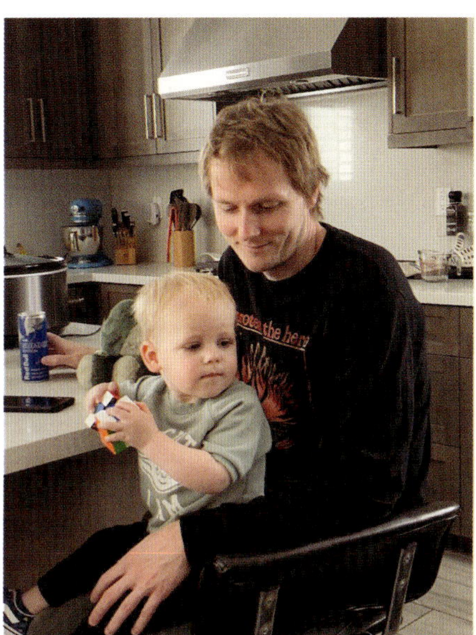

FIGURE 3.5 Child playing with a toy while enjoying the comfort of his father. (Courtesy of P. Kramer.)

The extended family is a group related through family ties or mutual consent that shares some part in child rearing. The extended or "multigenerational" family is a complex combination of family configurations, involving a nuclear family, children, and significant others from previous relationships (Taylor et al., 2010). The single-parent household is one in which an adult assumes all the parental responsibilities. All family members' needs are recognized and supported in a well-functioning, healthy family.

The fourth category of environmental factors is attitudes, which includes individual attitudes of immediate family members; extended family members; friends; acquaintances, peers, colleagues, neighbors, and community members; people in positions of authority; people in subordinate positions; personal care providers and personal assistants; strangers; health professionals; and other professionals. In addition, the attitudes category includes societal attitudes and social norms, practices, and ideologies. Attitudes—which include customs, beliefs, behavior standards, and expectations—have an impact on the child's expectations of self and the parents' expectations of the child. Subsequently, cultural attitudes may reflect on the child's functioning. For example, in some cultures, it is acceptable for a child to use a bottle until they are ready to enter preschool, whereas in other cultures, a child is weaned from the bottle once they become a toddler. This would impact on the child's exposure to a cup and their ability to drink from it. This is an example of a cultural attitude that affects functioning. In some cultures, the use of technology is highly valued, whereas in others, it is not accepted, especially at younger ages. Throughout life, attitudes influence what a person considers to be typical and what constitutes expected patterns of behavior. Within the process of intervention, the practitioner needs to be aware of and sensitive to the cultural background and attitudes of each child and their family that is encountered.

The fifth category is services, systems, and policies. Services may include benefits, programs, and operations; they are public, private, or voluntary by nature and are established by individuals, groups, organizations, or governments. Systems, usually established by governmental entities, provide organizational control to organize and monitor services. Policies that govern the systems are the rules, regulations, and standards established by various levels of government. A good example of services, systems, and policies in action and across time is the way in which pediatric occupational therapy has evolved and flourished since the 1970s because of changes in federal legislation in the United States.

Personal factors, the other part of Part 2: Contextual Factors are not formally defined or classified by the *International Classification of Function*. Recognized as contributing to the outcome of various interventions, personal factors encompass any aspect of the particular background of an individual's life and living and include gender, race, age, fitness, lifestyle, habits, upbringing, coping styles, social background, as can be seen in the Personal Factors section of *Context* within the *OTPF4*. Personal factors also encompass the individualized aspects of a person that an occupational therapy practitioner addresses during client-centered service provision.

The effects of personal factors on intervention are multifaceted. An individual's social background is a primary example of one aspect of personal factors a practitioner must consider. Views on health and illness may be influenced by a child's cultural background, which is consistent with social background within personal factors. How people feel and act toward persons who have disabilities reflect cultural views or biases. This may be true of family members and therapists alike. It is critical for the therapist to become as aware as possible of personal biases. The practitioner must be sensitive to cultural background identity. One way is to delineate how cultural background affects the selection of goals and the establishment of rapport (Agner, 2020; Beagan, 2015). Embracing the concept of cultural humility as part of understanding a child's context will help practitioners to reflexively evaluate their own cultural biases and recognize how their own values impact their interactions and clinical reasoning process (Beagan, 2015). For the pediatric occupational therapy practitioner, culture must be considered when assessing and providing intervention during the practitioner–child–parent interaction. Culture determines the choice of goals and the selection of legitimate tools and activities. "In every culture, some activities are regarded as proper, some inappropriate, and other unacceptable for specific ages, social status, economic class, men or women, times of day, days of the week, or seasons of the year" (Cynkin & Robinson, 1990, p. 10). The social background of the child also determines acceptable levels of functioning so that the therapist can collaboratively establish expected outcomes.

THE RELATIONSHIP OF THE OCCUPATIONAL THERAPY DOMAIN OF CONCERN TO INTERVENTION

The domain of concern of a profession defines the scope and focus of practice. The *International Classification of Function*, and by extension the OTPF4, only provide an outline of the occupational therapy domain of concern. This classification system does not provide any in-depth information on the theoretical knowledge that underlies the practice of occupational therapy. By looking at the broad aspects of the *International Classification of Function,* a therapist can identify occupation-based life areas, foundational body-level components, and contextual factors that require further assessment and possible attention. Once the therapist has identified these areas, components, and factors, the therapist can clinically reason which frame of reference would appropriately address these specific concerns. Frames of reference address different domains of concern specific or related to the context of the target population for intervention. No one frame of reference addresses all aspects of practice fully. Some frames of reference focus more on occupation-based life areas (*International Classification of Function* activities and participation domains), some on foundational components at the body level, and some on contextual factors. Consequently, to treat all areas of concern with a particular child and family, the therapist may have to use more than one frame of reference.

Regardless of the specific frame of reference chosen when working with a particular child, a pediatric occupational therapist draws from their expertise to view the child from various theoretical perspectives. This involves looking at a child relative to typical development and relative to that individual child's mastery of developmental milestones, which involves considering the child's chronologic and developmental age. In addition, the contextual factors affecting development must also be considered as part of the clinical reasoning process when assessing development.

The pediatric occupational therapist often begins by attending to the developmental aspects of the foundational body-level components affecting participation that are important in determining the frame of reference used to guide intervention. This attention to foundational components is based on the therapist's understanding and appreciation for typical development. As defined by the *International Classification of Function*, the body-level components (body functions and structures) are broad categories, sometimes too broad for dealing with an individual child. Because of the specific types of intervention, a therapist needs to divide these components into even smaller entities. When a therapist deals with a child who has grasp problems, for example, the categories of gross and fine coordination are not sufficient to understand and analyze these deficits. In this situation, the therapist needs to divide the child's functioning into even more discrete and specific aspects subcomponents.

Other times, therapists begin by focusing on the occupation-based life areas level—the activities and participation domains of the *International Classification of Function*. This requires looking at the overall functioning and determining areas in which the child is functioning well and areas in which the child may need assistance. To some, this is considered a more holistic or global view of the child's functioning. In addition, some frames of reference concentrate on specific activities and participation domains more than others or to the exclusion of others. Again, a therapist is concerned about the child's functioning within the *International Classification of Function* life areas, which are based on occupation, relative to their chronologic and developmental levels. For example, the therapist may first determine how the child is performing in self-care and how that functioning relates to the child's chronologic and developmental level and then explore which foundational body-level components may be contributing to any deficits in functioning. In this situation, the therapist again understands that functioning within the *ICF* life areas are not independent of foundational body-level components.

Finally, therapists may focus on contextual factors. When looking at the context, the therapist may first determine the demands on the child based on a particular environment or how a specific diagnosis, condition, or specific disability status may impact functioning overall. Once the therapist has determined the relationship of context to the child's functioning, then they can focus more specifically on occupation-based life areas or foundational body-level components. Pediatric occupational therapists are primarily concerned with the child's ability to function within their own contexts. Therefore, a therapist acknowledges that foundational body-level components and contextual factors interact and have an impact on occupation-based life areas.

When an occupational therapist uses a specific frame of reference, they focus on certain aspects of the professional domain of concern. More discrete and specific foundational body-level components, occupation-based life areas, or contextual factors serve a specific need for a therapists' understanding of the child with whom they work. These arbitrary divisions of human functioning allow therapists to understand the parts of the whole to which a child responds and then interacts with their environments. A therapist has a better perspective for analyzing the child's overall functioning by understanding the interplay of occupation-based life areas, foundational components, and contextual factors. This information gives the therapist a clear picture of how the child responds to situations and interacts with their environment.

Summary

All helping professions must evolve and change to meet the needs of society, otherwise the profession stagnates and becomes irrelevant. Within each of these professions, the profession's areas of expertise are considered their domain of concern. The domain of concern is often defined by the scope of practice which delineates what practitioners can do as part of their assessment and interventions. Professions use a common language to define and explain their scope of practice and this language becomes as essential tool used to explain the profession to external stakeholders as well as provide a common language among providers. This text has used the World Health Organization's *International Classification of Function (WHO, 2001)* and the closely aligned American Occupational Therapy Association's *OTPF4* (AOTA, 2020) as a means of providing a common language for understanding the children with whom we work and our areas of expertise and intervention as occupational therapists. Based on this common lexicon, we note how occupational therapy encompasses foundational body-level components serving as the basis of occupation-based life areas. These foundational components and life areas are influenced strongly by contextual factors.

In pediatric practice, the therapist is frequently concerned with three foundational body-level (*ICF* and the *OTPF4* body functions and structures) components: mental function, sensory functions and pain, and neuromusculoskeletal and movement-related functions. Foundational body-level components are an important factor considered in the clinical reasoning process. Although these components are essential to intervention, the therapist should always maintain the perspective of viewing the total child and how the child's strengths and challenges in these areas affect their ability to engage and participate in meaningful life areas.

Life areas, the occupation-based activities and participation domains of the *International Classification of Function*, include learning and applying knowledge; general tasks and demands; communication; mobility; self-care; domestic life; interpersonal interactions and relationships; major life areas (such as education, work and employment, and economic life), and community, social, and civic life. Occupational therapists are always concerned with client engagement and participation in meaningful occupation-based activities. Understanding how the foundational skills of the child provide opportunities or challenges to participation in their meaningful occupations provides the therapist with the tools to provide meaningful interventions.

The focus in pediatric occupational therapy is the child's functioning within various environments. The child's culture provides that setting or context for intervention and must be taken into account by the therapist to provide a holistic intervention.

The practitioner's ability to clearly identify the domain of concern and relevant areas within the scope of practice to guide clinical reasoning is an essential skill. Pediatric therapists combine their rich understanding of underlying component skills found in the body structures and function domain with contextual analysis as a means of determining appropriate interventions to improve participation and engagement in meaningful life activities. The analysis of these areas within the occupational therapy scope of practice guides practitioners to select appropriate frames of reference to theoretically guide interventions.

REFERENCES

Agner, J. (2020). Moving from cultural competence to cultural humility in occupational therapy: A paradigm shift. *The American Journal of Occupational Therapy, 74*(4), 7404347010p1-7404347010p7. https://doi.org/10.5014/ajot.2020.038067

American Occupational Therapy Association. (2020). Occupational therapy practice framework: Domain and process (4th ed.). *American Journal of Occupational Therapy, 74*(Suppl 2), 7412410010. https://doi. org/10.5014/ajot.2020.74S2001

Beagan, B. L. (2015). Approaches to culture and diversity: A critical synthesis of occupational therapy literature. *Canadian Journal of Occupational Therapy, 82*(5), 272–282. https://doi.org/10.1177/0008417414567530

Christiansen, C., Clark, F., Kielhofner, G., Rogers, J., & Nelson, D. (1995). Position paper: Occupation. *American Journal of Occupational Therapy, 49*(10), 1015–1018. https://doi.org/10.5014/ajot.49.10.1015

Cynkin, S., & Robinson, A. M. (1990). *Occupational therapy and activities health: Towards health through activities*. Little, Brown and Company.

Hinojosa, J., & Kramer, P. (1997). Statement: Fundamental concepts of occupational therapy: Occupation, purposeful activity, and function. *American Journal of Occupational Therapy, 51*, 864–866. https://doi.org/10.5014/ajot.51.10.864

Seligman, M., & Darling, R. B. (2017). *Ordinary families, special children: A systems approach to childhood disability* (3rd ed.). Guilford Publications.

Sharma, R. (2013). The family and family structure classification redefined for the current times. *Journal of Family Medicine and Primary Care, 2*(4), 306–310. https://doi.org/10.4103/2249-4863.123774

Taylor, P., Passel, J., Fry, R., Morin, R., Wang, W., Velasco, G., & Dockterman, D. (2010). The return of the multi-generational family household. *Pew Research Center Social and Demographic Report. 2010-03-18. Retrieved September 25, 2023 www.pewsocialtrends.org*

Turnbull, A. P., Summers, J. A., & Brotherson, M. J. (1986). Family life cycle: Theoretical and empirical implications and future directions for families with mentally retarded members. In J. J. Gallagher & P. M. Vietze (Eds), *Families of handicapped persons* (pp. 45–65). Paul H. Brookes Publishing.

World Health Organization (WHO). (2001). *International classification of functioning, disability and health*. World Health Organization.

World Health Organization (WHO). (2016b). *Classifications: International classification of function*. Retrieved from http://www.who.int/classifications/International Classification of Function/en/

4 Pediatric Occupational Therapy's Contemporary Tools for Intervention

Tsu-Hsin Howe ▪ Paula Kramer ▪ Francine M. Seruya

Every health profession has a specific set of tools, techniques, methods, instruments, or modalities that a practitioner in that profession claims to have expertise and uses in creating a therapeutic milieu. One way of referring to these therapeutic means is as the legitimate tools of the profession (Mosey, 1986, 1996). We have updated this terminology to contemporary tools for intervention. They are the professional's intervention tools because society accepts the practitioner as an expert in the use of these specific therapeutic methods or modalities. They are used as a means to accomplish goals. In occupational therapy, the tools of intervention are the specific methods, modalities, and techniques an entry-level occupational therapy practitioner is competent to use therapeutically. Competence comes from knowledge and skills learned and practiced in school and in fieldwork within the scope of practice that is defined by the profession, laws, and standard practice. As professions change and evolve, the scope of practice redefines, research defines some changes and the intervention tools transform accordingly. Practitioners stop using some tools and adopt others based on the needs of the clients they serve and changes in society. Intervention tools are also modified based on new knowledge and technologic advances. Additionally, the needs and values of the profession and society influence how a practitioner uses an intervention tool.

Most occupational therapy practitioners hold the specific intervention tools they use in high regard. For some occupational therapy practitioners, the professional's therapeutic methods, modalities, and techniques are symbolic of occupational therapy. Many occupational therapy practitioners feel that the intervention tools of occupational therapy are unique, and, in some cases, this may be true. However, professions share tools for intervention. The uniqueness lies in the way a profession uses the intervention tools. In occupational therapy, the frame of reference often describes how an occupational therapy practitioner uses a specific tool for intervention.

Each frame of reference addresses the process of change or the way in which the occupational therapy practitioner promotes change in the client. Occupational therapy has a variety of frames of reference that relate to many areas of practice. Intervention tools are chosen by occupational therapy practitioners to match the particular frame of reference that they have determined to be appropriate for a particular client. All practitioners in a profession are aware of its intervention tools; however, different tools are used with different clients. Furthermore, a specific intervention tool is chosen based on its compatibility with the client's developmental level and the environment in which intervention is provided. Some tools are applied uniquely in pediatric occupational therapy or other specialty practice areas. There have been extensive textbook discussions about the tools of the profession related to the profession and specific areas of practice (e.g., Bundy, & Lane, 2020; Evetts & Peloquin, 2017; Blount et al., 2023; Mosey, 1986; Pendleton & Schultz-Krohn, 2024; Dirette & Gutman, 2021; Gillen, & Brown, 2024). The ultimate goal in using intervention tools is engaging our clients (persons, groups, populations) in occupations. The application to practice section of the frame of reference delineates and defines the use of tools of occupational therapy for intervention.

When treating a child, an occupational therapy practitioner utilizes a wide range of intervention tools. This chapter presents an overview of selected therapeutic methods, modalities, and techniques for pediatric practice. The contemporary intervention tools in occupational therapy include activities and occupations, advocacy, critical reasoning, conscious use of self, nonhuman environment, physical modalities, sensory–response interactions, and teaching–learning process. In addition to those presented here, other tools exist. Some are specialized and may be specific to one frame of reference. These tools may be discussed in the application to practice section of each frame of reference. Some specialized tools require advanced education and training and, therefore, are beyond the scope of this book.

OCCUPATIONS AND ACTIVITIES

Occupation and activity are two core concepts of occupational therapy. They are often used interchangeably (Golledge, 1998). In this book, we present occupation and activity as two distinct concepts.

Occupations

While an activity is a culturally defined and general class of human action, the occupations refers specifically to everyday activities that people do as individuals, in families, and with communities to occupy time and bring meaning and purpose to life (AOTA, 2020) including looking after themselves (self-care), enjoying life (leisure), and contributing to the social and economic fabric of their communities (productivity) (Townsend & Polatajko, 2013). Pierce (2001) defined occupation is "a specific individual's personally constructed, nonrepeatable experience. That is, an occupation is a subjective event in perceived temporal, spatial, and sociocultural conditions that are unique to that one-time occurrence" (p. 139).

The concept of occupation has evolved over the course of the profession's history, as has been used to organize and define the profession's domain of concern. Occupations are categorized as activities of daily living, instrumental activities of daily living, health management, rest and sleep, education, work, play, leisure, and social participation.

One of the major ways that a pediatric occupational therapy practitioner uses occupation as a tool is through play. For play to be an occupation, it must be meaningful to the child. Ideally, the child should choose the particular play activity. All too often the practitioner, not the child, determines toys and play activities that fit the needs of the child and the goals of intervention. Another type of occupation that is often used in intervention is self-care. However, the specific play or self-care activity used in intervention must be meaningful to the child to be classified as an occupation (Hinojosa & Kramer, 1997). There are vast varieties of occupations that a therapist can use in therapy; however, it is incumbent on the therapist to ensure that the specific activity chosen is meaningful to the child, and not just meaningful to the therapist as a way to achieve therapeutic goals.

An occupational therapy practitioner needs to keep a child's occupations in the forefront of their thoughts when using any interventional tool. Interventions are always directed toward improving a child's ability to function within their occupations and in the roles as family member, sibling, player, or student. However, within the context of using any frame of reference, it is important to address the overall occupations of the child and to focus on the occupations of the particular child (Hinojosa & Kramer, 1997).

Play

Play is the most common occupation of children and the primary means for occupational therapy intervention with children to achieving other developmental goals. Erikson (1963) proposed the idea that play is the work of the child. A child learns through play (Parham & Fazio, 2008; Reilly, 1974). The various types of play activities in which children engage include sensorimotor play, constructional play, imaginary and symbolic play, and group play (team sports). Sensorimotor play is characterized by the use of sensory stimulation with a motor component. Constructional play promotes pleasure through building and creating things. Imaginary and symbolic play entails cognition combined with fantasy and creativity. Computer and video games, and costume play are also ways of engaging in imaginary and symbolic play. Group play is an interactional process where a child works with another child together with a relatively common theme. Team sports or games with rules provide a different form of group play. Based on the developmental level, culture, and needs of the child, the pediatric occupational therapist uses and adapts the types of therapeutic experiences to the benefit of that child (Parham & Fazio, 2008). Through the skilled therapeutic use of play as a tool, the therapist can enhance the child's enjoyment and success in therapy.

The ability to use play as an occupation requires specific knowledge and skills when therapy occurs around child-selected activities. A practitioner constructs therapeutic environments that allow the child to lead the direction of a therapy session. For example, a child might be working on increasing attention to task in socially appropriate situations. In advance of a therapy session, the therapist prepares the environment with several appropriate options based on the child's preferences, and their stage of development. When the child enters the therapy environment, the practitioner responds to the child's directives and, often, becomes a playmate within the child's world. Each activity is personally meaningful for the child and leads to the achievement of a therapeutic goal.

Another classification of occupation is the wide range of activities used to assist the child in the development of self-care skills. Frequently, it is a challenge for a therapist to engage a child in personally meaningful activities aimed at developing specific self-care skills. An occupational therapy practitioner frequently uses play such as dressing the doll or dressing up to develop these skills. Here again, it is the child's choice and participation in a fun meaningful activity that makes it an occupation. As a child matures, the motivation for attaining self-care skills may be self-motivated through peer pressure or parental concern. At this time, practice and repetition of specific activities themselves are attached with subjective meaning.

Activities

The term activity was defined as a set of tasks with a specific end point or outcome and not related to a specific client's engagement or context (Schell et al., 2019). The activities can be selected and designed to enhance occupational engagement by supporting the development of performance skills and performance patterns (AOTA, 2020). In occupational therapy, activities have been a therapeutic medium since the profession's beginning. An occupational therapy practitioner is concerned with a person's ability to engage in daily life occupations. Inherent in this concern is the ability to complete activities associated with and foundational to the various occupations. The goal of occupational therapy has always been to provide a person with the knowledge and skills to participate in the numerous activities that are part of daily life. Activities include the numerous things that people do as they live their lives (Hinojosa & Blount, 2014). Therapeutic use of activities is selecting the most appropriate activity for the client to create an environment within which the client can learn, develop skills, express feelings, and act on the environments toward a positive outcome (Evetts & Peloquin, 2017; Hinojosa & Blount, 2014). The practitioner needs to be skilled in activity analysis and activity synthesis.

The purpose of an activity can also be defined by the therapist. Frequently, a practitioner selects activities because of their therapeutic value. The practitioner presents the activity to the child because it has the greatest potential as a therapeutic medium. The practitioner often does not consider whether the child finds the activity personally meaningful. The major criterion for selecting activity is that participation in that activity will lead to a projected outcome or address specific deficit. At times, the child may even consider the activity unpleasant or boring. For example, if the child needs to learn to dress themselves, the practitioner might select a frame of reference that requires practice and repetition. In this scenario, the practitioner may have the child repeat putting on, taking off their shoes and socks, and tying their shoes. The child may not be interested in completing the activity without considerable encouragement and reinforcement by the therapist. To encourage participation, the practitioner may use another more desired activity as a reward. At other times, the practitioner might use other methods of manipulating the child's participation.

Activities that are defined and directed by a practitioner are an important part of occupational therapy intervention with child because the intervention directly relates to the therapy goals. A practitioner uses their knowledge and skills about working with pediatric clientele to motivate the child to participate in activities. Social interactions with the practitioner or another child may facilitate participation. When the child engages in the practitioner-directed activity, the practitioner is focusing on the goals associated with the activity as an end product. In other words, participating in the activity is just a means to an end. While this practice may not be desired by the child at times, it is sometimes entirely necessary to achieve therapeutic goals. Often, the physical environment and the context are important elements to be manipulated by the therapist when presenting practitioner-directed activities.

Activity Analysis

Occupational therapy practitioners learn about the value and importance of activities as a core aspect of practice. The use of activities as a therapeutic tool requires that a practitioner understand the activities of people and the multiple factors that influence them. Some factors are age, culture, ethnicity, gender, physical environment, and personal preferences. An occupational therapy practitioner's knowledge and use of activity analysis and synthesis are basic to the use of activities as a therapeutic medium.

Activity analysis is the identification of the component parts of an activity (Buckley & Poole, 2014; Buckley et al., 2023; Dancza & Rodger, 2018). It is an important tool used by the occupational therapy practitioner. The practitioner is continually fascinated by the parts that make up an activity. Even activities that seem simple because of their familiarity may actually be complex. The occupational therapy practitioner analyzes activities for use with client intervention. Through the use of this tool, the practitioner identifies whether the child has the necessary skills to perform or complete the activity. Activity analysis also enables the practitioner to teach the activity more successfully through a clear understanding of its component parts.

When working with a child, activity analysis is a constant focus of the intervention process. The pediatric occupational therapy practitioner continually divides activities into smaller parts to determine which skills are necessary to complete the task or activity. This is just the first step in the intervention process. The next step involves observation of how the child reacts and interacts with the activity or its component tasks. The practitioner then analyzes the activity and the child's participation in and reaction to it. This process provides the practitioner with the information they need to adapt, grade, or combine activities to make them effective in intervention (Hinojosa et al., 1993).

The simple activity of stacking blocks illustrates the complexity of the activity analysis process. The preliminary analysis entails gaining an understanding of the skills required for the child to stack blocks. The child needs to have beginning fine motor skills, the ability to grasp the blocks, and controlled release for stacking the blocks. Then, as the child begins to stack the blocks, the practitioner observes the child's behavior and response to the blocks. The next step involves analyzing the child and activity in combination. The questions that follow are examples of what the therapist may ask to start this analysis:

1. Can the child pick up the blocks?
2. Can the child place the blocks neatly on the stack?
3. Does the child have difficulty letting go of or releasing the blocks?
4. Does the child exhibit other compensatory body movements when engaged in the task?
5. Is the child more interested in building the tower or knocking it down?
6. What is the level of the child's fine motor skills in this task?

The practitioner answers these questions based on their preliminary analysis combined with the knowledge gained from observing the child perform the activity. The practitioner needs to look at the answers to all these questions before they proceed to know how to modify this activity to make it therapeutic for the child. Furthermore, the same activity may be different with another child because the reactions of the child and the answers to the previously stated questions would be different. Any activity becomes modified by the way a particular child interacts with the environment and how they perform the activity.

Activity Synthesis

> The magician's sleight of hand is smooth and sinuous, creating an illusion which is not really there. The audience watches in awe, trying to reconcile the reality that they know exists, with what they think they are seeing. It seems so simple, and yet creating the illusion is actually very complex (Hunt, 1997). In many ways, this is much like the activity synthesis created by the occupational therapy practitioner (Kramer & Hinojosa, 2014).

Activity synthesis for an occupational therapy practitioner is changing or creating an activity so that it meets therapeutic goals and the child can participate in it. The theoretical base of the specific frame of reference base guides the occupational therapy practitioner synthesis of an activity (Kramer & Hinojosa, 2014; Kramer & Walsh, 2023).

A practitioner begins to use activity synthesis when they consider how to adapt or modify an activity so that the child can participate in the activity. Activity synthesis begins with the therapy practitioner having completed a comprehensive activity analysis. The practitioner combines this knowledge about the activity with the specific child's situation and therapeutic goals. Important considerations are the child's personal goals and desires, capacities, and limitations. Fundamental to activity synthesis is a clear understanding of the child and the activities in which the practitioner expects the child to participate. At this point, the specific frame of reference guides the activity synthesis within the context of the frame of reference.

Before an activity can be synthesized, a practitioner must decide on the key elements that define the activity. For example, if someone is going to make chocolate chip cookies, what are the component parts of making the cookies? The activity must have chocolate chips, dough, and a means of baking. Missing any one of these, the activity would not be making chocolate chip cookies. With this knowledge, a practitioner begins to think about how they can synthesize the activity to meet therapeutic goals by adaptation or changing the activity. Activity adaptation means elements of the activity are modified to meet the needs of the client and to facilitate positive change. Activities can be adapted through alterations in the child's positioning, the way materials are presented, or by changing the characteristics of the materials such as their shape, size, weight, or texture. Adaptation may also involve modifying the procedure or sequence of events for the activity, nature, and degree of interpersonal contact (Hinojosa et al., 1993).

Activity synthesis occurs within the parameters of the dynamic theory of the theoretical base. The practitioner, guided by the dynamic theory, synthesizes or adapts the activity so that the child can successfully complete it. Using synthesis, the practitioner reconstructs activities taking into consideration the child's therapeutic goals and the child's strengths and limitations. Reconfiguration of the activities creates a situation where the child can engage in the activity with minimum fear of failure and probable success. The practitioner continually adapts activities for the child. As discussed previously, an example of adaptation is the modification of stacking blocks. The practitioner may use larger blocks, seat the child at a small table rather than on the floor, present one block at a time, or add Velcro to the blocks so that they may be attached more easily to each other. The possibilities of adaptation for this activity are endless, limited only by the practitioner's creativity.

The frame of reference guiding the intervention will determine how the adaptation is made to the environment or the activity. Adaptations do not change the person (Kramer & Hinojosa, 2014). The child changes as a result of interacting in the controlled environment.

The occupational therapy practitioner's skills and abilities, their understanding of the child, their appreciation of the context, and knowledge of the frame of reference are critical to activity synthesis. The theoretical base and the postulates regarding change in a frame of reference guide the synthesis; the frame of reference outlines how a practitioner uses, adapts, modifies, or creates activities (Kramer & Hinojosa, 2014).

Activity Groups

Activity groups are those that have a common goal that involves activities (Howe & Schwartzberg, 2001; Mosey, 1986). As an interventional tool, activity groups are used more often in some frames of reference than in others. In pediatric occupational therapy, a practitioner uses activity groups as a tool to promote age-appropriate peer interaction in a therapeutic environment. The occupational therapy practitioner designs activity groups based on the knowledge of child development, group dynamics, and a firm understanding of activities. Activity groups are used to develop play, social, and physical skills. The involvement of peers can be useful for facilitating motivation when it is developmentally appropriate. The occupational therapy practitioner fosters group interaction in a safe and supportive environment. Activity groups can be organized in various ways, including situations where a child works with another child side by side on similar projects (known as a parallel group), instances in which children work together on a common project (known as a cooperative group), and scenarios in which children develop a project and implement it together (known as a higher-level cooperative group). There are various taxonomies for activity groups that are used in occupational therapy (e.g., Mosey, 1986).

CRITICAL REASONING

Critical reasoning refers to a cognitive or metacognitive process that serves as a guiding force in practice (Schell & Benfield, 2024). It is the ability to actively and skillfully conceptualize, synthesize, analyze, question, and evaluate ideas and beliefs. As delineated by Fleming (1991), the process is intricate and dynamic, encompassing various dimensions including procedural, interactive, conditional, narrative, and pragmatic reasoning. Building upon this framework, Schell and Benfield (2024) further extended the facets by introducing scientific and ethical reasoning. Occupational therapy practitioners employ this process to effectively plan, direct, execute, and reflect on client care. The process has been referred to with different terms such as therapeutic reasoning, clinical reasoning, and professional reasoning. Critical reasoning is informed reasoning, and critical reasoning is critical self-reflection. A practitioner continually needs to do both: reason and reflect to effectively work with a client. To engage in effective practice, a practitioner must use multiple thinking strategies and consider multiple perspectives when determining suitable frame(s) of reference for intervention, as well as throughout the intervention process.

When a practitioner selects a frame of reference, they must possess an understanding of the child, the challenges they are encountering, and the broad array of factors within the child's environment that can influence them. This takes into account the totality of the child, including background and culture, the home and social environment, presenting problems, possible diagnosis and medical condition, and the context for intervention. Based on this information and possible additional information that may come from screening, observation, or discussions with other health care personnel, the practitioner chooses a frame of reference (Hinojosa, 2017). Once the therapist selects a frame of reference, they begin with a comprehensive evaluation (Hinojosa, Kramer, & Crist, 2014). Based on the results of the assessments, the critical reasoning process becomes more intense as the practitioner needs to consider a multitude of factors to develop a plan for intervention.

First, the practitioner explores whether this is the proper frame of reference to use with the child based on the problem areas that have been identified through the evaluation, the practitioner's own competence, the ethical circumstances, the empirical evidence available, and the available theoretical information (Hinojosa, 2017). If the practitioner determines that this may not be the best frame of reference for the child, additional assessments may be needed from the perspective of another frame of reference. Once the practitioner is comfortable that a particular frame of reference (or in some cases, multiple frames of reference) is the most effective way to intervene the child's identified problems, the therapist develops a plan for intervention. The development of the plan for intervention requires the practitioner to reflect on all the various pieces of information about the child. The plan for intervention involves more than just planning for care and developing an intervention strategy; it requires being able to separate critical information from information that is of lesser importance at any given time.

CONSCIOUS USE OF SELF

Conscious use of self involves the occupational therapy practitioner's use of themselves as an agent to effect positive change within the therapeutic process (Solman & Clouston, 2016; Taylor, 2008;

Taylor & Van Puymbroeck, 2013). Although sometimes called the therapeutic use of self, the term *conscious use of self* "allows occupational therapy practitioners to develop and manage their therapeutic relationship with clients by using narrative and clinical reasoning; empathy; and a client-centered, collaborative approach to service delivery" (AOTA, 2014, p. S12). Conscious use of self involves entering the child's world and relating to a child at their own level using emotional, cognitive, physical, and sensory components.

Establishing a positive therapeutic relationship between the practitioner and the child is an essential result of the emotional component of the conscious use of self. A principal characteristic of this relationship is the practitioner's ability to communicate and to develop rapport. Developing rapport involves making a child aware that the practitioner cares and accepts the child at a current level of performance. In addition, establishing rapport requires that a practitioner control their responses in a way that promotes a child's ability to function or operate in their own world.

In many cases, conscious use of self is expanded to interactions beyond the child to the caregivers. Often, the practitioner includes parents, siblings, teachers, other classroom personnel, and other health care providers within the therapeutic relationship. To collaborate successfully, the practitioner needs to interact with others positively and gauge the caregiver's understanding of the child. The practitioner should not dictate to caregivers, talk down to them, or be judgmental. This entails language, posture, gestures, and tone of voice that engages caregivers, ensuring that everyone can be an effective part of the therapeutic process. The conscious use of self in this sense, therefore, may mean that the practitioner provides an appropriate role model for the family or classroom. The practitioner's role with caregivers should be flexible and needs to be open to change over time, depending on need and context.

A practitioner can utilize conscious use of self with a developmental and cognitive component. For example, objects and directions may have to be presented in a specific and concrete manner so that the child can understand them and respond. The conscious use of self in this example is the practitioner's awareness of the child's level and practitioner's ability to adapt their behavior to that level. Toys and therapeutic tools also need to be at the child's developmental and cognitive level or slightly higher to stimulate the child's growth. The practitioner has to have a clear understanding of the child's levels and skills to intervene at that same level or higher; otherwise, the intervention may be less than successful.

In the intervention process, a practitioner can also provide conscious use of self with a physical component. If the child spends most of their time on the floor, for example, then the practitioner needs to work with the child on the floor. Another example of the physical component is holding a toy to the side and above a child's head while encouraging reaching and opening an involved hand. Another physical example is the practitioner who uses their body as a positioning device. For instance, a practitioner in tailor-sitting can use their legs to enhance an infant's tolerance to being positioned prone, or add a dynamic balance element for a toddler seated in their lap. Some frames of reference make extensive utilization of the physical aspects of conscious use of self; for instance, handling and some of the neuromuscular facilitation techniques are used in the neurodevelopmental treatment frame of reference.

A practitioner can also incorporate a sensory component into the conscious use of self. When working with infants, for example, a practitioner with blonde hair may choose to wear a black or navy shirt to provide color contrast. For a child who is working on sensory processing issues, a therapist may select clothing to assist in the therapeutic session. For instance, a sweatshirt worn inside out provides extra softness, and wool pants add a scratchy aspect in a therapeutic encounter. The therapist also can use scent (or the lack of scent) consciously. Wearing the same combination of soap, shampoo, and lotion can provide consistency in olfactory sensation for a child who is blind, and using fragrant-free products may help a child who is hypersensitive to odors. In addition, a practitioner can also utilize the conscious of self with a culture component. For example, a practitioner incorporates culturally appropriate foods into the child's feeding program during their intervention.

The skillful application of the conscious use of self develops with practice. A competent practitioner builds a conscious use of self-repertoire that has various emotional, cognitive, physical, and sensory components. Being an agent who affects positive therapeutic change is the reason why the conscious use of self is a core contemporary legitimate tool of occupational therapy.

THE NONHUMAN ENVIRONMENT

Life is contextual for everyone, including a child. In fact, Humphrey and Wakeford (2006) advocated shifting to a contextual perspective to deliver pediatric occupational therapy services. Context includes both nonhuman and human environments, which are named, defined, and grouped slightly differently in three classification systems: the World Health Organization's International Classification of Functioning, Disability and Health (World Health Organization, 2001), the American Occupational Therapy Association's Practice Framework (AOTA, 2020), and Uniform Terminology III (AOTA, 1994). In this chapter, the term *nonhuman environment* is utilized in the manner of Mosey (1986) based on the work of Searles (1960). An occupational therapy practitioner uses the nonhuman environment as an intervention tool of pediatric practice.

The nonhuman environment involves elements of space and time, is composed of the natural environment and human-made changes in the environment, and includes products and technology. The nonhuman environment can be physical or virtual. The nonhuman environment may be different within the various spaces a child occupies and across time. For instance, a little Midwestern girl in a rural setting during a typical summer week may be at home, her grandparents' house, or Sunday school. In March, her weekly routine might also include school, Brownies, and soccer. The little girl's nonhuman environment includes natural environment (trees in the backyard, the state park she visits with her troop) and human-made changes in the environment (her home, school, a soccer field converted from prairie grass). She uses various products and technology; for example, she plays with toys, talks or face times on a cell phone with her grandmother, watches her favorite television show, and uses a computer for homework. Some products act to ease transitions, from one stage of development to another or from one setting to the next. For example, a favorite teddy bear assisted this child's transition from a crib to a big girl bed, from her own room to her grandmother's spare bedroom, or to a hotel for a family vacation. The teddy bear also eased her transition during her daily routine. Although much of her context is physical, the girl's nonhuman environment may become virtual if she becomes absorbed in a book, a movie, or a computer game. From a temporal standpoint, the girl's nonhuman environment will vary as her abilities, interests, family situation—her overall life—changes across time.

Because using the nonhuman environment as an intervention tool varies among practitioners, this section provides a focus on three kinds of nonhuman environment commonly used by the pediatric practitioners. The three categories of the nonhuman environment are toys, domestic animals, and technology.

Toys

If we view play as a child's main occupation, then toys become crucial instrument that support in nurturing and advancing this occupation. In this chapter, the term "toys" includes both traditional toys and playthings (objects to play with), even though certain researchers regard them as distinct categories. Toys are particularly important learning tools in the nonhuman environment for children used to facilitate play. Although many researchers argue that play holds greater significance than toys and playthings, many of them emphasize the crucial role of toys, particularly for children with severe and profound disabilities (Brodin, 1999).

With toys, a child can find basic stimulation, comfort, enjoyment and fun, and a sense of competency. Many commercial toys are available that provide basic stimulation. Some toys have been designed to stimulate single senses, such as auditory, visual, vestibular, or tactile systems; other toys have multiple sensory components. There are commercially available baby toys that provide soothing sounds, vibrate, light up, and move, singularly or in combination. While teenagers may not use traditional toys in the same way as younger children, there are several types of items and activities that can be considered "toys" for this age group catering to their specific interests, hobbies, and developmental needs. These may include electronic gadgets and video games, sports equipment, art supplies, musical instruments, books and graphic novels, etc.

A child of any age can find comfort in toys, both emotionally and physically. A favorite blanket, a stuffed animal, or a doll may become a companion for a child, providing continuity across different routines and various developmental stages. A much-loved doll, for instance, could go from the nursery to a dorm room.

Toys can create feelings of excitement, causing a child to lose track of time. In fact, using the word "toy" as an intervention tool usually signifies a sense of enjoyment or fun from the child's. Toys may "grow" with the child, having different meanings at various ages and stages. For example, large brick-type blocks can be wrapped with towels and used as positioning devices early in life. The child may learn to throw blocks, then begin stacking the blocks, and at a later stage build structures used in imaginary play (Figure 4.1).

In pediatrics, almost every frame of reference uses toys as intervention tools. Toys most often form the basis for play, a fundamental concept in an occupation-based frame of reference. Certain toys, a miniature piano, for example, are designed to work on foundational skills such as fine motor coordination. Other toys, such as a swing set, designed for whole-body movement, may have therapeutic parallels in equipment used for specific frames of reference such as sensory integration. A practitioner who uses a teaching–learning frame of reference may sometimes use toys to provide practice and repetition to learn a specific skill; other times, they may use toys as positive reinforcement or negative reinforcement. A pediatric practitioner who uses a biomechanical frame of reference may use toys as positioning devices. Across frames of reference, toys are often a universal learning tool and an important part of the nonhuman environment.

Domestic Animals

Children and animals always form an incredible partnership. Animals have been reported to improve the emotional and functional status of children since the ancient time of Greeks. Pets are a specific category of domestic animals. Pets are significant parts of the nonhuman environment, and can be a source of pleasure and companionship for a child of any age. A pet can help a young child move beyond the natural egocentrism of early childhood to relate to other living organisms. An older child can learn to take care of pets. An occupational therapy

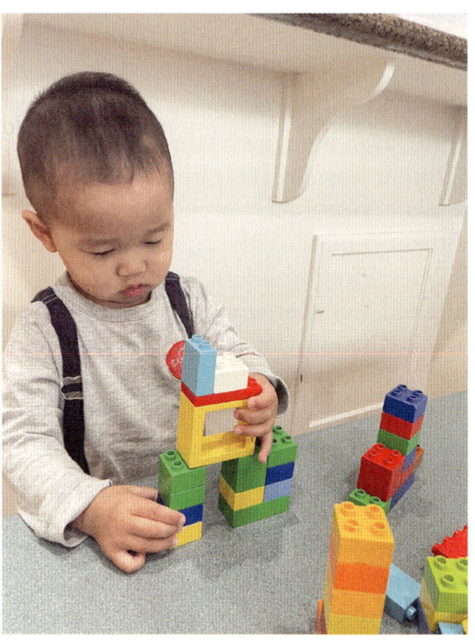

FIGURE 4.1 Child develops a sense of competency from playing with a toy. (Courtesy of J. Hsu.)

practitioner can use pets as a nonhuman environmental intervention tool for multiple purposes, including a source of pleasure, companionship, a nurturing relationship, and a responsibility (Figure 4.2).

In some frames of reference, such as those that use teaching-learning for example, the pleasure of spending time with a pet could be a reward (positive reinforcement) for completing a task. For other frame of reference, incorporating a pet into the environment during therapeutic intervention

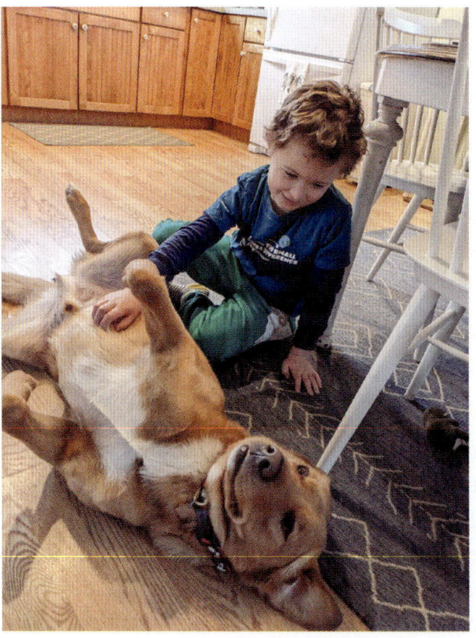

FIGURE 4.2 A child is in the company of his dearest dog pal. (Courtesy of C. A. Colangelo.)

can provide companionship for a particularly difficult activity or a task a child considers not very fun. For instance, a young boy, typically prefers indoor video games, is currently working on improving his outdoor mobility and safety, can find a faithful companion in his dog, who joins him as an intrepid sidekick on their daily hikes. The occupational therapy practitioner could upgrade the hike's challenge by introducing a leash and incorporating basic commands like "stop" and "heel."

A pet can teach a child how to relate to other living beings, helping to develop a nurturing relationship that is respectful and caring. A practitioner can work with the child to recognize a pet's nonverbal and verbal communication, by learning the meaning of a cat that circles and rubs against the legs or purring versus loud meowing, a dog with a wagging tail or barking at various pitches and instance levels, or a turtle retreating entirely into a shell. Looking for and assigning meaning to pet nonverbal and verbal cues can be generalized to interactions and relationships with persons.

With a pet, a child can learn responsibility and the importance of providing care to another living thing. Using an occupation-based frame of reference, for example, a pediatric therapy practitioner can recommend that a child have a chore of making sure a pet has water. A younger child (or a child with physical disabilities) could take responsibility for checking to see if water is in the pet bowl and notifying a caregiver if the bowl is empty. A practitioner could work with a family to have the child complete additional steps of the task or activity as the child assumes more responsibilities such as washing the bowl with soap, rinsing the bowl making sure that it is squeaky clean, refilling the bowl with water, and setting the filled bowl into place.

Animal-Assisted Therapy

Domestic animals are not merely pets. They are being used more often for therapeutic purposes to assist clients decreasing stress, improve physical and emotional conditions. The positive results using animals in the health care environment led health professionals to incorporate animals into their treatment sessions through animal-assisted therapy (AAT). AAT is defined as a goal-directed intervention that utilizes the human–animal bond as an integral part of treatment (Macauley, 2023). AAT involving dogs, horses, cats, guinea pigs, and elephants have been reported with positive effects in children across different age groups. These benefits include:

- Enhanced emotional well-being: such as improve the emotional state of children, reduced anxiety, and alleviating pain, particularly in hospital settings.
- Strengthen relationship: AAT has been found to foster improved relationships, higher self-esteem, increased confidence, and decrease problem behaviors in incarcerated youth, at-risk youth, and children with history of posttraumatic stress disorder, substance, physical or sexual abuse.
- Physical development: children have experienced advancements in their motor control, walking abilities, and balance through AAT interventions (Charry-Sanchez et al., 2018, Macauley, 2023).

This contributes to increased engagement and participation in various activities in their life. The use of domestic animals as an intervention tool of the nonhuman environment is limited only by the imagination of the practitioner.

Technology

Technology, characterized as a form of the nonhuman environment, has become an integral part of our daily lives, reshaping the way we communicate, work, learn and entertain ourselves. In the wake of onset of the COVID-19 pandemic in 2020, we have witnessed an ever-increasing dependence on technology to learn, live, and stay connected.

Technology has been used in treatment as in video games with children with perceptual problems. Many occupational therapy frames of reference utilized technology further and expanded it to enhance functions and to enable community participation which usually described as assistive technology (AT). AT is a subset of technology. It encompasses mainstream technologies tailored to cater to the unique requirements of individuals with disabilities. Its primary objective is to enhance their functional capabilities, foster independence, and improve accessibility. AT can also play a role in other selected pediatric intervention tools discussed in this chapter; however, this specialized type of technology is most often characterized as the nonhuman environment.

The ATs that assist individuals with disabilities come from two main sources, mainstream products developed with universal design principles, and those designed specifically for individuals with disabilities. Practitioners should thoroughly explore both sources to make informed choices, which can be especially beneficial in attaining cost-effective solutions, especially in resource-limited environments.

A smartphone can exemplify the integration of stand-alone AT products. A typical smartphone has a touchscreen for entering information or scrolling through menu choices. Many smartphones offer users the option to input data through typing or speaking, and they also include a speaker to provide auditory information, making them accessible to individuals with different sensory needs. Using these existing accessibility features (physical, auditory, visual, etc.) of the smart phone might be a more affordable solution to assist child with learning needs such as spelling, grammar, and word finding than developing a specific AT device for that purpose (Figure 4.3).

AT devices include a wide range of tools, equipment or product system, whether brought off the shelf, modified, or personalized, that is used to enhance, sustain, or improve functional abilities of individuals with disabilities (AT Act of 2004). They are usually categorized in three general groups: speech-generating devices (often referred to as augmentative communication systems), mobility systems (including wheelchairs and other similar devices), and

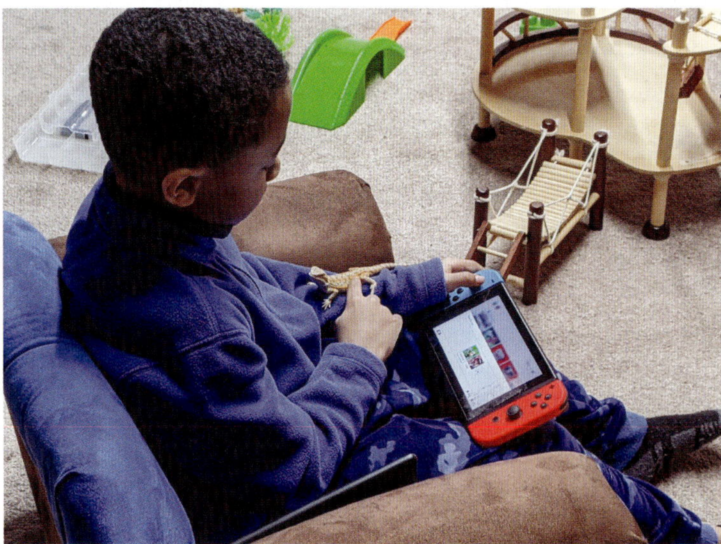

FIGURE 4.3 Child is enjoying a tablet game alongside his bearded dragon companion, who goes by the name Raptor. (Courtesy of G. John.)

electronic aids to daily living (EADL) (e.g., environmental control, computer access, etc.). Devices within the AT categories are available across a spectrum of levels from high tech to low tech.

For most people, the phrase "high tech" is synonymous with electronics-based devices. Electronic augmentative communication systems can assist a child in functional communication, power mobility systems can help with functional mobility, and bionic prosthetics can enhance a child's functionality in performing more complex tasks. Computers often provide assistance to enhance children's participation in a variety area of occupational performance including education, communication, and play (Chantry & Dunford, 2010). Another example of high-tech EADL devices is environmental control systems. These EADL devices can help children with disabilities control their surroundings. For example, a child with limited mobility can use voice-activated system to turn lights on and off or operate a television set to watch their favorite movies. Because an occupational therapy practitioner requires specialized backgrounds to work with high-tech equipment (which is beyond the scope of this chapter), additional AT information can be found in Cook et al. (2020) and Carpenter et al. (2015).

At the other end of the spectrum, less-expensive nonelectronic (low) technology continues to provide functional solutions for a child. Low-tech devices, under the guise of adaptive equipment, have been a primary staple in the occupational therapist's practice repertoire for decades. A child might use a picture board to aid in communication, don clothing with Velcro closures, or magnetic buttons, to dress independently, and/or use a walker to improve mobility. Adaptive equipment catalogs are packed with low-tech equipment, primarily related to self-care. Catalogs have numerous pages of spoons and forks with built-up handles, nonspill drinking cups, and one-way straws to assist in feeding and eating; button hooks, elastic shoe laces, and long-handled shoe horns for dressing as well as various devices for grooming, oral hygiene, bathing and showering, and toileting. Many school-based, work-related, play, leisure, and recreational low-tech devices are also available.

Technology can create a virtual environment. For centuries, readers experienced the virtual environments of books. Today, technology makes available a wide variety of virtual environments in both scheduled format (e.g., televised cartoon) and on-demand (subscribed streaming services such as Apple TV, Netflix). Gaming creates new worlds where a child can interact in large social networks and competitions, using avatars and code names to represent themselves. A child can go to school online and children can work on paying jobs without leaving home. With the AT available, people in virtual worlds may not realize a child with severe disabilities is participating in the same activities as everybody else.

A pediatric occupational therapy practitioner may recommend technology to be used as a virtual environment to keep a child safe. Using a virtual environment such as a favorite, recorded movie can help ease plane trips, or visits to the doctor's office. Telehealth and mobile health (mHealth) are examples of incorporating technology in health care. A practitioner using a teaching–learning frame of reference sometimes uses technology, especially technology that creates virtual environments, as rewards or positive reinforcement for completing specified tasks. One should remember that technology is only an intervention tool to be used as a mean to reach the end. It is not the outcome itself.

Using the nonhuman environment is essential to providing a contextual perspective in the delivery of pediatric occupational therapy services. Although toys, pets, and technology provided the focus for this section, there are unlimited ways the occupational therapist uses the nonhuman environment as a legitimate tool for pediatric practice.

PHYSICAL MODALITIES

Physical modalities encompass atmospheric elements and physical agents. The atmospheric elements include space, light, color, temperature and sounds, and physical agents include heat, cold, pressure, water, or electricity.

Pediatric occupational therapy practitioners may use physical modalities to prepare the child for occupational performance as part of a treatment session in preparation for or concurrently with occupations and activities. For example, practitioners may create a simulated sensory environment involving movements, tactile sensations, or scents to promote children's alertness and improve their self-regulation before they participate in a school-based activity (AOTA, 2020, OTPF-4).

SENSORY–RESPONSE INTERACTION

Many of the activities used in occupational therapy involve the use of sensory-response interaction as a tool including sensory stimulation, biofeedback, and handling. For example, the practitioner often chooses blocks that are soft and fuzzy because of their tactile properties in addition to their use as a building tool. They use different tactile materials with a child to determine how the child will respond and to provoke a specific adaptive response. Adaptive responses are responses that change over time based on the child's exposure to and integration of sensory input. The practitioner needs to observe and understand the child's ability to process sensory information in order to use this as a tool in treatment effectively. Sensory stimuli are not limited to the tactile realm but may also include visual, auditory, gustatory, and olfactory stimulation to produce a response (Figure 4.4). Stimulation applied by the practitioner, such as joint compression (or other physical

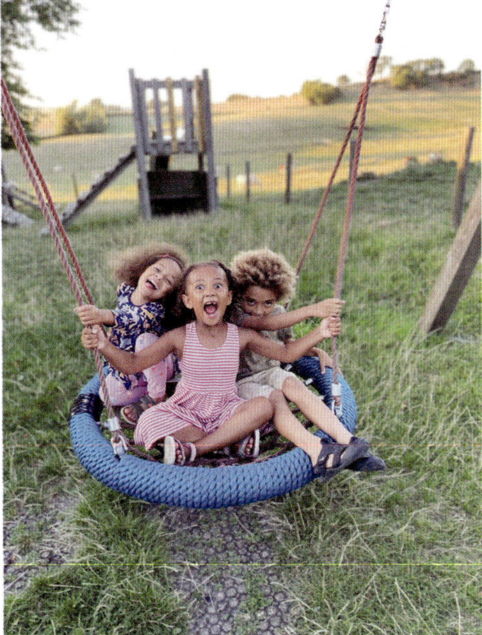

FIGURE 4.4 Children on the swing enjoying a multisensory experience involving visual, auditory, vestibular and physical sensations. (Courtesy of Janet E. Njelesani.)

modalities) and positioning in a way to allow for improved engagement in a task, is also part of the sensory stimulation tool. Gross and fine motor activities may also include aspects of sensory stimulation to bring about a particular adaptive response. Examples of this might include using a jumping activity to affect a neuromuscular response of increasing muscle tone or using scented markers to reinforce a child's associations between colors and fruits when coloring.

The practitioner creates environments that use sensory stimulation to provoke adaptive responses. Manipulating elements of the environments can elicit specific responses in a child. It is often used in conjunctions with atmospheric elements of physical modalities. For instance, the practitioner may adjust the light or temperature of the room, put on music, or use a variety of visually, auditory, olfactory, and room temperature to either stimulate or inhibit the adaptive responses of the child. A practitioner skillfully matches the environment of the treatment setting to obtain specific types of adaptive responses.

TEACHING–LEARNING PROCESS

Occupational therapy practitioners use the teaching–learning process as a significant intervention tool in just about every therapeutic encounter, even if they don't consciously acknowledge it. Providing feedback to a child based on their performance is a prime example of the teaching–learning process in action. A pediatric therapy practitioner, even when they are not using the teaching–learning process directly with a child, often engage in the teaching–learning process as part of caregiver education. Caregiver education has become increasingly important to ensure follow through from specific therapy sessions and provide overall continuity of care.

Although both teaching and learning involve active doing, it may appear different throughout the process. In its most fundamental form, the practitioner engages in the teaching component and the child is involved in the learning component. Teaching usually consists of giving instruction and providing demonstration, but often teaching is expanded to designing opportunities for active learning. Designing active learning opportunities involves creating contexts that are conducive for learning and planning therapeutic activities that allow exploration and discovery and then practice of new performance skills. The outcome of the teaching–learning process is learning that results in a relatively permanent positive change in behavior and performance.

Because the teaching–learning process has a grounding in behavioral approaches, teaching and learning are most often associated with frames of reference that include the word acquisitional or learning in the theoretical base or title. Any other frame of reference, however, that uses terminology such as trial and error, shaping, modeling, repetition, practice, coaching and discovery is using the teaching–learning process as a contemporary intervention tool to effect positive change in occupational performance.

Coaching

Coaching is identified as a core enabling skill of occupational therapy (Townsend & Polatajko, 2013). It is often used in the context of family centered approach to support children's occupational performance, maximizing parent choice and developing collaborative parent–practitioner relationship (Graham et al., 2013, Kessler & Graham, 2015). Despite various models of coaching used in the practice, the principles and techniques of coaching are mostly derived from theories of behaviorism such as adult learning theory, and guided discovery (Kessler & Graham, 2015).

Summary

This chapter has outlined the contemporary major intervention tools for pediatric occupational therapy. Other intervention tools exist that have not been presented here, however those are often specific to one frame of reference and may be highly specialized. These specialized tools often require advanced education and training. The tools of the profession can change over time, just as practice changes over time. Because these tools are used within a frame of reference to create an environment for change, each frame of reference has tools that are more relevant and acceptable to it than to others. Within each frame of reference, the change process is outlined, delimiting the tools that are preferable for effective intervention.

REFERENCES

Assistive Technology Act of 2004, Pub. L. No. 108–364 (2004), https://www.govinfo.gov/app/details/PLAW-108publ364

American Occupational Therapy Association. (1994). Uniform terminology for occupational therapy—third edition. *American Journal of Occupational Therapy, 48*, 1047–1054. https://doi.org/10.5014/ajot.48.11.1047

American Occupational Therapy Association. (2020). Occupational therapy practice framework; Domain and process (4th ed.). *American Journal of Occupational Therapy, 74*(Suppl. 2), 7412410010. https://doi.org/10.5014/ajot.2020.74S2001

American Occupational Therapy Association. (2014). Occupational therapy practice framework: Domain and process (3rd ed.). *American Journal of Occupational Therapy, 68*(Suppl. 1), S1–S48. https://doi.org/10.5014/ajot.2014.682006

Brodin, J. (1999) Play in children with severe multiple disabilities: play with toys – a review, *International Journal of Disability, Development and Education*, *46*(1), 25–34, https://doi.org/10.1080/103491299100704

Buckley, K., & Poole, S. E. (2014). Activity analysis. In Hinojosa, J. & Blount, M.-L. (Eds.), *Texture of life: Occupation and related activities* (4th ed., pp. 55–102). AOTA Press.

Buckley, K., Poole, S. E. & Wong, D. C. (2023). Occupation and activity analysis. In Blount, M.-L. & P. Kramer (Eds.), *Texture of life: Occupation and related activities* (5th ed., pp. 33–68). AOTA Press.

Bundy, A. C., & Lane, S. J. (Eds.). (2020). *Sensory integration: Theory and practice* (3rd ed.). F.A. Davis.

Carpenter, L. A. B., Johnston, L. B., & Beard, L. A. (2015). *Assistive technology: Access for all students* (2nd ed.). Pearson Higher Education.

Chantry, J., & Dunford, C. (2010). How do computer assistive technologies enhance participation in childhood occupations for children with multiple and complex disabilities? A review of the current literature. *British Journal of Occupational Therapy, 73*(8), 351–365. https://doi.org/10.4276/030802210X12813483277107

Charry-Sánchez, J. D., Pradilla, I., & Talero-Gutiérrez, C. (2018). Effectiveness of animal-assisted therapy in the pediatric population: systematic review and meta-analysis of controlled studies. *Journal of Developmental & Behavioral Pediatrics, 39*(7), 580–590, https://doi.org/10.1097/DBP.0000000000000594

Cook, A. M., Polgar, J. M., & Encarnacao, P. (2020). *Assistive technologies: Principles and practice* (5th ed.). Elsevier/Mosby.

Dancza, K., & Rodger, S. (2018). *Implementing occupation-centred practice: A practical guide for occupational therapy practice learning*. Routledge.

Dirette, D. P., & Gutman, S. A. (Eds.). (2021). *Occupational therapy for physical dysfunction* (8th ed.). Wolters Kluwer Health/Lippincott Williams & Wilkins.

Erikson, E. H. (1963). *Childhood and society* (2nd ed.). Norton.

Evetts, C. L., & Peloquin, S. M. (2017). *Mindful crafts as therapy: Engaging more than hands*. FA Davis.

Fleming, M. H. (1991). The therapist with the three-track mind. *American Journal of Occupational Therapy, 45*(11), 1007–1014. https://doi.org/10.5014/ajot.45.11.1007

Gillen, G., & Brown, C. (2024). *Willard and Spackman's occupational therapy* (14th ed.). Wolters Kluwer Health/Lippincott Williams & Wilkins.

Golledge, J. (1998). Distinguishing between occupation, purposeful activity and activity, part 1: Review and explanation. *British Journal of Occupational Therapy, 61,* 100–105.

Graham, F., Rodger, S., & Ziviani, J. (2013). Effectiveness of occupational performance coaching in improving children's and mothers' performance and mothers' self-competence. *American Journal of Occupational Therapy, 67*, 10–18. https://doi.org/10.5014/ajot.2013.004648

Hinojosa, J. (2017). How society's philosophy has shaped occupational therapy practice for the past 100 years. *The Open Journal of Occupational Therapy, 5*(2), https://doi.org/10.15453/2168-6408.1325

Hinojosa, J., & Kramer, P. (1997). Statement: Fundamental concepts of occupational therapy: Occupation, purposeful activity, and function. *American Journal of Occupational Therapy, 51*, 864–866. https://doi.org/10.5014/ajot.51.10.864

Hinojosa, J., Kramer, P., & Crist, P. (2014). Evaluation: Where do we begin? In Hinojosa, J., & Kramer, P. (Eds.), *Occupational therapy evaluation: Obtaining and interpreting data* (4th ed., pp. 1–18). AOTA Press.

Hinojosa, J., Sabari, J., & Pedretti, L. (1993). Position paper: Purposeful activity. *American Journal of Occupational Therapy, 47*, 1081–1082. https://doi.org/10.5014/ajot.47.12.1081

Howe, M. C., & Schwartzberg, S. L. (2001). *A functional approach to group work in occupational therapy*. Lippincott Williams & Wilkins.

Humphrey, R., & Wakeford, L. (2006). An occupation-centered discussion of development and implications for practice. *American Journal of Occupational Therapy, 60*, 258–267. https://doi.org/10.5014/ajot.60.3.258

Hunt, D. (1997). *The magician's tale*. Putnam.

Kessler, D., & Graham, F. (2015). The use of coaching in occupational therapy: An integrative review. *Australian Occupational Therapy Journal, 62*, 160–176. https://doi.org/10.1111/1440-1630.12175

Kramer, P., Blount, M.-L., & Blount, W. (2023). Occupation and occupational therapy. In Blount, M.-L., Kramer, P. & Blount, W. (Eds.), *The texture of life* (5th ed., pp. 1–10). AOTA Press.

Kramer, P., & Hinojosa, J. (2014). Activity synthesis as a means to structure occupation. In Hinojosa, J., & Blount, M. L. (Eds.), *Texture of life: Occupation and related activities* (4th ed., pp. 119–138). AOTA Press.

Kramer, P., & Walsh, W. E. (2023). Activity synthesis as a means to structure occupation. In Blount, M.-L., Kramer, P. & Blount, W. (Eds.), *The texture of life* (5th ed., pp. 87–106). AOTA Press.

Macauley, B. L. (2023). Animal-assisted therapy for pediatric patients. In E. Altschuler (Ed.), *Animal assisted therapy use application by condition* (pp. 119–145). Academic Press

Mosey, A. C. (1986). *Psychosocial components of occupational therapy*. Raven Press.

Mosey, A. C. (1996). *Applied scientific inquiry in the health professions: An epistemological orientation* (2nd ed.). American Occupational Therapy Association.

Parham, L. D., & Fazio, L. S. (2008). *Play in occupational therapy for children* (2nd ed.). Elsevier.

Pendleton, H. M., & Schultz-Krohn, W. (2024). *Pedretti's occupational therapy: Practice skills for physical dysfunction* (9th ed.). Elsevier.

Reilly, M. (1974). *Play as exploratory learning: Studies of curiosity behavior*. Sage.

Pierce, D. (2001). Untangling occupation and activity. *American Journal of Occupational Therapy, 55*, 138–146. https://doi.org/10.5014/ajot.55.2.138

Schell, B. A. B., Gillen, G., Crepeau, E., & Scaffa, M. (2018). Analyzing occupations and activity. In B. A. B. Schell & G. Gillen (Eds.), *Willard and Spackman's occupational therapy* (13th ed., pp. 320–333). Wolters Kluwer.

Schell, B. A. B., & Benfield, A. M. (2024). Professional reasoning in practice. In G. Gillen & C. Brown (Eds.), *Willard and Spackman's occupational therapy* (14th ed., pp. 420–437). Wolters Kluwer.

Searles, H. F. (1960). *The non-human environment*. International Universities Press.

Solman, B., & Clouston, T. (2016). Occupational therapy and the therapeutic use of self. *British Journal of Occupational Therapy, 79*(8), 514–516. https://doi.org/10.1177/0308022616638675

Taylor, R. R. (2008). *The intentional relationship: Occupational therapy and use of self.* F.A. Davis.

Taylor, R. R., & Van Puymbroeck, L. (2013). Therapeutic use of self: Applying the intentional relationship model in group therapy. In O'Brien, J. C. & Solomon, J. W. (Eds.), *Occupational analysis and group process* (pp. 36–52). Elsevier.

Townsend, E. A., & Polatajko, H. J. (2013). *Enabling occupation II: Advancing an occupational therapy vision for health, well-being, & justice through occupation*. CAOT Publications ACE.

World Health Organization. (2001). *ICF: International classification of functioning, disability and health*. WHO.

5 Contextual Factors Shaping Pediatric Practice

Janet Njelesani

The contexts in which children reside influence their functioning, engagement in meaningful activities, and how pediatric occupational therapy services are provided. To carry out occupational therapy practice that is equitable, family-centered, and evidence-based, occupational therapy practitioners must understand the breadth of contextual factors of the systems in which they practice and use this information as they consider how to link theory to frames of reference to guide their evaluations and interventions.

Occupational therapy practitioners scope of practice in pediatrics involves working with children and families to address concerns in function and/or occupational participation (AOTA, 2020). Occupational therapy practitioners also have a role in advocating for children's rights to inclusion and children's rights to a safe, supportive, and healthy environment to optimize occupational participation (Rodger & Kennedy-Behr, 2017). The focus on the child participating in their occupations within their contexts is core to occupational therapy's distinct role and value in pediatrics. A contextual factor that often impacts the delivery of services and focus of intervention is that of practice setting. Practitioners need to consider the particular local, federal, and insurance guidelines when providing services to children. This chapter explores the concept of context, the variety of contexts in which occupational therapy practitioners typically provide services, and discusses how contexts guide the occupational therapy process, including the influence on practitioners' use of frames of reference to structure pediatric practice.

DEFINING CONTEXT

According to the American Occupational Therapy Association's (AOTA) Occupational Therapy Practice Framework: Domain and Practice (4th ed.; AOTA, 2020), occupational therapy practitioners "use their knowledge of the transactional relationship among the client, the client's engagement in valuable occupations, and the context to design occupation-based intervention plans" (AOTA, 2020, p. 1). The current 4th edition of AOTA's Practice Framework uses the overarching term "context" to represent the former "contexts and environments" by adopting the World Health Organization (WHO, 2001) taxonomy from the International Classification of Functioning, Disability and Health (ICF). This change in terms of AOTA aims to establish standardized and widely accepted definitions across occupational therapy, with which this chapter aligns.

"Context" is described as a comprehensive concept encompassing the environmental and personal factors that impact the involvement and participation of each client, whether it is a person, a group, or a population (AOTA, 2020). Occupational therapy practitioners need to understand how the context and embedded environmental and personal factors influence clients' abilities to engage in occupations and services delivered within a practice setting (Njelesani et al., 2011). Environmental factors are "the physical, social, and attitudinal surroundings in which people live and conduct their lives," including the physical environment, products and technology, personal support and relationships, attitudes and services, systems, and policies (AOTA, 2020, p. S10). Environmental factors can facilitate or hinder a client's occupational participation and the services carried out in practice. "Personal factors are the unique features of a person that are not part of a health condition or health state and that constitute the particular background of the person's life and living" (AOTA, 2020, p. S10). These factors reflect the essence of a person, including age, sexual orientation, gender, race, ethnicity, socioeconomic status, education, customs, beliefs, activity patterns, behavioral standards, and expectations. They are not to be perceived as inherently positive or negative by practitioners. Practitioners must consider how these factors can influence occupational therapy practice and resulting occupational participation. Therefore, occupational therapy practitioners must consider the client's occupational engagement within their specific contexts (environmental and personal factors) when delivering interventions aligned with the chosen frames of reference.

BRONFENBRENNER'S ECOLOGICAL SYSTEMS THEORY

Children grow, develop, and change through the influence of their own personal factors as well as from surrounding environmental factors. Multiple environmental factors within and outside practice settings shape and define access to services and the variety, quality, and cost of services provided. Bronfenbrenner's ecological systems theory offers a framework for understanding these relationships (Figure 5.1). Bronfenbrenner's ecological systems theory sees child development as a multifaceted process shaped by numerous layers of the surrounding environment, encompassing immediate family and school environments and broader cultural values, laws, and customs. Human development is explained through episodes of both stability and change in the biopsychological characteristics of the individual, together with reciprocal relationships between the individual and their environments over time (Bronfenbrenner, 2005). These interactions, occurring regularly, are referred to as "proximal processes" and are the "primary engines of development" (Bronfenbrenner, 2005, p. 6). Throughout a child's life, these processes become increasingly more complex. Parent–infant daily bottle-feeding experiences, attending an older sibling's basketball games, outdoor play with neighborhood peers, and completing a group project during a classroom work period are some examples of situations and opportunities in which proximal processes abound.

According to Bronfenbrenner, the child's environment is composed of multiple layers, each a system of relationships that influences their growth and performance over their life span. The theory divides the person's environment into five different systems: the microsystem, the mesosystem, the exosystem, the macrosystem, and the chronosystem, with the five systems being interrelated, so the influence of one system on a child's development depends on its relationship with the others. Bronfenbrenner's ecological systems theory aligns with AOTA's Practice Framework's description of context. It acknowledges the contextual dimensions surrounding the child and family, how they influence the child's occupations, and how the child grows and matures.

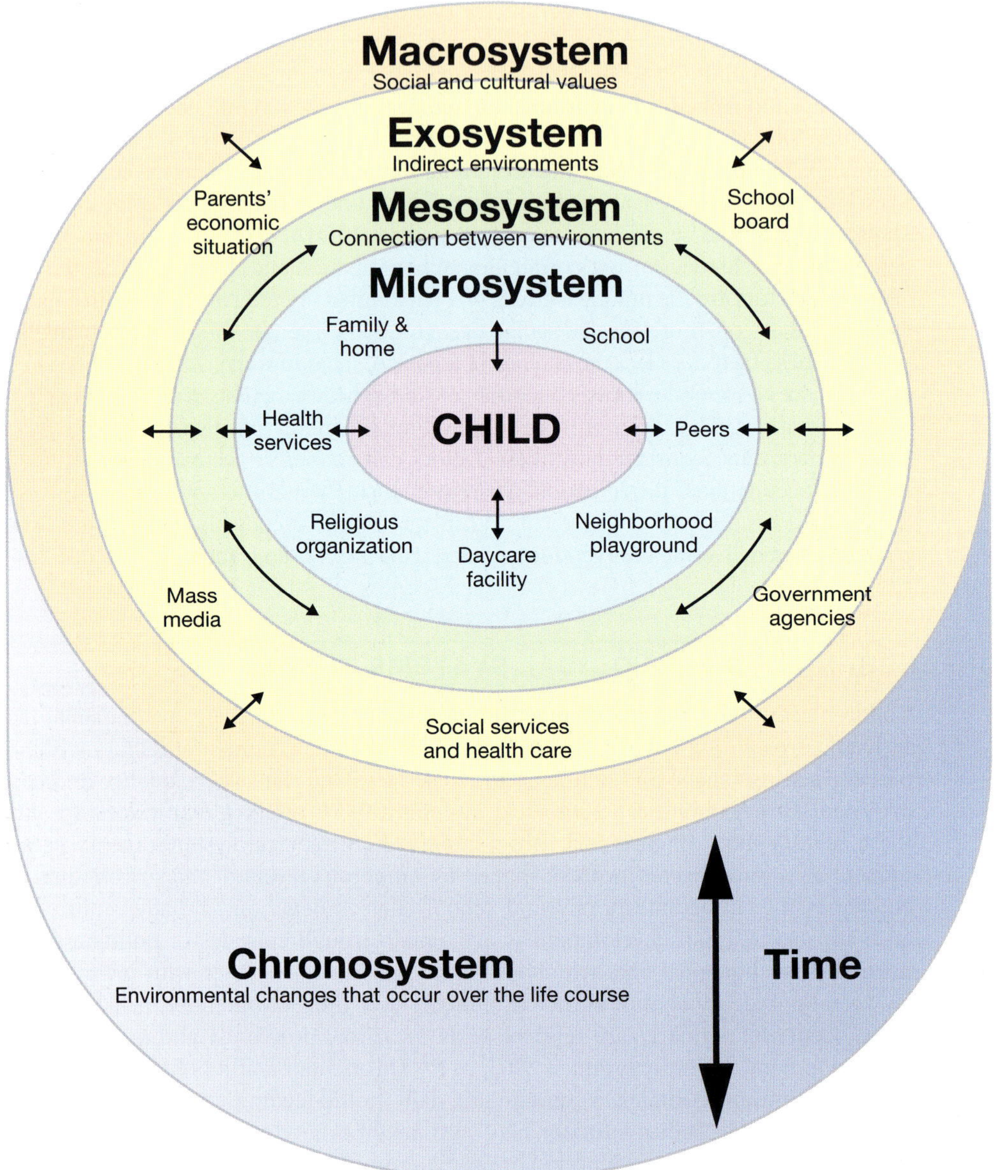

FIGURE 5.1 Bronfenbrenner's Ecological Systems Theory. (Adapted from Bronfenbrenner, U. (1979). *The ecology of human development: Experiments by nature and design.* Harvard University Press.)

Microsystem

The most proximal microsystem is defined as "a pattern of activities, roles, and interpersonal relations experienced by the developing person in a given face-to-face setting with particular physical and material features and containing other persons with distinctive characteristics of temperament, personality, and systems of belief" (Bronfenbrenner, 2005, p. 148). The family and

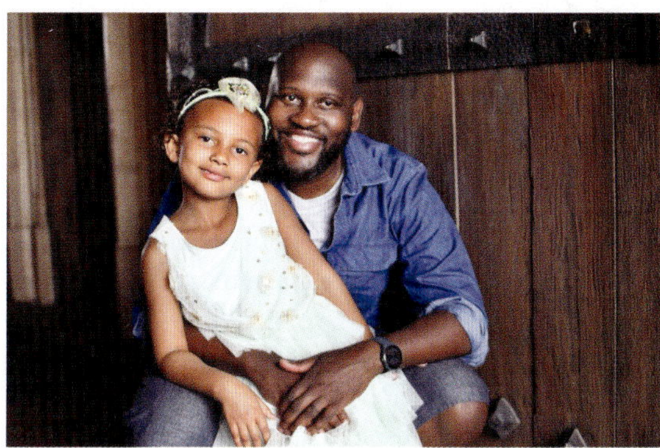

FIGURE 5.2 Photo of father and child.

the home environment represent an early microsystem for young children. The young child who attends a community child-care setting for part of the week experiences two different microsystems. As children grow, the number of microsystems present in their lives increases. School, home, religious organizations, and sports clubs are examples for teenagers. The activities, experiences, relationships, and even the distinct characteristics of persons in each of these settings are recognized as essential influences on the child's development.

The primary function of the family is to provide a supportive and nurturing environment for the child's development. A variety of features characterize families, including membership (single or dual-parent households, the inclusion of extended family members, siblings, and pets), size, ethnicity, socioeconomic status, traditions, and lifestyle preferences. Diverse combinations of beliefs, resources, and interests contribute to the nature of each family. As a social system, connectedness, relationships, and interdependence patterns are essential to the family's function (Jaffe & Cosper, 2015). Subsystems within families, such as parent–parent, parent–child, parent–sibling, and family–extended family, add to the dynamics and complexities of the family unit (Figure 5.2).

Mesosystem

Moving away from the child's immediate context, Bronfenbrenner (2005) identifies several dimensions that influence proximal processes and thus impact development. The mesosystem comprises connections and relationships between a child's microsystems (e.g., interactions between parents and teachers). Essentially, the mesosystem is a system of microsystems.

Exosystem

The exosystem comprises formal and informal social structures that do not directly involve the child but indirectly influence them through their impact on one of the microsystems. This system includes settings where the child's surrounding adults engage (e.g., parent's workplace) and the child's neighborhood. An instance of exosystems affecting a child's development could be a parent working in a job with long hours and limited flexibility, thereby reducing the quality and quantity of interaction they have with their child. The child may, therefore, experience less parental involvement in their daily life, such as help with homework, attendance at school events, or spending quality time together. This reduced parental involvement could impact the child's emotional well-being and academic performance.

Macrosystem

At the next level, the macrosystem includes cultural belief systems, societal patterns of behavior, and resources. This system differs from the previous ecosystems in that it does not pertain to the specific environments of an individual child but rather to the pre-existing societal and cultural contexts within which the child is growing up. An example of this system is if the child is raised in a society that places an extremely high value on academic achievement, leading to increased pressure and expectations for academic performance from parents, which may influence the child's well-being.

For occupational therapy practitioners, federal and state education regulations and state curriculum standards developed at the level of the macrosystem guide intervention and special education programs (Bazyk & Cahill, 2015). These present specific requirements and subtle distinctions that define the education system and influence the direction and expectations of occupational therapy services. The American Occupational Therapy guidelines for early intervention and school-based services (American Occupational Therapy Association, 2017) are updated as the education system evolves. Hence, the organization continuously provides a focus for occupational therapy practice.

Chronosystem

The fifth and final level of Bronfenbrenner's ecological systems theory is known as the chronosystem. This system encompasses all the environmental changes, spanning a lifetime, that shape development, including significant life transitions and historical events.

Life Transitions

Families and their children encounter numerous transitions from infancy through young adulthood, including changes in services, programs, providers, and locations. Effective family and professional partnerships during transition help parents and children prepare, adjust to new situations, and succeed in the process. Open communication, with opportunities to ask questions and discuss options, characterizes supportive interactions and information-sharing efforts.

Many of these changes are systemic. Some significant transitions are associated with age-related developmental stages, such as moving from early intervention to preschool special education when the child reaches age three, the start of kindergarten, and the move to middle school, high school, higher education, or employment. Leaving familiar surroundings and beginning in a new situation comes with many unknowns that can be stressful for the child and family. Changing a method of service delivery, such as beginning a center-based preschool following a home-based infant/toddler program, involves meeting new program personnel. Similarly, supporting a teenager's autonomy and self-advocacy when planning the high school transition are some challenges parents may face. Active participation by parents is an expectation of the Individualized Education Program (IEP) process. It is recommended that the student also participate once they are in high school. However, it is critical that both the parent and student participate in the transition process at age 16. At these team meetings, efforts focus on encouraging students, according to their strengths, to help plan transitions throughout service provision. Families need information to understand the process and their evolving responsibilities and know what they can expect from other team members. A defined transition planning process (Rehfeldt et al., 2012), occupational practitioners' knowledge about the transition process, and communication between the sending and receiving programs (Myers et al., 2011) can support positive transition planning outcomes. Keep in mind that this part of the educational system in the United States and may be different in other countries. Additionally, moving out of high school and into higher education requires complete change, where there is no longer an IEP and, instead, the need to self-advocate for accommodations. Moving into the working world from high school requires a whole different set of considerations.

PEDIATRIC PRACTICE SETTINGS

Medically Based Settings

Pediatric practice areas typically include medically-based settings, such as neonatal intensive care units, pediatric acute-care and rehabilitation units, intermediate and long-term health care facilities, and outpatient clinics (Table 5.1). Frames of reference that represent a curative view may be applied more successfully within these settings that are medically oriented or in instances of acute problems or other conditions that are likely to be resolved (e.g., recovery following a broken arm or rehabilitation for a child with Guillain–Barré syndrome). In these settings, groups of practitioners often constitute the "therapy department." Separate physical, occupational, and speech therapy divisions may be differentiated.

As such, the occupational therapy practitioner may complete the evaluation in isolation, summarizing findings in a written report. Alternately, the occupational, physical, and speech therapists may each evaluate distinct aspects of the child's performance, integrating perspectives from all three therapists into one report. During the team meeting, each professional presents their evaluation results for review and discussion by all team members. The departmentalized arrangement provides the occupational therapy practitioner with direction and supervision concerning care. There is ample opportunity for practitioners to interact and collaborate with others who "speak the same language" and share similar interests. Occupational therapy practitioners may involve another department colleague to review the case and treatment regimen so that they can consider additional or revised intervention strategies. The peer support provided through these exchanges is particularly valuable to entry-level practitioners. The collaborative opportunity is also rewarding for practitioners who enjoy mentoring with colleagues. Department members often acquire a similar knowledge base about interventions relevant to the population served by the agency.

Center-Based and Private Practices

Independently managed private practices offer center-based and itinerant services within the community. In a practice example, occupational therapy practitioners working at a private practice clinic select a frame of reference based on theories explaining causal relationships between component systems within the human organism, such as neurodevelopmental treatment. Evaluation of the child's posture and quality of movement during floor play with toys is completed independently, often in a specialized environment (e.g., the individual provider's office, examination room) rather than in the child's home or natural environment. The practitioner uses evaluation results to develop a care plan, summarizing findings and recommendations at a team meeting or through a written report. The occupational therapy practitioner implements intervention primarily through direct interaction with the child, either in a dyad or sometimes

Table 5.1 Distinguishing Features of Pediatric Service Settings

	Hospital	School System	Home Based	Private Practice	Child-care Center
Governance	Health care, managed care organization, board of trustees	State Education Department, local Board of Education, building administration	Family culture and norms	Independent corporation, partnership, or individual owner	Corporation, partnership, individual owner, or sponsoring agency
Funding	Public, private funds, endowment, charities	State and federal government, local taxpayers	Third-party payment, medical insurance, federal and state funding, out of pocket	Third-party payment, private insurance, out of pocket	Medical insurance, federal/state subsidies, early intervention programs, out-of-pocket
Focus of Care	Treating acute or chronic disease/dysfunction/conditions	Student's participation and progression within the education curriculum, preparation for higher education, employment, independent living	Family system and child as part of the family	Specific to agency's mission	Nurturance, health and safety, developmental progression
Peer Relations/Supervision	Therapy department with director and hierarchical supervision by medical and administrative staff, interprofessional collaboration	Principal is administrator of multidisciplined staff. Practitioner as employee or contractor	Employee or agency contractor traveling to homes on itinerant basis. Supervision from building administration and home agency personnel	Practitioner functions solo or with group of related professionals	Practitioner as contractor into child-care center. Administrative supervision from building administration and home agency personnel
Intervention setting	Simulated environment structured around dispensing care as a priority	Multiple school-based and community-based environments (least restrictive settings), as determined by educational team	Natural home and family settings, activities, and routines	Simulated settings in center-based practice may include home and community-based settings	Caregiver-child/children in settings that simulate home and preschool environments
Provider/Consumer relations	Brief, intermittent contact, episodic care in 1:1 relationship	Practitioner works with system, programs, education staff, students, and parents, short- to long-term contracts	Practitioner in 1:1 relationship with family/child, short- to long-term contracts	Practitioner in 1:1 relationship with family/child, short- to long-term contracts	Practitioner in direct relationship with child-care provider and may include direct relationship with child, short- to long-term contracts

with a small group of several children. Typically, these practitioners use space and equipment for child-centered intervention. For example, a spacious environment with a supply of various-sized positioning aids and an obstacle-free area to use when handling the child in various movement planes is well suited for therapy based on neurodevelopmental treatment. The practitioner shares progress updates with family and other team members through meetings and written summaries.

School-Based Settings

The priorities and concerns of the child, family, caretakers, and other significant adults are important in any practice setting. However, in the school system, the classroom teacher is very important and can help guide the occupational therapy process. Because the environment is valued as a context that influences behavior, the settings, activities, and routines that represent the child's everyday experiences are also a focus. While the practitioner might not work directly with the parents, they need to understand the family's concerns, and in a school setting, they may need to support the teacher, as well as the child. Evaluation and intervention approaches address child capacities, skills, and participation in occupation, environment, and context. In this setting, the occupational therapy practitioner selects from various frames of reference that emphasize theories, such as the biomechanical frame of reference, to promote the student's participation in school activities. Practitioners prefer strategies easily embedded into regular routines to increase opportunities for the child to participate in everyday experiences. For example, with a slant board placed on the desk, the student holds a pencil and writes for the duration of each classroom lesson, affording increased opportunities to practice penmanship skills. A phone interview with parents and a meeting with teachers are completed to gather information about their concerns and priorities and to learn about the context and environments in which the child is expected to participate. Practitioners might evaluate the student's ability to purchase and eat lunch in the school cafeteria during the scheduled lunch period. When this type of contextual opportunity is not available, practitioners may use simulated environments to evaluate performance areas. Practitioners identify opportunities already available in the child's environment that support participation and reinforce their benefit. Additionally, they plan strategies to enhance participation in areas where limitations exist.

Occupational therapy practitioners also provide services in families' homes, child-care centers, or in other community-based settings, such as the library's weekly parent–child music group, after-school programs, or a summer day camp as examples. Intervention visits to the settings where children grow, learn, and develop, such as home or the child-care center, are the optimal venue for service delivery. Periodic use of alternate settings designed for specific procedures may be required (e.g., a specialized location to fabricate a hand orthosis to support function in the child whose motor skills limit participation in tasks). Interventions may be directed toward the caregivers or teachers, offering support and specific strategies they implement in their ongoing interactions with the child. Intervention strategies may include developmental, remedial, and compensatory approaches. When therapist–child activity is indicated, consideration is given to how the involvement occurs so that it does not disrupt the naturally occurring context.

CONSIDERING CONTEXT WHEN PLANNING OCCUPATIONAL THERAPY SERVICE

The child, family, caregivers, and other persons essential in the child's life, along with multiple contextual factors within and surrounding the child, are important in occupational therapy programs. Occupational therapy practitioners contextualize services within the child's daily activities and experiences. The successful outcome is the child's occupational engagement and participation, which provides the most advantageous opportunities for learning and development. Effective occupational therapy services in pediatric settings require practitioners to be aware of and sensitive to the child's unique contexts. When practitioners conduct an evaluation or plan intervention without these considerations or including critical people in the child's environment, the evaluation is incomplete, and subsequent intervention recommendations may not be appropriate. While entry-level occupational therapy practitioners in pediatric settings have a solid knowledge base, they will need to learn more about the contexts within which they work and the communities in which their clients live. It is beyond the scope of this text to cover in-depth material related to working with children and their families; however, the following issues are essential whenever occupational therapy practitioners apply any frame of reference in pediatric settings.

Family-Centered Care

Occupational therapy practitioners utilize effective communication and interpersonal skills in their work with children and families. Families value reciprocal communication with their children's service providers and desire to participate in decision-making concerning their child's care (An et al., 2017; Jaffe & Cosper, 2015). To be responsive, practitioners must approach the family as a partner in this endeavor. Each family has its own needs and concerns. Practitioners must listen to parents' perspectives, interests, and priorities throughout all phases of the occupational therapy process. A family's or caregiver's ability and willingness to contribute information may vary throughout their involvement in programs and services that support their child's development. They should have multiple opportunities to communicate with the professionals involved in their child's life. These interactions should be nonjudgmental to meet the needs of all participating family members. Practitioners and family members should openly discuss issues related to the child and family through a relationship based on mutual trust. This collaboration can give practitioners a clear perspective of the real-life demands faced by the family and child. It also helps practitioners learn about how the child's specific needs impact the family and the family's ability to support their child within their context.

In any setting, occupational therapy practitioners should try to develop open and sustained communication with the individuals who are the child's primary caregivers, discussing goals and types of interventions that may be implemented and responding to questions that arise. For example, in school system practice, while teachers are often the practitioners' primary contact on a day-to-day basis, practitioners need to make efforts to reach out to parents through phone, e-mail, written notes, or face-to-face meetings. Practitioners solicit information from families and provide regular reports about the child's progress and participation in school activities and routines. Practitioners should include parents in discussions and decisions regarding changes in their child's program.

Some frames of reference, such as Chapter 14 on social participation, enhance childhood occupation and include the family and the human environment as aspects of the theoretical bases. These frames of reference involve family members or caregivers directly or indicate their influence in the application to practice. Alternately, the neurodevelopmental treatment frame of reference (Chapter 8) does not directly address family issues. Practitioners who use the neurodevelopmental treatment frame of reference need to consider family support and education when implementing intervention, as they recognize that their interventions will only be effective if they are reinforced frequently during the family's routine activity.

Depending on the frame of reference chosen, practitioners must be realistic about the family's role in the intervention process. Furthermore, they must recognize that family members are not experts in using the profession's therapeutic modalities. Despite all efforts to plan an effective intervention, occupational therapy practitioners accept that they do not have all the answers, and some intervention plans do not achieve the desired outcomes. Reasons for unsatisfied outcomes may include incomplete essential information regarding the child, changes in priorities, the choice of the frame of reference, unrealistic expectations by either practitioners or the family, the fit between the intervention and contextual factors, or other factors. Regardless of the reasons, occupational therapy practitioners should seek needed information from family members or other sources and engage in self-reflection to understand the breakdown. Practitioners ensure that adjustments are made promptly to implement an effective intervention plan to achieve shared goals.

Sometimes, practitioners are apprehensive about working directly with parents and other family members. They may not feel adequately prepared to support families or uncomfortable with a parent's distress, frustration, or feelings of elation over achievements. Experience in working with families and sensitivity to the parenting process is helpful. Being reflexive of one's feelings makes it easier for practitioners to understand their range of emotions and contributes to their ability to develop working relationships with families.

Intersectionality

To work effectively with families, practitioners need to understand the concept of intersectionality. Intersectionality, coined by Kimberlé Crenshaw in 1989, illuminates how various identities like gender, race, class, ability, sexuality, religion, age, nationality, intersect and mutually influence one another, resulting in multifaceted experiences of oppression. It is important to understand that these many identities do not exist independently, but rather, each informs the others (Figure 5.3). Many of the children and families occupational therapy practitioners work with have multiple identities to consider that impact their access to services and occupational engagement. Families of children with disabilities living in the United States often experience oppression on multiple levels at the intersection of disability, race, ethnicity, and socioeconomic status. For example, families of children with disabilities living in the United States are more likely to be at risk for poverty than families with no disabled members (Creamer, et al., 2022).

Considerations of intersectionality are well-established within the field of occupational therapy, as outlined by Trentham et al. (2007), and they represent fundamental elements of the AOTA's Vision 2025. Occupational therapy practitioners can consider intersectionality when working with children and families by recognizing and valuing the diverse identities and experiences that each individual brings to the therapy session. They can foster open and inclusive communication, creating a safe space where children and families feel heard and understood, regardless of their backgrounds. Additionally, practitioners can tailor their interventions to consider the unique cultural, social, and economic factors that may influence a child's needs and occupational goals, thereby promoting equitable care. In addition to understanding intersectionality, practitioners must recognize the potential influence their power, life experience, assumptions, and biases have on their work, as discussed in the section on cultural humility.

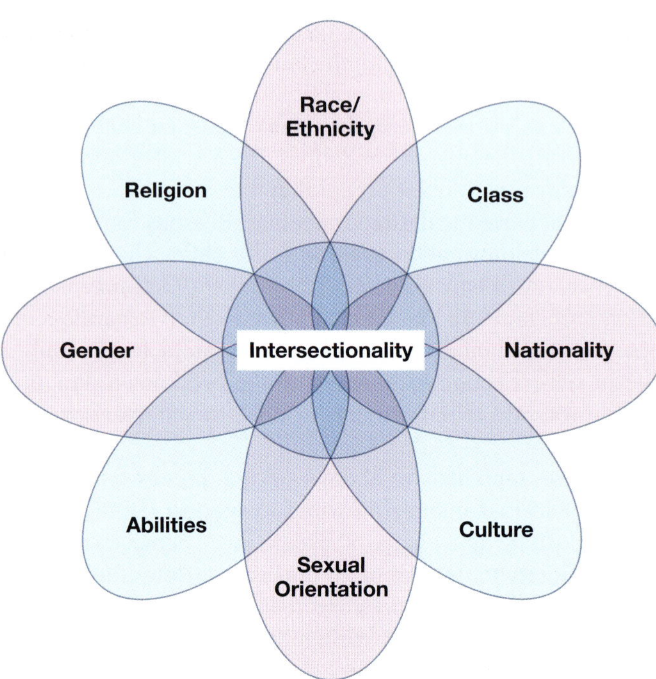

FIGURE 5.3 Intersectionality Identities. (Adapted from Crenshaw, K. W. (1989). Demarginalizing the Intersection of Race and Sex: A Black Feminist Critique of Antidiscrimination Doctrine, Feminist Theory and Antiracist Politics. *University of Chicago Legal Forum, 1989,* 139–167.)

Professional Relationships

Children who receive occupational therapy services have contact with various other professionals who address their health and medical needs and who administer or implement programs to support their growth and development. As discussed earlier, professionals have distinct beliefs, values, and attitudes. In addition, each brings a preconceived view of their role and the roles and responsibilities of other professionals involved. Consequently, despite a common interest in helping the child to grow, develop, and participate in relevant activities and environments, each lends a different viewpoint to the situation, and their unique perspectives generate individual concerns and goals for the child. However, pediatric occupational therapy practitioners and other children's developmental specialists can take advantage of various processes so that they do not operate in isolation. Professionals must communicate with each other and be willing to learn from one another. They must recognize and solve problems that arise when professionals from multiple disciplines interact and participate effectively in teams. The collaborative partnership between families and pediatric professionals is one of the foundations for effective services for children (Bazyk & Cahill, 2015).

Many entry-level occupational therapy practitioners initially feel insecure about working as a full-fledged team member. It takes skills to collaborate effectively with other professionals. All occupational therapy practitioners in pediatric practice need to become confident in their roles to participate successfully with other professionals who work with children. To do so, they must understand their profession, the structure of pediatric frames of reference, and how they may fit within different systems and contexts. Then, they must select and apply frames of reference in practice and teach other team members about occupational therapy perspectives. Occupational therapy practitioners can draw from their educational background concerning psychosocial functioning to understand the workings of the team and become important contributing members. Coursework related to facilitating the group process is also helpful for practitioners to be an effective, active team member.

CULTURAL HUMILITY

Social paradigms influence occupational therapy professional training, as they exist within the sponsoring educational institution. Coursework may be aligned with a perspective that reflects any of the views discussed in this chapter. Learning is assimilated with students' values, beliefs, and ways of thinking. Clinical or field-based training further contributes to students' experience, understanding, and points of view. Entry-level practitioners bring these influences into the practice setting, integrating their perspectives with those of the system as they apply the occupational therapy process to benefit the clients served. Within the practice setting, practitioners need to be aware of the position of authority implied by the role of being a health care provider, and they must be careful not to use that power in a negative way in relationships with families.

Furthermore, practitioners must be concerned with the expectations and responsibilities that they impose on families. Consistency between the paradigm that characterizes the setting, the practitioners' perspective, and the chosen frame of reference is important. It may contribute to the success of the intervention and the understanding of the occupational therapy process by family members, administrators, and other professionals in the program. These considerations in practice may be guided by an approach to practice that includes cultural humility. Cultural humility involves continuously engaging, questioning assumptions, and remaining open to learning about other cultures. It is not about achieving complete competence but fostering an ongoing process (Beagan, 2015). This approach can help reduce stereotyping by acknowledging that individuals can experience their culture in various and evolving ways (Agner, 2020). When applied in practice, cultural humility includes evaluating and modifying the assessment environment to accommodate cultural needs.

Reflexivity

Reflexivity is a crucial starting point for engaging in cultural humility and antiracism efforts (Sterman & Njelesani, 2021). Occupational therapy practitioners should engage in self-reflection regarding their cultural backgrounds, personal identities, perceptions of racism and prejudice, and areas of privilege. They should consider how these factors influence their views of valued occupations and their attitudes and behaviors toward individuals with different backgrounds than their own (Sterman et al., 2022). By practicing reflexivity, professionals can examine their cultural perspectives and how these perspectives impact their relationships with clients. Failure to engage in critical self-reflection can potentially harm the health and well-being of clients, particularly when working with children and families from Black and Indigenous communities (Jull & Giles, 2012). Further, professionals should be aware of their actions and behaviors with any client who comes from a different background than their own.

When choosing frames of reference, reflexivity involves questioning the values inherent in theories and frames of reference, recognizing that most were developed from Euro/Western viewpoints. Therefore they may perpetuate inequities for Black, Indigenous, and People of Color (BIPOC) clients and privilege goals of becoming an independent adult or participating in occupations seen as the expected norm within cultures. Again, this may occur with any clients from different cultures than those we are familiar with. In practical terms, this means adopting strengths-based frames of reference that build on clients' abilities instead of focusing solely on deficits (refer to Chapter 15 as a potential example of this). It also entails fostering collaborative engagement with BIPOC clients, where occupational therapy practitioners learn from families rather than solely dictating to them what they should do. By approaching conversations about families' values and health beliefs as opportunities for mutual learning, trust and collaboration can be nurtured, and stereotypes can be reduced.

APPLYING FRAMES OF REFERENCE IN CONTEXT

Practitioners should always consider family and child contextual factors and priorities when applying frames of reference throughout the occupational therapy process. Practitioners must also consider the congruity between their views and those that characterize the settings in which their service is provided and carefully select and apply frames of reference in practice. Practitioners must consider appropriate ways to incorporate the chosen frame of reference with the setting to provide interventions within the system's context. These considerations help practitioners effectively integrate occupational therapy evaluation principles, program planning, implementation, and outcome assessment for relevant and meaningful pediatric services.

For example, occupational practitioners may select a frame of reference based on person, environment, and occupation relationships, such as the frame of reference to enhance social participation. Through interviews, practitioners would learn about parents' and teachers' concerns and priorities. Teachers familiar with the student may meet and complete sections of the *School Function Assessment* (Coster et al., 1998). The parent may complete the *Participation and Environment Measure—Children and Youth* (Coster et al., 2012). Occupational practitioners observe the child during outdoor recess and indoor physical education classes to assess the student's social participation in varied contexts. Team members, including the parent, review and discuss the child's participation and performance from different perspectives and identify the child's strengths and needs. Together, they agree on outcomes that enable the child's social participation in the activities and situations within school routines, documenting evaluation findings and program recommendations into a summary report.

Evidence supports the utility of frames of reference to apply theory to guide practice. In a small exploratory study (Towns & Ashby, 2017), it was found that when fieldwork supervisors valued theory, articulated theory and frames of reference used with specific clients, and used theory in course assignments, fieldwork students felt they could apply it to practice. When fieldwork supervisors did not explicitly describe the theories used and explain how they guided the occupational therapy process for their clients, fieldwork students seemed to have less ability to do so. Nash and Mitchell (2017) reported that students placed increased value on frames of reference and tended to combine frames of reference for more holistic approaches when their fieldwork supervisors discussed how theory and frames of reference guided clients' occupational therapy interventions.

Occupational therapy practitioners identify strategies that promote the child's social participationin the activities and situations that ordinarily exist and serve as natural learning opportunities. Intervention includes collaboration with team members to help recess staff learn new methods and prompts they can use to support and facilitate the student's participation with classmates on the playground.

Once interventions are implemented, occupational practitioners need to ensure that the child's performance is assessed. If the desired change in targeted behavior is not evident, practitioners must ask questions. Is the planned intervention being used? Does the child have enough opportunities to participate in the intervention? Is the intensity of the intervention sufficient? A variety of issues need to be explored. This requires communication with the family, the child, and other team members and may require a review of the specific intervention, or another frame of reference may be used. With cultural humility and being reflexive of their interactions, practitioners are important team members. The following are important points to consider when using any frame of reference:

- Team members include the family and the child. All have a contribution and should work toward facilitating the discussed goals for the child and their family.
- Occupational therapy practitioners should be concerned about how they are communicating. Each frame of reference has its own jargon, which should be translated for mutual understanding by all who participate in the team, including family members and the child.
- Occupational therapy practitioners cannot see themselves as the only service provider to all children. They need to understand the essential contributions other professionals can make and discuss these openly with the family and other team members.
- Occupational therapy practitioners should be aware of the strengths and limitations of their profession and the frames of reference they use. They must be willing to examine their plans, adjust or even change the frame of reference, and modify their interventions to meet the child and family goals within the context in which they live.
- When following the guidelines within a frame of reference, occupational therapy practitioners must use culturally appropriate and meaningful activities in the client's context.

Summary

Occupational therapy practitioners must recognize that the effectiveness of their interventions hinges on a comprehensive understanding of the environmental and personal factors affecting their clients. These contexts, encompassing everything from physical surroundings to personal attributes, impact all phases of the occupational therapy process—from initial referral, selection of an appropriate frame of reference, throughout the evaluation and program planning, program implementation, progress monitoring, discharge planning, and discontinuation of services. To meet clients' rights and offer relevant and valued service in ever-changing health care and education systems, occupational therapy practitioners need to learn about the multiple contextual factors that uniquely influence each child they serve. Therefore, a thorough understanding of clients' contexts informs the therapeutic strategies employed and enhances the likelihood of achieving meaningful outcomes in pediatric occupational therapy.

REFERENCES

Agner, J. (2020). Moving from cultural competence to cultural humility in occupational therapy: A paradigm shift. *The American Journal of Occupational Therapy*, *74*(4), 7404347010p1–7404347010p7. https://doi.org/10.5014/ajot.2020.038067

American Occupational Therapy Association. (2017). Guidelines for occupational therapy services in early intervention and schools. *American Journal of Occupational Therapy*, *71*(Suppl. 2), 7112410010p1–7112410010p10. https://doi.org/10.5014/ajot.2017.716S01

American Occupational Therapy Association. (2020). Occupational therapy practice framework: Domain and process (4th ed.), *The American Journal of Occupational Therapy*, *74*(Suppl. 2), 7412410010p1.

An, M., Palisano, R., Yi, C., Chiarello, L., Dunst, C., & Gracely, E. (2017). Effects of a collaborative intervention process on parent empowerment and child performance: A randomized controlled trial. *Physical & Occupational Therapy in Pediatrics*, 1–15. https://doi.org/10.1080/01942638.2017.1365324

Bazyk, S., & Cahill, S. (2015). School-based therapy. In Case-Smith, J., & O'Brien, B. J. (Eds.), *Occupational therapy for children and adolescents* (7th ed., pp. 664–703). Elsevier.

Beagan, B. L. (2015). Approaches to culture and diversity: A critical synthesis of occupational therapy literature. *Canadian Journal of Occupational Therapy*, *82*(5), 272–282. https://doi.org/10.1177/0008417414567530

Bronfenbrenner, U. (2005). The bioecological theory of human development. In Bronfenbrenner, U. (Ed.), *Making human beings human: Bioecological perspectives on human development* (pp. 3–15). Sage Publications.

Coster, W., Deeney, T., Haltiwanger, J., & Haley, S. (1998). *School function assessment*. Psychological Corporation.

Coster, W., Law, M., Bedell, G., Khetani, M., Cousins, M., & Teplicky, R. (2012). Development of the participation and environment measure for children and youth: Conceptual basis. *Disability & Rehabilitation, 34*(3), 238–246. https://doi.org/10.3109/09638288.2011.603017

Creamer, J., Shrider, E. A., Burns, K., & Chen, F. (2022). *Poverty in the United States: 2021. US Census Bureau.*

Jaffe, L., & Cosper, S. (2015). Working with families. In Case-Smith, J., & O'Brien, J. (Eds.), *Occupational therapy for children and adolescents* (7th ed., pp. 129–162). Mosby.

Jull, J. E., & Giles, A. R. (2012). Health equity, aboriginal peoples and occupational therapy. *Canadian Journal of Occupational Therapy*, *79*(2), 70–76. https://doi.org/10.2182/cjot.2012.79.2.2

Myers, C., Schneck, C., Effgen, S., McCormick, K., Shasby, S., Nash, B., & Mitchell, A. (2011). Factors associated with therapists' involvement in children's transition to preschool. *American Journal of Occupational Therapy, 65*, 86–94. https://doi.org/10.5014/ajot.2011.09060

Nash, B., & Mitchell, A. (2017). Longitudinal study of changes in occupational therapy students' perspectives on frames of reference. *American Journal of Occupational Therapy, 71*, 7105230010p1–7105230010p7. https://doi.org/10.5014/ajot.2017.024455

Njelesani, J., Sedgwick, A., Davis, J. A., & Polatajko, H. J. (2011). The influence of context: a naturalistic study of Ugandan children's doings in outdoor spaces. *Occupational Therapy International*, *18*(3), 124–132.

Rehfeldt, J., Clark, G., & Lee, S. (2012). The effects of using the transition planning inventory and a structured IEP process as a transition planning intervention on IEP meeting outcomes. *Remedial and Special Education, 33*(1), 48–58. https://doi.org/10.1177/0741932510366038

Rodger, S., & Kennedy-Behr, A. (2017). *Occupation-centred practice with children: A practical guide for occupational therapists* (2nd ed). Wiley.

Sterman J, & Njelesani J. (2021). Becoming anti-racist occupational therapy practitioners: A scoping study. *OTJR: Occupation, Participation and Health*. https://doi.org/10.1177/15394492211019931

Sterman, J., Njelesani, J., & Carr, S. (2022). Anti-racism and occupational therapy education: Beyond diversity and inclusion. *Journal of Occupational Therapy Education*, *6*(1). https://doi.org/10.26681/jote.2022.060103

Towns, E. & Ashby, S. (2017). The influence of practice educators on occupational therapy students' understanding of the practical applications of theoretical knowledge: A phenomenological study into student experiences of practice education. *Australian Journal of Occupational Therapy, 61*(5), 344–352. https://doi.org/10.1111/1440-1630.12134

Trentham, B., Cockburn, L., Cameron, D., & Iwama, M. (2007). Diversity and inclusion within an occupational therapy curriculum. *Australian Occupational Therapy Journal, 54*, S49–S57. https://doi.org/10.1111/j.1440-1630.2006.00605

World Health Organization. (2001). *International classification of functioning, disability, and health: ICF*. World Health Organization.

SECTION II

Section II

Commonly Used Frames of Reference

This section of the book contains the most commonly used frames of reference in pediatric settings. Understanding and being able to use these frames of reference will make you, either as a student or practitioner, a theoretically grounded practitioner. Keep in mind that the importance of the frame of reference is that it is an intentional way of organizing theoretical material so that you can put it into practice. As you see children in schools, in a clinic or in private practice, some of this knowledge will become very familiar and may eventually seem instinctive to you. However, remember that even if your practice may seem automatic, it is rooted in complex theoretical knowledge. Each child is unique, so it is crucial to adapt your interventions to the specific needs of that child.

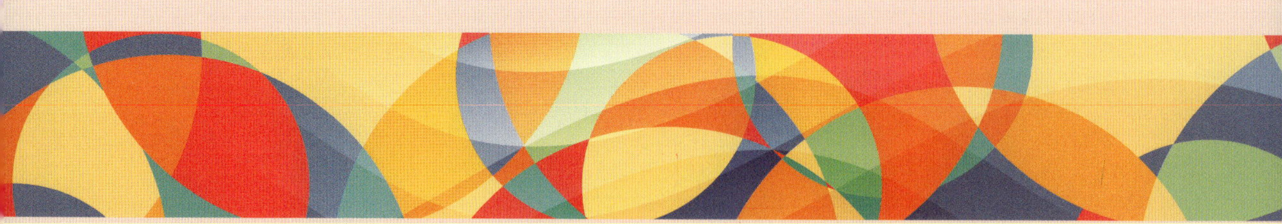

Ayres Sensory Integration Frame of Reference

Susanne Smith Roley ■ Roseann C. Schaaf ■ Annie Baltazar-Mori

Occupational therapy using a sensory integration frame of reference is the most investigated of any individual approach in occupational therapy (Parham & Mailloux, 2015). A. Jean Ayres, an occupational therapist with postdoctoral training in educational psychology and neuroscience, developed the sensory integration frame of reference that includes a scientific theory, standardized and observational assessments, intervention methods, and much of the equipment that is now iconic and often equated with pediatric occupational therapy (Sieg, 1988). Ayres's work in sensory integration affected occupational therapy by its scientific foundation and the scope of its theoretical construct. Furthermore, validation of her ideas was the foundation for clinical problem identification, instrument development, innovation in approach and equipment, efficacy studies, and educational efforts. Sensory integration methods within professional therapy practice are applied across the life span and with varying diagnoses following a comprehensive assessment in which sensory challenges are confirmed (Schaaf & Mailloux, 2015; Schaaf & Smith Roley, 2006; Smith Roley et al., 2001). Steeped within a tradition in scholarship and research, the work in sensory integration continues to be an important frame of reference in pediatric occupational therapy, currently meeting the criteria as an evidence-based practice (Schaaf et al., 2018; Schoen et al., 2019; Steinbrenner et al., 2020) that is feasible, acceptable and replicable (Schaaf et al., 2012).

To preserve the rights to the term "sensory integration," and the integrity of the use of the term along with Ayres' images and works, the Ayres family registered the trademark, Ayres Sensory Integration (ASI), which designates Ayres' seminal work and the ongoing development of sensory integration including its theory, assessments, intervention methods, and participation-related outcomes (Smith Roley et al., 2007). While occupational therapists are the primary contributors to the original and ongoing research and practice in sensory integration, ASI is also applied by other disciplines, such as physical therapy, speech pathology, and psychology.

THEORETICAL BASE

Sensory integration theory explains the way in which "integrative processes result in perception and other types of synthesis of sensory data that enable (people) to interact effectively in the environment" (Ayres, 1972, p. 1). Sensory integration is a brain-behavior process "that organizes sensations from one's body and from the environment and makes it possible to use the body

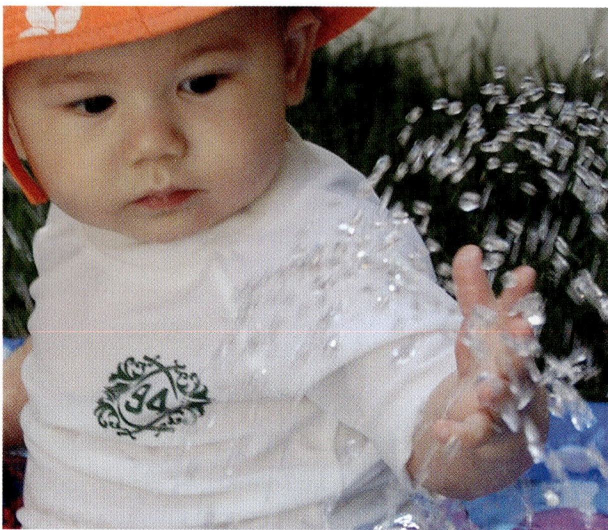

FIGURE 6.1 Children learn to coordinate their actions through exploring with their senses.

effectively in the environment" (Ayres, 1989, p. 22). As such, sensation provides the essential information needed for learning to occur (Figure 6.1). Challenges in organizing and integrating the masses of sensory information a child encounters every day from the body and the environment are often "hidden deficits" that are poorly understood and can profoundly interfere with learning and performance (Ayres, 2005; Parham, 2022; Schaaf et al., 2011, 2015).

Ayres created a model to depict her theory, illustrated in Figure 6.2—The senses, integration of their inputs and their end products (Ayres, 2005).

The model shows how the interactions between the sensory systems—the auditory, vestibular, proprioceptive, tactile, and visual systems—provide integrated information that contributes to increasingly complex learning and behaviors or "end products" (Ayres, 2005). For example, the vestibular and proprioceptive systems contribute to the ability to develop adequate posture, balance, muscle tone, gravitational security, and movement of the eyes in coordination with head and body movements. These, in turn, interact with the tactile system to provide an important foundation for adequate body awareness, coordination of the two sides of the body and praxis. Together, these sensory–motor skills form the foundation for eye–hand coordination, visual perceptual skills, and engagement in purposeful activity. In combination with the auditory system, the sensory systems contribute to speech and language development and provide an important foundation for behaviors needed for learning, such as maintaining an appropriate level of activity and emotional stability as well as the ability to concentrate or organize behavior for paying attention in the classroom.

Assumptions

- Learning is a brain function, dependent on sensory information.
- Sensory integration is a developmental and dynamic process.

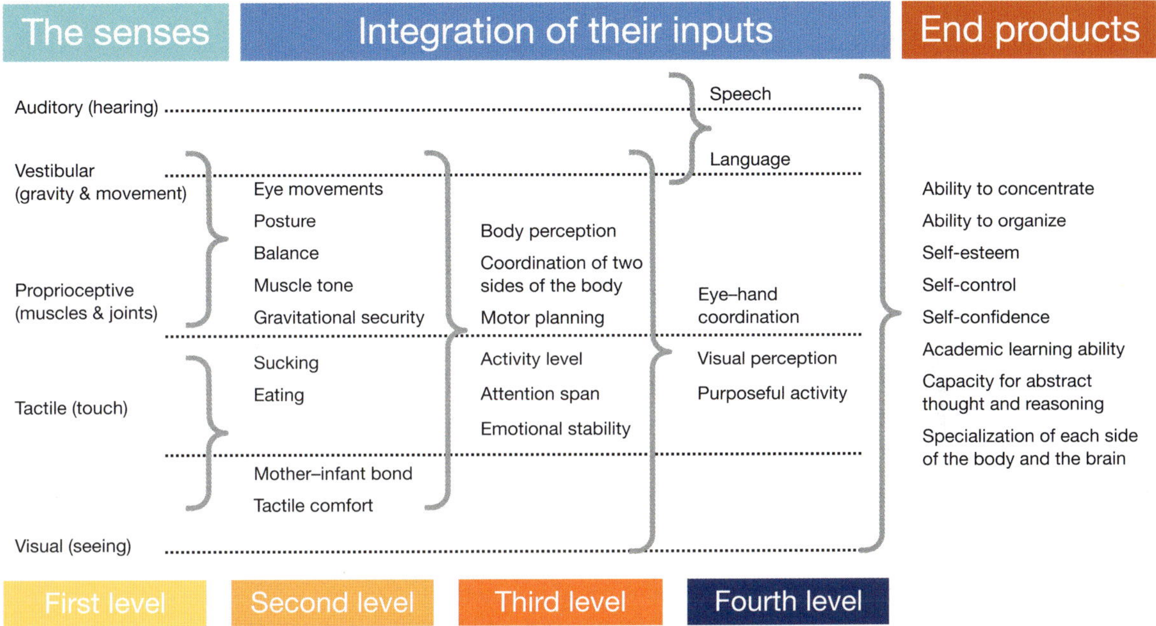

FIGURE 6.2 The senses, integration of their inputs, and their end products. (Reprinted with permission from Ayres, A. J. (2005). *Sensory integration and the child* (25th Anniversary Ed., p. 55). Copyright © 2005 by Western Psychological Services. Reproduced by Wolters Kluwer, with permission of the Publisher, WPS. All rights reserved.)

- Successful integration and organization of sensory information results in and is further developed by adaptive responses.
- Enriched experiences effect changes in the nervous system due to experience-dependent neuroplasticity.
- Sensory integration is a foundation for participation.

Each assumption will be elaborated upon in the following sections.

Learning Is a Brain Function, Dependent on Sensory Information

The theory of sensory integration evolves as new evidence emerges (Kilroy et al., 2019; Lane et al., 2019); however, the basic premise that the sensory systems and the integration of their inputs are important contributors to learning and behavior remains the key assumptions of sensory integration theory (Bundy & Lane, 2020; Lane et al., 2013; Smith Roley et al., 2001). The unique contribution of the sensory integration theory is its emphasis on the "body-related" senses—tactile, vestibular, and proprioceptive sensations. According to the theory of sensory integration, these body-related senses provide the reference point about the body relative to the environment, critical to all learning and behavior. For example, in order to move one's body effectively to accomplish a task, sensory integration theory posits that the brain must receive and integrate proprioceptive, tactile, and vestibular information about the position and location of the body. Current sensory information is checked against the existing "body sensory map" developed from previous sensory and motor experiences to continually update the brain's knowledge about the body. This information is used to plan and execute movements. Knowledge and feedback from successful movement experiences provide increasingly complex perceptions and enhance the child's ability to act and interact effectively in response to environmental demands. Table 6.1 describes the senses, their receptor end points in the nervous system, and their posited contributions to development and learning.

Several aspects of central nervous system function are critical to one's ability to integrate and use sensation adaptively (Ayres, 1972). They are:

- the integration of two or more processes affects the way the brain adapts;
- intermodality associations allow rapid convergence of information leading to a perception of wholeness, interaction between higher and lower neural centers that exert inhibitory influences, thereby affecting the way in which sensory information is processed;
- accurate sensory feedback results from actions and interactions; and
- neural inhibition is a critical component in the complex organization of sensory experiences and the resulting adaptive response.

Neuroscience research has confirmed that brain structure and function contribute to neural integration (Mesulam, 1998; Stein et al., 2020) because Ayres early work on sensorimotor processes occurred in a more dynamic fashion than previously understood, thus laying the foundation for complex emotion, praxis, and social interactions (Bear et al., 2016). Integrating sensory information is essential to perception, emotion, and behavior (Gingras et al., 2009). In addition, the synthesis of sensory information is attenuated by modulatory dynamics that allow for predictions (Smyre et al., 2023). These predictions based on sensory integration inform future actions and interactions (Berthoz, 2000), fundamental to praxis (Ayres, 1972; Ayres & Cermak, 2011).

Sensory Integration Is a Developmental and Dynamic Process

Sensory integration is based on the understanding that development unfolds in a sequence and is influenced by the experiences children have during development (Ayres, 2005). According to Ayres (1972), "(the) environment acts upon the innate tendencies...and molds and modifies them" (p. 6). Ayres believed that children have an innate drive to explore, interact with, and master their environments. Nowhere is this more evident than during early development as the infant first experiences touch from the caregiver and responds with visual regard and a smile! These early sensory experiences and simple motor responses of the infant, combined with the caring, nurturing responses of the caregiver, begin a process of neuronal integration that will lay the foundation for higher-level sensory–motor activity, emotional regulation, and social skills (Figure 6.3).

ASI intervention utilizes sensory–motor activities in the context of play building on the child's current abilities and interests, scaffolding to support the emergence of more complex actions and interactions. The practitioner provides the context and affordances that ignite the child's desire, that is, "innate drive," to act and interact with the people and objects in their environment. In this way, the child's innate/inherent motivation to participate and gain mastery is stimulated in concert with crafting activities that encourage the emergence of more complex skills and abilities at the just right challenge.

Table 6.1 The Sensory Systems

Sensory System	Pathway	Receptors	Sensation Detected	Features and Functions	Organization	Primary Central Projection(s)	Cortical Projections	Links to Sensory Integration Theory
Somatosensory								
	Dorsal column-medial lemniscus pathway (DCML)	• Muscle spindle • Golgi tendon organ • Meissner corpuscle • Merkel receptor • Pacinian corpuscle • Ruffini ending • Hair receptor	• Touch on the skin • Vibration • Movement of touch on skin	• Transmit information related to object/surface size, form, texture • Convey spatial and temporal aspects of touch • Input is fast, direct	• Precise somatotopic organization throughout • Little convergence • Few relays • Processing of information takes place at each synapse	• Ventral posterior lateral nucleus of thalamus • Reticular formation	• Primary and secondary somatic cortex • Areas 5 and 7 of parietal lobe	• Activity in anterolateral pathways can be decreased by simultaneous activation in low threshold mechanoreceptors that feed DCML • Projections from anterolateral pathways to reticular formation important for emotional and arousal aspects of touch • Projections from intralaminar thalamic nuclei are reflected broadly in cortex, also linked to behavioral arousal • Integration of discriminative inputs leads to perception of self and interpretation of tactile environment; lays foundation for praxis and organization of behavior
	Anterolateral (spinothalamic, spinoreticular, spinomesencephalic)	• Free nerve endings	• Pain, crude touch, temperature, tickle, neutral warmth, itch	• Signal to CNS that body tissue is at risk of damage • Transmission has both fast and slow aspects	• Somatotopic, but less specific • More convergence	• Ventral posterior lateral, intralaminar, and medial nuclei of the thalamus • Reticular formation • Periaqueductal gray • Tectum • Hypothalamus	• Primary and Secondary somatosensory cortex • Other thalamic nuclei	
	Trigeminothalamic		• Discriminative touch, proprioception from face and mouth • Pain, temperature, nondiscriminative touch of the face		• Somatotopic	• Principal sensory nucleus of the trigeminal nerve • Spinal nucleus of the trigeminal nerve • Trigeminal nuclei project to ventral posterior medial nucleus of thalamus	• Primary somatosensory cortex	

(*continued*)

Table 6.1 The Sensory Systems (Continued)

Sensory System	Pathway	Receptors	Sensation Detected	Features and Functions	Organization	Primary Central Projection(s)	Cortical Projections	Links to Sensory Integration Theory
Vestibular	Vestibular	• Hair cells in the utricle and saccule • Hair cells in the semicircular canals	• Linear and angular (rotary) movement of the head	• Position and movement of the head in space • Maintenance of balance, equilibrium • Coordination of the head and eyes; gaze stabilization during movement • Detection of speed and direction of movement • Maintain muscle tone	• Otolith organs: hair cells oriented either toward or away from striola, within utricle (horizontal) and saccule (vertical); orientation results in ability to transmit information about linear movement in all directions • Semicircular canals: hair cells embedded in cupula • Hair cells in both structures are tonically active. Displacement either increases or decreases activity, information CNS of movement	• Vestibular nuclei • Cerebellum	• Area 3a (region near face representation in SII), 2v of the cortex • Posterior parietal (area 5)	• Vestibular nuclei are important integrative centers, receiving input from cerebellum, visual and somatosensory pathways, as well as ipsilateral and contralateral vestibular information • Cortical region 3a also receives proprioceptive and visual information; linked to perception of body orientation in extrapersonal space • Critical in maintenance of upright, antigravity posture • Working with visual system, determines movement of self in space, and detects movement of self vs. objects

Auditory	Audition	• Hair cells in the organ of corti, within the cochlea	• Sound detection, localization	• Combination of different sound wave frequencies and intensities gives sound the qualities we recognize • Response to sound is function of fact that basilar membrane is wider and more flexible at apex • Perception requires simultaneous action of many cortical regions	• Tonotopic • Amplitude tuning curve	• Ventral and dorsal cochlear nuclei • Ventral nucleus bilateral projections to superior olive, to inferior colliculus • Dorsal nucleus to inferior colliculus • Multiple parallel pathways project from nuclei	• MGN to auditory cortex	• Superior colliculus projections role in for integration of visual and auditory information • Sound interpretation results in auditory map of space, development of sense of location • Interpretation of spoken words assists in understanding emotional meaning of communication • Considered "higher-level" sensory processing system within sensory integrative theory base; very complex cortical representation and interpretation

(*continued*)

Table 6.1 The Sensory Systems (Continued)

Sensory System	Pathway	Receptors	Sensation Detected	Features and Functions	Organization	Primary Central Projection(s)	Cortical Projections	Links to Sensory Integration Theory
Visual	Visual	• Rods and cones in the retina	• Cones: day vision, color • Rods: night vision	• Identify objects, position in space, movement through space, color, shape • Contrast and movement detection	• Much integration within layers of retina • Receptors project to bipolar cells; these project to ganglion cells • Ganglion cells form optic tract • Cones: little convergence onto ganglion cells, resulting in high degree of spatial resolution; found primarily in central retina • Rods: significant convergence, high light reactivity, low resolution; absent from central retina, found in periphery • Substantial interaction between receptor cells and other retinal cells prior to transmission to CNS • Detailed organization of information carried throughout this system (retinotopic)	• Majority of ganglion cells project to the lateral geniculate nucleus of the thalamus; primary processing center and gateway to cortex • Optic tract fibers also project to hypothalamus, pretectum, superior colliculus	• Primary visual cortex • Primary visual cortex projects to extrastriate regions, dorsal and ventral streams • Response to new visual stimuli • Lateral geniculate is primary processing center; receives streams of information • Lateral geniculate also receives input from reticular formation, regulating alertness and attention; this link modulates visual input	• Dorsal stream: analyzes visual motion and responsible for visual control of action, navigation through space • Ventral stream involved with perception of visual world and object and face recognition (shape, color) • Hypothalamic projections have role in synchronizing biologic rhythms (i.e., wake/sleep) • Tectal projections responsible for directing eye and head movements that bring image into central retina for optimal resolution; thus role in orienting eyes and head in • Considered "higher-level" sensory processing system within sensory integrative theory base; very complex cortical representation and interpretation and beyond …

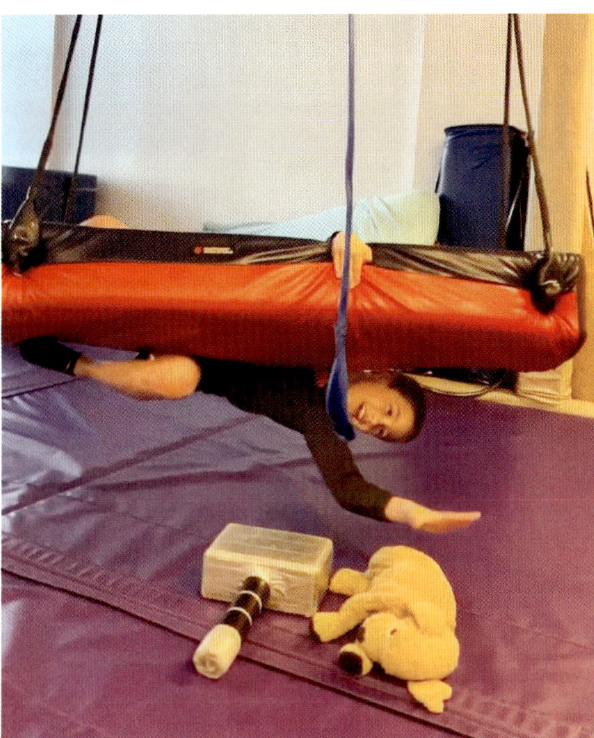

FIGURE 6.3 The therapist sets up an achievable challenge so that the child is motivated to try activities that may be beyond their current skill level.

Successful Integration and Organization of Sensory Information Results in and Is Further Developed by Adaptive Responses

Sensory integration provides the foundation for building increasingly complex and efficient neuronal schemas, which enhances the central nervous system's adaptive capacity. Every aspect of life requires adaptation to a constant barrage of sensations from the body and the environment in order to figure out what to do and to participate in an ever-changing environment. In order to act and interact in the world, the child must filter and organize countless bits of information entering the brain and respond to the changing environment. The child's ability to make adaptive responses to constantly changing sensory environments is a pivotal consideration in the sensory integration frame of reference. Ayres (1972) defined an adaptive response as an "appropriate action in which the individual responds successfully to some environmental demand" and stated that "the action of the environment upon the organism, and the reaction of that organism upon the environment…constitutes the essence of a sensory integrative and sensorimotor response" (Ayres, 1972, p. 22). Therefore, when encountering a new situation, the child draws upon a previous understanding of their abilities and competencies and modifies them accordingly to organize new behavior and meet the current demand. Successfully adapting to ongoing challenges provides increased motivation and skill to engage in further complex, challenging activities. For example, while playing in a safe environment, the child discovers new ways to play with objects and people and thus exhibits adaptive responses (see Figure 6.3). Subsequently, these adaptive responses create the foundation for further, more complex, play actions and interactions. The sensory integrative process, therefore, facilitates successful responses to environmental demands, resulting in adaptive responses. Furthermore, increasingly complex adaptive responses are both an indicator of ongoing sensory integration and an outcome of sensory integration.

Sensory Integration Promotes Neuroplasticity

Sensory integration theory is built on this principle of neuroplasticity and proposes that optimal sensory experiences that invite action and active participation influence the growth and development of the nervous system and subsequently behavior (Ayres, 1979). Neuroplasticity, defined as the nervous system's ability to change in response to environmental input and demands, is one of the key theoretical concepts of the sensory integration frame of reference. New findings and knowledge demonstrate that the nervous system is even more plastic, complex, and integrated than what Ayres and others believed at the time, and thus, the principles upon which the theory of sensory integration was built are still held in high regard in the scientific community (Jacobs & Schneider, 2001; Kramer, 2001).

Research on the mechanisms of neuroplasticity demonstrates that structural, molecular, and cellular changes in neural functions are possible and that meaningful sensory–motor activities are mediators of these changes (Greenough et al., 1987; Kandel et al., 2013; Kemperman & Gage, 1999; Merzenich et al., 1984). Environmental enrichment studies in both animals and humans support this concept and show that rich, meaningful sensory–motor experiences promote neuronal processing. For example, classic studies of primates show that there is an increase in the cortical representation of fingers when they are provided enriched opportunities for manual tactile exploration (Jenkins et al., 2013) as cited in (Kandel et al., 2021). Similarly, classic enriched environment studies on rodents, from Greenough et al. (1973, 1978, 1987), show that enhanced sensory–motor opportunities result in increased synaptic density and efficiency.

Contemporary research continues to validate these findings. Brown et al. (2003), for example, show that rodents involved in active sensory–motor activities, such as running in a wheel cage, demonstrate better ability to learn maze tasks. Furthermore, changes in the hippocampus area of the brain in these same animals were potentially linked to this enhanced learning and memory. Environmental enrichment and neuroplasticity studies inform ASI intervention (Ayres, 1972; Lane & Schaaf, 2010; Reynolds et al., 2010). By providing enriched sensory opportunities processed at the level of the brain stem and stimulating the child's motivation via the limbic system with the "just right" sensory and motor challenges, change will occur both neurologically and behaviorally as the child makes higher-level adaptive responses and is more willing to tackle challenges in everyday life (Schaaf & Smith Roley, 2006).

Sensory Integration Supports Participation in Life Activities

Sensory integration provides an important foundation for participation in meaningful, health-promoting activities that support participation in life (Ismael et al., 2018; Schaaf et al., 2011; Schaaf et al., 2012; Schaaf et al., 2015). As such, occupational therapy using a sensory integration frame of reference is designed to improve sensory integration as a basis for enhancing successful participation in daily occupations (Parham & Mailloux, 2015; Smith Roley et al., 2001). Sensory integration considers the dynamic interactions between the child's abilities or disabilities and the environment from an occupational science perspective as illustrated in Figure 6.4 (Spitzer & Smith Roley, 2001).

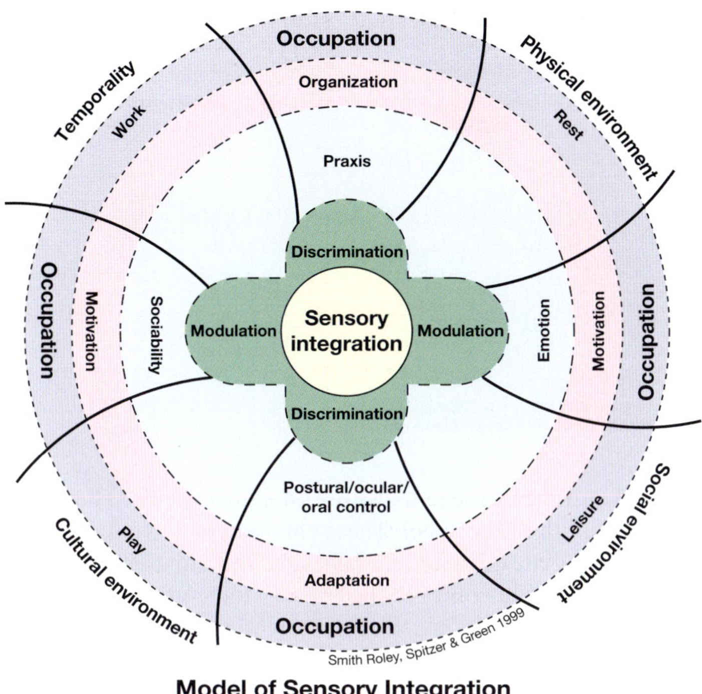

FIGURE 6.4 The dynamic process of sensory integration. (From Roley, S. S., Blanche, E. I., & Schaaf, R. C. (2001). *Understanding the nature of sensory integration with diverse populations* (p. 5). PRO-ED. Copyright 2001 by PRO-ED, Inc. Reprinted with permission.)

This figure shows the interaction between sensory integration and occupation, illustrating how the basic processes of sensory modulation and sensory discrimination interact to support praxis, postural/ocular/oral control, and social–emotional development. These processes subsequently form the basis for organized behavior, motivation to act and interact in the environment, and adaptation to environmental demands. These, in turn, support occupational engagement in multiple areas, such as work, play, leisure, and rest within the social, physical, and cultural contexts.

Sensory integration deficits disrupt the child and their family's ability to participate in daily routines, such as mealtimes, grooming, and bedtime routines; social activities such as family gatherings and shopping trips; and community activities such as school and organized sports. Commonly, during self-care routines, slow, imprecise, and poorly regulated reactivity to sensations makes dressing, eating, and grooming habits difficult for the child (Figure 6.5).

While participating at school, a child with sensory integrative dysfunction may be distracted by the variety and intensity of sensations in areas, such as the classroom, playground, and lunchroom, and have trouble paying attention and participating appropriately with the other children. The child with poor somatosensory feedback in the hands may have difficulty with handwriting, whereas the child with poor vestibular-mediated postural control will have difficulty maintaining a comfortable static posture while seated or standing. Also, social participation, which involves navigation of a vastly complex world of sensory and motor demands, is often difficult for a child with sensory integration problems. The child who has difficulty perceiving, tolerating, and

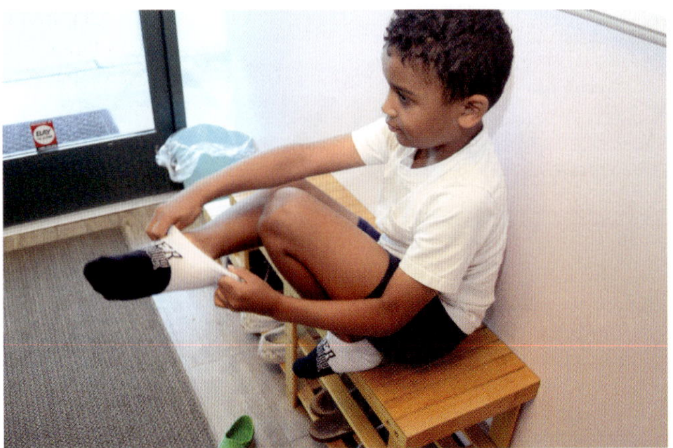

FIGURE 6.5 Adequate integration of tactile, proprioceptive, and vestibular systems allows for successful participation in daily activities.

integrating sensations also has difficulty negotiating the unpredictable and changing stimuli associated with social activities (Smith Roley, 2006). These children tend to fall out of step with their peers and demonstrate inappropriate or immature behavior. Participation issues are discussed in more detail in the section entitled "Outcomes of the Sensory Integrative Process."

Major Concepts and Definitions

Sensory integration theory combines concepts from human development, neuroscience, psychology, and occupational therapy into a holistic framework for viewing behavior and learning. Ayres identified the concepts of sensory integration from her review of the literature, developed assessments that could objectively measure these constructs, and then examined the relationship between the constructs (Ayres, 1989; Parham & Mailloux, 2015; Schaaf et al., 2022). The key concepts included in the sensory integration frame of reference are sensory reactivity, sensory perception (primarily tactile, vestibular, and proprioceptive as well as auditory, visual, taste, and smell), postural–ocular control, bilateral integration and sequencing, and praxis.

Sensory Reactivity

Sensory reactivity refers to the child's individual abilities to respond adaptively to sensation over a broad range of intensity and duration (Lane et al., 2022) serving a regulatory function (Lane et al., 2019). The ability to modulate sensation is a complex process of filtering perceived sensory information and regulating the response. "Modulation is the ability of the brain to regulate inhibition or propagation of neural signaling. Sensory modulation reflects adjustments made in response to continual physiologic processes to ensure adaptation to new or changing sensory information" (Kilroy et al., 2019, p. 3). Response to one or more sensations contributes to the capability to sustain engagement, despite variability in the intensity of sensations from the body or environment, and contributes to emotional stability, behavior, arousal, activity level, and attention (Bar-Shalita et al., 2008; Kilroy et al., 2019; Lane et al., 2019). Unusual sensory responses can be sensory or situation specific and vary according to the well-being of a child and the external environmental or social supports. Atypical sensory reactivity (over, under, or fluctuating reactions) occurs when the child routinely shows dysregulated responses to typical sensory experiences (Figure 6.6).

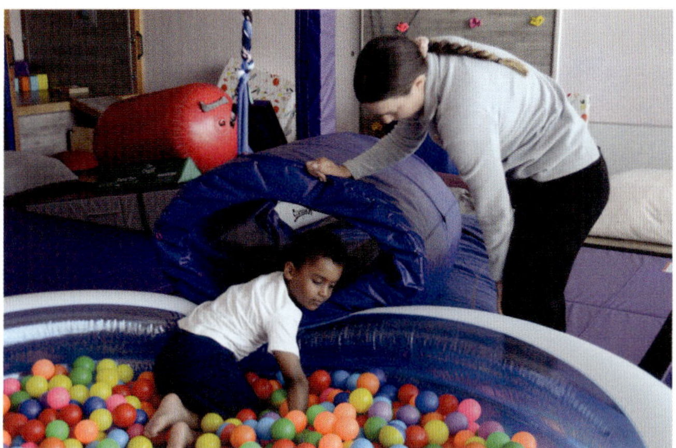

FIGURE 6.6 Children with adequate sensory modulation are able to tolerate the variety of sensations offered in the environment.

Sensory Perception

Sensory perception is the result of decoding one or more sensations into a perceptual whole. Sensory perception or sensory discrimination refers to the individual's ability to interpret and differentiate between the spatial and temporal qualities of sensory information—or the "where is it," "what is it," and "when did it occur" response (Wolfe et al., 2020). The ability to discriminate sensory information allows the development of perceptions of events and self in action and contributes to skill development, learning, social interactions, and play especially play that involves fine, discrete responses such as object manipulation. Sensation can originate from the interoceptors (inside the body), proprioceptors or somatosensation (by and about the body), or exteroceptors (external to the body) (Sherrington, 1906). Each individual sensory system has discriminative functions that contribute to the individual's knowledge of sensory input and preparation for a response. The timing of sensations, the child's interest, attention, memory, and motivation affect the ability to process data that leads to perception and participation (Schmitt & Schoen, 2022) (Figure 6.7).

- Interoception includes internal sensations from the viscera that inform an individual of physiologic conditions, such as heart and respiratory rate, pain, and temperature, as well as basic bodily needs such as hunger, thirst, or a full bladder. Perception of interoceptive information is linked to emotional awareness (Chen et al., 2021; Craig, 2003; Quigley et al., 2020).
- Somatosensation (the larger classification of proprioception according to Sherrington) includes information from the body, primarily touch and proprioceptive stimuli, and sometimes includes vestibular information.
  - Tactile discrimination provides information about the spatial and temporal qualities of the environment by perceiving the qualities of information from skin receptors essential for body awareness (Deflorio et al., 2022). Importantly, somatosensation provides an important foundation for social perception (Keysers et al., 2010).
  - Proprioceptive discrimination provides an understanding of the body's (muscles, joints, and tendons) position and the load or tension on muscles and joints. Together tactile and proprioceptive information provide important information that helps the child develop a "body awareness" or "body scheme" which provides the foundation for efficient motor planning (praxis) (Abrams et al., 2024; Ayres & Cermak, 2011).

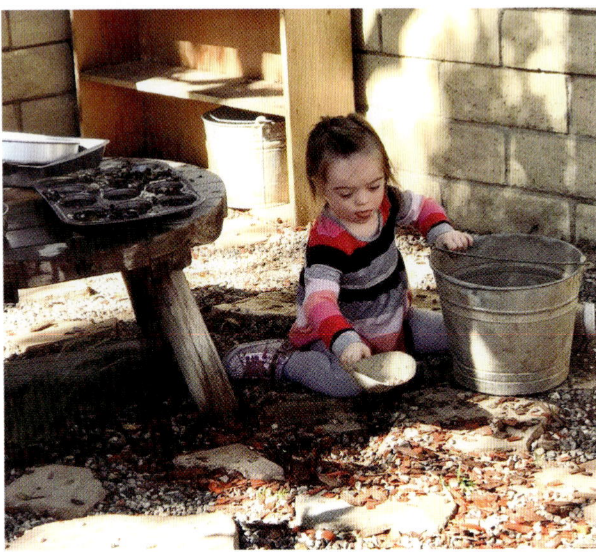

FIGURE 6.7 Adequate sensory discrimination provides an important foundation for successful actions in the environment.

- Discrimination of vestibular stimuli allows children to know where their head is in relation to the rest of their body and in relation to the environment at large by providing information about the position of the head relative to gravity, and the speed and direction of body movements (Berthoz et al., 1992). Vestibular discrimination works with somatosensory discrimination and contributes to postural control, balance, and equilibrium.
- Exteroceptors include auditory and visual sensations which are the only noncontact receptors along with taste, touch, and smell that require contact with the receptor on the body.
- Visual discrimination is incredibly complex and provides the foundation for spatial recognition including the distance, position, and location of objects and people and details that inform cognition, including recognition of form, shape, size, etc. There are many kinds of visual discrimination, such as visual figure-ground perception, visual rotation, and visual–motor abilities, that allow one to find hidden pictures on a page (figure ground) or tell the difference between the letters "b" and "d." Form constancy is being able to visually interpret an image even if it is turned upside down. Ocular motor skills are necessary to support a stable visual field and to move the head and eyes in a coordinated fashion to follow a written line across the page of a book (visual motor) or watch the teacher while she is lecturing. Visual discrimination interfaces with vestibular, proprioceptive, and auditory information to coordinate eye and head movements and to provide a map of the three-dimensional world relative to the body's position in space.
- Auditory discrimination is also complex and enables the child to detect the location of sounds and to differentiate sounds including those used in speech so that one can interpret the difference between a "p" and "t" in words such as "sheep" versus "sheet." Auditory discrimination is essential for orienting oneself relative to sounds within the environment essential for safety awareness, identifying sounds, understanding spoken language, following directions, and learning to read or write.
- Taste and smell perceptions work together to provide sensory perception of location, identification, safety, and emotional connections. Most frequently connected with eating, taste, and smell perceptions are critical in social interactions including family meals.

Postural Control

Postural–ocular control involves activating and coordinating muscles in response to sustained positions or dynamic movements of the body during transitions and while moving relative to gravity. Postural responses are required for any action needed during physical engagement. Postural control emerges as the child develops activation and coactivation of muscle groups that support movement. Postural control is dependent not only on adequate muscle strength, endurance, or the ability to coactivate muscle synergies but also on the integration of multisensory information before and during movement from the vestibular, proprioceptive, tactile, visual, and auditory systems. For example, antigravity postures, such as prone extension and supine flexion, develop to support the infant's ability to raise their head against gravity and initiate movement. These provide the basis for more complex postural mechanisms that allow a child to move in and out of a midline position and maintain balance and equilibrium. Balance and equilibrium are components of postural control that are modulated by the vestibular, proprioceptive, and visual systems. Daily activities require coordinating the position of the body relative to gravity by organizing not only upright posture also the coordination of the two sides of the body. These repetitive daily actions that are part of postural–ocular control and bilateral integration and sequencing are reliant on accurate and integrated sensory information to be executed well.

Bilateral Integration

Bilateral integration is the ability to coordinate the lateralized sensory information and motor functions from both sides of the body. Lateralized sensory information is linked to a lateralized motor skill such as handedness. For example, in right-handers, the right ear has slightly faster and better hearing than the left, although they work together to provide the perception of a single event. Bilateral motor control emerges as a function of refined postural control. Bilateral motor control relies on the immediate perception of the body's position or movement in space and the ability to use the two sides of the body together (Figure 6.8). Early bilateral coordination is typical symmetrical use of both sides such as hands to midline and development of a preferred hand for writing and throwing. More sophisticated bilateral tasks require disassociated or rotational movements, including cooperative hand use for bimanual tasks such as opening water bottles or managing fasteners on clothes, coordinated bilateral symmetrical tasks such as jumping, and bilateral asymmetrical tasks such as skipping. Bilateral integration forms the foundation for projected action sequences, that is, a sequence of motor acts put together to accomplish a goal in future time and space such as running to catch or kick a ball or coordinating the position and time to kick a soccer goal or make a basket.

Praxis

Praxis is the ability to conceive of, plan, and organize goal-directed actions. It is a cognitive, perceptual ability that requires adequate sensory integration to create and update the somatic map or schema of the body (Ayres & Cermak, 2011). Praxis enables people to adapt and react quickly to novel environmental demands in a meaningful and efficient manner. Praxis allows the child to plan and organize future actions by figuring out what the body can do relative to the perception of the external environment through auditory, visual, or tactile information. Praxis provides children with information about how to effectively use objects as tools, how to organize time and space, and how to adapt to changing or unpredictable environmental demands including social interactions.

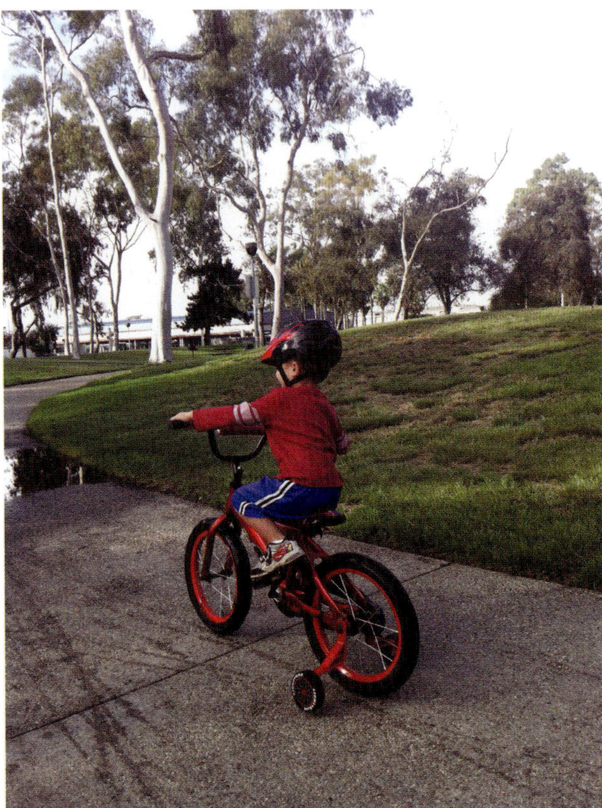

FIGURE 6.8 Adequate perception of one's body and movements through space allows for coordinated bilateral and postural–ocular abilities required for many childhood occupations.

Praxis is developed through meaningful and successful motor interactions with the world, and the ability to modify existing motor plans and link chains of action sequences together to do increasingly complex series of actions automatically. Once routinized daily life activities become automatic, they no longer require praxis. However, when something new or unexpected occurs, praxis is again required. This might be something like a growth spurt that changes the size and strength of the body during a task, a missing object, a change in the routine, unexpected life events, or the desire to learn something new.

Hypotheses on Sensory Integration's Contributions to Development

Sensory integration is a complex neurobiologic process that provides a critical foundation for successful participation. The way in which sensation affects function is well identified through the sensory integration patterns, which allow therapists to predict the impact of integrating sensory information that includes:

- rapid and accurate sensory integration including regulating and discriminating sensory information from the body and from the environment;
- self-regulation, which is the ability to sustain homeostasis and maintain regulated states of arousal, emotional responses, activity level, and attention/focus as appropriate for the demands of the task or activity;

- sensorimotor skills including postural, ocular, and oral–motor control; righting and equilibrium; and bilateral integration including lateralized sensory and motor functions such as hand preference;
- praxis including coming up with ideas about what to do and planning and organizing new and novel ways of interacting including tool use and figuring out what to do socially to sustain engagement with peers;
- resilience that includes a sense of being an effective actor in the world, thereby building self-esteem and self-efficacy; and ultimately;
- the ability of children to participate in their needed and desired life occupations and co-occupations.

When sensory integration works well, it provides the solid foundation upon which these other skills and abilities can emerge, exemplified in Figure 6.9.

One of the most notable childhood occupations is play. The way in which play is manifested varies depending on the age of the child, with the earliest play interactions observed via social imitation that requires somatic awareness and imitation abilities (Neumann, 1971). The complexity of play and playfulness encompasses contextual factors, developmental play capacities (cognitive, physical, and social play skills) individual preferences along with internal control, freedom to suspend reality, and intrinsic motivation (Bundy, 1997). Sensorimotor play requires an ability to defy gravity and build a body scheme that is constantly changing as the child grows and their physical proportions change. Object play emerges from perceptual motor exploration of

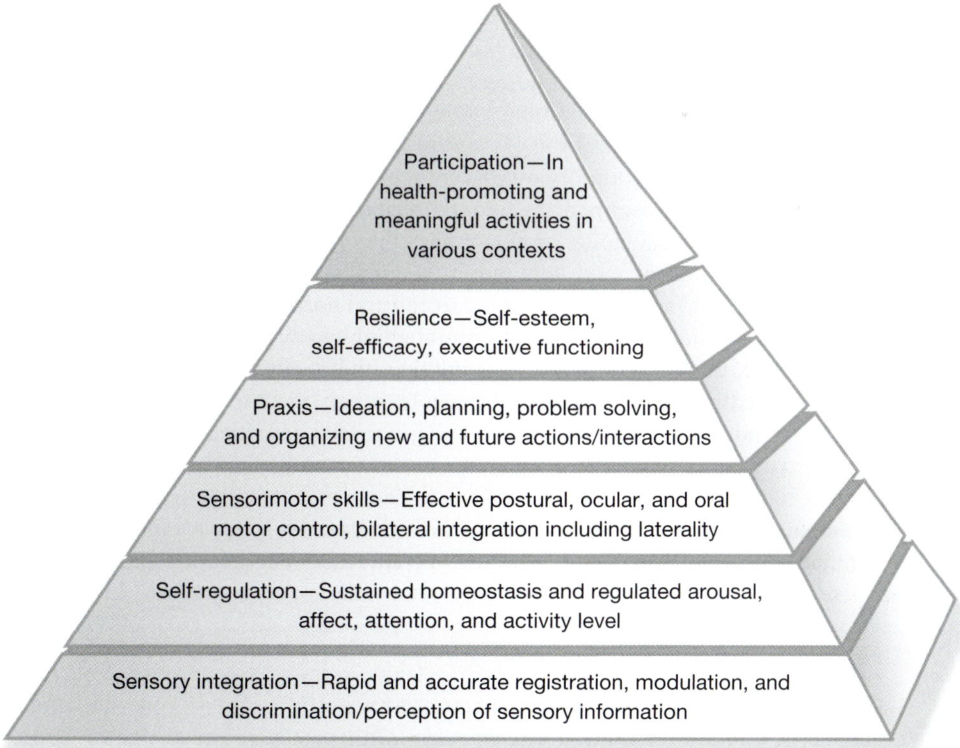

FIGURE 6.9 Sensory Integration Foundation for Participation. (Adapted from Schaaf et al. 2010, p. 127.)

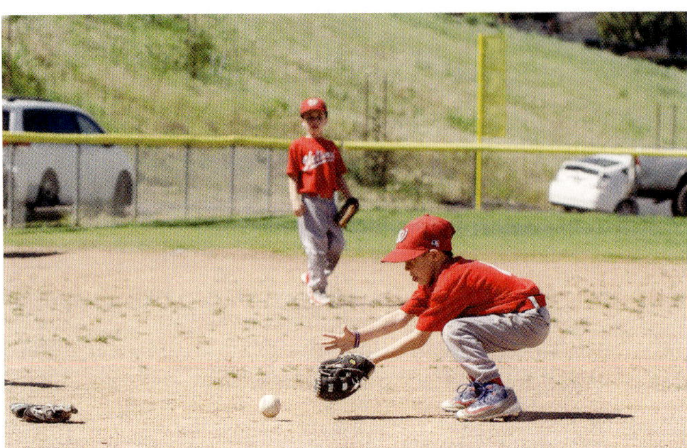

FIGURE 6.10 Adequate sensory integration allows the child to navigate both the physical and social world for meaningful social participation.

things or affordances around them. Play is subjective and therefore relies on intrinsic motivation to play as well as the ability to share control with a play companion, and the ability to engage in fantasy and pretend. Interactive play requires the ability to regulate sensory responses to unexpected sensations, body awareness, postural and motor control, as well as the ability to rapidly figure out what the other children are doing, planning how to act and react, and come up with new ideas about what to do next or in the future.

To participate at school and access the curriculum, children must manage the movement of their bodies, materials, and time while conforming to the direction of the teacher, rules, and school culture, in addition to building academic skills. This includes tolerating the noise and the sounds of a lunchroom, maintaining appropriate posture in a chair for prolonged periods, watching the teacher move around the classroom while taking notes, paying attention to noise going on around them, or negotiating objects in one's desk. Accordingly, adequate academic skills are at least partly dependent upon the foundational sensory integration and praxis.

Ultimately, sensory integration supports the child's ability to engage and interact meaningfully with peers, family, and community (Figure 6.10). Successful social participation can be described as a child's ability to conform to cultural norms in the context of daily life (Cohn et al., 2000). Social participation varies from interactions with familiar adults, which may be the easiest for a child, to interactions with unfamiliar children and adults and from interactions with an individual to different-sized groups of people. It can encompass routine daily activities that are scheduled and predicted to the nested and embedded activities that groups of people are doing. Social participation can take place in quiet and controlled environments, those that have strict rules of conformity, and open or unpredictable environments with limited rules. Importantly, as a foundation for all social participation, individuals must interpret and regulate sensory information and utilize praxis to figure out how to create and enact plans for social participation.

FUNCTION/DYSFUNCTION CONTINUA

Given the understanding of the way sensory integration supports participation, it follows that deficits in sensory integration will interfere with participation in one or more aspects of life (Figure 6.11). Numerous factor analysis studies with typical and atypical samples of children over the past 50 years have validated the different patterns of sensory integrative functions and

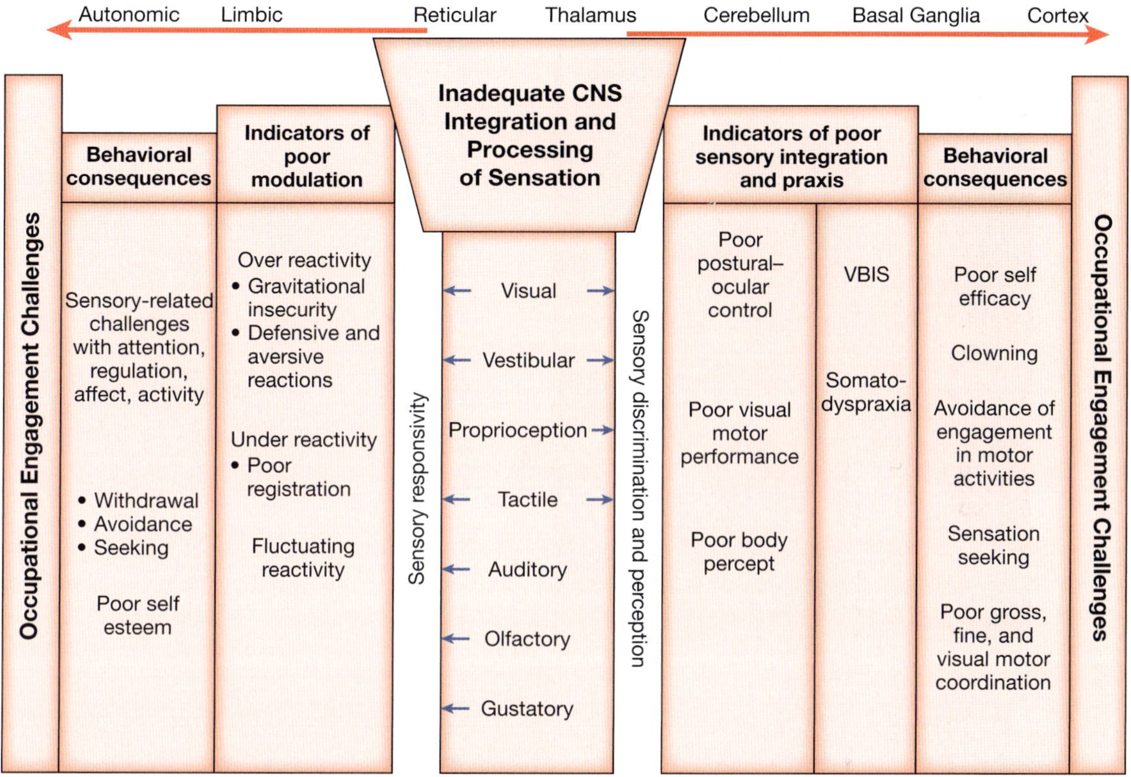

FIGURE 6.11 Sensory Integration Model of Dysfunction (Bundy & Lane, 2020).

dysfunction (Ayres, 1965, 1976, 1978; Ayers et al., 1989; Mailloux et al., 2011; Mulligan, 1998a, 1998b; Van Jaarsveld et al., 2015). What emerged from many studies was evidence supporting that sensory integrative functions are heterogeneous and involve multisensory systems. Although the factors differ slightly in various analyses, there is consistency of sensory integration patterns across research findings with both typical and atypical samples, specifically sensory reactivity, somatosensory, somatopraxis, visuopraxis, vestibular bilateral integration and sequencing, and language-based praxis (Bundy et al., 2020; Parham & Mailloux, 2015). Additional studies have identified sensory integration deficits in children without additional diagnoses (Mailloux et al., 2011; McIntosh et al., 1999; Mulligan, 1998b; Van Jaarsveld et al., 2015) and those with diagnoses such as autism, speech and language disorder, hearing impairment, attention deficit, and environmental deprivation (Smith Roley et al., 2001). A thorough evaluation of these patterns ensures that the sensory integration intervention is explicitly provided for those individuals with learning and behavior difficulties who demonstrate sensory integration deficits.

The following are the consistent patterns of sensory integrative deficits identified through research:

- Somatosensory perception deficits: poor body awareness from tactile and proprioceptive sensations and sometimes vestibular information that informs the development of a body schema essential to performing skilled tasks and social–emotional interactions.

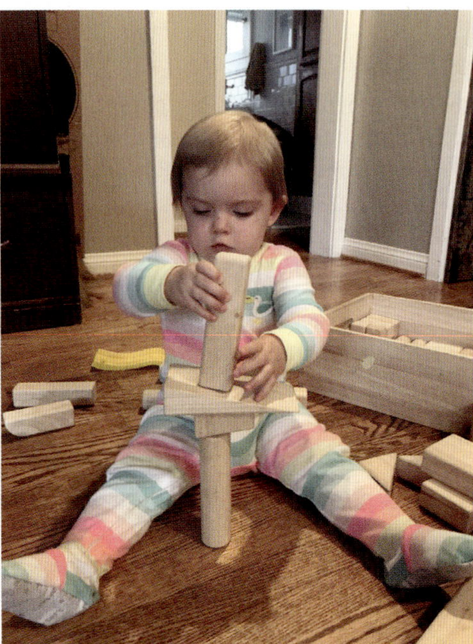

FIGURE 6.12 Visuopraxis supports the use of visual information to plan for using objects and forms, to manage school materials and toys for play.

- Vestibular bilateral integration and sequencing deficit: poor vestibular–proprioceptive processing essential to rapid and accurate processing of gravity and movement and the ability to stabilize one's posture and exert efficient postural control essential to balance. The automatic understanding of verticality in concert with the ability to move in and out of midline supports the coordinated use of both sides of the body, coordination of head, neck, and eye control, and dynamic sequential movements.
- Dyspraxia:
  - Visuodyspraxia: poor use of visual information to guide the planning and organization of self, objects, and space such as needed for construction or spatial arrangement of objects for use (Figure 6.12).
  - Somatodyspraxia: difficulty perceiving somatosensory information from the body and integrating it with information from the tactile system about things or people that are touching the body and their qualities; visual information about space, people, and objects; and auditory information about space, objects, and language that allows someone to conceptualize, plan, and organize motor actions and interactions.
  - Language-based dyspraxia: difficulty planning and organizing actions and interactions based on following written or verbal instructions from others and using one's own language to sequence and organize an activity or project, including writing lists or creating schedules.
  - Ideational dyspraxia: difficulty coming up with an idea or ideas about what to do and how to do it.
- Atypical sensory reactivity: unusual responses (over, under, or fluctuating responses) to the sensory aspects of materials, activities, or situations, also known as sensory modulation disorder.

Somatosensory Perception Deficits

Ayres (1972) proposed that the ability to motor plan movements depends on the development of an internal representation of the body. This unconscious knowledge of the body was theorized to be the result of somatosensory information coming from the skin, joints, and muscles. Thus, when information from the somatosensory system is inaccurate or imprecise, there will be a deficit in children's abilities to develop and utilize motor memories to guide future planned movements. Somatosensory deficits also interfere with interpersonal skills particularly related to accepting nurturing touch and giving affection as appropriate to the relationship. Consequently, social consequences include poor understanding of the nature and intent of interpersonal touch and the ability to communicate well nonverbally through touch. They may be too vigorous in their play or clumsy when interacting with other children, leading to rejection, misinterpretation of their intentions, leaving them vulnerable to being ostracized or bullied (Table 6.2).

Vestibular Bilateral Integration and Sequencing Deficits

Ayres identified this pattern by different names over different studies, including postural–ocular control, postural bilateral integration, bilateral vestibular integration, and bilateral integration and sequencing (Parham & Mailloux, 2015). Children with this discrete pattern of sensory integrative deficit tend to be bright and relatively typically developing but may be clumsy and underachieving academically with poor reading and writing (Ayres, 1976).

Ayres hypothesized that the relationship between poor vestibular functioning and academic abilities was due to the pivotal role of the vestibular system in integration of information at the brain stem level that enabled specialization of functioning at the cerebral level (Ayres, 1972). The vestibular system is like the heartbeat of the sensory systems, always working to inform the body about position and movement relative to gravity. When it is not working well, it impacts regulatory functions, postural and ocular control, and bilateral integration, including laterality and lateralized specialization, that allow complex reading and other academic abilities (Ayres, 1989).

Laterality is most apparent by observing a child's hand preference for writing. Bilateral motor control is related to these lateralized functions in the ability to use the two sides of the body cooperatively during skilled tasks, such as jumping, hopping, skipping, riding a bike, or cutting with scissors. The difficulty in rapidly perceiving and responding to vestibular information interferes with anticipatory actions, refined timing, and spatial coordination of movements. Problems with skilled coordination of sequential actions that require crossing the midline, smooth and efficient timing, and spatial accuracy are commonly manifested during sports activities such as soccer.

Because the vestibular, visual, and proprioceptive systems are intimately linked any time the head moves, these sensations work together to ensure smooth, coordinated movements. Therefore, postural and ocular-motor difficulties often accompany bilateral integration and sequencing problems and may further compromise a child's ability to perform skillful actions. Difficulties in these areas may also be associated with poor visual–motor skills and poor oral–motor skills. This can result in projected action sequence problems such as a sequence of motor acts put together to accomplish a goal in future time and space, such as running to catch or kick a ball or coordinating the position and time to kick a soccer goal or make a basket (Table 6.3).

Table 6.2 Indicators of Function: Somatosensory Perception

Touch	
Function	**Dysfunction**
Able to recognize and interpret tactile sensation	Difficulty recognizing and interpreting tactile sensation Poor body awareness and praxis is often present as well.
Indicators of Function	**Indicators of Dysfunction**
Recognizes whether the tactile sensation is on oneself vs. other person or object	Poor social recognition related to touch/affection with self/others
Identifies the type and location of touch	Misinterprets the type and location of touch
Identifies objects by their tactile properties such as size, shape, contour, weight, and texture	Unable to identify objects by their tactile properties such as size, shape, contour, weight, and texture
Identifies the origin, location, duration of transient touch on the hand, face, or body	Poor localization of touch including something on the face or correct orientation of clothing
Able to attach emotional meaning to the type of touch received, given, or perceived by others	Misunderstands emotional meaning to the type of touch received, given, or perceived by others
Uses appropriate pressure to grasp pencils and hugs with gentle contact	Uses too much pressure for a task such as a pencil grip or gives hugs that are too hard
Performs fine motor tasks without looking	Has trouble performing fine motor tasks without looking
Age-appropriate hygiene after toileting	Poor hygiene especially after toileting
Easily finds object in backpack without looking	Has trouble finding items in a backpack without looking
Writes name without looking	Cannot write name without looking
Proprioception	
Function	**Dysfunction**
Awareness of body position and alignment of body parts	Poor awareness of body position and postural alignment Poor body awareness and praxis is often present as well
Indicators of Function	**Indicators of Dysfunction**
Able to grade force, direction, and timing of movements	Difficulty judging the timing and distance for throwing and catching a ball
Able to sustain positions with midrange control such as core stability when sitting or standing	Difficulty with reactive postural control seems weak and lacks endurance; hyperextended joints
Shows strength and endurance during physical activities; moves smoothly and fluidly (Smith et al., 2001)	Poor timing of actions creates accidents, such as dropping, hitting, tripping, or running into things
Motivated to engage in physical activities at various intervals during the day	Refuses to engage in physical activities
Full use and range of upper extremities	Tends to hold limbs at end range rather than at midrange such as dragging a backpack with a straight arm or against chest

Table 6.3 Indicators of Function: Vestibular Bilateral Integration and Sequencing

Function	Dysfunction
Detection of movement of the head and postural adjustments to keep oneself upright when equilibrium is disrupted.	**Poor awareness of head position, decreased ability to keep body upright against gravity (poor antigravity posture), poor balance**
Indicators of Function	**Indicators of Dysfunction**
Automatically orients the head in midline	Difficulty maintaining vertical head alignment
Sustains an upright sitting posture: can stabilize the visual field during head movements	Props head when sitting
Automatically orients the head vertically when upright	Poor postural extension including head/neck control
Smoothly tracks objects	Poor ability to track or locate objects, especially those that are moving
Freely moves the head/eyes while stabilizing the trunk	Poor balance, righting, and equilibrium, so falls over easily
Good ocular motor control and able to stabilize head while moving eyes	Poor ocular motor control stabilizing head during eye movements or stabilizing eyes during head movements
Moves in diagonal and rotary planes while sustaining balance	Jumps around when trying to balance rather than holding still
Can disassociate head and body movements gracefully such as during dance or sport	Poor coordination of the head, neck, and eyes
Can shift gaze between horizontal and vertical planes and between near and far while stabilizing the posture or while moving	Difficulty sitting or standing up straight while holding still
Distinguishes movement of self from external movement	Poor postural background movements
Can freely move the head while coordinating the use of both hands	Has difficulty moving the head while coordinating the use of both hands
Moves in and out of midline during transitional movements gracefully without falling	Poor bilateral integration including lack of coordinated use of the two sides of the body, that is, jumping, skipping, hopping, catching or throwing a ball; right/left confusion; lateralized hand skills; crossing midline; and cooperative hand use
Completes bimanual tasks like tying shoes, holding paper while writing	Difficulty with bimanual tasks like tying shoes, holding paper, and writing
Completes projected action sequences	Difficulty with projected action sequences (anticipatory postural control) while sustaining postural–ocular control
Comfortable moving in different environments	Disorganized or uncomfortable while moving or needs to go very slowly
Good balance	Loss of balance during head movements especially when looking at something besides where they are going
Can utilize movement to change arousal, such as rocking for calming and rolling or jumping for alerting	Unable to use movement to change arousal, such as rocking for calming and rolling or jumping for alerting

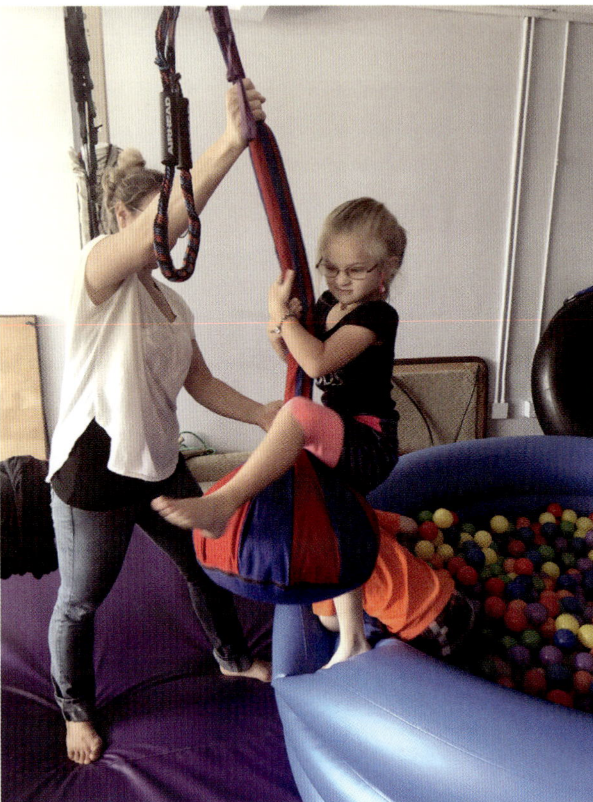

FIGURE 6.13 Praxis allows the identification and planning of how to make an effective goal-directed motor response to a specific situation.

Dyspraxia

Praxis is the ability to figure out how to adapt to novelty and challenges, including doing something new and different, or doing something in a new way or with a different person (Figure 6.13). Dyspraxia can be identified in children when they have difficulty conceptualizing and planning needed and desired actions and interactions (Ayres, 1985). First identified in adult patients with known brain damage, this problem was referred to as apraxia (Ayres & Cermak, 2011). In children with no known brain damage, this problem is called dyspraxia. Ayres identified several types of dyspraxia in children including visuodyspraxia—reflecting problems in using vision to guide planning and construction; somatodyspraxia—reflecting problems in motor planning and tool use; and language-based dyspraxia—including following the directions of others (Ayres & Cermak, 2011). Ideational dyspraxia reflects specific difficulties with conceptualizing motor actions (May-Benson, 2001; May-Benson & Cermak, 2007). Indicators of dyspraxia may be observed in the areas of generation of new ideas, planning, problem solving, sequencing, and updating and refining plans based on the sensory feedback from one's actions. Dyspraxia may be observed in conjunction with other concerns such as sensory modulation (Ringold et al., 2022), and impact not only motor performance but also social participation (Smith Roley et al., 2015).

Visuodyspraxia: Vision is the most complex of the sensory systems, providing the ability to perceive detail and gestalt simultaneously at the speed of light (Smith Roley et al., 2001). Vision provides critical information about the affordances available, the space in which to do something, and those things in the physical and social environments. Children rely on visual perception to plan what to do relative to the perception of the bodies and what is possible to do with their bodies. Visuodyspraxia occurs when visual perception is faulty or when someone is unable to figure out how to use visual information to plan and organize what to do and where to do it (Table 6.4).

Table 6.4 Indicators of Function: Visuopraxis

Visual Form and Space Perception	
Function	**Dysfunction**
Able to figure out how to use visual information to plan and organize what to do and where to do it	Unable to figure out how to use visual information to plan and organize what to do and where to do it
Indicators of Function	**Indicators of Dysfunction**
Demonstrates understanding of shape constancy	Does not demonstrate understanding of shape consistency
Matches shapes regardless of orientation in space, size, or color	Cannot match shapes regardless of orientation in space, size, or color
Matches objects by spatial orientation	Difficulty matching objects by spatial orientation
Figure-Ground Perception	
Function	**Dysfunction**
Able to find an object hidden in a distracting background	Cannot find an object hidden in a distracting background
Indicators of Function	**Indicators of Dysfunction**
Able to focus on a visual target in the midst of a complex visual background such as the teacher in the classroom	Has difficulty focusing on a visual target in the midst of a complex visual background such as the teacher in the classroom
Locates objects or people in a busy visual environment	Trouble visually locating objects or people in a busy visual environment
Visual–Motor Integration	
Function	**Dysfunction**
Able to coordinate vision with motor actions	Cannot coordinate vision with motor actions
Indicators of Function	**Indicators of Dysfunction**
Coordinated eye–hand movements in concert with a goal-directed task	Difficult coordinating eye–hand movements in concert with a goal-directed task
Copy by imitation	Difficulty imitating including tracing
Copy of model	Difficulty copying a model
Copy from memory (i.e., shapes, letter, numbers)	Difficulty drawing or writing from memory
Positions self well relative to table, chair, paper, and visual materials	Has difficulty positioning one-self relative to table, chair, paper, and visual material

(*continued*)

Table 6.4 Indicators of Function: Visuopraxis (Continued)

Visual–Spatial Planning	
Function	**Dysfunction**
Visually orients to surroundings	Unable to visually orient to surroundings efficiently
Indicators of Function	**Indicators of Dysfunction**
Puts objects in order relative to size, weight, shape, and accessibility	Difficulty organizing objects from large to small or by shape or weight
Creates an organizational system in which it is easy to locate things visually	Unable to create an organizational system in which it is easy to locate things visually
Leaves sufficient space to move about without hitting things or people	Difficulty calculating the space needed such as walking between desks without bumping into them
Organizes objects efficiently relative to how the child will use them	Difficulty organizing objects such as the book on the left, paper in the middle, and pencil on the right
Calculates the speed and distance of moving trajectories relative to the speed of one's movement	Difficulty calculating the speed of one's movement relative to something that is moving in the visual field such as crossing the street or avoiding being hit by a ball on the playground

Language-Based Dyspraxia

Ayres (1972) believed the auditory system was central to learning and an important contributor to sensory integration. The physical proximity of the auditory system to the vestibular apparatus suggests a reciprocal and complementary functional relationship between the two systems. Ayres found a pattern of discrete language-based dyspraxia, specifically without other signs of sensory integrative deficits that she felt was likely due more to speech and language deficits than a sensory integration problem. Often, language-based praxis deficits are observed in children with other sensory integrative patterns such as a more global dyspraxia (Mulligan, 1998b) and diagnoses such as autism (Smith Roley et al., 2015). Children with these deficits are likely to have difficulty planning based on verbal cues. They may understand the words but do not know how to respond with their bodies. This is particularly difficult with unfamiliar and multistep instructions. These children are often misunderstood as noncompliant when they do not follow directions properly (Table 6.5).

Somatodyspraxia

Difficulty learning new motor skills, planning new motor actions, and generalizing motor plans are hallmarks of somatodyspraxia. Ayres' unique contribution to the understanding of somatodyspraxia was the importance of somatosensory perception to the formation of efficient action plans. Action plans built on faulty sensory information, especially tactile and proprioceptive perception, lead to imprecise feedback about one's body movements, and therefore, the development of body schemas and motor memories will be compromised. Modifying motor plans based on faulty sensory feedback further compromises the ability to update and formulate more complex

Table 6.5 Indicators of Function: Language-Based Praxis

Auditory Sequential Memory	
Function	**Dysfunction**
Retains what is heard or said	Hears or remembers only a portion of what is said
Indicators of Function	**Indicators of Dysfunction**
Repeats the verbal sequence in the correct order	Recalls information but not in the correct sequence or correct tense
Completes several steps of a sequence	Completes only one step of a sequence
Does not require prompts for a required action	Requires prompts for each required action
Following Verbal Directions	
Function	**Dysfunction**
Interprets verbal instructions as intended	Seems confused by what is said
Indicators of Function	**Indicators of Dysfunction**
Follows instructions even when there is competing noise	Follows instructions sometimes and not others
Responds to instructions correctly	Responds to instructions incorrectly
Seeks out clarification when the instructions are not clear	Does not seek out clarification when the instructions are not clear
Compliant and attentive	Appears noncompliant, inattentive, or distracted
Using Language to Organize Tasks	
Function	**Dysfunction**
Able to recall a series of actions and recount them	Has difficulty recalling a series of actions and recounting them
Indicators of Function	**Indicators of Dysfunction**
Speaks than acts	Acts before speaking
Easily finds words to express what they want to do	Cannot find the words for what they want to do
Able to relate action sequences that are clearly linked to past, present, or future	Confuses action sequences and cannot link them to past, present, or future
Recounts the day's activities	Unable to recount the day's activities
Communicating Plans With Others	
Function	**Dysfunction**
Able to say what they are going to do when asked	Unable to say what they are going to do when asked

(*continued*)

Table 6.5 Indicators of Function: Language-Based Praxis (Continued)

Indicators of Function	Indicators of Dysfunction
Able to let others know what they are thinking or doing before doing it	Does not let others know what they are thinking or doing
Works with others	Appears to prefer doing things on one's own
Following Written Instructions	
Function	**Dysfunction**
Follows a visual or written schedule	Fails to read or follow written instructions
Indicators of Function	**Indicators of Dysfunction**
Can access instructions when needed	Requires additional caregiver support to figure out what to do
Can create lists to support getting a task done or reaching a goal	Unable to create lists to support getting a task done or reaching a goal
Remembers what to do	Difficulty remembering what to do
Uses a planner effectively	Does not use a planner effectively

plans. Finally, poor perception of the outcomes of actions leads to decreased awareness of the impact of one's actions on the environment, which further contributes to difficulties in adapting or modifying plans for success. The ability to build and retrieve accurate action schemas or motor plans is key to somatopraxis and central to the child's ability to make adaptive responses to new and novel environmental demands.

Children with somatodyspraxia who cannot easily motor plan demonstrate difficulties even in routine daily life activities, such as dressing, bathing, eating, or playing with toys or other people. They struggle to learn and complete new or complex motor tasks. Consequently, these children often avoid externally directed activities. Ayres & Cermak (2011) wrote that children who have trouble controlling their own bodies will have even more difficulty trying to figure out how to do what someone else wants them to do with their bodies. Avoidance of doing things planned by others results in the appearance of noncompliance, willfulness, lack of interest in peers, or a need to control the materials or direction of an activity. Transitions are often difficult. As children get older and the complexity of life is compounded, many of these children struggle to gain skills typical of their age group, such as driving for adolescents, or the multitude of activities that must be organized to maintain a family and job during adulthood (Table 6.6).

Ideational Dyspraxia

Ideation reflects the ability to generate ideas to initiate actions, figure out what to do based on prior experience, and respond effectively to new situations. For example, when ideation abilities are working well, a child can explore the possibilities for play with a new object by perceiving and acting on object affordances and by demonstrating a variety of actions with the object. Ideation allows a child to conceptualize new interactions and develop a wide repertoire of possible actions

Table 6.6 Indicators of Function: Somatopraxis

Body Scheme	
Function	**Dysfunction**
Aware of their body and moves body smoothly through space	Limited awareness of their body and does not move body smoothly through space
Indicators of Function	**Indicators of Dysfunction**
Moves smoothly and fluidly in, around, and through spaces	Clumsy, bumps into things
Positions self appropriately relative to people and objects	Sits or stands too close or too far away for the task or interaction
Handles objects with ease	Poor approximation of the need for strength or the way to position the body in preparation
Motor Planning—body	
Function	**Dysfunction**
Organization of actions to perform purposeful movements	Poor organization of actions and challenges planning and organizing purposeful movements.
Motor Planning—upper body	
Indicators of Function	**Indicators of Dysfunction**
Uses hands as tools to reach, manipulate, and modify objects	Poor use of hands to accomplish tasks such as opening containers or manipulating objects
Accesses objects as tools to extend what the body can do	Decreased object manipulation such as scissors or shoelaces
Figures out where to go to navigate around obstacles without getting stuck	Accident prone due to not anticipating the result of their actions, such as running into poles, tripping over objects, or running into people
Changes strategy to get something done if something is not working	Easily frustrated if their attempt to complete something does not work
Anticipates the result of the action sequence before starting	Refuses to attempt new tasks or imitate others
Fluidly executes a series/sequence of actions without needing to pause after each one	Slow to complete steps toward a goal by doing one thing at a time
Smooth sequencing and timing of actions, such as when playing ball with another person	Poor timing and sequencing of actions such as when playing a ball game with another person
Execution	
Function	**Dysfunction**
Modification of the plan based on knowledge of results	Unable to modify plan based on knowledge of results
Indicators of Function	**Indicators of Dysfunction**
Aware of the consequences of actions	Lack of awareness of impact of actions on people, objects, and space around them
Reflects on the success toward meeting the goal of an intended action	Poor awareness of goal-directed actions
Modifies motor plan for the next time it is used to be more effective	Repeats actions without correcting for errors
Plans action and strategies based on the situation; actions and strategies are not stereotypical	Uses same plans/strategies for many actions, even those that are not appropriate or will lead to failure

Table 6.7 Indicators of Function: Ideation

Function	Dysfunction
Conceptualization of a goal and some idea of the steps necessary to achieve that goal	Unable to conceptualize a goal or some idea of the steps necessary to achieve the goal
Indicators of function	**Indicators of dysfunction**
Initiating and proposing ideas about what to do; recognizing possibilities of things to do with objects/affordances in the environment	Poor initiation of tasks
Generating multiple ideas for things to do with other children during play	Difficulty knowing what actions are appropriate to use with a given object
Figuring out how to use objects in novel ways or adapt familiar objects as tools for which they were not originally intended	Uses objects in ways that are inefficient, ineffective, or unsafe due to poor foresight about their properties relative to their abilities
Can conceptualize a goal and initiate steps to accomplish that goal	Difficulty conceptualizing a goal and initiating steps to accomplish the goal
Responds easily to changes in routines	Difficulty modifying routines
Makes transitions easily	Poor transitions

and interactions with people and things in the environment, including those that a person may not have done before.

Children with poor ideation have difficulty knowing where to start, often relying on others for ideas or solutions. They may have difficulty generating or holding a mental image of previous actions and therefore cannot remember what they have done in the past that might help them plan for the future. Difficulties in ideation may result in repetitive inflexible behavior as the child is unable to "see" what is going to happen next. Play skills are characterized by a limited repertoire of simple interactions. These children may engage in repetitive activities, relying heavily on routines, or engaging in "scripted" behavior from reenacting stories, movies, or books (Table 6.7).

Atypical Sensory Reactivity

On a daily basis, individuals are bombarded by massive amounts of sensory information, most of which we tend to automatically inhibit and only some of which require attention. The way children respond to sensations depends on the state of their nervous system, personal preferences, and external regulators. Everyone has their own pain–pleasure continuum, with likes and dislikes for certain stimuli but can tolerate a range of experiences in daily life. Dysfunction occurs when people cannot tolerate sensations that are usual or necessary in their lives or when they do not notice critical sensory information that can keep them safe.

Most children, however, register some sensations depending on the type and intensity, but if they are hyporeactive, it is likely that they will have poor perception such as noted in the patterns above. These children often are slow and inaccurate in their responses; may seek out additional sensory feedback through sound, touch, or movement; or may appear apathetic, lethargic, unmotivated, and self-absorbed. Dunn (2014) found that children who were underresponsive could behave in a manner that was either lacking in orientation to the environment or seeking additional sensations.

Children who are sensory overreactive may demonstrate an excessive or exaggerated response to sensory stimuli that are not typically perceived as threatening, harmful, or noxious (Ayres & Tickle, 1980). Hyperreactivity to sensations is observed with dysregulation that can be identified at a physiologic level and at a behavioral level in humans (Brown & Dunn, 2002; Davies et al., 2010; McIntosh et al., 1999; Schaaf et al., 2010), and primates (Schneider et al., 2008, 2016). Characteristically, children with hyperreactivity to sensation, respond behaviorally with heightened fight, flight, fright, or freeze reactions that are manifested in dysregulated arousal, emotion, activity level, and attention (DeGangi, 2017).

It is common that children with atypical sensory reactivity may respond differently to different sensory experiences, at different times, with different people, or in different environments. Therefore, children may have fluctuating or inconsistent reactions to various stimuli. In practice as well as on questionnaire data, such as the *Sensory Processing Measure-2* (Parham et al., 2021), there may be significant differences in reporting sensory responses between parents, or the school setting and home. The variability or unpredictability of sensory reactivity is likely part of the deficit (Table 6.8).

Table 6.8 Indicators of Function: Sensory Reactivity

Touch		
Function	**Hyporeactive**	**Hyperreactive**
Accepts touch in activities and tasks and accepts nurturing touch and giving affection as appropriate to the relationship	Poor understanding of the nature and intent of interpersonal touch	Too vigorous in their play or clumsy when interacting with others
	Indicators of Dysfunction	
Indicators of Function	**Hyporeactive**	**Hyperreactive**
Accepts touch input during tasks and activities; gives and receives nurturing touch	Does not notice when touched	Pulls away from touch in activities, tasks, and gestures of tactile affection
Knows when touching something or someone	Encroaches on others' space without seeming to notice that they are touching them	Complains about things that touch the skin
Moves away when touching something that can cause pain such as prickles or heat	Does not respond to pain, such as bumping, falling cuts, or bruises	Overreacts to minor scrapes and bruises
Touches messy materials for cooking or play activities	Seeks certain textures especially lumpy, slimy, or soft	Avoids certain textures especially lumpy, slimy, or soft
Eats textured foods	Eats everything	Picky about foods

(*continued*)

Table 6.8 Indicators of Function: Sensory Reactivity (Continued)

	Indicators of Dysfunction	
Indicators of Function	**Hyporeactive**	**Hyperreactive**
Responds to temperatures	Does not distinguish between hot or cold	Upset by the temperature of the bath water if not exactly "right"
Wipes face when wet or dirty	Does not notice when face such as mouth and nose is dirty from food or saliva	Oversensitive to something on face such as food or saliva
Plays in sand or grass	Enjoys playing in sand or grass	Refuses to play in sand or grass
Wears all types of textured clothing	Does not notice when clothes are askew	Fussy about clothing
Cleans self thoroughly after a bowel movement	Cannot clean well after a bowel movement	Excessive cleaning after a bowel movement
Auditory		
Function	**Hyperreactive**	**Hyporeactive**
Able to orient relative to sounds within the environment	Overly responsive to sounds in the environment	Lack of response to sounds in the environment
	Indicators of Dysfunction	
Indicators of Function	**Hyporeactive**	**Hyperreactive**
Turns to person who is talking	Does not respond when name is called, says "what?" a lot	Feels like people are yelling when talking in a typical voice tone
Responds to person talking	Does not respond to verbal directions given only once	Distressed by environmental noises (vacuum cleaner, blender, siren, toilet flush)
Able to determine the location and source of sounds	Does not appear to know the location or source of a sound	Frightened of sounds that others do not notice
Not bothered by sounds that occur in daily activities	Seems not to notice noises	Dislikes the sound of laughter and singing
Participates readily in noisy community activities	Unresponsive at large gatherings such as parties or large spaces such as malls	Dislikes large gatherings such as parties or large spaces such as malls
Enjoys music, laughter, and nature sounds	Does not respond to unexpected loud sounds	Highly selective about types of music
Do not need to repeat words and phrases for understanding	Needs words and phrases repeated before showing understanding	Always attentive to someone speaking
Relies on hearing to obtain information	Relies on vision rather than hearing	Ineffectively use of visual and auditory input
Visual		
Function	**Hyporeactive**	**Hyperreactive**
Able to use functional visual skills in the environment	Not aware of the visual environment	Overly distracted by the visual environment

Table 6.8 Indicators of Function: Sensory Reactivity (Continued)

	Indicators of Dysfunction	
Indicators of Function	**Hyporeactive**	**Hyperreactive**
Makes direct eye contact	Seems to look through people rather than at them	Dislikes or avoids making direct eye contact
Watches things in environment	Does not pick up on nonverbal cues	Highly distracted by visual movement in the environment
Enjoys a variety of colors, patterns	Cannot see things right in front of them	Bothered by brightly colored or patterned materials
Comfortable in variably lighted areas	Cannot find things or people in a crowded visual field	Poor tolerance of certain types of lighting
Enjoys a variety of colors and patterns	Does not relate to colors or patterns in the environment	Strong preference and dislike of certain colors or patterns
Attentive to items in the environment appropriately	Seems vague when looking at something	Will focus visually on one thing to the exclusion of other
Appropriately attentive to thing in the environment	Runs into things that they know are there as if they do not see them	Bothered by visually cluttered environments
Vestibular		
Function	**Hyporeactive**	**Hyperreactive**
Enjoys and is aware of normal movement	Seeks out and craves excessive movement	Does not enjoy any type of movement, tends to be sedentary
	Indicators of Dysfunction	
Indicators of Function	**Hyporeactive**	**Hyperreactive**
Lifts up head easily	Loves and seeks movement opportunity	As an infant did not like lying on back for diapering or in stroller
Holds head in vertical position	Moves head a lot	Avoids moving head
Sustains antigravity positions	Hangs head to the side or back when resting	Avoids playground swings, slides, or climbing activities
Enjoys movement in all planes of space and in a variety of directions (up/down; back/forth, rotary)	Is not aware of movement and may crave additional movement	Dislikes movement play such as being thrown up in air, twirling, or dancing
Sustains and regains balance while moving	Not aware when he or she is losing his or her balance	Often off balance and feel as if he or she is falling
Appropriately aware of movement in the environment of the self and things around him or her	Does not seem to notice when the elevator is moving	Dislikes elevators and escalators, may be fearful of heights
Appropriately aware of movement inside and outside when riding in a car	Appears unaware of things outside when riding in the car	Is hyperaware of movement outside when riding in a car, get carsick

(*continued*)

Table 6.8 Indicators of Function: Sensory Reactivity (Continued)

Proprioception		
	Indicators of Dysfunction	
Function	**Hyporeactive**	**Hyperreactive**
Uses body with appropriate force and fluidity to accomplish purposeful movement Stands and move appropriately through the environment	Appears to have challenges adjusting the force and fluidity of movement Moves sluggishly, appears weak, and has poor posture	Rarely seen, see examples below
	Indicators of Dysfunction	
Indicators of Function	**Hyporeactive**	**Hyperreactive**
Sits and stands up straight	Poor posture Seems excessively tired	Hyperreactivity to proprioception is rare, but when present, the child avoids movement or pressure to the joints
Picks up objects without straining	Drags belongings rather than picking them up, often drops things	May overload him or herself when picking things up
Stable joints	Hyperextended joints, appear weak	Flexed joints
Moves precisely to given target	Moves slowly, taking forever to do things	May move randomly when moving toward a target
Does not bump into things except by accident	Breaks things due to poor grading of force, hugs too tightly	May hug too loosely, may drop things because of inadequate force
Likes to exert self through physical activities such as running, jumping, pushing, and pulling during play	Avoids all physical activity	Like a lot of physical activity without focus
Smell		
Function	**Hyporeactive**	**Hyperreactive**
Responds appropriately to good and bad smells	Is unaware of smells in the environment	Hypersensitive to smells
	Indicators of Dysfunction	
Indicators of Function	**Hyporeactive**	**Hyperreactive**
Enjoys pleasant smells of food, soaps, laundry, familiar people, and foliage around the home	Indifferent to odors of hygiene or cleaning products	Bothered by food smells, smell of household or hygiene products
Distinguishes between smells such as spices	Is unaware of smells in the environment	Avoids some environments because of smells
Can identify the location and source of smell such as what is cooking for dinner	Cannot distinguish foods by their smell	Nauseous at perfumes and smells in the environment

Table 6.8 Indicators of Function: Sensory Reactivity (Continued)

	Indicators of Dysfunction	
Indicators of Function	**Hyporeactive**	**Hyperreactive**
Notices strong or noxious smells	Does not notice strong or noxious odors	Overly sensitive to noxious odors, such as in some public restrooms
Taste		
Function	**Hyporeactive**	**Hyperreactive**
Enjoys a variety of tastes	Seems unaware of strong tastes	Very sensitive to tastes that are unfamiliar
	Indicators of Dysfunction	
Indicators of Function	**Hyporeactive**	**Hyperreactive**
Puts things in mouth appropriately	Does not seek food when hungry	Refuses to mouth toys
Eats when hungry	Will eat a wide variety of things	Picky about food, refuses to try new foods
Eats a variety of flavors; enjoys a range of spicy to bland foods	Able to tolerate extremely spicy foods—more than cultural norm	Avoids spicy or salty foods, avoids mixed flavors
Notices when something is sweet, sour, bitter, and salty	Does not seem to notice that food is excessively sweet, salty, bitter, or sour	Tastes certain foods such as vegetables even when they are hidden in a dish

GUIDE FOR EVALUATION

The provision of pediatric occupational therapy is based on an evaluation of the child and family's needs and concerns in the domain of concern of occupational therapy, without bias on age or diagnosis (American Occupational Therapy Association [AOTA], 2020). The process of occupational therapy includes analyses of health and participation and factors that might contribute to performance patterns and skills (AOTA, 2020). Through interviews, questionnaires, and chart reviews, the occupational therapist applies clinical reasoning to inform the selection of a frame of reference, and in this case, the sensory integrative frame of reference and the selection of assessments that are specific to the age and abilities of the child including sensory functions (Burke, 2001). Assessment data further informs the therapist's clinical reasoning about the relationship between underlying factors and the child's ability to meet desired expectations in one or more areas including participation in occupations such as activities of daily living, education, play, sleep, and leisure activities at home and in the community; social participation; and performance skills and patterns, including habits and routines (Schaaf & Smith Roley, 2006; Schaaf & Mailloux, 2015). Areas of occupation related to participation are both the reason for referral and the goal of intervention (Schaaf & Smith Roley, 2006). When sensory-related concerns are suspected, it is recommended that the therapist should have postgraduate specialized knowledge and skills to apply the sensory integrative frame of reference with fidelity to the method (Parham et al., 2007, 2011; May-Benson et al., 2014).

Key Component: Identifying the Child's Strengths and Participation Challenges

Objective: Familiarity with the client is critical to assessment and goal setting.
Objectives: To identify areas of strength and need in the child's daily life: to establish a therapeutic alliance with parents and other active participants in the child's life; and to gather data about the child's participation in various contexts that guide the goal setting and intervention process.

Gathering data from significant individuals, including caregivers, teachers, and other service providers, helps to provide a clearer picture of the child's strengths and challenges. The therapist uses reflective questions to gather needed information and frame the child's strengths and needs:

- What are the child's areas of competency and strength with the key daily life activities encountered?
- What are the child's areas of need that can be addressed by occupational therapy?
- Do I understand the family's priorities for their child?
- Does the ASI framework seem an appropriate theoretical approach for this child?
- What can I do to meet the needs of the child as well as of family members?

Key Component: Conducting the Comprehensive Assessment

Objective: To identify areas of strengths and deficits in sensory reactivity, sensory perception, postural and motor skills, and praxis that may be affecting the child's participation challenges; to identify potential sensory targets for intervention.

Specific Assessments

A therapist often employs multiple methods of assessment to identify the child's area of strength and need, including interview, observation, record review, and structured and unstructured observations, and standardized assessments (Smith Roley & Schneck, 2006). The therapist uses clinical reasoning to determine which assessments will provide reliable and valid data to guide recommendations for intervention. The therapist's knowledge and skills in administering and interpreting the data relative to sensory integration as well as the evidence to support the use of sensory integration methods during intervention for participation-related outcomes is essential.

Beginning in the 1960s, Ayres created a series of norm-referenced standardized performance assessments designed to evaluate sensory and motor processes (including tactile perception and discrimination, visual perception, motor planning, vestibular processing, and bilateral motor skills) culminating in the *Southern California Sensory Integration Tests*, revised and published as the *Sensory Integration and Praxis Tests* (SIPT). The SIPT consists of 17 computer-scored tests, standardized on children aged 4 to 8 years 11 months, designed to assess the various constructs, that is, visual and tactile perception and discrimination, visual–motor skills, bilateral integration and sequencing, praxis including construction, imitation, facial gestures, and sequencing, visual–spatial planning and following unfamiliar verbal directions, and vestibular–proprioceptive functions such as standing and walking balance, that identify sensory integration strengths and deficits (Table 6.9; Figure 6.14). The *Test of Sensory Functions in Infants* was developed within that time period as a performance assessment for children aged 4 to 18 months (DeGangi & Greenspan, 1989).

Table 6.9 Sensory Integration and Praxis Tests (SIPT) and Evaluation in Ayres Sensory Integration (EASI) Tests—Comparison

SIPT Test	EASI Test	Notes
VISUAL PERCEPTION		
Space Visualization (SV)	Visual Praxis: Construction (VPr:C)	No specific EASI equivalent, but we have orientation on VPr:C
Figure-Ground Perception (FG)	Visual Praxis: Search (VP:S)	
Constructional Praxis (CPr)	Visual Praxis: Construction (VPr:C)	Make a Silly Room most similar; tearing, folding, and puzzle items are new
Motor (MAc)		No specific EASI equivalent
TACTILE DISCRIMINATION		
Manual Form Perception (MFP)	Tactile Perception: Shapes (TP: S)	
Finger Identification (FI)	Tactile Perception: Localization (TP: L)	TP:L incorporates both FI and LTS
Graphesthesia (GRA)	Tactile Perception: Designs (TP: D)	
Localization of Tactile Stimuli (LTS)	Tactile Perception: Localization (TP: L)	TP:L incorporates both FI and LTS
PROPRIOCEPTIVE DISCRIMINATION		
Kinesthesia (KIN)	Proprioception: Joint Position (Prop: JP)	
	Praxis: Ideation (Pr:I)	No specific SIPT equivalent
	Proprioception: Force (Prop:F)	No specific SIPT equivalent
PRAXIS		
Praxis on Verbal Command (PrVC)	Praxis: Following Directions (Pr: FD)	
Postural Praxis (PPr)	Praxis: (Pr: P)	Body and Hands items on EASI
Oral Praxis (OPr)	Praxis: Positions (Pr:P); Praxis Sequences (Pr: S)	Face items for both EASI tests
Sequencing Praxis (SPr)	Praxis: Sequences (Pr: S)	Hand items on EASI
VESTIBULAR		
Postrotary Nystagmus (PRN)	Vestibular: Nystagmus (V:N)	
POSTURAL, OCULAR, BILATERAL CONTROL		
	Postural Control (PC)	No specific SIPT equivalent
	Ocular Motor and Ocular Praxis (O:M&Pr)	No specific SIPT equivalent
Bilateral Motor Coordination (BMC)	Bilateral Integration (BI)	
Standing and Walking Balance (SWB)	Balance (Bal)	
AUDITORY LOCALIZATION		
	Auditory Localization (A:L)	No specific SIPT equivalent

(*continued*)

Table 6.9 Sensory Integration and Praxis Tests (SIPT) and Evaluation in Ayres Sensory Integration (EASI) Tests—Comparison (Continued)

SIPT Test	EASI Test	Notes
SENSORY REACTIVITY		
Localization of Tactile Stimuli (LTS)-observation on response to pin-point touch	Tactile Perception: Localization, Directions, Shapes and Oral (TP: L; TP:D; TP:S; TP:O)	EASI Tactile Perception Tests include scores for both hyper and hypo tactile reactivity
	Auditory Localization (A:L)	No specific SIPT equivalent; EASI Hyper and Hypo auditory reactivity
	Postural Control (PC)	No specific SIPT equivalent; EASI Hyper gravitational reactivity (gravitational insecurity)
	Sensory Reactivity (SR)	Hyper tactile, auditory, olfactory, and gravitational reactivity; No specific SIPT equivalent

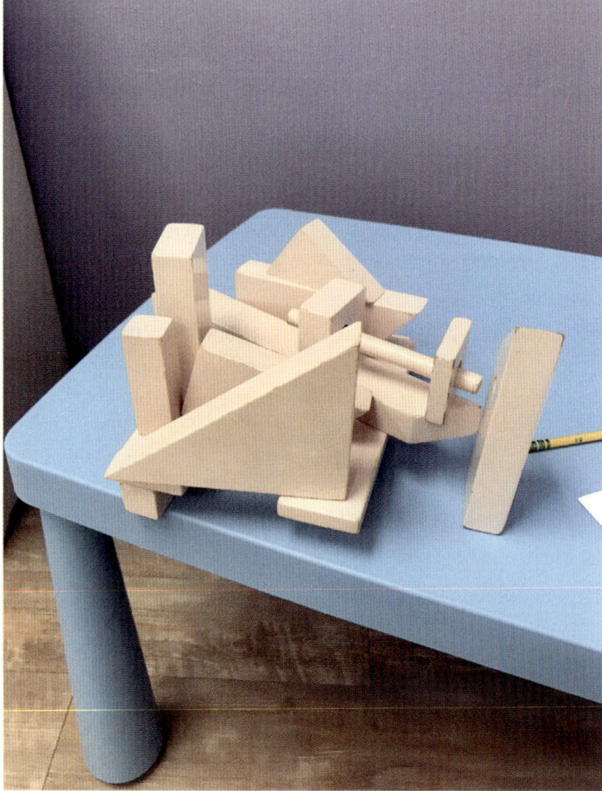

FIGURE 6.14 The Constructional Praxis Test of the Sensory Integration and Praxis Test provides details of visual praxis abilities.

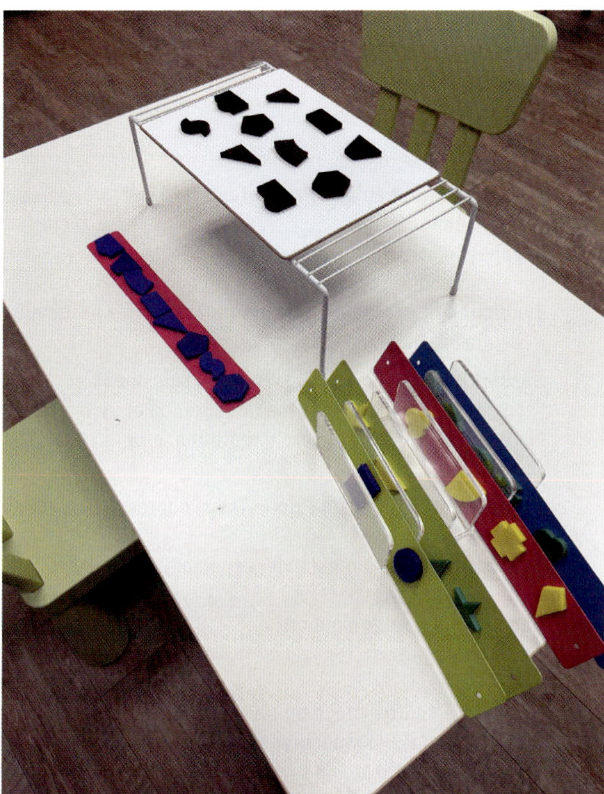

FIGURE 6.15 "The Evaluation in Ayres Sensory Integration" (EASI) the tactile perception: Shapes test of the EASI measures touch discrimination.

The *Evaluation in Ayres Sensory Integration (EASI)* (Mailloux et al., 2017) is a newly developed set of 20 standardized performance assessments that evaluate sensory hyper and hyporeactivity; sensory perception including visual, auditory, tactile, proprioceptive, and vestibular functions; postural and ocular motor control, balance, visual–motor and bilateral motor skills; and praxis including ideation, sequencing, imitation, and following directions. The *EASI* was standardized on a normative population of approximately 9,000 children ages 3 to 12 years, from over more than 80 countries and in the primary language of the region. The EASI is available to qualified therapists via online access, at a nominal annual fee for scoring (Figure 6.15). The tests have been analyzed for cultural competency (Gándara-Gafo et al., 2021; Holmlund & Orban, 2021); reliability and validity of the following constructs—tactile discrimination (Schaaf et al., 2023), praxis (Lamash et al., 2022), and vestibular and proprioception (Mailloux et al., 2021); and construct validity and internal reliability (Mailloux et al., 2023).

Performance testing is often complimented by the use of standardized questionnaires that examine sensory responses and related abilities via caregiver or self-report including the *Sensory Processing Measure-2* with versions available for ages 4 months through 87 years (Parham et al., 2021), the *Sensory Profile-2* with various versions from birth to 15 years (Dunn, 2014), and the *Sensory Experiences Questionnaire* ages 2 to 12 years for children with autism (Little et al., 2011).

A range of assessments yield information on the various sensory integrative constructs (Table 6.10).

Table 6.10 Assessments for Specific Areas of Function and Dysfunction

Function/Dysfunction Continua	Sensory Area	Specific Assessments
Somatosensory perception	Touch	Poor tactile perception **Sensory Integration and Praxis Tests**: manual form perception Finger identification Graphesthesia Localization of tactile stimuli **Evaluation in Ayres Sensory Integration**: tactile perception, shapes, discrimination, and localization
	Proprioception	**Sensory Integration and Praxis Tests**: kinesthesia Standing and walking balance (localization of tactile stimuli) **Evaluation in Ayres Sensory Integration**: proprioception force and direction
Vestibular bilateral integration and sequencing		**Sensory Integration and Praxis Tests**: depressed postrotary nystagmus (6 s or less) Standing and walking balance, especially with eyes closed Motor accuracy test Bilateral motor coordination Sequencing praxis Graphesthesia Lateralized scores including reversals, inversions, right-to-left errors **Evaluation of Ayres Sensory Integration:** Ocular–motor and praxis Postural control Bilateral integration
Visuopraxis	Visual form and space perception	**Sensory Integration and Praxis Tests**: space visualization **Evaluation in Ayres Sensory Integration**: visual perception, shapes Developmental Test of Visual Perception or Test of Visual Perception Skills
	Figure–ground perception	**Sensory Integration and Praxis Tests**: figure ground **Evaluation in Ayres Sensory Integration**: visual closure
	Visual–motor integration	**Sensory Integration and Praxis Tests**: design copying
	Visual–spatial planning	**Evaluation in Ayres Sensory Integration**: visual perception object interactions
Language-based praxis	Auditory sequential memory	**Sensory Integration and Praxis Tests**: sequencing praxis
	Following verbal directions	**Sensory Integration and Praxis Tests**: praxis on verbal command (especially when the postrotary nystagmus is typical (approximately 10 s or prolonged, more than 14 s) **Evaluation in Ayres Sensory Integration**: following directions

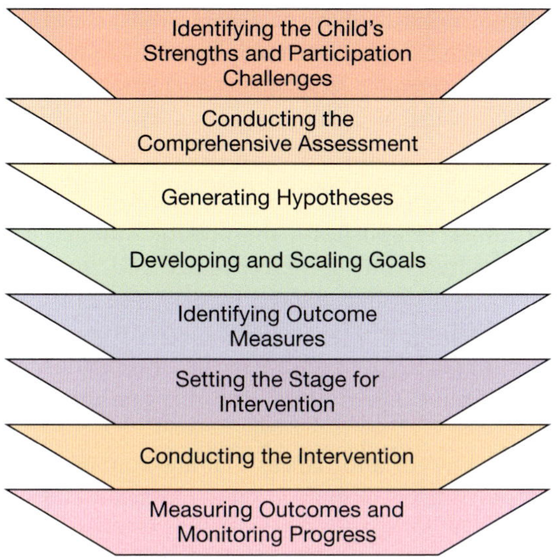

FIGURE 6.16 Data-Driven Decision-Making Model.

Schaaf and Mailloux (2015) proposed and tested a systematic framework, the Data-Driven Decision-Making Model (DDDM) that operationalized the concepts of ASI; the key components are listed in Figure 6.16.

Following the comprehensive evaluation, it is important for the occupational therapist to work together with the parents and family to determine the best way to collaborate with to share clinical observations and develop an intervention plan.

The therapist must be prepared to answer questions about the way in which occupational therapy can support the child and family and whether sensory integration is the appropriate frame of reference for this child. If sensory integration does not appear to be the appropriate approach for the child, the therapist must be prepared to make referrals for other disciplines or to use other frames of reference as appropriate.

POSTULATES REGARDING CHANGE

General Postulate Regarding Change

Occupational therapy practitioners should communicate with caregivers so that they understand their child's sensory and motor needs and how to craft daily routines and activities to address these including using the child's stronger sensory learning channels to facilitate function and participation.

- This includes helping the caregivers understand how to reframe behaviors to consider the sensory and motor components impacting behavior. Additionally, practitioners need to update the child and caregiver's occupational narrative as the child gains competencies.

Directional Postulate Regarding Change

The practitioner uses assessment data to tailor the intervention to address the child's areas of sensory and motor needs. Activities are directed at the "just right level of challenge," starting with the child's strengths, and increasing the complexity of the challenge so that the child will be able to master the challenge and accomplish increasingly more complex adaptive responses.

Specific Postulates Regarding Change

The sensory integration frame of reference has seven specific postulates regarding change:

- If the occupational therapy practitioner establishes a therapeutic alliance with the child that goes beyond pleasantries and feedback on the performance and supports the child's ability to collaborate in the activity choice and engage in play, the child is motivated, engaged, and supported. Therefore, learning will occur within a positive atmosphere, there will be a greater likelihood of the child participating fully in the intervention, and the child will be more likely to participate in similar activities across other settings and with others (Figure 6.17).
- If a therapy room is rich in sensory and motor affordances that are available to the child, the environment will engage the child's "inner drive" or motivation to physically engage in challenging and therapeutic activities that facilitate an adaptive response. In this way, the activities are their own reward, and the practitioner supports an internal locus of control for engagement in the activities (Figure 6.18).

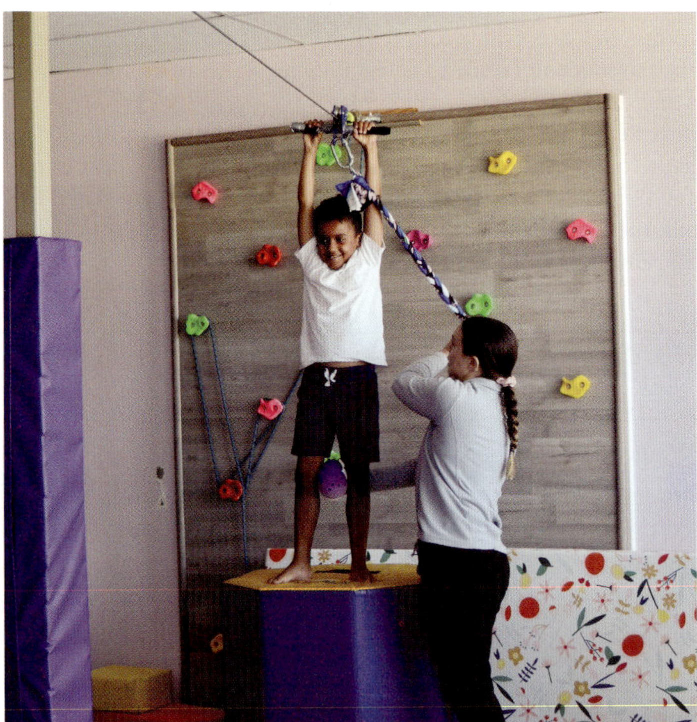

FIGURE 6.17 Establishing a partnership with the child and the family builds trust and collaboration in meaningful activity choices.

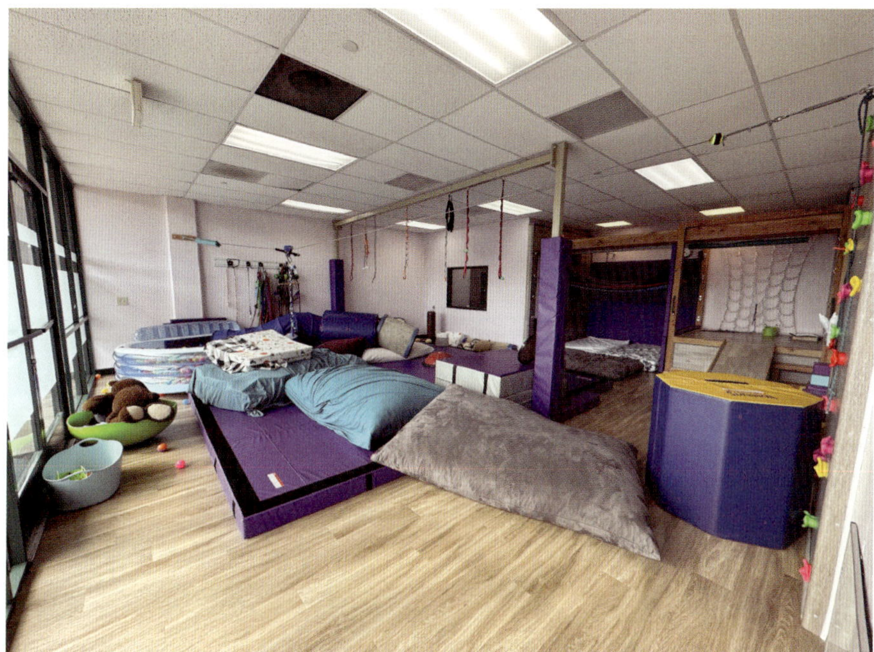

FIGURE 6.18 The therapeutic environment is designed to evoke creative problem solving in the child, while moving through and manipulating a fun environment.

- If the practitioner provides sensory opportunities in at least two of the three sensory systems (tactile, vestibular, proprioceptive), the child will build better body awareness and interactions that include regulated responses and speed and accuracy of sensory information processing relative to perception of people, space, and objects in the environment.
- If the practitioner engages the child in physical sensory and motor activities that are safe, motivating, fun, and yet challenging in the areas of needed growth and development, the child will build a foundation for increasingly complex adaptive skills and abilities.
- If the practitioner provides support for the child's self-regulation by providing specifically tailored intensities of sensory and motor activity, the child will demonstrate improved emotion regulation, behavior regulation, and cognitive regulation, and the ability to sustain engagement therapeutic activities.
- If the practitioner creates and offers a range of appropriate activities and challenges to the child's ability to discriminate and perceive body-centered sensory information (i.e., proprioceptive, vestibular, and tactile) and provides anticipatory and reactive postural, ocular, and bilateral motor challenges, the child will develop an improved ability for sustained and dynamic postural, ocular, and bilateral motor control. Furthermore, the child will then be more skillful with the use of their body during fine and gross motor tasks.
- If the practitioner provides challenges to the child's ability to conceptualize and plan novel actions and interactions, then the child will be more likely to develop praxis with the body, objects, time, and space; and organization, sequencing, imitation, following other-directed tasks, and construction (Figure 6.19).

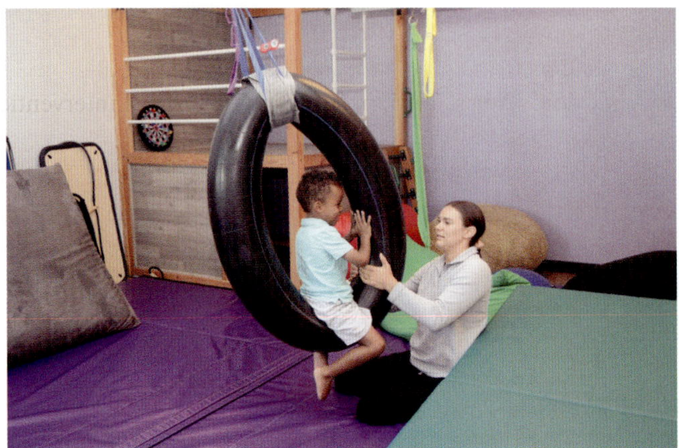

FIGURE 6.19 This approach is active and child directed, with the therapist seeking the just right challenge. In this situation, the therapist is using vestibular, proprioceptive, and tactile experiences to facilitate postural–ocular skills.

- If the practitioner communicates with parents and caregivers, then the generalizability of occupational therapy intervention will be increased across settings and with different people.

APPLICATION TO PRACTICE

Occupational therapy using an ASI frame of reference is a dynamic, process-oriented, and strength-based intervention. The intervention is unique in that it addresses the child's integration of sensory–motor foundations for learning and behavior. It specifically supports self-regulation, perception, and cognition through more efficient central nervous system information processing, rather than being a skill-building model of intervention. The active ingredients of the intervention are individually tailored, sensory–motor activities, contextualized in play at the just-right challenge designed to improve adaptive responses for participation in activities, tasks, and occupations (Schaaf & Mailloux, 2015). The sensory integrative frame of reference is intended to be part of a comprehensive intervention program. The intervention does not follow a specific or prearranged set of therapeutic activities directed by the practitioner but instead includes a dynamic process of cocreating activities with the child and collaborating with the primary caregivers, including education and support. Therapy is not prescriptive but rather it is individualized to meet the specific needs of each child and family toward improved participation (Bundy & Szklut, 2020; Koomar & Bundy, 2002). Traditionally, occupational therapy using sensory integration occurs in a 1:1 practitioner-to-child ratio in a clinic setting but also has applicability in other settings. May-Benson et al. (2014) found that practitioners who indicated that they used ASI in their practice also found fidelity in schools, clinics, hospitals, and community settings. Whiting et al. (2023) reported improved school performance and participation for children with sensory integration and processing challenges when provided sensory integration intervention with consultation in an educational setting. Odom et al. (2021) in a review of educational interventions for autism advised that ASI can be effective if provided by trained practitioners (Schaaf et al., 2014) and cautioned that a variety of other "sensory" interventions such as weighted vests, sensory diets, or sensory rooms have little evidence of effectiveness (Case-Smith et al., 2015).

Play

"When the therapist is doing her job effectively, and the child is organizing his nervous system, it looks as if the child is merely playing" (Ayres, 2005, p. 142). Intrinsic to ASI intervention, the practitioner and child are partners in the cocreation of therapeutic activities, thus engendering the child's intrinsic motivation to engage in activities in which they have the possibility for success.

Play is to sensory integration intervention as water is to swimming. Through the medium of play, the child finds joy in the somatomotor adaptive response thereby achieving therapeutic aims. Play for play's sake is supported as a way to enjoy the moment rather than a means to an end. Children's play choices often include sensory–motor activities including crashing and hanging, providing proprioception, swinging providing vestibular sensations, and immersion in a ball pool or Lycra swing that provides tactile input. The practitioner scaffolds the child's interests and abilities by ensuring safe, regulated, and adaptive responses within the session. The positive emotional state of the child becomes the state for learning and motivation to engage in activities that may appear at first too difficult, sustain the child's attention, and support their play skills outside of the therapy arena. Modeling cooperative play and teaching fun activities support the child to be a more interesting play partner to other children, often an area of concern for children with sensory integration deficits.

Fun and Inviting Environment

Sensory integration intervention typically utilizes "simple and versatile equipment" designed to engage the child in active sensory–motor play (Ayres, 1972, p. 260). Whether the therapy is provided in contrived spaces such as clinics or natural spaces such as the neighborhood playground, the physical environment must have adequate space and surfaces to safely allow for the flow of vigorous sensory–motor activities and several pieces of novel equipment that provide the affordance for creating activities (Ayres, 1972; Parham et al., 2011). There should also be a quiet space such as a tent, adjacent room, or partially enclosed area to allow opportunities for less distraction as needed. The arrangement of the equipment and materials needs to be flexible enough to allow for rapid changes in configuration during an intervention session. Physical safety is ensured using mats, cushions, and pillows that are used to pad the floor underneath all suspended and climbing equipment. Equipment should be adjustable to the size of the child. Suspended equipment that allows for single- and dual-point suspension for swings and related equipment is important so that there is opportunity for movement in all directions. The Ayres Sensory Integration Fidelity Measure (Parham et al., 2011) recommends a minimum of three hooks in the ceiling from which to suspend hanging equipment with a minimal distance of 2.5 to 3 feet between hooks. The hooks should have one or more rotational devices attached to the ceiling support to allow for 360 degrees of rotation. The use of bungee cords with the hanging suspended equipment allows for increased vertical and horizontal movements. All equipment must be routinely monitored for safety (Table 6.11).

Physical Engagement in Motivating and Fun Sensory–Motor Activities

The practitioner provides the milieu for developmentally appropriate sensory–motor play activities using novel affordances, with an emphasis on regulating and discriminating body-centered senses, and engagement with the practitioner. The practitioner observes the child's responses

Table 6.11 A List of Recommended Items for an Occupational Therapy Clinic That Uses the Sensory Integration Frame of Reference

- Bouncing equipment
- Rubber strips or ropes for pulling
- Therapy balls
- Platform swing
- Platform glider
- Frog swing
- Scooter board and ramp
- Flexion disc
- Bolster swing
- Tire swing
- Weighted objects such as balls or bean bags in a variety of sizes
- Inner tubes
- Spandex fabric
- Crash pillows
- Ball pit
- Vibrating toys or massagers
- Variety of tactile material
- Visual targets
- Climbing equipment
- Barrel
- Props to support engagement in play (dress-up clothes, sports equipment dolls, puppets)
- Materials for practicing daily living skills (school tools, clothing, hygiene, and other home-related objects)

during the activity and makes changes in the environment, intensity of the sensory experiences, and social interactions to increase or decrease the sensory and motor demands. The practitioner also makes environmental modifications as necessary in order to support the child's comfort and self-regulation.

Communication With Significant Caregivers

Collaboration with caregivers is an essential step toward a deeper understanding of the child and their engagement in the family and community. The reframing behavior to an understanding of the hidden difficulties is an initial step to altering the narrative about the child's engagement. Communication throughout the therapeutic process ensures that the practitioner and caregivers are appraised of the child's progress as well as ongoing concerns to update goals and better improve participation in home, school, and community activities, and assists the generalizability of the occupational therapy intervention across settings and with different people.

Schaaf and Mailloux (2015) provide a guide for caregiver education during ASI that includes parent education, a sampling of home and community activities, and materials helpful for interacting with families (Roan et al., 2022). The practitioner discusses with the parents the importance of play, and how sensory and motor activities can provide a foundation for participation in activities, tasks, and occupations, and collaborates with the parents to integrate these into their daily routines. Suggestions for adaptations to tasks, routines, and the environment to address the child's needs are also provided. The practitioner's insights about the hidden sensory strengths and challenges can reframe the perspective and help them understand that some behaviors that may be viewed as "negative behaviors" can be related to challenges in sensory integration. This understanding yields a value for sensory–motor strategies that can be employed in various settings to approach the presenting concerns from a sensory integrative point of view, that make daily life easier and more productive. Caregivers as partners in the intervention help to embed sensory–motor activities into the daily routine of the child and family and to better understand the child's unique sensory needs that support their development and reduce the impact of sensory integration challenges on learning and behavior. As the child gains competencies, the practitioner supports a positively changing narrative about the child and family's engagement in needed and desired occupations and co-occupations. As intervention proceeds and the child gains adaptive skills, the narrative during play and with the caregivers becomes more and more positive improving self-esteem and self-advocacy.

Generating Hypotheses for Intervention Planning

Interpretation of the assessment results provides the foundation for hypotheses that inform clinical reasoning regarding the impact of sensory integration on actions and interactions. Hypothesis generation requires knowledge and skills of typical and atypical development as well as ASI and patterns of function and dysfunction as it relates to adaptive skills. The therapist can utilize the Ayres Sensory Integration Assessment Interpretation Tool (Schaaf & Mailloux, 2015) to assist with analysis of assessment data and identification of sensory integration patterns of function and dysfunction. These will be used to tailor the intervention to the child's specific needs.

Once the therapist has gathered adequate assessment data, including specific sensory integrative, functions, medical and contextual background, and adaptive skill levels, the therapist synthesizes the data to decide whether a sensory integrative approach is warranted. The data synthesis is critical in determining the next steps including whether occupational therapy is warranted and if so, the frames of reference including ASI will support participation-related outcomes (Schaaf & Mailloux, 2015). Importantly, if there is insufficient assessment data in one or more of the sensory integrative areas, such as tactile perception or praxis, or a skewed perception of what is typical, the therapist may miss critical areas that hinder the child's participation that could be addressed by occupational therapy. Understanding the child's strengths is as important in decision making as identifying the deficit areas and should be a consideration when making service recommendations and designing interventions. ASI considers the individual's strengths in various sensory, motor, and related functions when setting goals, consulting, and designing the therapeutic activities that support participation in a variety of occupations.

Developing and Scaling Goals and Identifying Outcome Measures

Objectives: To identify specific goals that will be targeted in the therapeutic process and to monitor success of intervention toward meeting these identified goals.

Goals represent the predicted areas for intervention and expected change resulting from the intensity and type of intervention. They articulate areas of development where occupational therapy can contribute, and ensure accountability based on the effectiveness of the chosen intervention strategies. Once the therapist gathers and interprets the assessment data, the decision must be made about the projected impact of occupational therapy on the priorities and concerns that initiated the referral to occupational therapy. These decisions are made together with the caregivers and teacher as appropriate. An estimate of degree of change is contingent on a recommended intensity and duration of occupational therapy service. In the process of establishing goals, the therapist can reflect upon the intermediary steps that need to occur for a goal to be realized by the child. Often called objectives, benchmarks, or short-term goals, these intermediary steps can help to identify the functions, components, steps, or foundation skills that need attention for the child to achieve broader goals (Schaaf & Mailloux, 2015; Schaaf et al., 2015).

The therapist begins the process of setting goals by identifying the presenting problem, current level of function in the identified goal, the underlying sensory integrative factors impacting the goal, and the desired outcome.

The presenting problem is the issue that brings the child to occupational therapy. For example, a common presenting problem for a school-age child is poor completion of a specific learning task such as participation in group learning activities. Using assessment data and thoughtful clinical reasoning grounded in this frame of reference, the therapist identifies the factors impacting participation in these activities. The specific ways that the child is performing this task at present are described in detail and this information helps set baseline and outcome points of measurement. In the sensory integration frame of reference, a presenting problem, such as difficulty sitting for participation in learning tasks may be the result of an underlying problem in somatosensory perception, praxis, or vestibular-postural control. Difficulties with visual perception may also play a role. The desired outcome is directly related to the presenting problem and is the same regardless of the underlying problem. However, intervention strategies are designed to reach the desired outcome using strategies that address the underlying problem.

Table 6.12 presents a sample format for goals in the sensory integration frame of reference, including the presenting problem, underlying problem, and desired functional outcome (Schaaf & Mailloux, 2015). This format is useful as it articulates the proposed underlying sensory basis of the child's participation difficulties and guides the therapist in the appropriate choice of intervention targets (in this case, a focus on improved vestibular processing and improved postural and ocular control). Measurement of outcome is focused on the goal (i.e., distal outcome) although the therapist may also be interested in measuring whether there are any changes in the specifically identified sensory and motor factors hypothesized to be impacting the goal (i.e., proximal factors). This is discussed in more detail below in the section on outcome measurement.

Goal attainment scaling provides a tool for creating and measuring customized client-centered goals (Mailloux et al., 2007). In a randomized clinical trial with children with autism,

Table 6.12 Example of Targets for Educationally Related Goals

Presenting Problem	Hypothesized Underlying Problem	Desired Functional Outcome
Difficulty in copying from the blackboard	Inefficient processing of vestibular sensory input that affects the ability to extend the neck and to keep the head up; to coordinate head and eye movements; and to use bilateral hand movements	Adequate ability to copy assignments from the blackboard

goal attainment scaling method showed significant gains in the children receiving sensory integration intervention methods (Omairi et al., 2022; Schaaf et al., 2014; Whiting et al., 2023).

Intervention Planning and Implementation

Recommendation for therapy using the sensory integration frame of reference includes a variety of service delivery options, including 1:1, direct intervention sessions with the child, consultation or collaboration with the family and other significant caregivers including the teacher, and environmental modifications. The best options are based on the child's needs and the intensity that will provide therapeutic benefits. Occupational therapists should also consider the key elements of the ASI approach when choosing service delivery options. Table 6.13 might be particularly helpful for novice therapists.

The primary outcome when using the sensory integration frame of reference is improved participation in tasks, activities, and occupations. During the treatment, the practitioner observes the child's level of adaptive response (Ayres, 1972) and supports increasing levels of adaptive responses accordingly. These may vary from simple to complex—simply responding to stimuli to performing complicated activities. By supporting the child's motivation for engagement in sensory–motor challenges rich in tactile, vestibular, and proprioceptive sensations the therapist facilitates the child's ability to meet the challenge adaptively.

The therapeutic environment is designed to spark the child's inner drive/motivation to play (Ayres, 1972). The practitioner uses keen observation skills to observe and interpret the child's behaviors and interests and then creates and activity modifies a playful environment in which the child actively pursues achievable challenges (Bundy et al., 2020; Schaaf & Smith Roley, 2006). For example, occupational therapy using a sensory integration frame of reference for a child with hyperreactivity to tactile and vestibular stimuli might include "enticing" opportunities for sensory-rich play such as heavy work proprioceptive activities or crashing for deep touch pressure that serve to regulate sensory reactivity while providing achievable challenges to experience sensory activities. Challenging sensory activities include climbing up a small platform, grabbing onto a trapeze bar, swinging, and then landing in a matted pit full of colorful balls. Thus, the intervention is child directed and practitioner guided through challenging and fun activities designed to modulate reactivity to sensation, enhance the speed and accuracy of interpreting multisensory information,

Table 6.13 Key Process Elements of the Sensory Integrative Approach

1. Practitioner ensures physical safety
2. Practitioner presents sensory opportunities from a combination of touch, proprioception, and vestibular sensations during therapeutic activities
3. Practitioner facilitates the child's sensory responses toward self-regulation of arousal, affect, attention, and activity level.
4. Practitioner challenges vestibular-related postural, ocular, and bilateral motor development
5. Practitioner promotes praxis and organization of behavior
6. Practitioner designs activity to present just-right challenge
7. Practitioner and child collaborate in activity choice, including self-directed activities by the child and scaffolding to ensure adaptive engagement by the therapist
8. Practitioner ensures that activities are successful for the child
9. The practitioner fosters a context of play
10. The practitioner fosters a therapeutic alliance with the child

stimulate and challenge sensory and motor systems, and facilitate the integration of adaptive higher-level sensory, motor, cognitive, social, emotional and perceptual skills. Child directed refers to following the child's interests, strengths, and motivational activities in the treatment.

Sample Intervention Session

The key components presented above represent a sophisticated blend of clinical reasoning embedded in the occupational therapy process and the theoretical principles of the sensory integration frame of reference. The intervention process is fluid and dynamic, as the practitioner constantly monitors the child's strengths, needs, and skills required for participation in life activities. Table 6.14 provides an example of a typical occupational therapy session using the sensory integration frame of reference.

Table 6.14 A Typical Occupational Therapy Session Using Sensory Integration Frame of Reference

Activity	Purpose	Example	Comments
Warm-up	To ensure that the child is comfortable and relaxed for play	Greeting and playful interactions: "Hi did you come to play with X today?" What would you like to play today?[a]	Favorite game is tossing beanbags at a large stuffed bear in an attempt to knock it over
Active sensory–motor play with a focus on multisensory input	To decrease sensory sensitivities and increase praxis	Swinging on space bag and crashing into large pillows and bolsters. Space bag is set low to ground to offset any fear that the child might have and to encourage independence during this activity	Therapist sets up the environment with the child's needs in mind and then observes the child, following the child's cues, to select an activity[b]
Active sensory–motor play with a focus on praxis	To decrease sensory sensitivities, improve awareness of body, and increase praxis	The therapist helps the child create a "bridge" (two triangular climbing devices with a flat bolster suspended between them). The child climbs up the ladder (with assistance), climbs onto bolster, and then dumps into large "crash pad" (pillows)[c]	Therapist vigilantly observes the child's reactions and actions, encouraging the child as needed but allowing for as much self-direction and independence as possible[d]
Snack with a focus on socialization	To decrease oral sensitivities, expand food repertoire, and enhance socialization	The child brings a snack to share with another child. The child sets up a snack, invites another child, and participates in a snack	Mother packs food and beverages that the child enjoys in addition to one or two foods that the child is not familiar with or usually avoids

[a]If no response: I have your favorite game ready. Do you want to play?

[b]Upgrade: add tactile and motor planning component (count to 3 and "crash" into pillows).

[c]If child is not willing to climb up to bridge, therapist downgrades by lowering ladder.

[d]Therapist uses playful language (singing) or pretend play (climbing into spaceship).

Activities are upgraded and downgraded to meet the child's needs and to ensure success.

Schaaf, R. C., & Nightlinger, K. M. (2007). Occupational therapy using a sensory integrative approach: A case study of effectiveness. *American Journal of Occupational Therapy, 61*, 239–246.

Therapy is contextualized in sensory-rich play and taps into the child's inner drive for competence (Ayres, 1979). The practitioner artfully and skillfully creates enticing, achievable challenges for the child to promote the ability to process and integrate sensory information and observes adaptive responses to these challenges (Schaaf & Nightlinger, 2007). During intervention, a practitioner records goals and progress by noting observable changes in the child's ability to participate in sensory-based activities, regulate arousal level, and increase repertoire of sensory–motor skills and improved ability to participate independently in daily life activities for example (Schaaf & Nightlinger, 2007). In addition to direct intervention with the child, the practitioner interacts and collaborates with parents, teachers, and others who are involved with the child to (1) help them understand and reframe the child's behavior from a sensory perspective, (2) adapt the environment to the needs of the child, (3) create needed sensory and motor experiences throughout their day in their natural environments, and (4) assure that therapy is helping the child become more functional in his or her daily life activities (Schaaf & Smith Roley, 2006).

CASE EXAMPLE

The following is a case study in which standardized assessment data informed the use of the ASI frame of reference by identifying strengths and weaknesses in various patterns of sensory integration and designing customized intervention strategies that yield salient participation-related outcomes in needed and desired actions and interactions.

Soraya: Vestibular Bilateral Integration and Sequencing Pattern

Referral: Soraya's parents describe her as a smart, hardworking, and helpful 9-year-old girl who is well-behaved, cautious, and active. She tires easily during sedentary tasks and has difficulty with reading, math, and penmanship. The diagnosis of attention-deficit hyperactivity disorder is suspected but not confirmed.

Medical history: Soraya had frequent ear infections requiring pressure equalization tubes at the age of 2 years and again at 9 years.

Educational history: Soraya repeated kindergarten. She qualified for special education services in second grade due to a specific learning disability. She attends general education classes with accommodations including extra time on writing assignments, preferential seating, copies of class notes, and 1 hour of resource support per week.

Developmental History (Parent Report)

State regulation: Soraya is a quiet, serious girl who is anxious unless she is in the presence of her mother.

Gross motor: Soraya sat at 8 months and did not crawl. With the aid of physical therapy, Soraya pulled to stand at 14 months and walked at 16 months.

Play and leisure: Soraya enjoys interacting with her friends and family. She is somewhat shy. She enjoys gymnastics, theater, and swimming but seems to run out of energy faster than her peers.

Assessment results: On the *Sensory Processing Measure-2*, Soraya's parents reported typical responses in all areas with the exception of Moderate Difficulties in Touch.

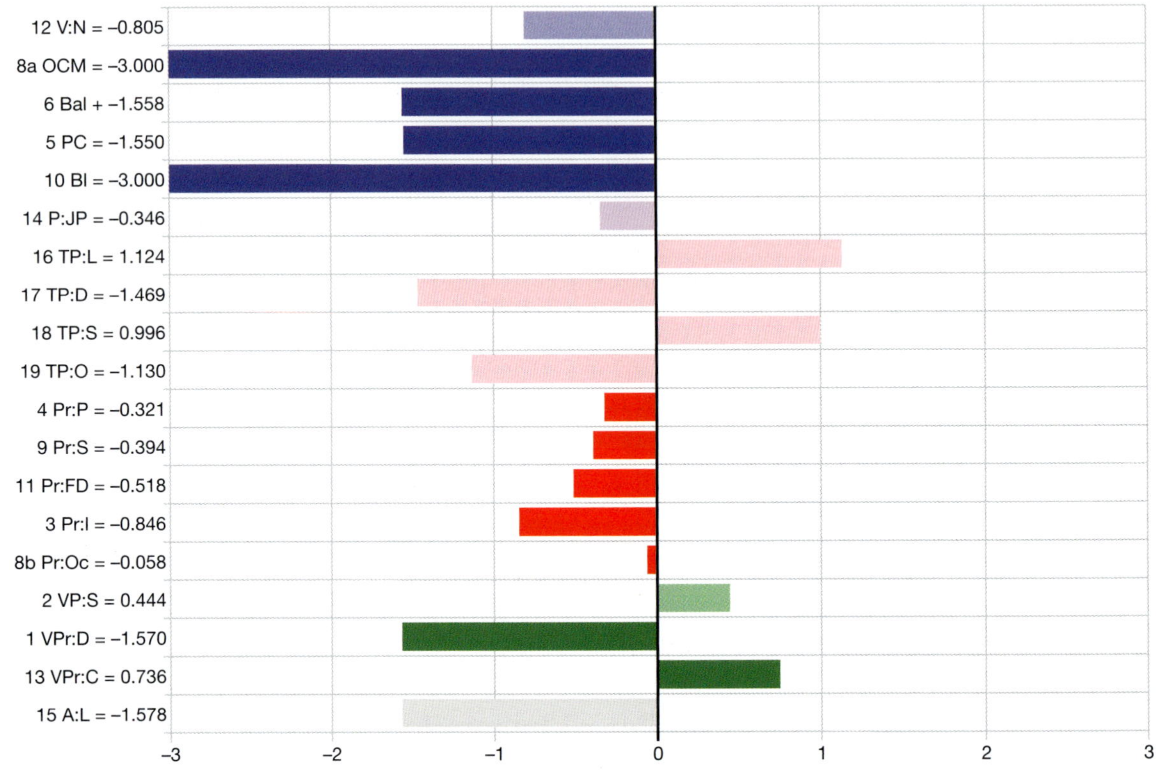

FIGURE 6.20 Soraya's Evaluation of Ayres Sensory Integration (EASI) scores.

Her teacher reported typical responses in Touch, Taste and Smell, and Balance and Motion. Moderate Difficulties were identified in Vision, Hearing, and Body Awareness. On the *EASI* tests Soraya obtained the following scores (score indicate standard deviation from the mean): Vestibular Nystagmus -0.80, Balance, -1.55, Ocular Motor -3.00, Bilateral Integration -3.00, and Postural Control -1.55. These scores are consistent with the scores on the *SIPT,* which revealed a pattern of scores consistent with vestibular bilateral integration and sequencing deficits predictive of postural control, handwriting, and learning difficulties (Figure 6.20) (EASI).

Impression: Soraya is a bright, pleasant, and cooperative girl who enjoys socializing with others. She has the diagnosis of specified learning disability with graphomotor and handwriting difficulties. She has vestibular–proprioceptive processing difficulties along with decreased balance and coordination that affect her speed and agility during sports activities and her ability to sustain her attention during prolonged sedentary tasks.

Recommendations: Occupational therapy is recommended as follows: 1:1, 1 h/wk, in a setting with specialized therapy equipment, for 1 year, by an occupational therapist, with an additional 15 min/mo collaboration with her caregivers.

Goals

1. Writing and copying: Given improved vestibular functioning, Soraya will show improved eye tracking, sitting in upright position, perception of directions such as "up and down" and right and left" as observed by the ability to copy two sentences from a visual model, without losing her place, with appropriate letter size, shape, formation, directionality, and spacing, remaining within 0.5-inch lines and correctly placing letters below the center dotted lines, utilizing adapted paper (e.g., raised-line, highlighted, bold lined paper), on three of four opportunities.
2. Manipulating materials: Soraya will demonstrate improved bilateral coordination during necessary tasks such as holding her paper while writing, opening containers, or folding and cutting without adult assist on four of five opportunities.

Intervention

The test scores provided a roadmap for providing sensory–motor activities that were engaging and fun, building on her strengths and guiding her into challenges that supported growth and development in her adaptive skills. The following are a few examples of activities to use in treatment:

1. Given her strengths in tactile and proprioceptive awareness informing body awareness and her ability to plan activities, we prepared a "circus performer" set of challenges that highlighted her gymnastic skills. She was excited to set up and go through an obstacle course, and provided challenges for her to sequence the equipment and her actions, sustain her grasp and flexion while on the zipline, to go from the zipline to the trapeze to the platform swing using bilateral hand skills, and incorporate targets such as holding beanbags with her knees and dropping them into a bucket while flying through the air. She identified where she would aim (higher/lower, i.e., "up and down" and over here/over there, i.e., "right and left"). At the end, she requested to do the performance for her mother and brother who had been in the waiting room.
2. Building on her strengths with creativity and her love of and need for movement, Soraya was eager to engage with the swinging and climbing equipment that supported her vestibular–proprioceptive processing. We set up an activity in which we could decorate this equipment with the colors and theme of her choice, using streamers, cut out snowflakes, labels, and signs, which she could then fly through the air and climb to the top in order to affix these decorations with string, rope or tape. She was able to take photos of her creations and take the decorations and supplies she wanted to recreate at home.

Suggested Classroom Accommodations

- Frequent movement opportunities and access to recess and other outdoor and movement-based periods. Breaks should not be removed for any reason such as to complete incomplete work.
- Option to stand rather than sit while working and access to dynamic or mobile seating devices such as a rocking or swivel chair, ball chair, sit-n-move cushion, or therapy ball to support her ability to pay attention, complete her school work, and benefit from her education.

POSTGRADUATE EDUCATION

Practitioners who wish to develop advance competence in sensory integration should strongly consider postgraduate training and mentorship in ASI theory, assessment, and intervention (Baltazar Mori et al., 2017; Parham et al., 2007a; Parham et al., 2011). Table 6.15 is the International Council for Education in ASI (ICEASI) guidelines for developing expertise.

Table 6.15 Proposed Pathways to Expertise in Ayres Sensory Integration

Levels	Knowledge and Skills
Level 1: Entry-level outcomes	1. Introduction to the seminal work of Dr. A. Jean Ayres 2. Sensory contributions to development including concepts of body-centered sensations, sensory–motor skills, and praxis 3. Sensory challenges including reactivity, perception, postural and motor skills, and praxis 4. When to refer to a professional with postgraduate specialization in Ayres Sensory Integration 5. Basic principles and equipment used in classic Ayres Sensory Integration intervention 6. Impact of sensory systems on the lived experience of people with sensory challenges
Level 2: Certificate-level outcomes Training programs typically consist of 120 contact hours or more	1. Historical and Current Foundations of Sensory Integration Theory 2. Foundations of Sensory Integration in Occupational Therapy and Occupational Science 3. Ayres Sensory Integration as Trademarked Term 4. Typical sensory integration development 5. The impact of sensory integration across the lifespan 6. Neurobiologic foundations for sensory integration 7. Models of sensory integration function and dysfunction 8. Terminology related to sensory integration 9. Reliability and validity of direct and indirect assessments of sensory integration and praxis 10. Research from factor analyses supporting knowledge of the patterns of sensory integration function and dysfunction 11. Evidence on sensory integration and praxis deficits in various populations 12. Clinical reasoning tools such as Data-Driven Decision-Making Model 13. Differentiating sensory integration deficits from other types of difficulties 14. Ayres Sensory Integration intervention planning based on systematic reasoning and hypothesis generation 15. Link engagement in occupation and participation with sensory integration for goal setting and outcomes measurement 16. Considerations of a manualized intervention 17. Structural and process elements of Ayres Sensory Integration intervention 18. Distinguishing Ayres Sensory Integration intervention methods from other interventions 19. Evidence on effectiveness of Ayres Sensory Integration methods 20. Benefits and limitations of the Ayres Sensory Integration approach

Table 6.15 Proposed Pathways to Expertise in Ayres Sensory Integration (Continued)

Levels	Knowledge and Skills
Level 2 Skills demonstrating the ability to	1. Choose and administer Ayres Sensory Integration assessments that inform understanding of participation challenges relevant to the profession 2. Administer assessments reliably 3. Support interpretation with objective data 4. Interpret, synthesize, and analyze assessment data and achieve meaningful goals 5. Communicate assessment results in a conclusive and understandable way 6. Relate sensory integration assessment finding to reasons for referral and participation 7. Make an impact and empower others to effect change for the person with sensory integration difficulties 8. Understand therapeutic use of self in Ayres Sensory Integration intervention 9. When sensory integration is warranted, meet criteria for fidelity in Ayres Sensory Integration intervention
Level 3 Advanced-level outcomes	1. Shows motivation to continue learning 2. Builds expertise in 1 or more areas of research, advocacy, education, and practice 3. Links with professionals with additional expertise within and outside of their own profession 4. Contributes to new knowledge and skills in Ayres Sensory Integration 5. Takes a leadership role in their community of practice 6. Shares knowledge, e.g., through publications or lectures
Level 4 Expert-level outcomes	Experts are identified as individuals with exemplary knowledge and skills who make substantial contributions to Ayres Sensory Integration research, advocacy, education, or practice

SUPPORTING EVIDENCE

Ayres was one of the first occupational therapists to build a model of evidence-based occupational therapy practice though the following essential steps: understanding the problem and its' causes through the scientific theory (Ayres, 1972; Bundy & Lane, 2020). She identified the factors that have the greatest scope for changes via standardized assessments (Ayres, 1989; Mailloux et al., 2017). Further, she identified postulates for change (Ayres, 1972; Lane & Schaaf, 2010). The manualized method that feasibly can deliver the change mechanism (Schaaf et al., 2012; Schaaf & Mailloux, 2015) with fidelity to ensure its replicability for research (Parham et al., 2011; May-Benson et al., 2014) was identified through conducting sufficient rigorous studies with meaningful positive outcomes. Some of these studies identified via goal attainment scaling (Mailloux et al., 2011; Schaaf & Mailloux, 2015), to justify the use of the intervention (Ayres, 1972, 1976, 1978, 1980) with increasing number of randomized clinical trials showing promising outcomes (Chan et al., 2022; Dunbar et al., 2012; Iwanaga et al., 2014; Kashefimehr et al., 2018; Omairi et al., 2022; Pfeiffer et al., 2011; Randell et al., 2022; Schaaf et al., 2014; Williams et al., 2023).

Building on the tradition of research starting in the 1960s, the ASI frame of reference is currently a manualized approach within occupational therapy (Schaaf & Mailloux, 2015) that meets the criteria as an evidence-based practice from multiple agencies (Council for Exceptional Children, 2014; Steinbrenner et al., 2020; The National Professional Development Center on ASD https://autismpdc.fpg.unc.edu/evidence-based-practices; U.S. Preventative Services Task Force Guidelines for Evidence Reviews https://uspreventiveservicestaskforce.org/uspstf/about-uspstf/methods-and-processes/procedure-manual/procedure-manual-section-4-evidence-review-development; National Clearinghouse on Autism Evidence an Practice https://ncaep.fpg.unc.edu/) and through systematic reviews (Odom et al., 2021; Schoen et al., 2019; Schaaf et al., 2018; Watling et al., 2018).

ASI is now recognized as an evidence-based practice for autistic children with autism (Steinbrenner et al., 2020), and one of the most commonly used occupational therapy interventions for this population (Case-Smith & Miller, 1999). Prevalence estimates of sensory differences in autism range between 74% (Kirby et al., 2022) and 80% to 90% (Kientz & Dunn, 1997; Rogers & Ozonoff, 2005; Tomcheck & Dunn, 2007) with excessive seeking of sensory stimuli with an unusual preoccupation with smells or visual stimuli and overengagement in activities that involve touch, sounds, or movement. Sensory integration and praxis deficits including somatopraxis, vestibular–postural and bilateral integration as well as sensory reactivity have been identified (Kilroy et al., 2019, 2020; Reynolds et al., 2011; Smith Roley et al., 2015) affecting participation in daily life activities, emotional regulation, and social participation at home, at school and in the community (Butera et al., 2020). Self-reports from individuals with autism spectrum disorder confirm these findings and are particularly potent in terms of describing the impact of sensory dysfunction on participation in daily life activities (Grandin, 1995; O'Neill & Jones, 1997; Williams, 1992, 1994). Despite the high prevalence of sensory features in autistic children and their sequelae, disparities in identification persist particularly among girls, children of color, and children of mothers with less education, indicating potential disparities in access to occupational therapy to provide this evidence-based intervention to address these sensory challenges.

Increasing evidence shows that children with attention deficits may benefit from a sensory integrative approach (Isaac et al. 2017; Lane et al., 2012; Miller et al., 2011) as well as those children with specific learning difficulties (Ayres, 1972, 1976, 1978), developmental coordination disorder (Kilroy et al., 2022; Ringold et al., 2022), and sensory reactivity differences with no other diagnosis (Miller et al., 2007a, 2007b).

Although sensory integration was never intended to explain the neuromotor or cognitive disorders evident in populations with cerebral palsy or Down syndrome, individuals with these and other disorders often exhibit sensory integration deficits. Thus, children with cerebral palsy and Down syndrome have benefitted from sensory integration–based interventions as an important adjunct to other therapeutic interventions (Schaaf & Miller, 2005; Schaaf & Smith Roley, 2006; Smith Roley et al., 2001). Practitioners have also found that therapy based on sensory integration theory is efficacious when working with infants born at risk or with regulatory disorders (DeGangi, 2017), fragile X syndrome (Hickman, 2001), and children from environmentally deprived situations (Cermak, 2001).

Summary

In conclusion, ASI intervention applied within occupational therapy is guided by assessment, using clinical reasoning informed by data which is analyzed based on decades of research on the patterns of sensory integrative function and dysfunction, and provided with fidelity by a qualified therapy professional with postgraduate training in ASI. As previously stated, any practitioner using this approach should obtain postgraduate training and mentorship, stay abreast of the literature, and critically analyze their practice relative to present and emergent research. In the meantime, practitioners are encouraged to follow the principles outlined in this chapter and systematically collect data to evaluate the effectiveness of their intervention as part of "best practice." Continued research will refine our understanding in all areas including the complexity of multisensory integration in the central nervous system and its impact on health and resilience, which clients benefit most, refining the dosage, duration, and delivery mechanism, and how to maximize cost-effectiveness while achieving consumer-driven participation-related outcomes.

ACKNOWLEDGMENT

All of the photos in the chapter were taken by Annie Baltazar-Mori.

REFERENCES

Abrams, G., Jayashankar, A., Kilroy, E., Butera, C., Harrison, L., Ring, P., Houssain, A., Nalbach, A., Cermak, S. A., & Aziz-Zadeh, L. (2024). Differences in praxis errors in autism spectrum disorder compared to developmental coordination disorder. *Journal of Autism and Developmental Disorders, 54*(3), 1113–1129. https://doi.org/10.1007/s10803-022-05858-8

American Occupational Therapy Association (AOTA). (2020). Occupational therapy practice framework: Domain and process (4th ed.). *The American Journal of Occupational Therapy, 74*(Suppl 2), 7412410010p1.

Ayres, A. J. (1965). Patterns of perceptual-motor dysfunction in children: A factor analytic study. *Perceptual & Motor Skills, 20*, 335–368. https://doi.org/10.2466/pms.1965.20.2.335

Ayres, A. J. (1972). *Sensory integration and learning disorders*. Western Psychological Services.

Ayres, A. J. (1976). *The effect of sensory integrative therapy on learning disabled children: The final report of a research project*. Center for the Study of Sensory Integrative Dysfunction.

Ayres, A. J. (1978). Learning disabilities and the vestibular system. *American Journal of Occupational Therapy, 11*, 33–40. https://doi.org/10.1177/002221947801100104

Ayres, A. J. (1979). *Sensory integration and the child*. Western Psychological Services.

Ayres, A. J. (1985). *Developmental dyspraxia and adult onset apraxia*. Sensory Integration International.

Ayres, A. J. (1989). *The sensory integration and praxis tests (SIPT)*. Western Psychological Services.

Ayres, A. J. (2005). *Sensory integration and the child* (25th anniversary ed.). Western Psychological Services.

Ayres, A. J., & Cermak, S. A. (2011). *Ayres dyspraxia monograph* (25th anniversary ed.). Pediatric Therapy Network.

Ayres, A. J., Mailloux, Z. K., & Wendler, C. L. W. (1987). Developmental dyspraxia: Is it a unitary function? *Occupational Therapy Journal of Research, 7*, 93–110. https://doi.org/10.1177/153944928700700203

Ayres, A. J., & Tickle, L. (1980). Hyperresponsivity to touch and vestibular stimuli as a predictor of positive response to sensory integration procedures by autistic children. *American Journal of Occupational Therapy, 34*, 375–381. https://doi.org/10.5014/ajot.34.6.375

Baltazar Mori, A., Carrasco Koester, A., Holland, D., Fernandes, P., Gray Rogers, R., Smith Roley, S., Smith Roley, S., Soechting, E., & VanJaarsveld, A. (2017). Building competency in SI: Evidence-based guidelines for occupational therapy using Ayres Sensory Integration®. *OT Practice, 22*(12), 8–13.

Bar-Shalita, T., Vatine, J. J., & Parush, S. (2008). Sensory modulation disorder: A risk factor for participation in daily life activities. *Developmental Medicine and Child Neurology, 50*(12), 932–937. https://doi.org/10.1111/j.1469-8749.2008.03095.x

Bear, M. F., Connors, B. W., & Paradiso, M. A. (2016). *Neuroscience: Exploring the brain* (4th ed.). Lippincott Williams & Wilkins.

Berthoz, A. (2000). *The brain's sense of movement*. Harvard University Press.

Berthoz, A., Graf, W., & Vidal P. P. (1992). *The head-neck sensory motor system*. Oxford University Press.

Brown, C., & Dunn, W. (2002). *Adolescent/adult sensory profile manual*. Psychological Corporation.

Brown, J., Cooper-Kuhn, C. M., Kempermann, G., Van Praag, H., Winkler, J., Gage, F. H., & Kuhn, H. G. (2003). Enriched environment and physical activity stimulate hippocampal but not olfactory bulb neurogenesis. *European Journal of Neuroscience, 17*, 2042–2046. https://doi.org/10.1046/j.1460-9568.2003.02647.x

Bundy, A. C. (1997). Play and playfulness: What to look for. In L. D. Parham & L. S. Fazio (Eds.), *Play in occupational therapy for children* (pp. 52–66). Mosby-Year Book Inc.

Bundy, A. C., & Lane, S. J. (2020). *Sensory integration: Theory and practice* (3rd ed.). F.A. Davis.

Bundy, A. C., Smith Roley, A., Mailloux, Z., & Parham, L. D. (2020). Interpreting and explaining evaluation data. In A. C. Bundy & S. J. Lane (Eds.), *Sensory integration: Theory and practice* (3rd ed., pp. 256–283). F.A. Davis.

Bundy, A. C., & Szklut, S. (2020). The science of intervention: Creating direct intervention from theory. In A. C. Bundy & S. Lane (Eds.), *Sensory integration: Theory and practice* (3rd ed., pp. 300–335). F.A. Davis.

Burke, J. P. (2001). Clinical reasoning and the use of narrative in sensory integration assessment and intervention. In S. Smith Roley, E. I. Blanche, & R. C. Schaaf (Eds.), *Understanding the nature of sensory integration with diverse populations* (pp. 203–214). ProEd, Inc.

Butera, C., Ring, P., Sideris, J., Jayashankar, A., Kilroy, E., Harrison, L., Cermak, S., & Aziz-Zadeh L. (2020). Impact of sensory processing on school performance outcomes in high functioning individuals with Autism spectrum disorder. *Mind, Brain, and Education*, *14*(3), 243–254.

Case-Smith, J., & Miller, H. (1999). Occupational therapy with children with pervasive developmental disorders. *The American Journal of Occupational Therapy*, *53*(5), 506–513. https://doi.org/10.5014/ajot.53.5.506

Case-Smith, J., Weaver, L. L., & Fristad, M. A. (2015). A systematic review of sensory processing interventions for children with autism spectrum disorders. *Autism, 19*(2), 133–148. https://doi.org/10.1177/1362361313517762

Cermak, S. (2001). The effects of deprivation on processing, play and praxis. In S. Smith Roley, E. I. Blanche & R. C. Schaaf (Eds.), *Understanding the nature of sensory integration with diverse populations* (pp. 385–408). Pro-Ed, Inc.

Chan, P. L. C., Poon, M. Y. C., Bux, V., Wong, S. K. F., Chu, A. W. Y., Louie, F. T. M., Wang, A. Q. L., Yang, H. L. C., Yu, E. L. M., & Fong, S. S. L. (2022). Occupational therapy using an Ayres Sensory integration® approach for school-age children – a randomized controlled trial. *World Federation of Occupational Therapists Bulletin*, 79, 228–235. https://doi.org/10.1080/14473828.2022.2097814

Chen, W. G., Schloesser, D., Arensdorf, A. M., Simmons, J. M., Cui, C., Valentino, R., Gnadt, J. W., Nielsen, L., St. Hillaire-Clarke, C., Spruance, V., Horowitz, T. S., Vallejo, Y. F., & Langevin, H. M. (2021). The emerging science of interoception: Sensing, integrating, interpreting, and regulating signals within the self. *Trends in Neurosciences, 44* (1), 3–16. https://doi.org/10.1016/j.tins.2020.10.007

Cohn, E. S., Miller, L. J., & Tickle-Degnan, L. (2000). Parental hopes for therapy outcomes: Children with sensory modulation disorders. *American Journal of Occupational Therapy, 54*, 36–43. https://doi.org/10.5014/ajot.54.1.36

Council for Exceptional Children. (2014). Council for exceptional children standards for evidence-based practices in special education. Council of Exceptional Children: Voice and Vision of Special Education. Retrieved from http://www.cec.sped.org/˜/media/Files/StandardscEvidence%20based%20Practices%20and%20Practice/EBP%20FINAL.pdf

Craig, A. D. (2003). Interoception: The sense of the physiological condition of the body. *Current Opinions in Neurobiology, 13*(4), 500–505. https://eric.ed.gov/?id=EJ1059294

Davies, P., Chang, W., & Gavin, W. (2010). Middle and late latency ERP components discriminate between adults, typical children, and children with sensory processing disorders, *Frontiers in Integrative Neuroscience, 4*, 1–9. https://doi.org/10.3389/fnint.2010.00016

Deflorio, D., Di Luca, M., & Wing, A. M. (2022). Skin and mechanoreceptor contribution to tactile input for perception: a review of simulation models. *Frontiers in Human Neuroscience, 16*, 862344. https://doi.org/10.3389/fnhum.2022.862344

DeGangi, G. (2017). *Pediatric disorders of regulation in affect and behavior: A therapist's guide to assessment and treatment* (2nd ed.). Elsevier.

DeGangi, G. A., & Greenspan, S. (1989). *Test of sensory functions in infants*. Western Psychological Services.

Dunbar, S. B., Carr-Hertel, J., Lieberman, H. A., Perez, B., & Ricks, K. (2012). A pilot study comparison of sensory integration treatment and integrated preschool activities for children with autism. *Internet Journal of Allied Health Sciences and Practice, 10*(3), 6.

Dunn, W. (2014). *The sensory profile 2 manual*. Pearson.

Gándara-Gafo, B., Beaudry-Bellefeuille, I., Mailloux, Z., Moriyón, T., Parham, D., Santos-del Riego, S., Smith Roley, S., Toledo, P., & Schaaf, R. C. (2021). Cultural adaptation of the Evaluation in Ayres Sensory Integration® (EASI) for Spanish speaking populations. *American Journal of Occupational Therapy, 7*(75), 7505205090. https://doi.org/10.5014/ajot.2021.044693

Gingras, G., Rowland, B. A., & Stein, B. E. (2009). The differing impact of multisensory and unisensory integration on behavior. *Journal of Neuroscience, 29*(15), 4897–4902. https://doi.org/10.1523/JNEUROSCI.4120-08.2009

Grandin, T. (1995). How people with autism think. In E. Schopler & G. B. Mesibov (Eds.), *Learning and cognition in autism* (pp. 137–156). Springer.

Greenough, W. T., Black, J. E., & Wallace, C. S. (1987). Experience and brain development. *Child Development, 58*(3), 539–559. http://www.jstor.org/stable/1130197

Greenough, W. T., Volkmar, F. R., & Juraska, J. M. (1973). Effects of rearing complexity on dendritic branching in frontolateral and temporal cortex of the rat. *Experimental Neurology, 41*, 371–378. https://doi.org/10.1016/0014-4886(73)90278-1

Greenough, W. T., West, R. W., & DeVoogd, T. J. (1978). Subsynaptic plate perforations: Changes with age and experience in the rat. *Science, 202*, 1096–1098. https://doi.org/10.1126/science.715459

Hickman, L. (2001). Sensory integration and fragile X syndrome. In S. Smith Roley, E. I. Blanche, & R. C. Schaaf (Eds.), *Understanding the nature of sensory integration with diverse populations* (pp. 409–420). Pro-Ed, Inc.

Holmlund, M., & Orban, K. (2021). Translation and cross-cultural adaptation of the performance-based test—Evaluation in Ayres Sensory Integration®, *Scandinavian Journal of Occupational Therapy, 28*(8), 609–620. https://doi.org/10.1080/11038128.2020.1831059

Isaac, V., Olmedo, D., Aboitiz, F., & Delano, P. H. (2017) Altered cervical vestibular-evoked myogenic potential in children with attention deficit and hyperactivity disorder. *Frontiers in Neurology, 8*, 90. doi:10.3389/fneur.2017.00090

Ismael, N., Lawson, L. M., & Hartwell, J. (2018). Relationship between sensory processing and participation in daily occupations for children with autism spectrum disorder: A systematic review of studies that used Dunn's sensory processing framework. *American Journal of Occupational Therapy, 72*, 7203205030. https://doi.org/10.5014/ajot.2018.024075

Iwanaga, R., Honda, S., Nakane, H., Tanaka, K., Toeda, H., & Tanaka, G. (2014). Pilot study: Efficacy of sensory integration therapy for Japanese children with high-functioning autism spectrum disorder. *Occupational Therapy International, 21*(1), 4–11. https://doi.org/10.1002/oti.1357

Jacobs, E., & Schneider, M. L. (2001). Neuroplasticity and the environment: Implication for sensory integration. In S. Smith Roley, E. I. Blanche, & R. C. Schaaf (Eds.), *Understanding the nature of sensory integration with diverse populations* (pp. 29–40). Pro-Ed, INc.

Jenkins, B. A., & Lumpkin, E. A. (2017). Developing a sense of touch. *Development, 144*(22), 4078–4090. https://doi.org/10.1242/dev.120402

Jenkins, et al. (1990) as cited in Kandel, E. R., Schwartz, J. H., Jessell, T. M., Seigelbaum, S. A., & Hudspeth, A. J. (2013). *Principles of neuroscience* (5th ed.). The McGraw Hill Companies.

Kandel, E. R., Koester, J. D., Mack, S. H., & Seigelbaum, S. A. (2021). *Principles of neuroscience* (6th ed.). The McGraw Hill Companies.

Kashefimehr, B., Kayihan, H., & Huri, M. (2018). The effect of sensory integration therapy on occupational performance in children with autism. *OTJR, 38*(2), 75–83. https://doi.org/10.1177/1539449217743456

Kemperman, G., & Gage, F. H. (1999). New nerve cells for the adult brain. *Scientific American, 280*, 48–53. http://www.jstor.org/stable/26058240

Keysers, C., Kaas, J., & Gazzola, V. (2010). Somatosensation in social perception. *Nat Rev Neuroscience, 11*, 417–428. https://doi.org/10.1038/nrn2833

Kientz, M. A., & Dunn, W. (1997). A comparison of the performance of children with and without autism on the sensory profile. *American Journal of Occupational Therapy, 51*(7), 530–537. https://doi.org/10.5014/ajot.51.7.530

Kilroy, E., Aziz-Zadeh, L., & Cermak, S. A. (2019a). Ayres theories of autism and sensory integration revisited: What contemporary neuroscience has to say. *Brain Sciences, 9*(3), 68.

Kilroy, E., Cermak, S. A., & Aziz-Zadeh, L. (2019b). A review of functional and structural neurobiology of the action observation network in autism spectrum disorder and developmental coordination disorder. *Brain Sciences, 9*(4), 75.

Kilroy, E., Harrison, L., Butera, C., Jayashankar, A., Cermak, S., Kaplan, J., Williams, M., Haranin, E., Bookheimer, S., Dapretto, M., & Aziz-Zadeh, L. (2020). Unique deficit in embodied simulation in autism: An fMRI study comparing autism and developmental coordination disorder. *Human Brain Mapping, 42*(5), 1532–1546.

Kilroy, E., Ring, P., Hossain, A., Nalbach, A., Butera, C., Harrison, L., Jayashankar, A., Vigen, C., Aziz-Zadeh, L., & Cermak, S. A. (2022). Motor performance, praxis, and social skills in autism spectrum disorder and developmental coordination disorder. *Autism Research, 15*(9), 1649–1664.

Kirby, A. V., Bilder, D. A., Wiggins, L. D., Hughes, M. M., Davis, J., Hall-Lande, J. A., Lee, L. C., McMahon, W. M., & Bakian, A. V. (2022). Sensory features in autism: Findings from a large population-based surveillance system. *Autism Res, 15*(4), 751–760. https://doi.org/10.1002/aur.2670

Koomar, J., & Bundy, A. (2002). Creating direct intervention from theory. In A. Bundy, S. Lane & E. Murray (Eds.), *Sensory integration theory and practice* (2nd ed., pp. 261–306). F. A. Davis.

Kramer, G. (2001). Developmental neuroplasticity. In S. Smith Roley, E. I. Blanche, & R. C. Schaaf (Eds.), *Understanding the nature of sensory integration with diverse populations* (pp. 43–55). Pro-Ed, I.

Lamash, L., Grady-Dominguez, P., Mailloux, Z., Parham, L. D., Schaaf, R. C., Smith Roley, S., & Gal, E. (2022). Brief Report—EASI Praxis tests: Age trends and internal consistency. *American Journal of Occupational Therapy, 76*, 7602345020. https://doi.org/10.5014/ajot.2022.049145

Lane, S. J., Leão, M. A., Spielmann, V. (2022). Sleep, sensory integration/processing, and autism: A scoping review. *Front Psychol, 13*, 877527. https://doi.org/10.3389/fpsyg.2022.877527

Lane, S. J., Mailloux, Z., Schoen, S., Bundy, A., May-Benson, T. A., Parham, L. D., Smith Roley, S., & Schaaf, R. C. (2019). Neural Foundations of Ayres Sensory Integration®. *Brain Science*, 9(7), 153. https://doi.org/10.3390/brainsci9070153

Lane, S. J., Reynolds, S., & Dumenci, L. (2012). Sensory overresponsivity and anxiety in typically developing children and children with autism and attention deficit hyperactivity disorder: Cause or coexistence? *American Journal of Occupational Therapy, 66*, 595–603. https://doi.org/10.5014/ajot.2012.004523

Lane, S. J., & Schaaf, R. C. (2010). Examining the neuroscience evidence for sensory-driven neuroplasticity: Implications for sensory-based occupational therapy for children and adolescents. *American Journal of Occupational Therapy, 64*, 375–390. https://doi.org/10.5014/ajot.2010.09069

Lane, S. J., Smith Roley, S., & Champagne, T. (2013). Sensory integration and processing: Theory and applications to occupational performance. In B. Schell & G. Gillen (Eds.), *Willard and Spackman's occupational therapy* (12th ed., pp. 816–868). Lippincott Williams & Wilkins.

Little, L. M., Freuler, A. C., Houser, M. B., Guckian, L., Carbine, K., David, F. J., & Baranek G. T. (2011). *Psychometric validation of the sensory experiences questionnaire*. *American Journal of Occupational Therapy, 65*, 207–210. https://doi.org/10.5014/ajot.2011.000844

Mailloux, Z., Grady, P., Petersen, J., Parham, L. D., Roley, S. S., Bundy, A., & Schaaf, R. C. (2021). Evaluation in Ayres Sensory Integration (EASI) vestibular and proprioceptive tests: Construct validity and internal consistency. *American Journal of Occupational Therapy, 75,* 1–11. https://doi.org/10.5014/ajot.2021.043166

Mailloux, Z., Grady, P., Petersen, J., Parham, L. D., Roley, S. S., Bundy, A., & Schaaf, R. C. (2023). Evaluation in Ayres Sensory Integration Praxis Tests: Construct validity and internal reliability. *American Journal of Occupational Therapy, 77*, 4.

Mailloux, Z. K., May-Benson, T. A., Summers, C. A., Miller, L. J., Burke, J. P., Brett-Green, B., Burke, J. P., Cohn, E. S., Koomar, J. A., Parham, L. D., Roley, S. S., Schaaf, R. C., & Schoen, S. A. (2007). Goal attainment scaling as a measure of meaningful outcomes for children with sensory integration disorders. *American Journal of Occupational Therapy, 61*(2), 254–259. https://doi.org/10.5014/ajot.61.2.254

Mailloux, Z., Mulligan, S., Smith Roley, S., Blanche, E., Cermak, S., Coleman, G. G., Bodison S., & Lane, C. J. (2011). Verification and clarification of patterns of sensory integrative dysfunction in a retrospective clinical sample. *American Journal of Occupational Therapy, 65*(2), 143–151. https://doi.org/10.5014/ajot.2011.000752

Mailloux, Z., Parham, L. D., Roley, S. S., Ruzzano, L., & Schaaf, R. C. (2017). Introduction to the evaluation in Ayres sensory Integration® (EASI). *American Journal of Occupational Therapy, 72*, 7201195030p1-7201195030p7. https://doi.org/10.5014/ajot.2018.028241

May-Benson, T. (2001). A theoretical model of ideation in praxis. In S. Smith Roley, E. I. Blanche, & R. C. Schaaf (Eds.), *Understanding the nature of sensory integration with diverse populations* (pp. 163–179). ProEd.

May-Benson, T. A., & Cermak, S. A. (2007). Development of an assessment for ideational praxis. *American Journal of Occupational Therapy, 61*, 148–153. https://doi.org/10.5014/ajot.61.2.148

May-Benson, T. A., Smith Roley, S., Mailloux, Z., Parham, L. D., Koomar, J., Schaaf, R. C., Van Jaarsveld, A. V., & Cohn, E. (2014). Interrater reliability and discriminative validity of the structural elements of the Ayres sensory integration® fidelity measure. *American Journal of Occupational Therapy, 68*, 506–513. https://doi.org/10.5014/ajot.2014.010652

McIntosh, D. N., Miller, L. J., Shyu, V., & Hagerman, R. (1999). Sensory-modulation disruption, electrodermal responses, and functional behaviors. *Developmental Medicine and Child Neurology, 41*(9), 608–615.

Merzenich, M. M., Nelson, R. J., Stryker, M. P., Cynader, M. S., Schoppmann, A., & Zook, J. M. (1984). Somatosensory cortical map changes following digit amputation in adult monkeys. *Journal of Comparative Neurology, 224*, 591–605. https://doi.org/10.1002/cne.902240408

Mesulam, M. M. (1998). From sensation to cognition. *Brain, 121*(Pt. 6), 1013–1052.

Miller, L. J., Coll, J. R., & Schoen, S. A. (2007a). A randomized controlled pilot study of the effectiveness of occupational therapy for children with sensory modulation disorder. *American Journal of Occupational Therapy, 61*(2), 228–238. https://doi.org/10.5014/ajot.61.2.228

Miller, L. J., Nielsen, D. M., & Schoen, S. A. (2011). Attention deficit hyperactivity disorder and sensory modulation disorder: A comparison of behavior and physiology. *Research in Developmental Disabilities, 33*(3), 804–818. https://doi.org/10.1016/j.ridd.2011.12.005

Miller, L. J., Schoen, S. A., James, K., & Schaaf, R. C. (2007b). Lessons learned: A pilot study on occupational therapy effectiveness for children with sensory modulation disorder. *American Journal of Occupational Therapy, 61*, 161–169. https://doi.org/10.5014/ajot.61.2.161

Mulligan, S. (1998a). Patterns of sensory integration dysfunction: A confirmatory factor analysis, *American Journal of Occupational Therapy, 52*, 819–828. https://doi.org/10.5014/ajot.52.10.829

Mulligan, S. (1998b). Application of structural equation modeling in occupational therapy research, *American Journal of Occupational Therapy, 52*, 829–834.

Neumann, E. A. (1971). *The elements of play*. MSS Information.

Odom, S. L. Hall, L. J., Morin, K. L., Kraemer, B. R., Hume, K. A., McIntyre, N. S., Nowell, S. W., Steinbrenner, J. R., Tomaszewski, B., Sam, A. M., & DeWalt, L. (2021). Educational interventions for Children with youth and autism: A 40-year perspective. *Journal of Autism and Developmental Disorders, 51(*12), 4354–4369. https://doi.org/10.1007/s10803-021-04990-1

Omairi, C., Mailloux, Z., Antoniuk, S. A., & Schaaf, R. (2022). Occupational therapy using Ayres sensory integration®: A randomized controlled trial in Brazil. *American Journal of Occupational Therapy*, *76*(4), 7604205160. https://doi.org/10.5014/ajot.2022.048249

O'Neill, M., & Jones, R. S. (1997). Sensory-perceptual abnormalities in autism: a case for more research? *Journal of Autism and Developmental Disorders, 27*(3), 283–293.

Parham, L. D. (2022). Sensory integration in everyday life. In A. C. Bundy, S. J. Lane, & E. A. Murray (Eds.), *Sensory integration: Theory and practice* (2nd ed., pp. 21–39). F. A. Davis.

Parham, L. D., Cohn, E. S., Spitzer, S., Koomar, J. A., Miller, L. J., Burke, J. P., Brett-Green, B., Mailloux, Z., May-Benson, T. A., Smith Roley, S., Schaaf, R. C., Schoen, S. A., & Summers, C. A. (2007). Fidelity in sensory integration intervention research. *American Journal of Occupational Therapy, 61*(2), 216–227. https://doi.org/10.5014/ajot.61.2.216

Parham, L. D., Ecker, C. L., Kuhaneck, H., Henry, D. A., & Glennon, T. J. (2021). *Sensory processing measure, second edition (SPM-2)*. Western Psychological Services.

Parham, L. D., & Mailloux, Z. (2015). Sensory integration. In J. Case-Smith & J. O'Brien (Eds.), *Occupational therapy for children and adolescents* (7th ed., pp. 258–303). Mosby Elsevier.

Parham, L. D., Roley, S. S., May-Benson, T. A., Koomar, J., Brett-Green, B., Burke, J. P., Cohn, E. S., Mailloux, Z., Miller, L. J., & Schaaf, R. C. (2011). Development of a fidelity measure for research on the effectiveness of the Ayres Sensory Integration® intervention. *American Journal of Occupational Therapy, 65*(2), 133–142. https://doi.org/10.5014/ajot.2011.000745

Pfeiffer, B. A., Koenig, K., Kinnealey, M., Sheppard, M., & Henderson, L. (2011). Effectiveness of sensory integration interventions in children with autism spectrum disorders: A pilot study. *American Journal of Occupational Therapy, 65*(1), 76–85. https://doi.org/10.5014/ajot.2011.09205

Quigley, K. S., Rogers, E. N., Kanoski, S., Grill, W. M., & Tsakiris, M. (2020). Functions of interoception: From energy regulation to experience of the self. *Trends Neuroscience, 44*(1), 29–38. https://doi.org/10.1016/j.tins.2020.09.008

Randell, E., Wright, M., Milosevic, S., Gillespie, D., Brookes-Howell, L., Busse-Morris, M., Hastings, R., Maboshe, W., Williams-Thomas, R., Mills, L., Romeo, R., Yaziji, N., McKigney, A. M., Ahuja, A., Warren, G., Glarou, E., Delport, S., & McNamara, R. (2022). Sensory integration therapy for children with autism and sensory processing difficulties: the SenITA RCT. *Health Technol Assess*, *26*(29), 1–140. https://doi.org/10.3310/TQGE0020

Reynolds, S., Bendixen, R. M., Lawrence, T., & Lane, S. J. (2011). A pilot study examining activity participation, sensory responsiveness, and competence in children with high functioning Autism Spectrum Disorder. *Journal of Autism and Developmental Disorders, 41*(11), 1496–1506. https://doi.org/10.1007/s10803-010-1173-x.

Reynolds, S., Lane, S. J., & Richards, L. (2010). Using animal models of enriched environments to inform research on sensory integration intervention for the rehabilitation of neurodevelopmental disorders. *Journal of Neurodevelopmental Disorders*, *2*, 120–132. https://doi.org/10.1007/s11689-010-9053-4

Ringold, S. M., McGuir, R. W., Jayasankar, A., Kilroy, E., Butera, C. D., Harrison, L., Cermak, S. A., & Aziz-Zah, L. (2022). Sensory modulation in children with developmental coordination disorder compared to autism spectrum disorder and typically developing children. *Brain Sciences, 12*(9), 1–24. https://doi.org/10.3390/brainsci12091171

Roan, C., Mailloux, Z., Carroll, A., & Schaaf, R. C. (2022). Brief Report—A parent guidebook for occupational therapy using Ayres Sensory® Integration. *American Journal of Occupational Therapy, 76*, 7605345020. https://doi.org/10.5014/ajot.2022.049419

Rogers, S. J., & Ozonoff, S. (2005). Annotation: What do we know about sensory dysfunction in autism? A critical review of the empirical evidence. *Journal of Child Psychology and Psychiatry, 46*(12), 1255–1268. https://doi.org/10.1111/j.1469-7610.2005.01431.x

Schaaf, R. C., Benevides, R. W., Kelly, D., & Mailloux, Z. (2012). Feasibility, safety, acceptability and fidelity study occupational therapy and sensory integration for children with autism: A feasibility, safety, acceptability, and fidelity study. *Autism, 16*(3), 321–327. https://doi.org/10.1177/1362361311435157

Schaaf, R. C., Benevides, T., Mailloux, Z., Faller, P., Hunt, J., van Hooydonk, E., Freeman, R., Leiby, B., Sendecki, J., & Kelly, D. (2014). An intervention for sensory difficulties in children with autism: A randomized trial. *Journal of Autism and Developmental Disorders, 44*, 1493–1506. https://doi.org/10.1007/s10803-013-1983-8

Schaaf, R. C., Cohn, E. S., Burke, J., Dumont, R., Miller, A., & Mailloux, Z. (2015). Linking sensory factors to participation: Establishing intervention goals with parents for children with autism spectrum disorder. *American Journal of Occupational Therapy, 69*, 6905185005.

Schaaf, R. C., Dumont, R. L., Arbesman, M., & May-Benson, T. A. (2018). Efficacy of occupational therapy using Ayres Sensory Integration®: A systematic review. *American Journal of Occupational Therapy, 72*, 7201190010.

Schaaf, R. C., Hunt, J., & Benevides, T. (2012). Occupational therapy using sensory integration to improve participation of a child with autism: A case report. *American Journal of Occupational Therapy, 66*, 547–555. http://dx.doi.org/10.5014/ajot.2012.004473

Schaaf, R. C., & Mailloux, Z. (2015). *Clinician's guide for implementing Ayres sensory integration®: Promoting participation for children with autism*. Bethesda, MD: AOTA Press.

Schaaf, R. C., Mailloux, Z., Ridgway, E., Berruti, A. S., Dumont, R., Jones, E. A., Leiby, B. E., Sancimino, C., Yi, M., & Molholm, S. (2022). Sensory phenotypes in Autism: Making a case for the inclusion of sensory integration functions. *Journal of Autism and Developmental Disorders, 53*(12), 4759–4771. https://doi.org/10.1007/s10803-022-05763-0

Schaaf, R. C., & Miller, L. J. (2005). Occupational therapy using a sensory integrative approach for children with developmental disabilities. *Mental Retardation and Developmental Disabilities Research Reserve, 11*(2), 143–148. https://doi.org/10.1002/mrdd.20067

Schaaf, R. C., & Nightlinger, K. M. (2007). Occupational therapy using a sensory integrative approach: A case study of effectiveness. *American Journal of Occupational Therapy, 61*, 239–246. https://doi.org/10.5014/ajot.61.2.239

Schaaf, R. C., Schoen, S. A., Smith Roley, S., Lane, S. J., Koomar, J. A., & May-Benson, T. A. (2010). A frame of reference for sensory integration. In P. Kramer & J. Hinojosa (Eds.), *Frames of reference for pediatric occupational therapy* (3rd ed., p. 127). Lippincott Williams & Wilkins.

Schaaf, R. C., & Smith Roley, S. (2006). *Sensory Integration: Applying clinical reasoning to practice with diverse populations*. Pro-Ed, Inc.

Schaaf, R. C., Toth-Cohen, S., Johnson, S. L., Outten, G., & Benevides, T. W. (2011). The everyday routines of families of children with autism: Examining the impact of sensory processing difficulties on the family. *Autism. 15*(3), 373–389. https://doi.org/10.1177/1362361310386505

Schaaf, R. C., Wright, K. A., Mailloux, Z., Grady, P., Parham, L. D., Roley, S. S., & Bundy, A. (2023). Evaluation in Ayres Sensory Integration® (EASI) Tactile Perception Tests: Construct validity and internal reliability. *American Journal of Occupational Therapy, 77*, 7701205050. doi:10.5014/ajot.2023.050053

Schmitt C. M., & Schoen, S. (2022). Interoception: A multi-sensory foundation of participation in daily life. *Frontiers in Neuroscience, 16*, 875200. https://doi.org/10.3389/fnins.2022.875200

Schneider, M. L., Moore, C. F., Adkins, M., Barr, C. S., Larson, J. A., Resch, L. M., & Roberts, A. (2016). Sensory processing in Rhesus monkeys: Developmental continuity, prenatal treatment, and genetic influences. *Child Development, 88*(1), 183–197. https://doi.org/10.1111/cdev.12572

Schneider, M. L., Moore, C. F., Gajewski, L. L., Laughlin, N. K., Larson, J. A., Gay, C. L., Roberts, A. D., Converse, A. K., & DeJesus, O. T. (2008). Sensory processing disorders in a nonhuman primate model: Evidence for occupational therapy practice. *American Journal of Occupational Therapy, 61*(2), 247–253. https://doi.org/10.5014/ajot.61.2.247

Schoen, S. A., Lane, S. J., Mailloux, Z., May-Benson, T., Parham, L. D., Smith Roley, S., Schaaf, R. C. (2019). A systematic review of ayres sensory integration intervention for children with autism. *Autism Research*, 1–14. https://doi.org/10.1002/aur.2046

Sherrington, C. S. (1906). *The integrative action of the nervous system*. Yale University Press.

Sieg, K. W. (1988). A. Jean Ayres. In B. R. J. Miller, K. W. Sieg, F. M. Ludwig, S. D. Shortridge, & J. V. Deuson (Eds.), *Six perspectives on theory for the practice of occupational therapy* (pp. 95–142). Aspen Publishers.

Smith Roley, S. (2006). Evaluating sensory integration function and dysfunction. In R. C. Schaaf & S. Smith Roley (Eds.), *Sensory Integration: Applying clinical reasoning to practice with diverse populations*. Pro-Ed, Inc.

Smith Roley, S., Blanche, E. I., & Schaaf, R. C, (Eds.). (2001). *Understanding the nature of sensory integration with diverse populations*. ProEd, Inc.

Smith Roley, S., Mailloux, Z., Miller-Kuhanek, H., & Glennon, T. (2007). Understanding Ayres sensory Integration®. *OT Practice, 12*(17), CE1–CE8.

Smith Roley, S., Mailloux, Z., Parham, L. D., Schaaf, R. C., Lane, C. J., & Cermak, S. (2015). Sensory integration and praxis patterns in children with autism. *American Journal of Occupational Therapy, 69*, 1–8. https://doi.org/10.5014/ajot.2015.012476

Smith Roley, S., & Schneck, C. (2006). Sensory integration for children with visual impairments including blindness. In R. C. Schaaf & S. Smith Roley (Eds.), *Sensory integration: Applying clinical reasoning to practice with diverse populations* (pp. 149–164). Pro-Ed, Inc.

Smyre, S. A., Bean, N. L., Stein, B. E., & Rowland, B. A. (2023). Predictability alters multisensory responses by modulating unisensory inputs. *Frontiers in Neuroscience, 17*, 1150168. https://doi.org/10.3389/fnins.2023.1150168

Spitzer, S., & Smith Roley, S. (2001). Sensory integration revisited: A philosophy of practice. In S. Smith Roley, E. I. Blanche, & R. C. Schaaf (Eds.), *Understanding the nature of sensory integration with diverse populations* (pp. 3–23). Pro-Ed, Inc.

Stein, B. E., Stanford, T. R., & Rowland, B. A. (2020). Multisensory integration and the Society for Neuroscience: Then and now. *Journal of Neuroscience*, *40*(1), 3–11. https://doi.org/10.1523/JNEUROSCI.0737-19.2019

Steinbrenner, J. R., Hume, K., Odom, S. L., Morin, K. L., Nowell, S. W., Tomaszewski, B., Szendrey, S., McIntyre, N. S., Yücesoy-Özkan, S., & Savage, M. N. (2020). *Evidence-based practices for children, youth, and young adults with Autism*. The University of North Carolina at Chapel Hill, Frank Porter Graham Child Development Institute, National Clearinghouse on Autism Evidence and Practice Review Team.

Tomcheck, S. D., & Dunn, W. (2007). Sensory processing in children with and without autism: A comparative study using a short sensory profile. *The American Journal of Occupational Therapy*, *61*(2), 190–200. https://doi.org/10.5014/ajot.61.2.190

Van Jaarsveld, A., Mailloux, Z., Smith Roley, S., & Raubenheimer, J. (2015). Patterns of sensory integration dysfunction in children from South Africa. *South African Journal of Occupational Therapy, 44*(2), 2–6.

Watling, R., Miller Kuhaneck, H., Parham, L. D., & Schaaf, R. (2018). *Occupational therapy practice guidelines for children and youth with challenges in sensory integration and sensory processing*. AOTA Press.

Whiting, C. C., Schoen, S. A., & Niemeyer, L. (2023). A sensory integration intervention in the school setting to support performance and participation: A multiple-baseline study. *American Journal of Occupational Therapy, 77*, 7702205060. https://doi.org/10.5014/ajot.2023.050135

Williams, D. (1992). *Nobody nowhere: The remarkable autobiography of an autistic girl*. Jessica Kingsley Publishers.

Williams, D. (1994). *Somebody somewhere*. Doubleday.

Williams, Z. J., Schaaf, R. C., Ausderau, K. K., Baranek, G. T., Barrett, D. J., Cascio, C. J., Dumont, R. L., Eyoh, E. E., Failla, M. D., Feldman, J. I., Foss-Feig, J. H., Green, H. L., Green, S. A., He, J. L., Kaplan-Kahn, E. A., Keçeli-Kaysılı, B., MacLennan, K., Mailloux, Z., Marco, E., ... Woynaroski, T. G. (2023). Examining the latent structure and correlates of sensory reactivity in Autism: A multi-site integrative data analysis by the Autism Sensory Research Consortium. *Research Square*, rs.3.rs-2447849. https://doi.org/10.21203/rs.3.rs-2447849/v1

Wolfe, J. M., Kluender, K. R., & Levi, D. M. (2020). *Sensation and perception* (6th ed.). Sinaur Associates, Inc.

7 A Frame of Reference for Sensory Integration and Processing Differences: Sensory Therapies and Research (STAR)

Virginia Spielmann ■ Sarah A. Schoen ■ Lisa M. Porter

Individuals with differences in the sensory integration process often require unique interventions designed to meet their individual needs. One such approach is the Sensory Therapies and Research (STAR) frame of reference. This frame of reference assumes the individual is a complex, dynamic system drawing on an amalgam of perspectives from humanistic psychology, neurobiology, developmental theory, a psycho-bio-socio-ecological (BPS-E) perspective of disability, relationship-based approaches including Developmental, Individual Differences, Relationship-based (DIR)/Floortime® and attachment theory (Greenspan & Wieder, 1998), and sensory integration theory as conceptualized by Ayres (Ayres, 1972, 1979). Although this chapter focuses on children, the STAR frame of reference is applicable across the lifespan and in varied contexts (Miller et al., 2023; Schoen et al., 2019, 2022). It has been adapted for use with adults and adolescents, and for use in group settings.

STAR is a family-centered approach that addresses the child's needs in three dimensions (1) through one-to-one occupational therapy with a relationship-based sensory integrative approach; (2) by focusing on the caregiver–child relationship and coaching parents in strategies designed to enhance sensory health and wellness; (3) through provision of environmental accommodations and adaptations. The central focus of the STAR frame of reference is the agency and autonomy of the child and the well-being of the entire family unit. STAR is flexible and individualized to the child and family's needs and priorities. Through parent education and collaboration supportive strategies and accommodations are integrated into the child's natural environments at home, at school, and in the community.

The STAR frame of reference provides a framework for understanding the sensory integration process and its dynamic relationship to occupation and family co-occupations. The intervention described is for individuals experiencing barriers to occupational engagement attributed to differences in the integration of internal and external sensory experiences. The STAR frame of reference is most commonly employed to support neurodivergent children and their families, this includes the following neurotypes: sensory processing disorder, autism spectrum disorders, attention-deficit hyperactivity disorder, generalized anxiety disorder, gifted and/or twice exceptional, developmental coordination disorder, fetal alcohol spectrum disorder, and other neurodevelopmental differences. The STAR frame of reference strives to be neurodiversity affirming which means that different neurotypes are *not* considered psychopathologies. Therefore, identity-first language is used wherever possible, and all practitioners are encouraged to engage in reflective supervision that supports unlearning of ableist assumptions, and postprofessional learning led by neurodivergent educators.

DEFINITIONS IMPORTANT TO THIS FRAME OF REFERENCE

Agency: The ability to make choices and successfully act on them to change your situation.
Autonomy: The freedom and/or ability to be driven by one's own interests and desires (intrinsic motivation) and the source of one's own behavior (self-organization).
Neurodiversity: The variety in how our brains work. In a neurodiversity-affirming frame of reference, these differences are recognized and respected as any other human variation.
Neurodivergence: Variations in the human brain regarding sensory processing, learning, attention, interpersonal style, and other neurodevelopmental functions.
Neurotype: Specific neurodivergences. These include, but are not limited to, Dyspraxia, Dyslexia, Attention-Deficit Hyperactivity Disorder, Autism, Tourette Syndrome, Anxiety, Sensory Processing Disorder.
Sensory Integration and Processing (SI-SP): For the purposes of this chapter, we will be using the term SI-SP (Watling et al., 2018). The terms Sensory Integration Dysfunction, Sensory Processing Disorder, and sensory processing differences frequently appear in the literature and are often used interchangeably. However, this chapter emphasizes the distinction between sensory processing differences and instances when these differences significantly impact an individual's daily life, carefully avoiding the use of "disorder" or "dysfunction" to acknowledge that not all sensory processing variations lead to difficulties or disabilities.

THEORETICAL BASE

The STAR frame of reference is a robust clinical reasoning tool that expertly combines the DIR model, sensory integration theory (as conceptualized by Ayres, see Chapter 6), theories of nervous system state regulation, attachment theory, and dynamic systems theory. It is client-centered, supports complex clinical reasoning, and is affirming of the neurodivergent lived experience.

The DIR model is centered on nurturing functional emotional developmental capacities and offers strategies to support growth in this area (Greenspan et al., 2001; Wieder, 2017). This approach emphasizes the power of sensory-affective communication between individuals, where interactions with attuned and attentive adults—often a practitioner working collaboratively with involved parents—can enhance these skills. The "I" in DIR stands for individual differences, and a large proportion of the "I" in the model relates to the sensory integration process. These individual differences wield significant influence over functional emotional development, potentially shaping it for better or for worse. Additionally, it is important to note the bidirectional relationship between these domains which means that enhancing functional emotional development may lead to growth in SI-SP capabilities. SI-SP differences significantly influence various aspects of human development, especially during co-occupations between caregivers and infants where continuous sociosensory signals are shared. These exchanges lay the foundation for secure attachment bonds and support coregulation, as caregivers and infants regulate arousal levels through their interactions. Sensory experiences play a key role in forming relationships, cultivating coregulation and fostering self-regulation. These interactions help infants learn about the *cause-and-effect* of their actions, nurturing a sense of agency. By simultaneously considering the social–emotional responses of caregivers and children along with the neurobiologic responses of the sensory system, a holistic and dynamic approach is taken to address the interconnected sensory–motor and social–emotional aspects of development.

Theories regarding the nervous system state regulation are outlined in the table below (Table 7.1). The collective insights from these theories converge to form a holistic understanding of well-being grounded in nervous system regulation, relationship dynamics, and the sensory integration process. This perspective emphasizes the interconnectedness of nervous system state regulation and social interactions, highlighting how the nervous system responds to external stimuli and interpersonal cues to shape individuals' regulation in the moment and the development of future regulation capacities. By recognizing the triad domains of relationships, regulation, and the sensory integration process, this approach underscores the importance of a balanced and connected nervous system in promoting well-being.

Attachment theory, as pioneered by John Bowlby (1969), Mary Ainsworth (1979), and Mary Main (1986), offers a foundational framework for understanding the formation of emotional bonds and their impact on development. The insights from attachment theory resonate with the collective perspectives of the theorists in Table 7.1, particularly in highlighting the significance of early relationships in shaping emotional regulation and well-being. Ayres' work on sensory integration further enriches this understanding by emphasizing how sensory experiences contribute to the child's psychic inner world, influencing their emotional responses and regulatory processes. Furthermore, DIR/Floortime® contributions to developmental psychology underscore the importance of emotional connections and attuned interactions in promoting healthy development, aligning closely with the principles of attachment theory. By integrating these perspectives, a comprehensive view emerges, emphasizing the intricate interplay between relationships, SI-SP, and regulation in fostering optimal development and well-being.

ASSUMPTIONS

The dynamic systems theory of human development sets the stage for the entire frame of reference. In keeping with dynamic systems thinking a BPS-E perspective of disability is also explicitly employed.

People are, and are part of, a dynamic system consisting of complex, adaptive, and interactive subsystems, which change over time (Arthur, 1999; Thelen, 2005). We consider the brain and body as parts of the system, unique to each individual. Furthermore, we recognize the essential role of external systems including the environment, relationships, and contexts of our immediate and extended communities. The dynamic systems perspective encompasses multiple levels when looking at the client. It provides a big picture view of the ecological context, zooms in to the more immediate level concerning caregiver relationships, home context, and other settings where the client spends time and interacts with others, and also delves into the intricate neurobiophysiologic client factors. Consequently, therapy stems from holistic analysis of the person with an in-depth analysis of changing domains, contexts, and systems within systems (Royeen, 2003). The four statements listed below are viewed as assumptions within the STAR frame of reference but are also noted as theoretical principles of dynamic systems theory.

- Nonlinear development: Development is a dynamic process that does not happen in an orderly straight line. The child is a system within many nested systems (family, community, state,

Table 7.1 Theories Underlying Nervous System Regulation and Relationship Dynamics

Theorist	Approx. Date	Main Proposal	Key Idea
Baumeister	1994	Self-regulation and social relationships	Emphasizes the role of self-regulation in social interactions and relationships
Beebe	1977	Infant–parent communication patterns and attachment dynamics	Early infant–caregiver interaction patterns and attachment dynamics influence the development of nervous system regulation in infants
Butler & Randall	2013	Embodied self-regulation theory	Focus on the role of the body in shaping self-regulation processes. Highlighting interconnectedness of physical and cognitive processes in the regulation of emotions and behaviors
Feldman (Ruth)	1996	Importance of social interactions in self-regulation and coregulation	Bidirectional influence of social cues on physiologic responses and emotional regulation; emphasis on coregulation in social contexts
Feldman Barrett (Lisa)	1997	Constructed emotion theory	Emphasis on the idea that emotions are constructed in the brain based on past experiences and context, influencing self-regulation and coregulation processes
Fogel	1980	Development of infant communication and social interaction	Emphasis on the role of social interactions in emotional development
Meltzoff	2007	"Like Me Theory," Importance of imitation in social cognition in infancy	Contributions to understanding how infants learn through imitation and social engagement, shaping cognitive, and emotional development; exploration of neural pathways related to social cognition and regulation
Niven	2009	Relation between stress regulation and emotion processing	Examines the interplay between stress regulation, emotion processing, and regulatory mechanisms in behavior and development, contributions to understanding how stress regulation and emotion processing are influenced by relational experiences
Porges	1995	Role of autonomic nervous system (ANS) in social engagement (and vice versa)	Hierarchical organization of ANS, highlighting bidirectional relationship between ANS function, regulation, and relationships
Shanker	2012	Individual regulation strategies with emphasis on coregulation	Focus on identifying and addressing stressors, personalized self-regulation, and the importance of coregulation in development
Siegel	1999	Relationship's impact on brain and emotional regulation	Integration of disciplines to understand mind, brain, and relationships
Trevarthen	1979	Early social interactions in emotional development	Emphasis on rhythmic patterns in infant communication and social engagement
Tronick & Cohn	1989	Reciprocal interactions in coregulating emotions	Focus on dynamic, moment-to-moment exchanges shaping emotional experiences and regulatory processes
Vygotsky	1930s	Sociocultural theory of development	Role of social interactions, cultural tools, and language in shaping cognitive development, self-regulation, and coregulation processes

federal environment etc.) and the child consists of multiple subsystems all acting at the same time and all influencing one another (sensory systems, homeostasis, respiratory, cardiac, etc.) (Fogel et al., 2008; Smith & Thelen, 2003).

- Interactions between systems: Interactions between external systems, including the family, teachers, school systems, cultural experiences, and larger community, can propel or hinder development. Likewise with development and function of the systems within the child. A change in one aspect of a system impacts other aspects of the system (Fogel et al., 2008; Thelen, 2005).
- Systems are self-organizing: Systems are self-organizing and evolve toward attractor states that are dynamically sustained much like a web or suspension bridge (Kamm et al., 1990; Thelen, 1995; Young, 2011). The whole system in combination with the coaction of every part within the system is what produces stability (Fogel et al., 2008). These states of self-organization are open to change. Development in dynamic systems is varied with multiple pathways to success.
- Nothing happens in isolation: Dynamic systems theory postulates that changes occur over time (Fogel et al., 2008) and nothing happens in isolation. Development represents a complex, adaptive interaction between genetics, the organism, the environment, experience, and culture (Bronfenbrenner & Ceci, 1994; Bronfenbrenner & Morris, 2007).

Additionally, the frame of reference is heavily influenced by the BPS-E model of health and disability (Stineman & Streim, 2010). This model recognizes that disability experiences are a result of myriad intersecting factors and considers the context of the client in their physical and cultural environments. It is a comprehensive view that includes relationships and home life as part of environment and context. During childhood, the parent–child relationship provides the most powerful context for intervention (Ainsworth, 1979; Beebe & Lachmann, 2015). The BPS-E model is cross disciplinary and rooted in dynamic systems thinking. Furthermore, it aligns with social models of disability, self-determination theory (Deci & Ryan, 2008), and advocacy work (Stineman & Streim, 2010).

Specifically, the ecological component considers the interaction between a person and their environment and suggests that by making environments more accommodating and inclusive, we can reduce or eradicate the disability experience. In keeping with a neurodiversity affirming perspective this standpoint promotes acceptance and accommodation of neurodivergent individuals, rather than trying to "fix" them to fit into a neuronormative mold.

Operating from these theoretical assumptions emphasizes viewing the client and client–family through a lens of multilayered systems and subsystems that interact in multiple directions. Even when the primary focus of intervention is sensory, the STAR frame of reference advocates for a continuous assessment of regulation, and relationships, in the context of mutable environments, social–emotional development, and attention (Figure 7.1).

THEORETICAL POSTULATES

The theoretical postulates of the STAR frame of reference have four sections. Theories related to (1) regulation, (2) relational health, (3) SI-SP, and (4) environment.

Regulation Is the Foundation of Development

The term regulation refers to nervous system state regulation, but it is not an individualistic phenomenon and can refer to coregulation, interactive regulation, *and* self-regulation. In the case of

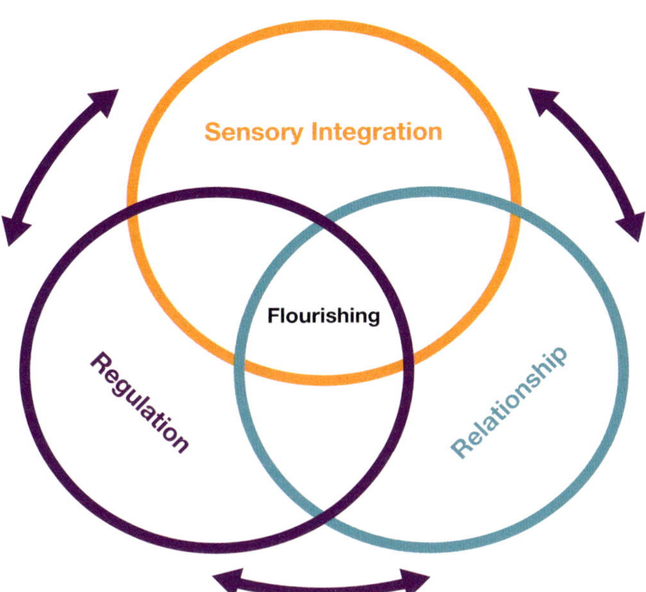

FIGURE 7.1 Three principal domains of human development. (Courtesy of STAR Institute, used with permission.)

infants, as Browne and Talmi (2015) pointed out, the ability to "regulate" is a precursor to the more conventional milestones of early childhood, developed across multiple domains, including:

- biologic/physiologic (respiration, thermoregulation, perfusion, digestion, and elimination),
- arousal (awake/alert cycle and circadian rhythm),
- body movement (tone, posture, motor control),
- interactions (availability, responsiveness, engagement), and
- eating and soothing (self-regulation, self-soothing, and coregulation).

Within the newborn and young infant period, the term regulation refers to the process of adjusting to life outside the womb when regulation is no longer provided by the mother's body. This requires maintaining homeostasis and the "just right" state of arousal by adapting to the current environment and task demands (Browne & Talmi, 2015; Papoušek, 2008; Szklut, 2014).

The parent must regulate self and coregulate the neonate, this involves a kind of *loaning* of the parents' more mature nervous system. As the neonate matures, they begin to develop self-regulation capacities with parent support (Fonagy, 2015). Within the context of daily co-occupations, millions of social exchanges occur and the development of the regulatory system takes place (Browne & Talmi, 2015). Indeed, in keeping with systems theory this relationship is bidirectional; as the caregiver's relationship supports the development of regulation, and that regulation feeds back into the parent's arousal and ability to coregulate. It is impossible to extract the relationship from the theory of regulation.

Early regulation is a foundational capacity for the development of later fundamental competencies (Greenspan & Greenspan, 2010; Greenspan et al., 2001; Greenspan & Wieder, 2006; Lillas & Turnbull, 2009; Wieder & Wachs, 2012). Regulation plays a pivotal role in the development of self and attachment to the primary caregiver(s) (Nugent et al., 2007) and has been linked to the development of cognitive processing, independent learning (Graziano et al., 2007), resiliency, and the skills necessary for school readiness and academic achievement (Spinrad et al., 2006). Self-regulation

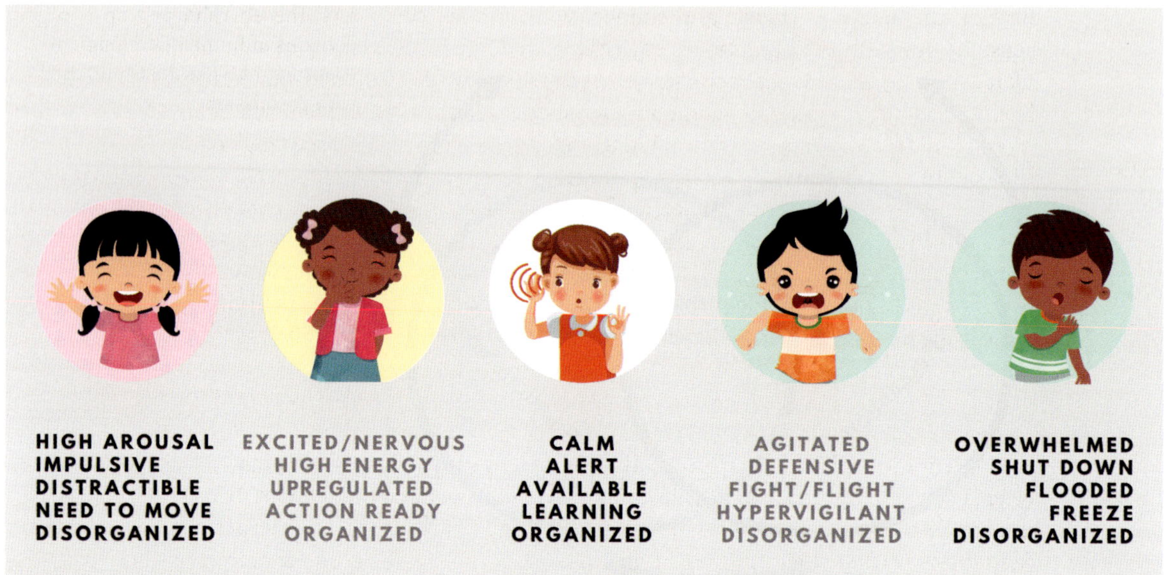

FIGURE 7.2 Regulation continuum. (Courtesy of STAR Institute, used with permission.)

and coregulation are circular causal processes. As infants initiate, maintain, and adjust to soothing interactions, they learn to repair, evade, and terminate uncomfortable and poorly attuned interactions; this is part of self-regulation (Beebe & Lachmann, 2015). The two processes of self-regulation and coregulation are integrated as both partners regulate their inner state and coordinate with the other (Fonagy, 2015; Harrison & Tronick, 2011). Mutually supportive interaction develops when caregivers can hold the children's mind in their adult minds, look beneath behaviors to the experience and regulation of the child (Figure 7.2), and demonstrate reflective caregiving (Kelly et al., 2005; Martinez-Torteya et al., 2014; Slade, 2005; Slade et al., 2005).

Relationships Drive Development

Human development occurs in the context of relationships from the moment of conception and throughout the lifespan (Greenspan & Shanker, 2004). In infancy, development is embedded within the context of the infant–caregiver dyad (Papoušek et al., 2008). We return to the co-occupations of family life within which infants internalize representations of themselves and their physiologic, social–emotional, sensory, and interoceptive (visceral) experiences. Papoušek et al. (2008) highlight the pivotal role of the parent–infant relationship in shaping infants' development, emphasizing that the core focus of therapy lies not just on the infants or caregivers individually, but on their relationship: the dynamic and crucial bond between caregivers and their infants. This perspective, once more in accordance with systems theory, posits that every therapeutic interaction involves three clients: the child, the caregivers, and the relationships between the child and caregivers, or the dyad (Greenspan & Wieder, 2006; Greenspan et al., 2001; Nugent et al., 2007; Papoušek et al., 2008).

The STAR frame of reference emphasis on relationships is grounded in early attachment research (Allen, 2023; Bowlby, 1969). As infants gain regulatory and attentional capacities, they develop the ability to engage and connect with primary caregivers, thereby shaping an evolving sense of safety in familiar sensory environments. Only in the context of safe, attuned, and coregulated relationships can attachment emerge within which children fully realize the paradox of feeling together and becoming unique (Lichtenberg, 2015). The development of an adaptive attachment pattern sets the stage for the child to engage in progressively more challenging sensory–motor exploration which in turn sets the stage for resiliency and establishing healthy stress responses.

Relationships are often disrupted when children have sensory differences (Ben-Avi et al., 2012; Thye et al., 2017) especially so when these are unidentified. Sensory processing differences can impact functioning in daily life, due to differences in underlying brain mechanism and/or because goodness of fit may be disrupted between parents, children, and the environment. Thus, development may be interrupted, stalled, or become uneven (Ben-Avi et al., 2012; Thye et al., 2017).

The Sensory Integration Process Organizes Development

The integration of sensory information is a developmental process that starts in utero and remains prominent in a child's life until around the age of 7 or 8 years. Sensory data provides information about the physical body as well as the physical and interpersonal environment. Sensations set the stage for body awareness, postural development, motor coordination, attention, activity level, and arousal regulation. As data from the sensory systems are registered and integrated the initial processes of learning about the world, ourselves, and each other, take place. The sensory integration process is a critical client factor that provides the building blocks for development and underlies function and participation in all areas of daily life.

"Sensory Processing is a means to an end and the end is quality of life." (Miller, 2018)

When children do not have organized sensory experiences, development is disrupted which hinders their ability to effectively organize behavior, concentrate, regulate, adapt to their ever-increasing world, and can undermine development of regulation and relationships. See Ayres Sensory Integration Frame of Reference (Chapter 6) for more details.

Bodily self-awareness originates in the interpretation of combined sensory data from external and internal sensation. Exteroceptive data comprises information from our distance senses like vision and sound, as well as our perception of bodily motion and position in relation to the environment (e.g., reaching for a light switch or kicking off your shoes without looking). Interoceptive data involves our awareness of internal bodily functions such as gut motility, a full bladder, or feelings of hunger, and somatic-affective sensations like experiencing butterflies in the stomach or a racing heart. An individual's big picture of the world and of themselves in the world constitutes composite data from multiple sensory systems including sensory data that is generated from their own bodily movements. The sensory integration process is a continuously layered and iterative one, it includes the response actions that we generate based on our perceptions *and* the interpretation of the data generated by those movements and actions (Figure 7.3).

The Environment

The environment provides a broader context in which the child and family exists. The familial environment can provide support and modifications for the child with disabilities and neurodiversity, though parents may need help and education in order to do so. Overall, the larger environment often provides barriers for those with disabilities, both from a physical and emotional perspective. Practitioners may suggest modifications that can be alleviated the barriers for those with disabilities.

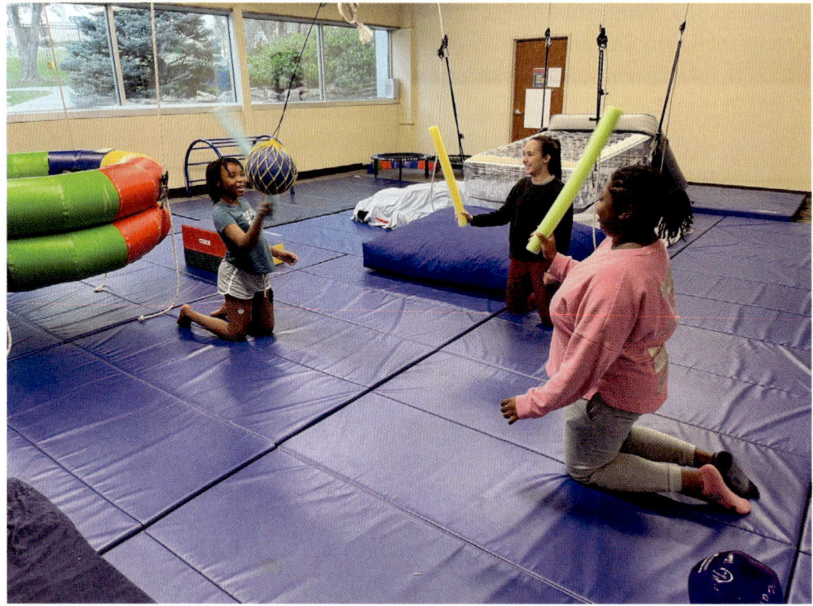

FIGURE 7.3 The sensory integration process organizes development. (Courtesy of STAR Institute, used with permission.)

FUNCTION/DYSFUNCTION CONTINUA

A function–dysfunction continuum facilitates identification of those in need of therapeutic support and facilitates the process of diagnostic clinical reasoning, however clinicians are encouraged to incorporate other perspectives of occupational well-being and occupational marginalization into their ways of thinking. Including the physical and social environment into our understanding of the phenomenon of daily life that those with differences in SI-SP experience could be represented in a quadrant chart (Figure 7.4).

Regulation

Regulation in the STAR frame of reference relates to brain–body readiness for sustaining attention and being in-sync with context while being aware and adaptively responsive to events in the environment. Regulation originates in the nervous system and is a process that supports function through constant adaptation to the ever-changing demands of both our body and surroundings. The process of regulation involves a shifting balance between conscious and unconscious effort, though it is generally perceived as less demanding for individuals with neurotypical responses.

Contextual factors such as temperature, sensory modulation differences, postural development, cultural expectations, interpersonal experiences, performance expectations and challenges, and academic expectations, can alter a person's regulation. One's achievement and maintenance of regulation—especially in childhood—is not considered volitional although conscious strategies to change our state of arousal can be taught and learned as clients develop higher-level executive

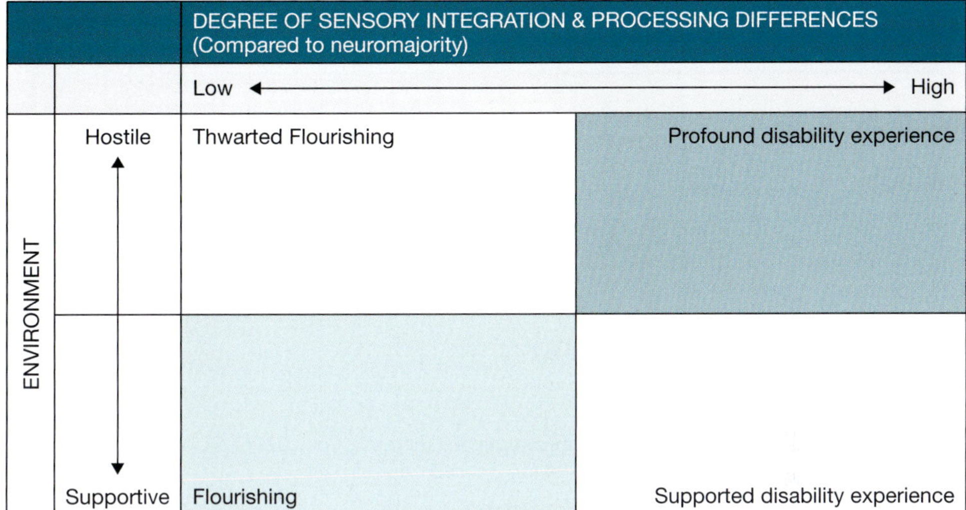

FIGURE 7.4 Quadrant chart representing interaction of the environment and differences in sensory integration and processing. (Courtesy of STAR Institute, used with permission.)

functions. In early life, however, it is generally the responsibility of a caregiving adult to support the child and ensure that they feel safe and available for activity and interaction.

Practitioners are encouraged to learn how to identify their own regulation needs and functional strategies, alongside developing refined attunement to signs of nervous system arousal and resulting regulation capacity in clients of all neurotypes. Adaptive coregulation refers to interpersonal neurobiologic supports that facilitate a state of optimal arousal resulting in regulation in the other person. It is a continuous part of therapy provision and requires constant monitoring and attention. See Figure 7.5 for an example of how a clinician might respond to fluctuating regulation states during a therapy session. As these capacities are cultivated through reflection in and on practice, they can move to supporting coregulation between the caregiver and child.

Children learn the experience of becoming regulated and initial self-regulation ability in the context of their caregiver's ability to coregulate. Sometimes, this process benefits from additional support, particularly when sensory profiles do not naturally match. When caregivers have difficulty matching their child's arousal and affect, intervention focuses on facilitating more accurate reading of their child's cues. For instance, if parents of a child who requires high affect and energy to engage are inactive, exhibit minimal emotional expression in their voice and face, frequently divide their attention, respond slowly, or prioritize other environmental issues over their child, direct coaching on attunement and active involvement in play and other activities become important. Part of the STAR frame of reference involves finding authentic ways for parents of all neurotypes to show sustained interest, follow the child's lead, honor the child's sociosensory needs and demonstrate regulated responses through varied environments and activities.

Relationship

This function relates to the child's relationship to parents and caregivers, other people in the environment, and with their ability to communicate with others (Table 7.2). Positive caregiver

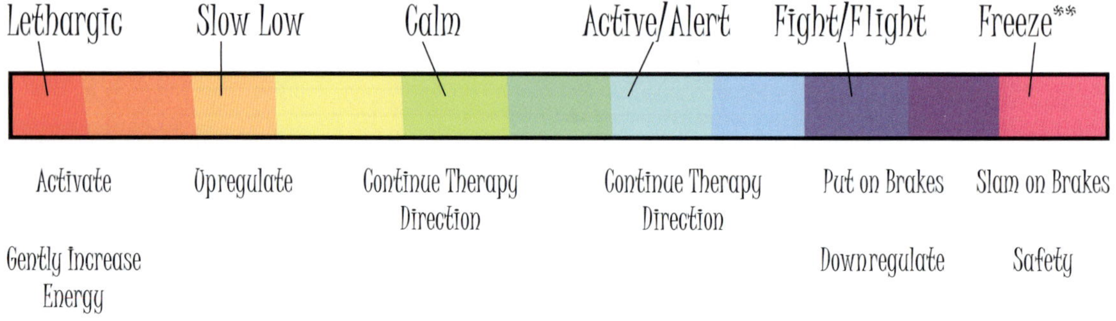

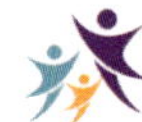

FIGURE 7.5 A regulation continuum with implications for therapy. (Courtesy of STAR Institute, used with permission.)

behaviors are the ability to maintain engagement, signal availability and interest, and notice distress. These caregivers support their child's strategies for recovery, support their child's emotional range in play, and expand play at the just right level. They also support play themes and elaborate on them, giving the child freedom to express themes. Some caregivers need support to give clear cues, to notice their child's response, and to join their child in their preferred activities. Others, who tend to use a more authoritative behavioral parenting style, may initially consider a relationship-based approach to be permissive and need support to focus on connection rather than correction. Caregivers who are overprotective may take time to focus on the flow of play and relax concerns regarding safety or social expectations (Table 7.3).

The Sensory Integration Process

The sensory integration process, as viewed in the STAR perspective, has four distinct sections, sensory modulation, sensory discrimination, posture, and praxis (Figure 7.6). Sensory modulation is how the child's nervous system regulates and responds to sensations. Sensory discrimination is how the child interprets the qualities of sensory information in their life. Posture allows the child to remain stable and upright when engaged in activities. Praxis is the ability to plan, sequence, and execute a motor action.

Table 7.2 Function/Dysfunction Continuum: Indicators for Regulation

Function—the child is able to regulate their behavior and be responsive to the environment	Dysfunction—the child has difficulty regulating behavior and is not generally responsive to the environment
Indicators of Function	**Indicators of Dysfunction**
Calm, attentive, well-modulated, in pace	Sluggish/withdrawn
Available, responsive, in-sync with environment	Agitated/hypervigilant
Activity/Arousal level recovers from distress	Fight/flight/freeze

Table 7.3 Function/Dysfunction Continuum: Relationship Indicators

	Indicators of Function	Indicators of Dysfunction
	Child engages with others and the environment in a confident self-organized manner	**Child has difficulty sustaining engagement with others and the environment**
Availability	Orients, responds, initiates, and shows emotional interest and connection with others	Self-absorbed, withdrawn, or passive. Agitated, fleeting attention to others, overly excited by interactions
Mutual engagement and attachment	Child initiates engagement through smiles, vocalizations, joyful looks and gestures, visual referencing, curiosity and excitement	Child is hypervigilant, constant talking/babbling, turns away, prolonged distress
Communication includes both parties	Child participates in opening and closing circles of communication, purposeful, intentional play, solicits help, variability in play	Child is aimless, impulsive, disorganized. Play is stereotypical or repetitive, does not notice responses
Gestures and problem solving	Child responds to another's lead and expands play, shows a range of emotional themes	Child has constricted themes of play, insists on being in control of play, impulsively changes play
Symbols used to express thoughts and feelings	Child participates in simple problem solving, engages in symbolic play, imitates parent/other, and uses pretend play to convey emotional themes. Allows parent or other to take the lead	Child does not show pleasure in playtime with others, insists on always taking the lead

Lillas, C., & Turnball, J. (2009). *Infant/child mental health, early intervention, and relationship-based therapies: A neurorelational framework for interdisciplnary practice*. Copyright © 2009 by Interdisciplinary Training Institute. Used by permission of W. W. Norton & Company, Inc.

Sensory Modulation

Sensory modulation is how the nervous system regulates and grades responses that are adaptive to sensory situations experienced in daily life. Intervention is indicated when heightened or lowered responsivity cannot be accommodated and interferes with daily life routines and roles. Differences in sensory modulation include sensory overresponsivity (also called hyperreactivity), and sensory underresponsivity (also called hyporeactivity). Sensory overresponsivity is an intense, exaggerated response to sensory events that lasts a long time and may result in anxiety, withdrawal, avoidance, or aggression. Sensory underresponsivity is characterized by muted or slow responses to sensory experiences that may look like lack of awareness, lethargy, or indifference.

Sensory Discrimination

Sensory discrimination (sometimes referred to as sensory perception) is the ability to discern and interpret the qualities of sensory information in daily life. Discrimination permits comparison of details and detection of similarities and differences in sensory features, for instance reaching in your pocket to pull out a key without looking, distinguishing the direction of your name being called, or judging the force required to wash a delicate glass. Sensory discrimination occurs in each of the sensory domains (auditory, tactile, visual, proprioceptive, vestibular, olfactory, gustatory) as well as within the multidimensional interoceptive system, that is, stimuli from gut and other internal organs.

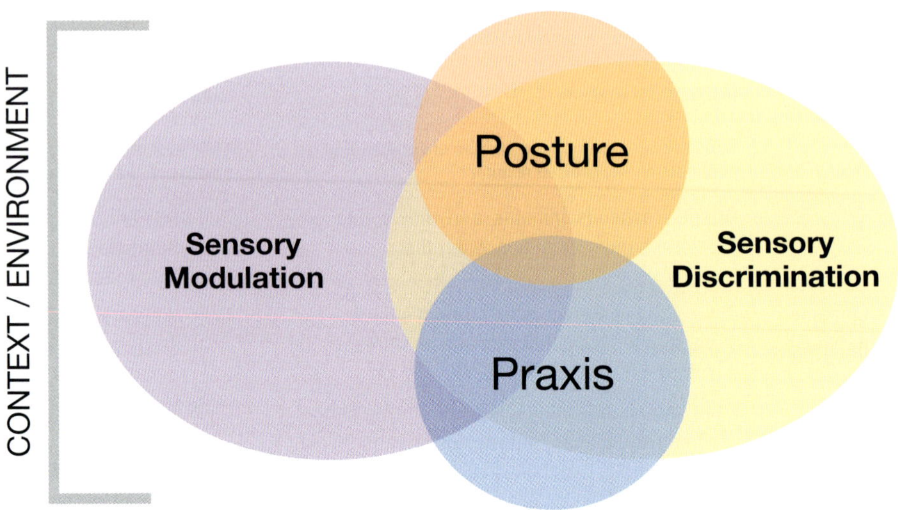

FIGURE 7.6 Topology of sensory integrative processes. (Courtesy of STAR Institute, used with permission.)

Posture

Postural abilities allow children to sustain muscle activation for the completion of daily life activities and routines. Posture serves to maximize endurance and support the ability to move the body and limbs in antigravity positions. Underlying the postural domain are discriminative functions in multisensory interpretation of vestibular and proprioceptive inputs. Without the provision of the "just right" experiences to develop postural abilities and sustain postural activation, children with these differences often present with immature postural development. Children with postural challenges use more effort to remain upright and work very hard to be "ready" for movement and sustain static positions of standing or sitting. They may "slump" when standing or sitting, be unable to adjust body positions for efficient and successful task performance, and/or experience problems with development of ocular-motor control. Low postural tone and impaired joint stability may underlie postural challenges resulting in difficulty with bilateral coordination, motor sequencing, rhythmic activities, and overall motor control. These postural challenges often co-occur with praxis differences.

Praxis

Praxis is characterized by the ability to conceptualize, plan, sequence, execute, evaluate, and problem-solve action. Praxis differences commonly occur in conjunction with lower tactile and proprioceptive responsivity, and/or sensory discrimination differences in the tactile, proprioceptive, and vestibular domains. Without provision of the "just right" experiences to support development of motor mastery, praxis skills will likely remain unexplored and underdeveloped. Children with praxis challenges seem unsure of where their body is in space and often have trouble judging their distance from objects, people, or both. They display difficulty with sequences of movement in which they must judge timing and spacing, particularly if they must mentally project forward to complete a task. Execution of discrete motor skills (e.g., standing, walking, pincer grasp) may

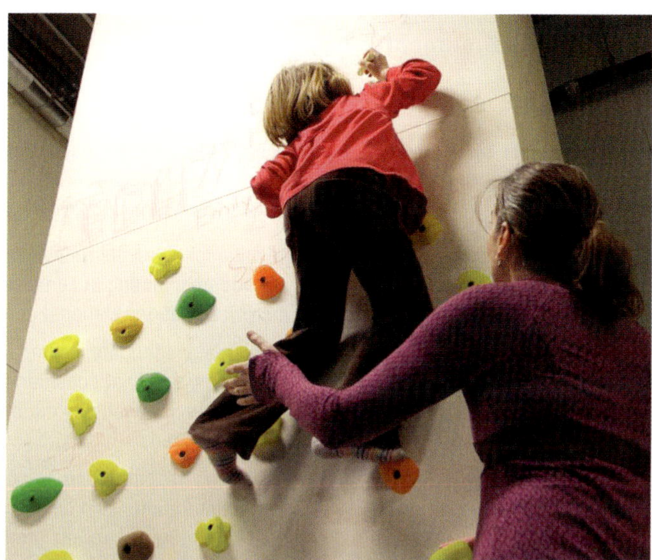

FIGURE 7.7 Ability to respond to novelty and perform activities. (Courtesy of Dr. Lisa Porter, used with permission.)

be age appropriate and adaptive. Splinter skills are skills specific to a few well-defined tasks under highly specific conditions, and these can also be learned by some children. However, the child's ability to respond to novelty and performance of more complex tasks as part of functional activities in a dynamic environment may be compromised (Figure 7.7).

When practic abilities are impacting function and participation, SI-SP should be the primary focus of intervention (Table 7.4).

Table 7.4 Indicators of Function: Sensory Integration and Processing

	Function	Dysfunction
Sensory modulation	The child is able to regulate and grade responses to sensory events to complete daily life activities with autonomy and agency	The child's responses to sensory situations are not adaptive to the situation, too intense or exaggerated The child's responses are muted or slow The child demonstrates disorganization/distress behaviors
	Indicators of Function	**Indicators of Dysfunction**
Sensory discrimination	The child is able to interpret sensory information for use in daily life	The child has difficulty differentiating and interpreting the characteristics and qualities of sensory stimuli within one or more sensory domains
	Indicators of Function	**Indicators of Dysfunction**
Posture	The child has acquired efficient motor skills for performance of daily activities and routines	The child demonstrates delayed/inefficient fine, gross, oral, or visual motor skills interfering with daily life
Praxis	The child is able to conceptualize, plan, organize, sequence, evaluate, and problem solve movements used in daily life	The child has problems conceptualizing, planning, organizing, sequencing, evaluating, and problem-solving movements in daily life

Table 7.5 Function/Dysfunction Continuum: Environmental Function/Dysfunction

	Indicators of Function	Indicators of Dysfunction
	Child is aware of and able to respond to the environment around them positively.	**Child has difficulty responding to the environment and to changes in the environment around them. This contributes to disability experience.**
Physical Environment	Flexible, responsive, supportive, individualized, and accommodating to sensory/sensory motor/regulation/relational differences.	Rigid, inhospitable, obstructive, standardized, nonaccommodating of sensory/sensory motor/regulation/relational differences.
Resource Environment	Diverse strategies, adaptations, and resources are accessible to the individual as needed and in real time to facilitate sensory modulation, sensory–motor success, engagement, and participation.	Unavailable, inadequate, limited access to resources, does not consider/or actively hinders sensory/sensory motor/regulation/relational needs.
Attitudinal Environment	Inclusive, understanding, embraces diversity, welcomes self-advocacy, adapts to accommodate individual differences. Promotes acceptance and support.	One-size-fits-all, pathologizing of sensory/regulation/relationship differences. Sink or swim, merit based, insists on conformity, ignores processing/learning styles.
Proximal/Peripersonal Environment	Individual knows what they need and advocates for their needs across all environments and contexts. Personalized, sensory-sensitive adaptations and accommodations enhancing comfort, engagement, and participation.	Nonadaptive, inaccessible environments lacking accommodation for sensory sensitivities, impedes engagement and function.

Environment

The experience of disability is significantly influenced by the environment, wherein the individual's interaction with societal and environmental barriers plays a crucial role. These barriers can be physical, such as inaccessible buildings or public transportation, or attitudinal, in the form of discrimination or stigma. Consequently, environmental modifications, such as enhanced accessibility or stigma reduction, can alleviate disability. From this standpoint, the practitioner aims to address remediable neurodevelopmental and environmental factors in line with the individual's specific activity limitations and participation constraints (Table 7.5).

GUIDE FOR EVALUATION

The therapist administers a comprehensive occupational therapy evaluation when a child is suspected of having sensory differences that interfere with regulation, relationships, or other aspects of daily life activities, routines, or occupations. The evaluation includes data from multiple sources (e.g., an examiner-administered scale, parent report, teacher report, and structured and unstructured observations in the clinic). The STAR frame of reference uses a process-based approach to evaluation. The evaluation seeks to answer how the child's sensory differences interact with environments and support or undermine their engagement in relationships, regulation, and functioning/participation in daily life. The goals that a therapist will develop at the end of the evaluation reflect the family's priorities and an understanding of the sensory, regulation, and relationship challenges revealed in the child's assessment.

Table 7.6 Linking Assessments to Presenting Problems

Name	Author	Publication Date
Tools for evaluating social–emotional development		
Social-Emotional Assessment/Evaluation Measure	Squires, Bricker, Waddell, Funk, Clifford, & Hoselton	2014
Infant-Toddler Social and Emotional Assessment	Carter, Briggs-Gowan	2006
Brief Infant Toddler Social	Carter, Briggs-Gowan	2006
Greenspan Social-Emotional Growth Chart	Greenspan	2004
Tools for evaluating relationship		
Parenting Interactions with Children: Checklist of Observations Linked to Outcomes	Roggman, Cook, Innocenti, Norman, & Christiansen	2013
Parenting Sense of Competence	Gibaud-Wallston & Wandersman	1978
Emotional Availability Self-Report	Biringen	2008
Tools for evaluating relationship and social–emotional development		
Ages & Stages Questionnaires®: Social-Emotional, Second Edition	Squires, Bricker, & Twombly	2015
Functional Emotional Assessment Scale	Greenspan, DeGangi, & Wieder	2001

The Process

The evaluation begins with the completion of an extensive history form and intake meeting. This preliminary information is obtained about the child and family and includes a developmental history, family history, medical information, and performance in school and the community. The process starts when the therapist meets the family and begins to collect data on the child's attention, activity level, and play preference. The therapist also assesses the child's ability to relate and engage with others and separate from the parent(s). The therapist reviews the presenting problems identified by the parents. This assessment includes administration of a standardized sensory–motor assessment, a SI-SP assessment, and structured and unstructured observations in the clinic (Table 7.6).

Specific Scales

The *Sensory Processing Three Dimensions Scales (SP3DS)* (Miller et al., 2018) is a standardized performance measure that assesses the child evaluating sensory processing. The subtests of the SP3DS measure the three primary patterns of sensory differences: sensory modulation, sensory discrimination, and sensory-based motor. The caregiver questionnaire parallels the structure of the performance assessment. Additionally, the following are included:

1. A caregiver questionnaire asks parents to answer questions about sensory-related behaviors in a child.
2. The *Occupational Performance Screening* captures the parents' perception of how the child's SI-SP challenges impact daily activities and routines and rates the priority for changing those issues in the parents' viewpoint.
3. A *Behavior During Testing Checklist* that evaluates the degree to which atypical sensory behaviors affect regulation and relationships.

It should be noted that a 2-to-3-hour evaluation is an important component of the STAR frame of reference, although it is often not funded by third-party payors. It is necessary to acknowledge to parents and caregivers the many barriers, most notably financial, that exist in the current healthcare system (see Table 7.6).

The assessment is followed by the parent feedback session, a 1-hour meeting with only the parents (no children) during which the therapist conveys the findings of the evaluation. During this session, the therapist shares the data in the form of hypotheses about the impact of sensory processing differences on daily life (e.g., participation, play, and social interaction). In the evaluation report, these hypotheses are conveyed in the form of impact statements, relating sensory challenges to presenting problems (i.e., the impact of challenges in postural control on being accident prone). The goal is to help parents reframe the child's functional challenges in terms of their sensory profile. Goal Attainment Scales (Kiresuk et al., 1994) are used to establish goals that are consistent with both the parents' and therapist views of the needs of the child. A sample is provided (Table 7.7).

An assessment of regulation and relationships is also critical. The therapist takes into account the child, the parent, and the parent–child relationship. Child and parental reciprocity are observable qualitatively during most interactions, starting in the waiting room and including gestural, nonverbal, affective, and more conventional communicative transactions. To a lesser degree, the same can be said of child–parent reciprocity. Considerations of both members of the dyad or triad include regulation, attunement, ability to communicate and interpret communications accurately, emotional availability, disruption and repair, and goodness of fit, including sensory preferences and profiles. When resources are available, the therapist should administer a formal assessment of these components. Structured and unstructured observations are used to confirm hypotheses made about the child during the standardized assessment and in relation to the presenting problems. The examiner observes the child's level of function and provides support to elicit optimal capacities in the areas of arousal, regulation, play, engagement, and participation.

POSTULATES REGARDING CHANGE

General Postulate Regarding Change

The therapeutic process takes place within the context of safety and trust in the sensory gym and the context of the child–caregiver relationship with carryover into home life. Safety and trust are established through genuinely listening to the child, presuming competence, and always honoring consent.

In this case, presuming competence means operating from the assumption that the child has boundless potential and is at least as cognitively able as their peers. Throughout the treatment process, essential components of the therapeutic environment are the practitioner, the parent or caregiver, and the adapted physical environments.

Directional Postulate Regarding Change

Intervention begins with acknowledgement of the child/family strengths and presuming competence. The practitioner then builds a trusting and safe relationship with listening and validation. From this safe space the practitioner then encourages brave exploration of my body, in space, with other people. In this way the child is able to move toward agency, autonomy, and community engagement on their own terms. A program is successful when the child experiences a sense of mastery, agency, and autonomy in life.

Table 7.7 An Example of Goal Attainment Scaling

#5 Functional Goal: Improve participation at mealtimes

Current Performance: Johnny can take up to an hour to eat his meals. He eats slowly and only a few bites. He becomes distracted, falling out of his chair, getting upset with his sister, and talking.

–2	–1	0	1	2
Johnny will stay seated to eat within 45 min with two prompts	Johnny will stay seated to eat within 45 min with one prompt	Johnny will stay seated to eat within 45 min independently	Johnny will stay seated to eat within 30 min independently	Johnny will stay seated to eat within 30 min without falling out of his chair

Sample ASECRET

Child's strengths: engaging and playful, great language skills, strong visual system, enjoys problem solving; loves sports and active play, loves and looks up to older siblings

Child's challenges that are barriers to function: poor attention; difficulty with maintaining posture (endurance); fluctuations in arousal state; challenges with sequencing multiple steps

Challenge Area	Attention	Sensation	Emotion Regulation	Culture	Relationship	Environment	Task
Poor independent completion of homework	Create schedule on a white board for after-school time period to include when homework will be done and use visuals of what makes sense to him (drawings or words)	Play interactive physical activity with parent or sibling before homework time; supportive seating with feet flat on floor and table surface that works for forearm support	Acknowledge homework can be hard!	Create a culture of joint problem solving; decide together when his body feels the most awake and ready to do homework—right after school, after dinner, before bed, after a shower, in the morning, etc.	Have siblings join him in deciding when homework time feels best and have everyone doing it at the same time and having breaks together to do something fun	Experiment with different homework environments and settings, have child engage in problem solving of what setting works best (desk in room, with quiet, desk in room with music on headphones, kitchen table with action going on around him)	Create positive reward system, to indicate how many days he was able to successfully complete homework on his own—working toward a goal

Specific Postulates Regarding Change

The STAR frame of reference focuses on each individual as a complex, dynamic system, and draws upon an amalgam of perspectives. In turn, postulates for change include multiple areas for facilitating growth and self-organization. This section of this frame of reference is divided into specific strategies, based on the individual needs of each child and family.

Regulation Strategies

The frame of reference has five postulates regarding change related to regulation strategies.

1. If a child has a problem with regulation, the practitioner must direct intervention toward facilitating an optimal level of arousal.
2. If the practitioner supports the child's experience of safety and joy, then the child will be more likely to participate fully in the intervention (Figure 7.8).
3. If the practitioner acknowledges the child's emotional state (verbally or nonverbally), builds emotion awareness, and grades emotional interactions, the child will develop greater emotional regulation.
4. If the practitioner uses attuned and authentic graded affect and anticipation and responds to child's cues, the child will experience greater self-regulation and be more likely to engage in increased circles of communication. Authenticity occurs when the therapist's affect, gestures, and words align.
5. If the practitioner supports the just right success, the child will be more likely to achieve the self-confidence and self-esteem necessary for participation in social interaction and play.

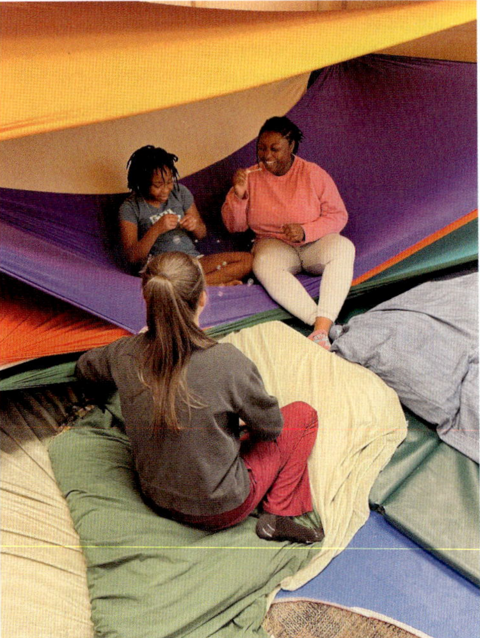

FIGURE 7.8 Practitioner providing regulation support. (Courtesy of STAR Institute, used with permission.)

Relationship Strategies

There are four postulates in this frame of reference that address relationship strategies.

1. If the practitioner authentically attunes to the child, then the child will be more likely to engage in higher-level play, social problem solving, and joyful interactions.
2. If the practitioner creates an atmosphere of trust, safety, and acceptance with the parent/caregiver, the parent will more likely accept coaching strategies and participate in therapy sessions.
3. If the practitioner supports the child's engagement and relationship with significant others, then the child will be more likely to attain higher-level capacities across their developmental profile.
4. If the practitioner follows the child's lead, focusing on the child's strengths, what gives the child joy and is most interested in, then therapy is more likely to sustain engagement in the process (Figure 7.9).

Sensory Integration Strategies

Seven postulates regarding change address SI-SP strategies.

1. If the practitioner provides sensory opportunities tailored to the child's responsivity preferences, then the child will be more likely to learn to self-regulate.
2. If the child addresses modulation, posture, discrimination, and praxis domains with graded support from the practitioner during therapy, the child will be more likely to acquire functional skills in daily life (Figure 7.10).
3. If the practitioner utilizes principles from sensory integration therapy (as conceptualized by Ayres), then the child will be more likely to develop adaptive capacities in sensory modulation, postural control, praxis, bilateral coordination, and discrimination.

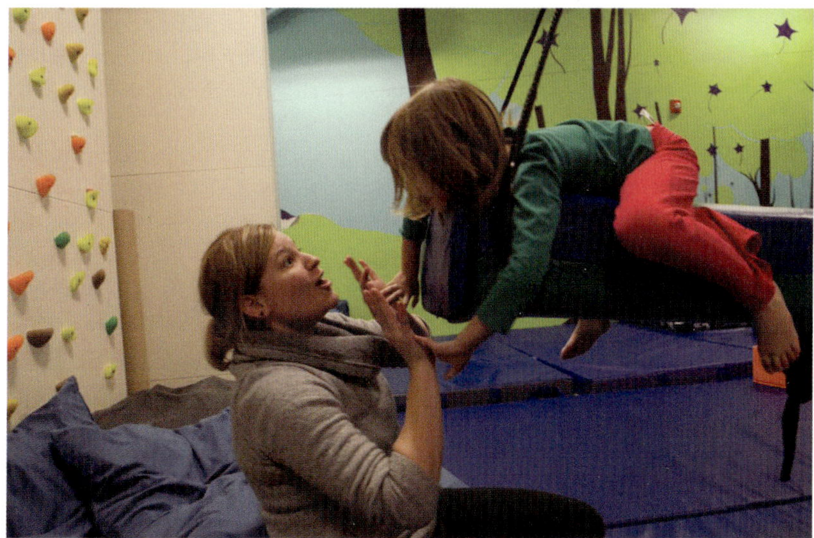

FIGURE 7.9 Practitioner building relationship with a child. (Courtesy of Dr. Lisa Porter, used with permission.)

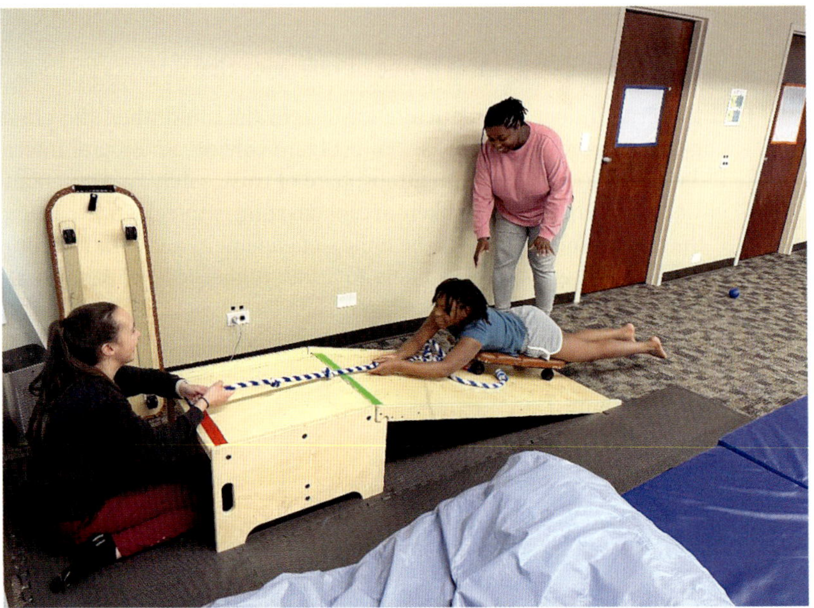

FIGURE 7.10 An example of a sensory integration activity. (Courtesy of STAR Institute, used with permission.)

4. If the practitioner joins and shares the sensory-affective experience and attunes to the child's sensory responsivity pattern, then the child will be more likely to engage in playful interactions.
5. If the practitioner provides the child with opportunities to develop interoceptive awareness, the child will likely develop emotional awareness and control of their body.
6. If the practitioner provides ongoing postural activities directed toward alignment, weight bearing and weight shifting, balance, antigravity control, core stability, strength, and endurance, the child will be better able to perform desired goal-directed, efficient gross and fine motor activities.
7. If the practitioner encourages repeated opportunities with graded support for planning, sequencing, execution, and problem solving, the child will develop foundational abilities that will insure better praxis and organization of behavior in daily life.

Environmental Strategies

Two of the postulates regarding change are related to environmental strategies.

1. If the practitioner collaborates with the parent/caregiver/family member or teacher in treatment, the child will be more likely to achieve carry over into the home, school, and community environments.
2. If the practitioner makes recommendations about potential environmental modifications for the child and those modifications can be implemented, the child will be more likely to achieve success in a broader environment.

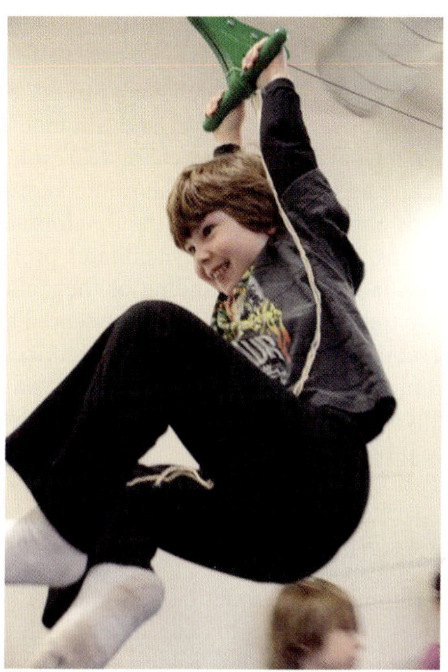

FIGURE 7.11 STAR PROCESS: Child showing joy, and success. (Courtesy of STAR Institute, used with permission.)

APPLICATION TO PRACTICE

The intervention in the STAR frame of reference is referred to as PROCESS. PROCESS stands for **P**lay, **R**elationships, **O**rganize, **C**ommunicate, **E**njoy, **S**ensation, **S**uccess, all key elements of the intervention process (Figure 7.11). Importantly, these elements intermingle and co-occur during treatment sessions such that the therapist, caregiver, child triad dances among these seven elements. The context of therapy is play during which the child experiences the parent/caregiver and practitioner relationship as play partners. The focus is on helping the child stay organized, reading child cues, and supporting their ability to express their needs and desires so that each encounter brings joy and success. Multisensory experiences are embedded within the environment and activities. Intervention reflects individual differences based on the child's distinct sensory, social, and emotional profile that when understood can guide a parent or teacher to implement sensory tools, and strategies across the day and across contexts.

Parent Education Modules

Central to the STAR frame of reference is the parents-only education sessions. The goal is to empower parents with the knowledge that will help them understand their child and ultimately advocate for their child. The exact content of the parent education sessions varies depending on parent's needs and wishes. However, the practitioner always provides the parent with information about the sensory preferences/patterns, the bell curve (to help interpret findings from standardized scales), the arousal continuum (see Figure 7.2) and the quadrant chart (see Figure 7.4). The first education session is the feedback meeting following the initial evaluation where the therapist links the child's evaluation findings to the parent's presenting concerns.

This session is followed by the goal-setting meeting during which goals are established based on the family's priorities. Goals are specific, objective, measurable, and attainable within the 20- to 30-session model utilizing the technique of Goal Attainment Scaling (Kiresuk et al., 1994). The next four to five meetings occur periodically across a 20–30 session intervention program. These are opportunities to discuss changes that have been seen and the development of strategies to support the parent's request and concerns. The practitioner facilitates problem solving, and various handouts are used to enhance the family's understanding of their child's sensory, emotional, or relational challenges. At the last parent meeting, the goals are scored and reviewed with the family, strategies are reviewed, and recommendations for follow-up services are made if necessary. Two online virtual sessions are recommended as a follow-up to in-person intervention during which the practitioner can address any remaining questions or concerns regarding the child's functioning after the completion of the program.

Attributes of the Practitioner

Integral to application of the STAR frame of reference is the practitioner's knowledge and ability to implement neurodiversity-affirming practices. This is a rights-based approach that respects individual differences and recognizes the child's autonomy, strengths, interests, and areas of need. Additionally, application relies on the practitioner's knowledge of clinical reasoning (Mattingly & Fleming, 1994; Schell & Schell, 2018). The practitioner uses various types of clinical reasoning to decide on the content of intervention, including procedural reasoning, interactive reasoning, and conditional reasoning. The process requires an understanding of the child's physiologic, social–emotional, and both interoceptive and exteroceptive sensory experiences that are "meaning making," those experiences that imbue a sense of meaning to their lives. The practitioner uses phenomenologic reasoning to understand people in terms of their daily practices, considering the facts of their life histories, and recognizing the importance of their social relationships (Mattingly & Fleming, 1994). Also, the practitioner attempts to understand the family's long-term goals.

The STAR approach also encourages ongoing mentorship and reflective practice for the treating practitioner through weekly/monthly supervision sessions. Separate spaces are provided for clinical, reflective, and administrative supervision, thus ensuring that reflective practice is intentionally cultivated as part of professional development. At least bimonthly, practitioners should meet with a supervisor to reflect on their own thoughts and feelings in the work as a clinician. Separate meetings with a clinical mentor focus on a review of treatment session videos for clinical reasoning support and to determine fidelity to the frame of reference. Peer collaboration within the multidisciplinary team can also support clinical reasoning. A practitioner using the STAR approach must have a background in sensory integration theory and relationship-based therapy. Participation in Level 1 Mentorship training at the STAR Institute is also highly recommended (see https://sensoryhealth.org/landing-page/education).

Additionally, the STAR frame of reference has developed a STAR PROCESS Fidelity Measure for use by the therapist. It can be especially helpful for novice practitioner and those who are not very familiar with this frame of reference. The Fidelity Measure can be found as Appendix 7.1 at the end of the chapter.

CASE EXAMPLE

Paul

Background

Paul is an American Filipino 4.5-year-old boy who lives with his parents in an urban area and attends a half-day program at a private preschool. Paul's birth and delivery were unremarkable. Milestones were achieved within age expectations. Parents described Paul's crawling like a worm before he progressed to 4-point crawling. Paul's identified strengths were his sense of humor, outgoing personality, and positive outlook.

Presenting problems

Parental concerns were tied to Paul's ability to participate and be successful at school and include:

1. attention to tasks and finishing tasks,
2. sitting still during lessons, and
3. using social skills appropriately in the classroom and playground at school.

Evaluation

Paul attended the assessment accompanied by his mother and father. He participated in a 2-hour comprehensive occupational evaluation which included standardized assessment, structured and unstructured observations in the clinic and standardized parent report measures.

- Standardized Scales Administered: *Sensory Processing Three Dimensions Scales* (SP3DS; Miller et al., 2018); *Miller Function and Participation Scales* (M-FUN; Miller, 2006); *Goodenough Harris Draw A Person* (Goodenough, 1963).
- Clinical Assessment: Comprehensive observations in the occupational therapy gym of engagement and relationship abilities, sensory and motor abilities, cognitive, participation and play abilities.
- Parent and Teacher Report Scales: *The Sensory Processing Measure -2 Preschool* Home and Teacher Scale (Parham et al., 2021), *Adaptive Assessment Scale, 2nd Edition* (ABAS): (Harrison & Oakland, 2003), *Behavior Assessment System for Children, 2nd Edition* (BASC-2): (Reynolds & Kamphaus, 2004).

Behavioral Observations During Assessment

Paul was eager to please and worked hard. He sought reassurance from his parents throughout the assessment by exchanging glances. He demonstrated a sweet sense of humor, was very quick to respond to verbal instructions, and asked pertinent questions and for clarification when necessary.

Results of Standardized Scales

Results of the *M-FUN* (Miller, 2006) indicated that Paul scored below average for fine motor development and well below average for gross motor ability. Results from the SP3DS (Miler et al., 2018) confirmed sensory differences that were affecting function including sensory over-responsivity and postural challenges. The draw-a-person test result was in the average range. Qualitative observations of posture and motor coordination, during the assessment, were further confirmed as a contributing factor to Paul's presenting concerns and are detailed below.

Clinical Assessment Findings

During the evaluation, Paul was observed to "W-sit," lean and prop himself on furniture using his extremities with very little evidence of recruitment of core muscles in any position. He used inefficient postural skills and preferred to stand rather than sit for tabletop work. Paul also demonstrated low postural tone and hypermobility throughout his joints. Observed play centered around the Star Wars theme was somewhat disorganized. Paul used very few words throughout this first meeting. When climbing and exploring in the gym, Paul demonstrated inefficient motor patterns, using his feet for prehension and his mouth and tongue stability when climbing and swinging. Paul's breathing appeared to be somewhat shallow. Much of his gross motor movements involved extension patterns, increased stiffness in his neck and shoulders, and end-of-range movements to achieve momentum and stability.

Paul enjoyed crashing and jumping. He became quickly overaroused by rotary vestibular input and required considerable scaffolding and use of heavy work activities to recover to a calm and alert state of arousal.

Results of Parent Report Scales

Parent report scales indicated sensory overresponsive patterns in auditory and visual processing. Behavioral scores on report measures were all within typical range and not consistent with teacher concerns about attention and social skills. Overall, Paul's parents did not have the same concerns as the school, and it was therefore determined that a school visit would be beneficial.

School Observation Findings

The therapist visited Paul's school, observing in the classroom, during a room transition, and a class library session. The therapist also interviewed the class teacher. Paul increasingly regarded people and objects with side-on gaze out of the extreme corner of his eyes, mostly to the right side and often did not look directly at his teacher or the story being read aloud. Paul moved between standing with his legs in wide straddle for tabletop work, high kneeling for carpet time, and other atypical positions throughout the observation. He oriented to the majority of environmental stimuli, including repeated and unchanging stimuli that he was unable to habituate to, at the expense of the task at hand.

Teacher report measures indicated overresponsivity to visual, auditory, and movement experiences and seeking certain movements like crashing and bumping, touching, and leaning against walls and people. Paul's teacher reported that he is an asset to the classroom and a "strong thinker." He takes pride in products of constructive play and participates in role-playing games. The teacher reported that she was aware of his need for a lot of support to be "calm enough to learn."

Strengths That Will Support Progress in Therapy

Paul was a positive, bright, and hardworking young boy who was eager to please and able to persist through difficult tasks. Functional, emotional development is age appropriate. His temperament and positive outlook support relationships with family and peers. Paul's strong relationship with his parents will support progress in therapy.

Impact Statements

The following impact statements link presenting problems to hypothesized sensory, relationship, and regulation challenges identified during the evaluation.

Impact of Sensory Overresponsivity on Activity Level and Attention at School

Paul is overresponsive to many movement experiences and the majority of sound and visual stimuli in his environment and his overresponsivity increases as the day progresses. Challenges with posture and discrimination place heavy demands on Paul, which impacts his ability to self-calming through the school day. At home, Paul is supported for success as his parents have intuitively provided calming daily routines and a physical environment that supports his sensory needs. Paul's difficulty with sensory modulation and his state of heightened arousal may be perceived as inattentiveness and distractibility and limits his ability to engage in the classroom curriculum.

Impact of Challenges in Postural Stability on Sitting for Circle Time and Tabletop Work in the Classroom

Paul has difficulty sustaining static positions due to his difficulty recruiting core postural muscles to keep him upright. He tends to lean on walls, the furniture, his limbs (rather than his core), and standing or moving to stay upright. This means that sitting or standing still is very effortful for Paul, which reduces his capacity to engage in learning activities and remain regulated. As a result, Paul may appear to be fidgety and disengaged from activities presented at school.

Impact of Challenges With Somatosensory Discrimination on Social Skills

Paul has difficulty moving around the classroom and navigating spaces due to his challenges with posture, regulation, and his poorly developed body map. In circle time, he may sit too close or lean onto his classmates; he leans across the table during tabletop activities and can knock over the work of other children. He stands too close to his peers when lining up and does not notice when he is standing on other people's feet. This has created some difficulty with social skills during group work and recess and results in Paul appearing "out of tune" with his environment and classmates.

Parent Meeting #1

Following the evaluation, the therapist met with Paul's parents to discuss the findings, including his sensory presentation and its impact on function. This helped his parents reframe challenges in terms of the SI-SP, understand the compensatory supports they were providing at home, and how postural differences explained challenges with sitting still. Parents were motivated to participate in therapy sessions and engage in follow-up at home. Goals were set collaboratively.

Treatment

The occupational therapist (OT) recommended that Paul participate in an intensive 20-session program with parents present, as much as possible, over the course of 2 months. Every fifth session was a parent education session with both parents attending and providing timely feedback on what worked and what did not. Over the course of the 20 sessions, the team was able to successfully create a "sensory lifestyle," including strategies and tools for home and school. This involved incorporating playground time, climbing on the monkey bars during the walk to the school bus each day, and adapting wrestling games at home with his father to provide organizing resistance and heavy work.

Problem Solving During Intervention

Initial observation during intervention showed Paul's motor inefficiencies resulted in him being excessively fatigued and dysregulated by the effort.

The therapist used Paul's interest in Star Wars to engage him in sessions. This preferred and well-established play schema allowed the therapist to follow Paul's lead while guiding him to create the just-right challenge. The therapist also emphasized "attunement" as part of the therapeutic process. This was achieved by allowing Paul time to express his thoughts without interruption or rushing him and by acknowledging the messages he was communicating through gestures, and other nonverbal communication. Paul's parents were coached to easily engage in play with him.

Through honoring Paul's play ideas, building connection and communication, and attuning to Paul, trust was built, and Paul's enjoyment of the sessions was enhanced. He was excited to be in the room each day and demonstrated measurable joy, which was observable not only in his words, tone of voice, and the way his face "lit up." He enthusiastically engaged with the games and motor challenges and demonstrated effort and perseverance. Being attuned and connected to a play partner provided opportunities for shared social problem solving.

These elements of shared joy, back-and-forth communication, and exchange of ideas, created ongoing opportunities for the therapist to optimize the positive potential of activities as they organically occurred in sessions. A wide variety of sensory opportunities, including vestibular and somatosensory experiences (e.g., running and crashing, climbing, and swinging) were made available to Paul, giving him information about where his body was in space. Using his interest in Star Wars to guide the play, the "just-right success" was regularly achieved. The play scheme lasted over multiple sessions during which the therapist introduced small changes, including different sensory equipment, to sustain elements of novelty and support Paul's ability to adapt to change and be flexible in the moment.

By allowing Paul's father to be the main play partner and facilitating his role as collaborator in the play, the therapist enabled this father–son dyad to celebrate victories and achievements as a team. This had a positive effect on their relationship. A strong therapeutic relationship was established between all members of Paul's team, and his parents were empowered to become experts in Paul's therapy experience. Honoring the principle of process over "goal-driven" intervention, Paul's regulation was always assessed and supported as a priority; this took place in the waiting room before a session started and throughout all sessions. Whenever necessary, the OT would adjust the session to support regulation before returning to a more sophisticated play scheme (and then only if Paul achieved a "just right" state of arousal).

Principles Guiding Therapy Sessions:

- Begin at the child's level and assess the state of arousal
- Provide a safe physical environment with sensory affordances
- Engage child in play choice and attune to the child
- Provide challenges for the child

Further Progress and Continuing Clinical Reasoning

Other questions and observations were generated during intervention including, visual motor coordination ability and overly gregarious greetings, limited ability to tune into interoceptive signals, highly detailed strong memory for games, and complex game ideas although within a limited repertoire of interests. Paul needed support to build flexibility until he was receptive to ideas from his father, his mother, and the OT. Deliberately adding visual motor aspects into therapy sessions also seemed to support ocular motor coordination, which initially had appeared challenging for Paul. Paul's tolerance for movement and specifically rotary vestibular experiences also changed noticeably from highly overresponsive to being able to remain organized and attentive.

Prior to the end of intervention, a meeting with his parents, teachers, special needs team, and the therapist was scheduled at school to discuss further goal setting and strategies that would benefit Paul. This meeting focused on advocacy for Paul and education around his sensory needs. Furthermore, Paul's very supportive classroom teacher incorporated sensory lifestyle adaptations into the school environment and spontaneously reported significant improvements at the school (Table 7.8).

Response to Intervention—Post Testing

The following tests were administered again:

- Standardized Scales Administered
  - *SP3DS* (Miller et al., 2018);
  - *M-FUN* (Miller, 2006);
  - *Goodenough Harris Draw A Person* (Goodenough, 1963).
- Clinical assessment which included
  - Comprehensive observations in the occupational therapy gym of engagement and relationship abilities; sensory and motor abilities; cognitive, participation, and play abilities.
- Parent and Report Scales
  - *ABAS* (Harrison & Oakland, 2003);
  - *BASC-2* (Reynolds & Kamphaus, 2004).

Improvements in Sensory Overresponsivity on Activity Level and Attention

Before coming to therapy, Paul's overresponsivity to movement, sound, and visual stimuli significantly impacted his ability to participate in school. Since intervention, Paul has shown outstanding progress in his ability to tolerate and process movement, sound, and visual input as well as to advocate for his wants and needs in relation to these sensations. Now, Paul can remain organized throughout the school day or, in collaboration with his teacher, is able to identify when he needs to change position or do some heavy work to get back into the "just right" state for learning. His teacher has reported improvements in both listening and social skills.

Improvements in Postural Stability for Sitting in Circle Time and Tabletop Work in the Classroom

Due to improved sensory discrimination, Paul is now better able to make the necessary postural adjustments to remain upright. He remained seated in his chair throughout 15 minutes of tabletop work during posttesting. He demonstrated less extraneous movement in order to keep a proper upright position. Improved postural stability and endurance will assist in Paul's attention and behavior in the classroom.

Table 7.8 Goal Attainment Scaling (Parent Meeting #2). Goal Setting Took Place at the Second Parent Meeting and in Collaboration With Both Parents

A. Functional Goal		**Increase Self-Regulation and Availability for Learning**		
Current Performance		Regulation and attention deteriorate rapidly over the course of the morning at school, toward the end of the day is unable to follow instructions and wanders around the classroom		
–2 Much less than expected	–1 Less than expected	0 Expected outcome	1 More than expected	2 Much more than expected
Paul will sustain appropriate attention to task for 2 min with two prompts from the teacher	Paul will sustain appropriate attention to task for 5 min with two prompts from the teacher	Paul will sustain appropriate attention to task for 10 min with two prompts from the teacher	Paul will sustain appropriate attention to a task for 10 min with one prompt	Paul will sustain appropriate attention to a task for 10–15 min independently
B. Functional Goal		**Increase Postural Control and Endurance for Sitting**		
Current Performance:		Unable to adopt a functional seated position at the tabletop		
–2 Much less than expected	–1 Less than expected	0 Expected outcome	1 More than expected	2 Much more than expected
Able to sit in classroom chair for 1 min with aligned posture, without propping	Able to sit in classroom chair for 3 min with aligned posture, without propping	Able to sit in classroom chair for 5 min with aligned posture, without propping	Able to sit in classroom chair for 8 min with aligned posture, without propping	Able to sit in classroom chair for 10 min with aligned posture, without propping
C. Functional Goal		**Improved Classroom Relationships as Measured by Classroom Teacher**		
Current Performance		Impulsive during recess and circle time often requires teacher intervention		
–2 Much less than expected	–1 Less than expected	0 Expected outcome	1 More than expected	2 Much more than expected
Able to successfully interact with peers in reciprocal turn-taking games for 1 out of 4 h of the school day with adult support	Able to successfully interact with peers in reciprocal turn-taking games for 2 out of 4 h of the school day with adult support	Able to successfully interact with peers in reciprocal turn-taking games for 2 out of 4 h of the school day	Able to successfully interact with peers in reciprocal turn-taking games for 3 out of 4 h of the school day	Able to successfully interact with peers in reciprocal turn-taking games throughout the school day with the same level of support as classmates

Improvements in Challenges With Somatosensory Discrimination on Social Skills

Paul's teacher reports that Paul's understanding of where his body is in space has improved considerably and that he is now able to stand in line or in circle time without any special support or considerations. He is also able to participate in peer group work with minimal teacher support.

Table 7.9 ASECRET for Paul

Child's Strengths: Outgoing, creative, well-connected to parents, engaging, motivated, playful
Child's Challenges that are barriers to function: overresponsive and often in a state of high arousal; difficulty with attaining and maintaining posture; challenges with body map and sense of self in space

Challenge Area	Attention	Sensation	Emotion Regulation	Culture	Relationship	Environment	Task
Difficulty following verbal instructions at school	Provide visual reinforces of verbal activities on the mini whiteboard on the table next to Paul. Use his strength in reading to provide simple written cues	Provide heavy work activities through recess and other parts of the day; consider making noise reduction headphones available to Paul and normalize this by making them available to the whole class	Support Paul's ability to tune into and acknowledge interoceptive signals by encouraging him to label and notice his own internal states; do the same for his emotional experiences and states of arousal. Use speedometers as visual props to support this	Create a culture of collaboration, joint problem solving—decide together when his body feels the most awake and ready to do work. Work together as a team to identify when Paul's arousal needs support and celebrate his successes	Take extra time to connect with Paul and join him when he is calming down, and when he is successfully working hard. This increases his tolerance for frustration and his ability to persevere significantly	Minimize extraneous sound (e.g., tannoy speakers) and visual stimuli—consider a desk shield to provide a visually "quiet" area; provide dynamic seating options	Provide Paul with positive feedback and appropriate classroom rewards when you see him working hard; encourage him to acknowledge his own effort; allow Paul to explore, enjoy, and celebrate work that is not perfect

Final Parent Meeting

A sensory lifestyle was discussed during the final parent meeting to ensure that Paul's parents felt prepared to continue to support changes at home and at school (Table 7.9).

Paul's standardized test results improved. Goal attainment scale review indicated positive outcomes; Paul demonstrated improvements in sustained attention, sitting in a classroom chair, and interacting with peers. Additionally, his classroom teacher noted improved awareness of space and turn-taking during the school day.

Paul was noted to have continued difficulty remaining regulated without the support of family members or therapist. It was recommended that his "sensory lifestyle" remain a priority to support him throughout each day across environments. A future Zoom consultation was recommended to monitor progress and support Paul's parents in the implementation of home strategies, tools, and resources.

SUPPORTING EVIDENCE

The first study of the STAR frame of reference was completed in 2007 by Miller and her team (Miller et al., 2007). This randomized controlled trial examined elements of the STAR PROCESS, related to intensity and duration of therapy, individualized goal setting, and adherence to principles of sensory integration. Twenty-four children participated in this study. They were randomly assigned to one of three groups: occupational therapy, activity protocol or a waitlist, and no treatment condition. The occupational therapy group showed the greatest improvements in goal achievement as measured via Goal Attainment Scaling, as well as on the attention and cognitive and social composites of the Leiter-R parent rating scale.

Following completion of this study, retrospective research was employed to study treatment effectiveness further. The benefit of this methodology is that it is more cost effective, provides easier access to data, and fully reflects what happens in day-to-day clinical practice. A retrospective chart review produced data from 179 clients who participated in the full STAR PROCESS program over a 5-year period (Schoen et al., 2018). Improvements were noted using parent report of adaptive behavior and problem behaviors. Areas of daily life functioning impacted were functional communication, self-direction, self-care, home living, health, safety, leisure, and social skills (Effect Size [ES] = .45 to .55). Additionally, there was a significant reduction in problematic behaviors associated with externalizing, internalizing, and other behavioral symptoms such as hyperactivity, aggression, anxiety, depression, withdrawal, and inattention (ES = .41 to .52). A decrease in sensory symptoms was reported on the Sensory Processing 3 Dimensional Inventory (Miller et al., 2018) (ES = .18 to .52) with individuals who displayed sensory craving symptoms showing the greatest reduction in externalizing and behavior problems after the intervention. There was evidence of improvement in fine motor, gross motor, and visual motor abilities as measured by examiner-administered scales. Although further research is needed, these studies provide preliminary evidence of the effectiveness of the STAR PROCESS.

Another methodology used to study treatment effectiveness is single subject research using a multiple baseline, and repeated-measures design. This methodology is also well suited for clinical settings, as it allows examination of individual differences that is often obscured in large group studies (Kennedy, 2005). A current study involves four participants during a baseline, no therapy condition, and then weekly over the course of participation in treatment. A coding system was used to record changes in play and social behavior observed with the parent (no therapist present) on a sensory-friendly playground. All participants showed improvements in cooperative play, and there was an increase in parent participation in the child's play activities. Parents not only more readily joined in the play but also supported their child to engage in higher levels of play behavior. Notably, there were also improvements in the novel use of playground equipment (Schoen et al., 2018).

Summary

The STAR frame of reference draws primarily on the work of A. Jean Ayres (1972, 1979) and Greenspan and Wieder (1998) and is committed to ongoing refinement based on new data, updated theories, and research findings (Miller et al., 2002; Miller et al., 2007). This approach has evolved over time through the integration of infant mental health, developmental theory, and neurobiology (including interpersonal neurobiology). The primary focus of the STAR frame of reference is to assess the impact of sensory differences on regulation, relationships, and engagement in daily activities, with a personalized approach tailored to each child's needs. While initially designed for children, the STAR frame of reference has been successfully adapted for use with groups, adolescents, and adults (Schoen et al., 2019, 2022; Miller et al., 2023), extending its application across the lifespan. Ongoing research aims to explore the utilization of the STAR frame of reference beyond pediatric settings.

STAR intervention is grounded in clinical reasoning and emphasizes three key continua related to SI-SP, regulation, and relationships. Therapy strategies are play-based and center on enhancing the interactions between the child, parent, and parent–child relationship. Mastery of the STAR frame of reference is best achieved through mentorship, ongoing education, and supervised practice under the guidance of experienced mentors. Advanced training in sensory integration and DIR/Floortime® is ideal. The overarching goal of the STAR approach is to foster autonomy, instill a sense of agency, and nurture a strong sense of self in individuals across the lifespan

Appendix 7.1 STAR PROCESS Fidelity Measure

Therapeutic Principles

1. Arousal regulation:
   - Therapist modulates voice to coregulate child
   - Therapist modulates affect to coregulate child
   - Therapist adapts sensory strategies to support arousal regulation
   - Therapist uses preferred objects, themes, ideas to support arousal regulation
   - Therapist adapts pacing to support arousal regulation
   - Therapist adapts environment to support arousal regulation
   - Therapist grades (increases or decreases challenge in) play in at least one of the following areas:
     - Posture
     - Praxis
     - Modulation
     - Social–emotional
     - Attention
     - Discrimination
2. Connect with attunement to create strong relationships and enjoyment (this is critically important).Therapist is in synchrony, mirroring affect, communication, and/or movement with the child.
   - Therapist adapts play to engage child, follow child's lead and increase interest
   - Therapist matches play to child's interests, desires, and developmental level (cognition, emotional, motor skills, sensory processing)
   - Therapist matches communication to child's level
   - Therapist supports child to share intents and ideas
   - Therapist demonstrates flexibility with activity choice facilitating social problem solving
   - Therapist (or parent) demonstrates genuinely fun and joyful interactions with child
3. Therapist establishes trust with child:
   - Therapist honors child's consent
   - Therapist and parent are near enough to the child that the child feels safe/protected
   - Therapist involves child in activity choice
   - Therapist creates a safe environment for the child
   - Therapist demonstrates flexibility, will repeat activity if needed to support automaticity, or will switch activities as needed
   - Therapist demonstrates awareness of child's individual sensory differences in adapting activity or environment (provide routine, visual cues and supports, rewards) to support child
4. Therapist establishes trust with parent:
   - Therapist provides time to listen to parent
   - Therapist creates a comfortable/safe environment for the parent
   - Parent is involved directly in play to the extent they are comfortable
   - Therapist coaches parent during play in order to set up parent–child connections during "magic moments" (moments when the child experiences joy and mastery)
   - Therapist models interaction or strategy with parent present
   - Therapist coaches interaction or strategy with parent present
   - Therapist sets up play to increase connection between child and parent
   - Parent and child demonstrate joyful interaction

(*continued*)

Appendix 7.1 STAR PROCESS Fidelity Measure (Continued)

Therapeutic Principles

5. Includes sensory integration principles: (at least two of the following)
   - At least two of three primary sensory opportunities available (tactile, vestibular, proprioceptive)
   - Challenges at "just right" level emotionally, physically, and interpersonally
   - Ensures that activities are successful
   - Prioritizes self-organization of child
   - "Just right" challenge is provided in at least one of the following areas:
     - Postural and/or postural-ocular-motor
     - Resistive whole body
     - Praxis and organization of behavior
     - Bilateral movement patterns
     - Feedforward, e.g., projected action sequence
     - Discrimination
6. The child experiences autonomy and agency while participating
   - Child is actively involved in choosing or planning activities
   - Child is engaged in process, not just motivated by the end result
   - Therapist supports child's ideas to facilitate success
7. Therapist acknowledges emotional regulation and needs (at least one of following):
   - Therapist verbalizes empathy for child's emotion
   - Therapist uses visual scale (e.g., 5-point scale, zones of regulation, Powerfully You, Autism Level Up, etc.) during play to draw awareness to child's emotional/energy state
   - Therapist uses character/symbolic play to engage child in emotion awareness and label emotions
   - Therapist uses interoception-based activities to enhance awareness of internal body state and relation to emotions
   - Therapist grades sensory and interaction opportunities to facilitate success, confidence, and internal motivation
   - Therapist incorporates one or more of the themes of attachment, separation, fears, bodily injury, good guy/bad guy (aggression), or reality testing
8. Facilitates circles of communication (this is critically important):
   - Joins the child (matches/imitates) rather than directs the child
   - Demonstrates comfort in waiting, watching, listening
   - Uses affect and anticipation to increase back-and-forth communication
   - Responds to child's cues, particularly when subtle (eye gaze, posture shift)
   - Uses pacing to allow time for child to respond
9. Discipline is kept to a minimum (at least one of the following, if needed):
   - Discipline used to ensure safety of self, child, or others
   - Uses "time-in" to support child during dysregulation
   - Visual supports and routine for transitions
   - Few or no power struggles
   - By correctly reading needs of child, therapist can provide easier or harder tasks to avoid power struggles most (>80%) of the time

Appendix 7.1 STAR PROCESS Fidelity Measure (Continued)

Content of Parent Education Meetings

1. Initial feedback meeting:
   - Starts by asking about child's strengths or what is special about the child
   - Uses lay terminology and takes time to check for parent understanding
   - Focuses on the quality of life (functional abilities)
   - Reports on strengths and challenges
   - Uses introduction to Sensory Integration and Processing parent education document
   - Reviews general findings without focus on scores
   - Shares findings from standardized testing (strengths and weaknesses)
   - Explains bell curve and how to transfer standard scores to bell
   - Facilitates generation of goal areas for next meeting (provides GA Scale handout if needed)
2. Goal setting meeting:
   - Helps generate appropriate (reachable) goal areas based on child and child–family priorities
   - Collaborates with parent to assure that parents and therapists are in agreement
   - Creates specific goals that describe current function and markers of change
   - Checks out accuracy of completed GA Scale with parents at start of therapy
   - Involves child whenever possible
3. Parent education meeting 2 (Session 8 or 9):
   - Starts by asking parents about changes they have seen
   - Discusses own (therapist) perspective on progress made by child and parents
   - Provides strategies to support parents' requests/concerns
   - Therapist educates parents regarding purpose and/or outcome of sessions

     Topics covered include:
     - Regulation
     - Neurodivergent communication and play styles
     - Possible communication supports (AAC)
     - Self-advocacy skills
     - Environmental accommodations
     - Parental attunement
4. Parent education meeting 3 (~Session 16–20 or before break):
   - Support development of home and school strategies, tools, and resources
   - Discuss strategies modeled and practiced in therapy
   - Provides strategies to support parents' requests/concerns
   - Therapist educates parents regarding purpose and/or outcome of sessions
   - Review Functional Emotional Developmental Levels handout
5. Parent education meeting 4 (after break—or combined with #3 if no break):
   - Gather feedback from family regarding child's function over break
   - Review home strategies used over the break
   - Discuss priorities for remaining sessions
   - Provides strategies to support parents' requests/concerns
   - Therapist educates parents regarding purpose and/or outcome of sessions.

(*continued*)

Appendix 7.1 STAR PROCESS Fidelity Measure (Continued)

Content of Parent Education Meetings

6. Parent education meeting 5:
   - Summarize progress
   - Review and score GA Scale
   - Emphasize strengths of child and family
   - Review findings of posttesting
   - Review modifications and additions (home, school, community)
   - Present home program written information or visuals as needed
   - Provide strategies to support parents' requests/concerns
7. Follow-up meetings via Zoom
   - Gather feedback from family regarding child's function after completion of program
   - Review strategies and other tools being used
   - Provide strategies to support parents' requests/concerns

Logistic Elements

- Intensive treatment—3 × 5 session/wk for 30 sessions
- Parent education
- Feedback meeting
- GAS meeting—parent is actively involved in goal setting
- Meeting every 6–7th session
- Parent participation (at least two of the following)
  - Parent participates in play
  - Parent coaching from the therapist
  - Therapist models strategies for parent
  - Parent observes and notes elements of Play
- Ongoing mentoring for treating therapist:
  - Weekly supervision meetings/mentoring for treating therapist
  - At least biweekly video review or session observation by mentor
  - Weekly transdisciplinary meetings
  - At least monthly group reflective supervision
- Therapist qualifications:
  - Pro Certification 1 in the STAR Frame of Reference
  - Sensory integration evaluation and treatment certification (Ayres)
  - At least basic DIR training or other relationship-based therapy
  - Training in neurodiversity affirming practice
  - Master's level or higher OT degree and licensure
- Environmental requirements
  - Access to a range of sensory and motor equipment (per Ayres Sensory Integration)
  - Access to a range of environmental spaces (small quiet spaces and large sensory-rich spaces)
  - Environment is safe for child (mats, pillows, etc.)
- Transition/discharge plan
- Begin talking about transition at least three sessions in advance
- Celebrate completion of program with special certificate/award/other (final session)
- Complete a project with child (final session)
- Have child/caregiver complete satisfaction survey (final session)

REFERENCES

Ainsworth, M. S. (1979). Infant-mother attachment. *American Psychologist, 34*(10), 932–937. https://doi.org/10.1037/0003-066X.34.10.932

Allen, B. (2023). The historical foundations of contemporary attachment theory: From John Bowlby to Mary Ainsworth. In B. Allen (Ed.), *The science and clinical practice of attachment theory: A guide from infancy to adulthood* (pp. 13–35). American Psychological Association. https://doi.org/10.1037/0000333-002

Arthur, W. B. (1999). Complexity and the economy. *Science, 284*(5411), 107–109. https://doi.org/10.1126/science.284.5411.107

Ayres, A. J. (1972). *Sensory integration and learning disorders*. Western Psychological Services.

Ayres, A. J. (1979). *Sensory integration and the child*. Western Psychological Services.

Beebe, B., & Lachmann, F. M. (2015). The expanding world of Edward Tronick. *Psychoanalytic Inquiry, 35*(4), 328–336. https://doi.org/10.1080/07351690.2015.1022476

Ben-Avi, N., Almagor, M., & Engel-Yeger, B. (2012). Sensory processing difficulties and interpersonal relationships in adults: An exploratory study. *Psychology, 3*(1), 70–77. https://doi.org/10.4236/psych.2012.31012

Bowlby, J. (1969). *Attachment and loss*. Pimlico.

Bronfenbrenner, U., & Ceci, S. J. (1994). Nature-nurture reconceptualized in developmental perspective: A bioecological model. *Psychological Review, 101*(4), 568–586. https://doi.org/10.1037/0033-295X.101.4.568

Bronfenbrenner, U., & Morris, P. A. (2007). The bioecological model of human development. In *Handbook of child psychology* (Vol. 1, pp. 793–827). John Wiley & Sons. https://doi.org/10.1002/9780470147658.chpsy0114

Browne, J. V., & Talmi, A. (2015). The BABIES © Model: Training for community professionals who work with newborns and young infants with special needs and their families, (September). *Occupational Therapy Journal of Research, 32*(2), 39–47. https://doi.org/10.1016/j.ridd.2011.01.033

Deci, E. L., & Ryan, R. M. (2008). Self-determination theory: A macrotheory of human motivation, development and health. *Canadian Psychological Association, 49*(3), 182–185. https://doi.org/10.1037/10012801

Fogel, A., Greenspan, S. I., King, B. J., Lickliter, R., Reygadas, P., & Shanker, S. G. (2008). A dynamic systems approach to the life sciences. In Fogel, A., & King, B. J. (Eds.), *Human development in the twenty-first century* (pp. 235–253). Cambridge University Press.

Fonagy, P. (2015). Mutual regulation, mentalization, and therapeutic action: A reflection on the contributions of Ed Tronick to developmental and psychotherapeutic thinking. *Psychoanalytic Inquiry, 35*(4), 355–369. https://doi.org/10.1080/07351690.2015.1022481

Goodenough, F. L. (1963). *Goodenough-Harris drawing test*. Harcourt Brace Jovanovich.

Graziano, P. A., Reavis, R. D., Keane, S. P., & Calkins, S. D. (2007). The role of emotion regulation and children's early academic success. *Journal of School Psychology, 45*(1), 3–19. https://doi.org/10.1016/j.jsp.2006.09.002

Greenspan, S. I., DeGangi, G., & Wieder, S. (2001). *The functional emotional assessment scale for infancy and early childhood: Clinical and research applications*. Interdisciplinary Council on Developmental and Learning Disorders.

Greenspan, S. I., & Greenspan, N. T. (2010). *The learning tree: Overcoming learning disabilities from the ground up*. De Capo Press/Lifelong Books.

Greenspan, S. I., & Shanker, S. G. (2004). *The first idea: How symbols, language, and intelligence evolved from our early primate ancestors to modern humans*. De Capo Press/Lifelong Books.

Greenspan, S. I., & Wieder, S. (1998). *The child with special needs: Encouraging intellectual and emotional growth*. Addison-Wesley/Addison Wesley Longman.

Greenspan, S. I., & Wieder, S. (2006). *Infant and early childhood mental health*. American Psychiatric Association.

Harrison, P., & Oakland, T. (2003). *Adaptive behavior assessment system*. The Psychological Corporation.

Harrison, A. M., & Tronick, E. Z. (2011). "The noise monitor": A developmental perspective on verbal and nonverbal meaning-making in psychoanalysis. *Journal of the American Psychoanalytic Association, 59*(5), 961–982. https://doi.org/10.1177/0003065111422539

Kamm, K., Thelen, E., & Jensen, J. L. (1990). Dynamical systems approach motor development. *Physical Therapy, 70*, 763–775. https://doi.org/10.1093/ptj/70.12.763

Kelly, K., Slade, A., & Grienenberger, J. F. (2005). Maternal reflective functioning, mother-infant affective communication, and infant attachment: Exploring the link between mental states and observed caregiving behavior in the intergenerational transmission of attachment. *Attachment & Human Development, 7*(3), 299–311. https://doi.org/10.1080/14616730500245963

Kennedy, C. H. (2005). *Single-case designs for educational research*. Pearson Education Inc.

Kiresuk, T. J., Smith, A., & Cardillo, J. E. (Eds.). (1994). *Goal attainment scaling: Applications, theory, and measurement*. Lawrence Erlbaum Associates, Inc.

Lichtenberg, J. (2015). *A developmentalist's approach to research, theory, and therapy: the selected works of Joseph Lichtenberg*. Routledge.

Lillas, C., & Turnbull, J. (2009). *Infant/child mental health, early intervention, and relationship-based therapies: A neurorelational framework for interdisciplinary practice*. WW Norton & Company.

Main, M., & Solomon, J. (1986). Discovery of a new insecure-disorganized/disoriented attachment pattern. In M. Yogman & T. B. Brazelton (Eds.), *Affective development in infancy* (pp. 95–124). Ablex.

Martinez-Torteya, C., Dayton, C. J., Beeghly, M., Seng, J. S., McGinnis, E., Broderick, A., Rosenblum, K., & Muzik, M. (2014). Maternal parenting predicts infant biobehavioral regulation among women with a history of childhood maltreatment. *Development and Psychopathology, 26*(2), 379–392. https://doi.org/10.1017/S0954579414000017

Mattingly, C., & Fleming, M. H. (1994). *Clinical reasoning: Forms of inquiry in a therapeutic practice*. F.A. Davis.

Miller, L. J. (2006). *Miller function and participation scale*. Harcourt Assessment.

Miller, L. J. (2018). The STAR Frame of Reference [PowerPoint Slides] *Mentorship Level 1* STAR Institute, Centennial CO.

Miller, L. J., Anzalone, M. E., Lane, J., Cermak, S. A., & Osten, E. T. (2007). Concept evolution in sensory integration: A proposed nosology for diagnosis. *American Journal of Occupational Therapy, 6*, 135–140.

Miller, L. J., Schoen, S., & Mulligan, S. (2018). *The sensory processing three dimensions inventory*, unpublished manuscript. Available from the STAR institute.

Miller, D., Schoen, S. A., Schmitt, C., & Porter, L. (2023). A qualitative analysis of adolescents and adults' perception of experiences of sensory-based interventions. *American Journal of Occupational Therapy, 77*, 5. https://doi.org/10.5014/ajot.2023.050198

Miller, L. J., Wilbarger, J., Stackhouse, T., & Trunnell, S. (2002). Use of clinical reasoning in occupational therapy: The STEP-SI model of intervention of sensory modulation dysfunction. In A. C. Bundy, S. J. Lane, E. A. Murray (Eds.), *Sensory integration theory and practice* (2nd ed.). F.A. Davis.

Nugent, J. K., Keefar, C. H., Minear, S., Johnson, L. C., & Blanchard, Y. (2007). *Understanding newborn behavior and early relationships*. Paul H. Brookes Publishing.

Papoušek, M. (2008). Disorders of behavioral and emotional regulation: Clinical evidence for a new diagnostic concept. In M. Papoušek, M. Scheiche, H. Wurmser (Eds.), *Disorders of behavioral and emotional regulation in the first years of life* (pp. 53–84). Zero to Three.

Papoušek, M., Scheiche, M., & Wurmser, H. (2008). *Disorders of behavioral and emotional regulation in the first years of life*. Zero to Three.

Parham, L. D., Ecker, C. L., Kuhaneck, H., Henry, D. A., & Glennon, T. J. (2021). *Sensory processing measure, second edition (SPM-2)*. Western Psychological Services.

Reynolds, C. R., & Kamphaus, R. W. (2004). *Behavior assessment system for children* (2nd ed.). American Guidance Service.

Royeen, C. B. (2003). The 2003 Eleanor Clarke Slagle lecture. Chaotic occupational therapy: Collective wisdom for a complex profession. *American Journal of Occupational Therapy, 57*, 609–624. https://doi.org/10.5014/ajot.57.6.609

Schell, B. A. B., & Schell, J. W. (2018). *Clinical and professional reasoning in occupational therapy* (2nd ed.). Wolters Kluwer Health.

Schoen, S. A., Ferrari, V. & Valdez, A. (2022). It's not just about bicycle riding: sensory-motor, social and emotional benefits for children with and without developmental disabilities. *Children,* 9, 1224. https://doi.org/10.3390/children9081224

Schoen, S. A., Eink, C., Valdez, A. Spielmann, V., & Miller, L. J. (2019). A trampoline group: Feasibility, implementation and outcomes. *Autism and Developmental Disorders, 17*, 58–86. https://doi.org/10.17759/autdd.2019170206

Schoen, S. A., Miller, L. J., & Flanagan, J. (2018). A retrospective pre post treatment study of occupational therapy intervention for children with sensory processing challenges. *The Open Journal of Occupational Therapy, 6*. https://doi.org/10.15453/2168-6408.1367

Slade, A. (2005). Parental reflective functioning: An introduction. *Attachment & Human Development,* 7(3), 269–281. https://doi.org/10.1080/14616730500245906

Slade, A., Sadler, L. S., De Dios-Kenn, C., Webb, D., Currier-Ezepchick, J., & Mayes, L. (2005). Minding the baby: A reflective parenting program. *Psychoanalytic Study of the Child, 60*, 74–100. https://doi.org/10.1017/CBO9781107415324.004

Smith, L. B., & Thelen, E. (2003). Development as a dynamic system. *Trends in Cognitive Sciences, 7*(8), 343–348. https://doi.org/10.1016/S1364-6613(03)00156-6

Spinrad, T. L., Eisenberg, N., Cumberland, A., Fabes, R. A., Valiente, C., Shepard, S. A., Reiser, M., Losoya, S. H., & Guthrie, I. K. (2006). Relation of emotion-related regulation to children's social competence: A longitudinal study. *Emotion, 6*(3), 498–510. https://doi.org/10.1037/1528-3542.6.3.498

Stineman, M. G., & Streim, J. E. (2010). The biopsycho-ecological paradigm: A foundational theory for medicine. *PM R: The Journal of Injury, Function and Rehabilitation*, *2*(11), 1035–1045. https://doi.org/10.1016/j-pmrj.2010.06.013

Szklut, S. (2014). Early identification and intervention of sensory issues in the birth to 3 years population. *OT Practice, 19*(19), CE-1–CE-8. Retrieved from http://ezproxy.usherbrooke.ca/login?url=https://search.ebscohost.com/login.aspx?direct=true&db=rzh& AN=2012775496&site=ehost-live

Thelen, E. (2005). Dynamic systems theory and the complexity of change. *Psychoanalytic Dialogues: The International Journal of Relational Perspectives, 15*(2), 255–283. https://doi.org/10.1080/10481881509348831

Thye, M. D., Bednarz, H. M., Herringshaw, A. J., Sartin, E. B., & Kana, R. K. (2017). The impact of atypical sensory processing on social impairments in autism spectrum disorder. *Developmental Cognitive Neuroscience, 29,* 151–167. https://doi.org/10.1016/j.dcn.2017.04.010

Watling, R., Miller-Kuhaneck, H., Parham, L. D., & Schaaf, R. (2018). *Occupational therapy practice guidelines for children and youth with challenges in sensory integration and sensory processing*. AOTA Press.

Wieder, S. (2017). The power of symbolic play in emotional development through the DIR lens. *Topics in Language Disorders*. *37*(3), 259–281. https://doi.org/10.1097/TLD.0000000000000126

Wieder, S., & Wachs, H. (2012). *Visual/spatial portals to thinking, feeling and movement*. Profectum.

Young, G. (2011). *Development and causality: Neo-piagetian perspectives*. Springer.

A Frame of Reference for Neurodevelopmental Treatment

Tina Weisman

Neurodevelopmental treatment (NDT), originally known as the Bobath approach, was developed by Berta and Karel Bobath in the mid-1940s. NDT is a clinically based frame of reference used by occupational, physical, and speech therapists worldwide treating individuals with neuropathology that primarily impacts their postural and movement systems. NDT is a clinical problem-solving approach that incorporates handling and facilitation of treatment intervention processes (Beirman, 2016).

Berta Bobath was a trained remedial gym teacher who had a private practice of massage and exercise. When approached to assist a prominent artist recovering from a left cerebrovascular accident (CVA) that affected his dominant right upper extremity, Bobath drew upon her expertise in physical education. Leveraging her understanding of typical movement patterns, she guided the client through motions diverging from his atypical postures. Through this approach, she successfully altered muscle tone, enabling the activation of more typical movements. After persistent persuasion, she managed to convince her husband Dr. Karel Bobath, a neuropsychiatrist, to observe her treatment. Intrigued by the results, he devoted the remainder of his career to collaborating with his wife, interpreting the effectiveness of her clinical discoveries within the context of neurophysiology of the time. Together, they created a practice model grounded in their findings. This practice model persists, undergoing continual updates and adaptations in alignment with the latest advancements in neurophysiologic theories.

During the mid-1900s, neuroscientists believed the central nervous system (CNS) was organized hierarchically. Dr. Bobath explained spasticity and tone based on the reflex hierarchical model. The neuroscience of motor control in the 1940s was based on Sherrington's theories of the reflex hierarchical model (Bierman, 2016). According to this model, higher centers of the CNS influence the inhibition or excitation of muscle activation needed for efficient movement patterns. An infarct to the CNS blocks the balance of inhibition and excitation resulting in atypical muscle tone, and therefore atypical movement. Primitive reflexes that were typical in infant development either become integrated or absolve as postural development matures. The child developing atypically, depending on the severity, maintains some or all of these reflexive movement patterns, which interfere with efficient gross, fine, and oral motor functioning.

Initially, the Bobaths highlighted the importance of the developmental sequence as a means of facilitating typical movement. The understanding of cephalocaudal and traditional development provided the means of understanding typical infant development, in comparison to children who develop atypically due to neuromotor impairments. This gave Mrs. Bobath the imputus to analyze the differences between typical and atypical motor development, enabling her to discern stereotypical movement patterns associated with children affected by cerebral palsy. She believed that atypical motor development impeded posture and movement (automatic movement patterns), which subsequently hindered an individual's functional roles in their daily life, family, and community. She observed how mothers handled their typically developing babies and modeled her handling accordingly. She incorporated how atypical development impedes posture and movement (automatic movement patterns) and impacts the person's functional roles within their daily life, family, and community. Later, the Bobaths shifted their teachings to facilitating the movement components that the child with neuropathology was not developing versus the actual sequence of developmental skill. For example, they no longer believed that a baby must crawl before they could walk. Instead, the skilled NDT therapist would analyze the motions the child practices in crawling and facilitates those components in higher age/stage-appropriate positions, such as climbing, cruising, and transitioning from the floor to sit or stance.

In its origin, NDT was developed as an intervention for adults who suffered a CVA and for children with cerebral palsy. Today NDT is a frame of reference for intervention applicable for all children that exhibit postural and movement impairments due to neuropathology. NDT has been primarily utilized as a frame of reference to address an individual's needs when there are neurologic deficits causing a change in their postural and movement systems. Diagnoses with neurologic deficits resulting in tonal abnormalities such as cerebral palsy, CVA, Down syndrome, traumatic brain injury (TBI), and other congenital disorders are more typically seen within the pediatric population.

According to Bierman (2016), contemporary NDT is characterized as a holistic and interdisciplinary clinical practice model. Informed by current and evolving research, it underscores individualized therapeutic handling based on movement analysis for the habilitation and rehabilitation of individuals with neurologic pathophysiology. NDT explains spasticity, tone, stiffness, dystonia, and hypotonia as movement characteristics of the variation of types of cerebral palsy, adult hemiplegia, and TBIs. A fundamental principle of NDT is the recognition of neuroplasticity and adaptability across all body systems throughout the lifespan. Flexibility, adaptability, and neuroplasticity addressed by NDT play a crucial role in determining the extent of occupational performance and participation across the lifespan and various settings. Enhancing the understanding of neurologic plasticity and musculoskeletal adaptive or maladaptive development aligns with clinical problem solving and handling approach of NDT. This alignment serves as a foundation for enhancing engagement and participation from birth to geriatrics.

In summary, NDT is an interdisciplinary, holistic, and client-centered approach that places emphasis on the individual, task, and the environment. It addresses primary sensorimotor impairments resulting from neurologic injuries while actively working to prevent common secondary impairments. Specifically, NDT is committed to optimizing a child's posture and movement patterns within their musculoskeletal alignment, utilizing techniques such as positioning, handling, adaptive equipment, and orthotics to promote their functional performance. The evolution of the Bobaths' living concept aligns with the contemporary sciences, including neurophysiology, kinesiology, biomechanics, and motor development. This chapter serves as a foundational guide to understanding of the NDT frame of reference.

THEORETICAL BASE

Assumptions

The theoretical base of the NDT adopts four core assumptions:

1. Individuals with neuromotor pathology contend with impaired patterns of postural control and movement coordination which are the primary problems in children with neuromotor pathology.
2. Identifiable sensorimotor impairments are changeable, and overall function improves when the problems of postural control and motor coordination are treated directly by addressing atypical neuromotor and postural control in a task-specific context.
3. The foundation for evaluating individuals' capacity to participate in age/stage-appropriate functional activities, as well as for clinical reasoning and planning intervention, is rooted in practitioners' understanding of typical motor development.
4. Movement is linked to sensory processing in two distinct ways (feedback and feedforward/anticipatory control).

Theoretical Foundations

NDT is focused on promoting motor efficiency of the postural and movement systems to optimize the clients' efficiency in daily life occupations. NDT emphasizes the importance of real time problem solving and analysis during treatment allowing for variation of NDT individualized treatment strategies. Neurologic insult is proposed to result in sensorimotor impairments of the postural and movement systems altering the musculoskeletal development of children with neuromotor pathology. Atypical muscle tone, dysfunction in their proprioception, feedforward and feedback systems, biomechanical alignment, and kinesthetic awareness are all contributing factors impacting the child's occupational performance. Dynamic Systems Theory of Motor Control, Neuronal Group Selection Theory (NGST), Motor Learning, Motor Control and Motor Developmental Theory, Kinesiology and Biomechanics form the theoretical foundation for understanding therapeutic principles impacting change in the postural and movement systems for function and to implement NDT interventions. The following section provides an overview of these theories and how they support the NDT frame of reference.

Dynamic Systems Theory of Motor Control

Dynamic systems theory (DST) is a top down model that postulates that motor learning, task performance, and skill acquisition are learned through the interaction between the individual, the task, and the environment. This theory examines all systems involved in movement production (Kamm et al., 1990; Smith & Thelan, 1993), describing each subsystem as an equal contributor to learning novel tasks within adaptive and flexible task performance and environmental factors (Darrah & Bartlett, 1995). Guided by the theoretical tenets of DST, practitioners can identify movement constraints and employ problem solving to select optimal treatment strategies. Factors constraining movement production may include bony restrictions, limited flexibility in soft tissues and fascia, varying levels of arousal, poor sensory processing, and movement impairments arising from faulty timing and a lack of coordinated firing of muscles attempting to work cooperatively together (Howle, 2002).

According to the DST, motor development is self-organizing and naturally occurs as children experience their environments. Through practice and repetition, different elements of the movement system come together, integrating information to form a distinct movement synergy. When learning new movements, children actively solve movement problems through their engagement with the environment, practicing a wide variety of movement strategies before selecting the single "best" solution to their movement problem. Children actively problem solve new movement opportunities by repeating and reinforcing new movements in a variety of contexts and tasks. Trial and error provides feedback to the system, allowing for adjustment and refinement of motor skills within a context. The development of and changes in function are connected to children's neural networks and distributed throughout their nervous systems. As such, the competences of all the other body systems interact dynamically with children's contexts and the task goals (Howle, 2016). Children with neuropathology, conversely, use compensatory motor synergies to problem solve when learning new movements due to their limited motor repertoire.

In summary, DST proposes that movement is organized around behavioral goals. In typically developing children, movements are guided by children's abilities to select and match the appropriate movements to the tasks. They can adjust their bodies to the forces of gravity and their musculoskeletal systems. Furthermore, they respond naturally and easily to environmental demands. In contrast, children with atypical development movements are restricted by the limitation of their body and limited abilities to adjust to environmental demands (Bierman, 2016). Consequently, the atypically developing child with neuromotor dysfunction exhibiting stereotypical movements have difficulty adapting or accommodating the task demands within their environmental constraints.

Neuronal Group Selection Theory

NGST proposes that the CNS is constantly adapting and changing in response to a variety of tasks and environmental factors. NDT incorporates the theoretical foundations of the NGST (Hadders-Algra, 2000), which emphasizes that function is the driving force of motor development. NGST provides practitioners with an understanding of the neuronal interactions inside the CNS contributing to movement production. According to this theory, the human brain is organized in a dynamically oriented set of neural networks or neuronal groups that share connections related to their function. These neuronal groups are shaped by engagement with the environment and various tasks. Repeated experiences create neural networks of hardwired neurons. These functional neuronal units "come online" jointly as a coded synergy of information, producing efficient and integrated interaction with the environment.

The nervous system possesses an inherent mechanism recognizing the distinct value of a particular movement or behavior to each individual. This built-in mechanism fuels the hardwiring process with neurochemistry, reinforcing the connection of these neural synergies within the CNS (Edelman, 1987). Cognition, motivation, and temperament are factors that prime the nervous system for this selective organizational process. The architecture of an individual's nervous system is shaped by their distinct and unique experiences, guided by a neurobiologic process known as pruning. Like pruning a hedge, the nervous system selectively trims unnecessary neural connections while organizing and preserving valuable ones.

NDT incorporates NGST by providing several opportunities to practice and perform task variation that promotes problem solving and engagement in meaningful tasks across different settings, within the context of the individual's child abilities. This allows for the child's CNS to organize neuronal pathways that meet their cognitive, sensorimotor, and musculoskeletal systems capabilities and constraints.

Motor Control, Motor Learning, and Motor Developmental Theory

Motor control theories have evolved significantly beyond Dr. Bobath's initial description of Sherrington's reflex hierarchical theory of motor control. The living concept of NDT remains dynamic, continuously integrating, and drawing upon contemporary theories of motor control. The following section will describe contemporary modern motoric theories and their relevance to NDT intervention.

Motor Control

Motor control is how the CNS organizes and directs functional motion. Motor control is a result of interactions among systems that are integral to posture and movement. Each system works interdependently with each other and there is variability within each system. The musculoskeletal system is responsible for implementing the motion that is person, task, and environmentally variable by the activation of specific muscles within the degrees of freedom respective to each joint recruited for efficiency of task performance.

The general assumptions of motor control include:

1. Motor behavior is a result of interaction among dynamic systems such as the person, task, and environment.
2. Systems are variable, flexible, and adaptable to person, task, and across different environments.
3. Motor dysfunction occurs when there is a lack of adaptability and environmental constraints.
4. Modification of task and environment, along with body systems may promote occupational participation and performance in meaningful daily activities.
5. Optimal motor learning occurs when the child is engaged in meaningful tasks within an environment that supports task performance and engagement.

(Adapted from O'Brien, J., Coker-Bolt, P., & Dimitropoulou, K. (2020). Application of motor control and motor learning, In O'Brien & Kuhaneck, H. (Eds.), *Case Smith's occupational therapy for children and adolescents.* Elsevier.)

Motor Learning

Motor learning is the process by which motor efficiency and coordination are developed. When a child reaches for their bottle or cup, the amount of force for grasp, orientation of their posture, and hand accommodation during reach and knowing when to terminate their reach displays their motor control for that task, in the specific environment of performance. Constraints to any systems, such as range of motion, weight, shape, or length of bottle and its placement in the environment will impact their level of motor performance.

NDT emphasizes facilitating client-centered, meaningful, functional task performance while addressing movement impairment with variation of task and environments with the assumption that increased opportunities of practice will promote generalization of skill acquisition across settings. Using NDT, the practitioner is able to identify and facilitate the initiation and activation of the movement components that are impairing the clients occupational performance within varying environmental contexts.

Motor Learning Theory

NDT integrates motor learning theory principles into its primary theoretical foundations (Barthel, 2020). Motor learning theory describes how one acquires motor efficiency in novel skill acquisition throughout the lifespan. The complexity of motor learning includes the interaction between the developing nervous system, musculoskeletal systems, sensory and cognitive systems working in tandem as the child engages in task participation within a variety of different environmental contexts. Motor learning theory proposes that factors such as goal-directed tasks, verbal and nonverbal feedback, the variability of practice, and context affect motor performance. Understanding the principles of motor learning significantly enhances the practitioners' ability to help children achieve carryover from therapy to everyday life (Howle, 2016).

Children learn by practicing tasks with variation and in different environments. Self-correction and efficiency occur through feedback mechanisms by generalizing skill development in familiar and unfamiliar environments. Children's motor performance occurs through purposeful, functional, and goal-directed task performances across a variety of settings allowing for generalization of motor learning. The NDT clinical framework aligns with the motor learning theory, emphasizing the creation of opportunities for functional activities' practice, novel environmental exposures, and hands-on facilitation of movement components that the child has difficulty initiating or activating independently. It is aimed to promote generalization of goal-directed functional tasks across environment for efficient motor learning and retention of skill acquisition (O'Brian et al., 2020). The practitioner's level of support varies moment to moment according to the task demands.

Motor learning theory provides the NDT therapist with a theoretical foundation to help children with neuromotor pathology learn novel, goal-directed functional tasks, such as feeding, self-care, play, and gross motor skills with the goal of generalization across environments for efficient motor learning and retention of skill acquisition (O'Brien et al., 2020). NDT promotes motor learning by engaging the child in purposeful activities within a supportive environment that promotes feedback for self-correction and problem solving to occur, allowing neurologic systems to work together in the development and generalization of novel skill acquisition.

Sensory Contributions to Motor Control and Motor Learning

Sensory information is an essential component to the development of motor learning, motor control, and ultimately efficient and coordinated motor performance due to the sensory feedback and feedforward systems. Somatosensory information also plays a role in motor learning, with emphasis on level of arousal and emotional state of being. Sensory processing is the process by which the CNS registers sensory information, processes and organizes that information into a meaningful output motor response. The CNS precisely filters out what is background information, with selection of meaningful information for an efficient motor response related to the individual's motor performance, the task, and the environment.

NDT recognizes the feedforward and the feedback systems of sensory systems contributing to the production of well-coordinated movements (Howle, 2002). The feedforward sensory system is a proactive sensory system that anticipates and initiates movements intrinsic to the person. In contrast, the complementary feedback sensory system reacts to the environment, regulating and adapting motor execution. Together, these sensory systems interact within the CNS informing the motor system with information about the movement, the task, and the environment.

The acquisition of sophisticated, intentional, and accurately coordinated movements requires precise registration and interpretation of sensory feedback derived from both the movement and the surrounding environment. The registration of this sensory information within the nervous system functions as an internal mechanism for detection of movement errors, learning new movements, engaging in motor planning, and executing skilled motor execution. When an individual's motor system generates movements in the absence of sensory feedback from the body or the environment, it relies on the feedforward sensory system. This feedforward system prepares the motor system with relevant sensory information prior to muscle recruitment. NDT provides the child with an enriched variety of sensorimotor experiences, and diverse range of opportunities to practice movements. NDT places an emphasis on sensorimotor feedback, enabling the development of problem-solving movement strategies through the application of anticipatory motor control (Barthel, 2020).

Motor Developmental Theory

Motor development theory provides a foundational framework for motor skills and behavior changes across the lifespan. A thorough understanding of motor development in infants and children is an essential prerequisite for assessing and treating those with neuromotor dysfunction.

Infants explore their world through their senses, interaction with people and objects in their environment and via their ability to efficiently transition from one position to another allowing for visual, sensorimotor exploration of the world around them. Although cognitive, behavioral, and social skills are all essential dynamic systems that develop and influence sensorimotor development, in this chapter we will be emphasizing motor development and control. It is, however, important to emphasize the occupational therapy practitioner's understanding of the influence of all systems when assessing the whole child. The infant's oral motor, fine, and gross motor development are intertwined and rely on the postural system to support the dynamically stable foundation for refined oral motor, visual, and fine motor dexterity in a variety of positions. In the context of the NDT frame of reference, practitioners typically assess a child's motor performance by observing them in age/stage-appropriate positions during activities like play, feeding, dressing, and transitional movements such as rolling, crawling, sitting, and walking. Typical developing children naturally refine motor skills through exploration and interaction with their environment, demonstrating variability in positions and movement patterns. The absence of such variability or the presence of stereotypical patterns often acts as a warning sign, prompting practitioners to conduct further investigation.

When considering typical development from a motor control perspective, NDT posits postural development occurs in a cephalocaudal (head to feet) progression. The infant is born in physiologic flexion. The infant exhibits a variety of random motions in their extremities with lack of volitional control of their body parts. Control of postural extension develops down the cervical spine before control of cervical flexion. As the baby gains control for thoracic extension, they begin to develop cervical flexion allowing for a chin tuck position.

The NDT practitioner may facilitate head control by encouraging use of tummy time while providing a visually engaging activity. The NDT occupational therapy practitioner may place their

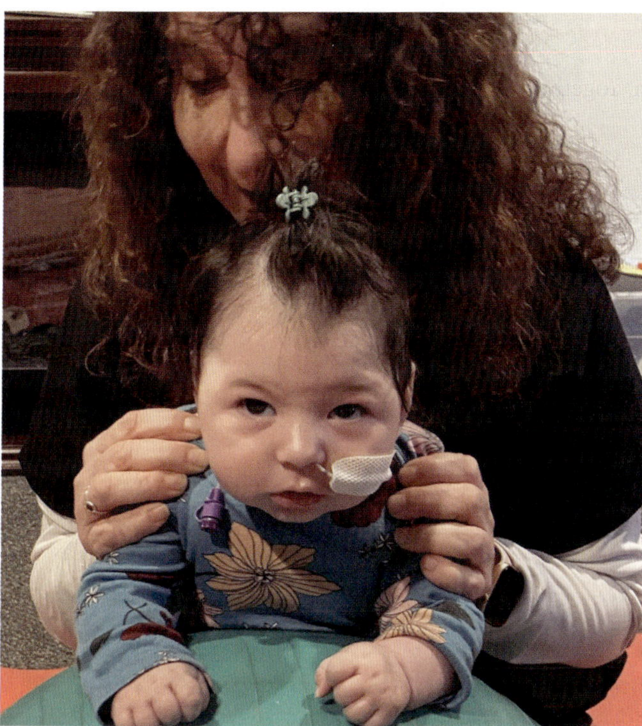

FIGURE 8.1 Three-month-old atypical baby in facilitated prone prop on a ball.

hands to promote motor activation in the components of motion needed to develop head control. The child with cerebral palsy may require hands on facilitation of their hip extensors and scapula to assist in activation of thoracic extension, scapula depression, and cervical elongation (Figure 8.1).

In the past, NDT proposed the necessity of progression through a developmental sequence of motion to master subsequent antigravity levels of motion. However, this treatment principle has evolved, recognizing the greater significance of focusing on the movement components of each developmental skill and their influence on upright functions. For example, the 4-month-old infant is developing symmetry and midrange control of the trunk and extremities. In the supine position, the infant brings hands and feet together with hips and knees in flexion (Figure 8.2). This activity involves working on eccentric hip extension and abduction, with isometric and concentric contractions of hip flexors and abdominals. These movement components are the same ones the child will need to maintain a sitting position at 6 months in upright vertical position (Figure 8.3).

A practitioner using an NDT frame of reference will focus on the movement components that the typical baby is practicing from 3 to 5 months of age that provides the postural and movement support the child needs to maintain unsupported ring sitting. Through handling and facilitation and environmental constructs incorporating meaningful task performance, the practitioner will facilitate the motor activation required for age/stage-appropriate skill acquisition in higher upright positions. In other words, NDT does not believe that one has to roll before they can sit. Instead, the therapist may facilitate the child to activate the motions practiced in earlier developmental stages while facilitating transitional movements in and out of sitting, while reaching, grasping, and manipulating toys in a variety of planes of motions. Handling

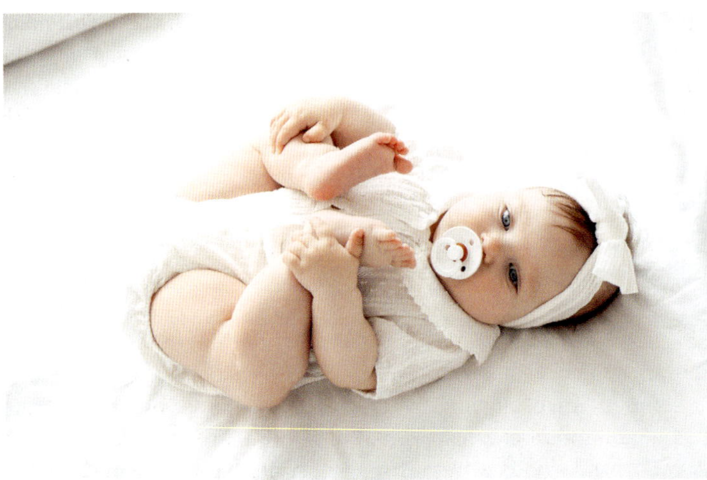

FIGURE 8.2 Four-month-old typical baby playing hands to feet in supine.

through exploratory play facilitates curiosity and engagement in person, task, and environmental constructs.

Within the context of the NDT frame of reference, practitioners observe and analyze any typical movement components that the child cannot initiate independently during play and age/stage-daily occupations. Movement during functional tasks is evaluated to identify atypical patterns of

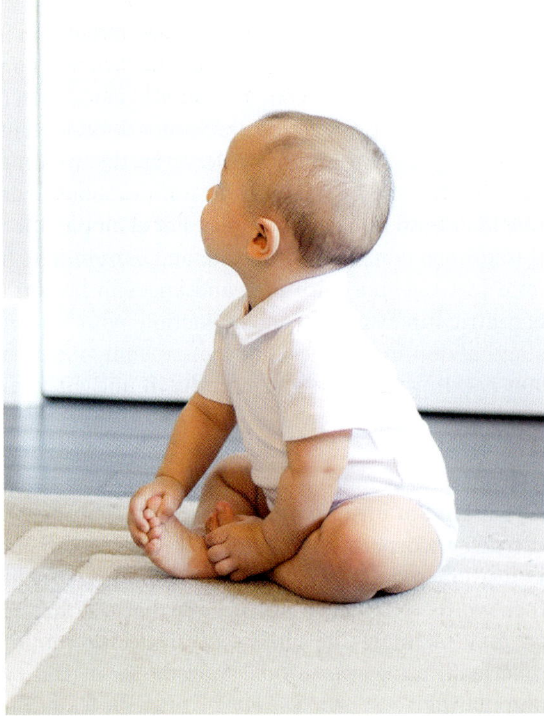

FIGURE 8.3 Six-month-old typical baby maintains a supported sit while bringing hands to feet, and visually looking at the environment.

motion contributing to motor inefficiency during task performance. A child with neuromotor dysfunction exhibits a deficiency in diverse movements, leading to a limited repertoire of movement patterns for practice, resulting in the development of compensatory stereotypical movement patterns limiting environmental exploration and motor efficiency. The development of their postural and movement systems is compromised, resulting in neuromotor dysfunction impacting muscle tone, forces, and motion activation.

Atypical development of the musculoskeletal systems occurs due to asymmetrical muscle forces around the developing skeletal joints and boney structures. Practitioners recognize the importance of anatomical alignment for the postural and movement systems' variation, adaptation, and efficiency. NDT assumes that without intervention, atypical compensatory movements will develop into habitual compensatory patterns of motion, limiting the child's movement repertoire and putting them at higher risk for developing musculoskeletal contractures and deformities. Facilitating the components of movements missing for task performance through handling strategies and environmental modifications are hallmarks of NDT strategies. NDT classifies atypical movements as primary or secondary impairments. Primary impairments are the components representing the significant constraints upon movement and posture. These impairments are a direct result of the original pathology. Examples of primary impairments may include stiffness, impaired muscle activation or motor unit recruitment, excessive muscle coactivation, ineffective, stereotyped muscle synergies, impaired motor execution, atypical scaling of muscle forces, and impairments with regulation or sensory impairments.

Evaluation of competing typical and atypical patterns of movement demonstrated by children with neuromotor impairment is fundamental to evaluation and treatment. Atypical movements resulting from CNS insults are diverse. Therefore, each child with different neuromotor disorders may demonstrate various atypical postural and movement patterns. NDT treatment planning strategies are based on facilitating the components of movements missing for task performance through handling strategies and environmental constructs. Gradation of support occurs throughout the session, intending to provide the least amount of support for postural control and motor activation during task performance. Facilitating the components of movements missing for task performance through handling strategies and environmental modifications are hallmarks of NDT treatment strategies. Gradation of support occurs throughout the session, with the goal of providing the least amount of support for postural control and motor activation during task performance.

Kinesiology and Biomechanical Concepts

NDT utilizes kinesiologic and biomechanical principles to examine and address issues related to posture and movement impairments. Key concepts include planes of movement, alignment of the body, range of motion, the base of support (BOS), muscle strength, postural control, weight shifts, and mobility.

Planes of movement refer to motor action in the anatomical planes of the body (Figure 8.4). The body exhibits movement in three spatial planes. The initiation of motor control occurs in the sagittal plane, where infants engage in flexion and extension movements against gravity. As the torso muscles of infants become active and proficient in generating forces against gravity, movements in the frontal plane begin to integrate with sagittal plane movements. Transverse plane movements represent the most advanced motor patterns in typical development, requiring coordination of the musculature developed in both the sagittal and frontal

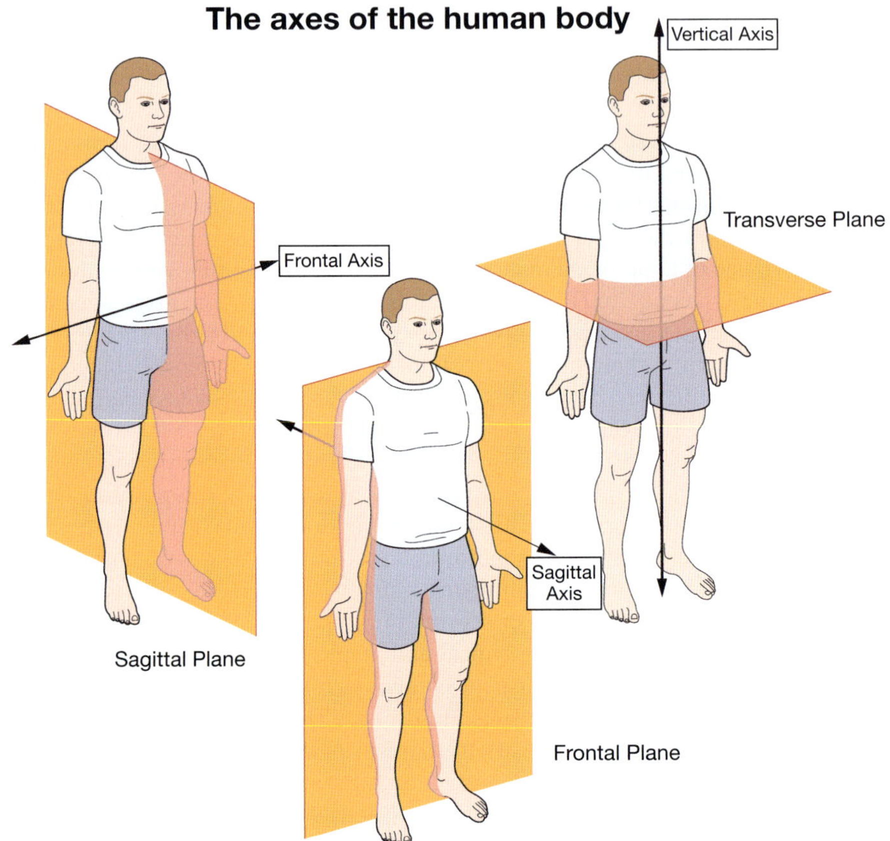

FIGURE 8.4 Planes of motion. (Based on image from Shutterstock.)

planes. These transverse plane movements enable rotation around the body axis, necessary for the development of balance and posture in space (Table 8.1). NDT intervention prioritizes facilitation and manipulation to improve postural control through involvement in weight-bearing activities, weight shifting, and guiding movement through space. Meanwhile, the practitioner focuses on elongating muscles and activating them while they are in a lengthened state during functional tasks.

Table 8.1 Planes of the Body and Associated Movements

Planes of Motion	Axis of Motion
Sagittal plane	Anterior and posterior
Frontal plane	Lateral motion of the trunk/abduction and adduction of extremities
Horizontal/Transverse plane	Rotation

FUNCTION AND DYSFUNCTION CONTINUA

Function/dysfunction continua provide practitioners with descriptions of clinically relevant observable behaviors and identify the presence of function and dysfunction of motor skills in children with neuropathology (Schoen & Anderson, 1999).

The following seven function/dysfunction continua are identified as key elements of NDT assessment process:

1. Postural muscle tone
2. Postural control
3. Range of motion
4. Musculoskeletal alignment and patterns of weight bearing and weight shifting
5. Dissociation of movement
6. Motor coordination and efficiency
7. Proprioception

Indicators of Postural Muscle Tone

Postural muscle tone is a widely utilized clinical term that is often misunderstood. The most recognized definition of muscle tone is the resistance to stretch during the muscles resting state (Lundy-Ekman, 2018). In other words, it reflects the preparedness of a muscle to initiate action potential. For example, upon waking up to your alarm clock, your postural muscle tone is in a lower state of readiness compared to a scenario where an expected fire drill occurs mid-morning in your clinical setting.

Postural muscle tone is a term that is commonly used among rehabilitation professionals, referring to the foundational postural background required to provide dynamic stability during antigravity or upright positioning. As previously described in this section, muscle tone is described as the force with which a muscle resists being lengthened, indicating the muscle's amount of stiffness. Table 8.2 identifies the continuum of tone in relation to its resistance to stretch. Functionally,

Table 8.2 Classification of Muscle Tone

Muscle Tone		
Typical Nomenclature of Muscle Tone	**Definition**	**Muscle Resistance During Passive Stretch**
Rigidity	Increase in resistance to stretch regardless of velocity/movement	Excess resistance that is present regardless of velocity or speed of stretch
Spasticity/Hypertonia	Increase in resistance to stretch dependent on movement/velocity	Excess resistance that increases with velocity or speed of stretch
Normal	Normal stretch resistance in a resting, normally innervated muscle	Typical resistance of muscles on passive stretch
Hypotonia	Atypically low muscular resistance to passive stretch	Less than typical resistance
Flaccidity	Complete lack of muscle tone	No resistance

Adapted from Lundy-Ekman, L. (2018). *Neuroscience fundamentals for rehabilitation* (5th ed.). Saunders Elsevier.

postural tone refers to the increase of activity in our postural muscle working to counteract the force of gravity. Studies have shown that tonic or postural muscles remain active throughout the body during periods of quiet or static stance (Ivanenko & Gurfinkel, 2018), challenging the perception that static stance is inert. Furthermore, studies suggest that "postural control involves active sensory processing with a constant mapping of perception to action, so that the postural system is able to calculate where the body is in space and can predict where it is going and what action will be necessary to control this movement" (Shumway-Cook & Woolcott, 2017, p. 170).

Postural muscle tone is influenced by the elastic characteristics of the muscle and connective tissue. Muscles that are overly stretched or muscles that are shortened in their resting state have differing responses to stretch. The elongated muscle may be characterized as hypotonic due to its decreased resistance to stretch, whereas the shortened or contracted muscle may have an elevated resistance to stretch. Muscle tone changes readily with position, posture, activity (resting or during movement), excitement, illness, and factors that affect overall state (Barthel, 2004).

The continuum of muscle tone ranges from flaccid, hypotonia (low muscle tone), normal muscle tone, spasticity to rigidity. Clinically muscle tone is assessed by the resting muscles resistance to stretch.

- **Flaccidity** is defined as the complete loss of muscle tone, with zero stretch resistance.
- **Hypotonia** is characterized by very low or minimal stretch resistance. Children with hypotonia exhibit a diminished resting muscle tension and decreased ability to generate voluntary muscle force. They often have excessive flexibility and postural instability.
- **Normal tone** is indicated by a typical or normal stretch resistance of the neuromuscular system.
- **Hypertonia** consists of two categories, spasticity and rigidity, both exhibiting an abnormally strong resistance to passive stretch. Individuals with hypertonicity exhibit overall neuromuscular excitability and is often a result of a lesion involving their spinal cord or motor cortex.
- **Spasticity or hypertonia** exhibits a velocity-dependent stretch resistance in the resting muscle. The resistance to slow stretch is low, however the resistance to quick or fast stretch is high and can be clinically felt by a "catch" in the muscle when the therapist provides a quick stretch.
- **Rigidity** is velocity independent, indicating that regardless of the speed of stretch, fast or slow, the muscle response remains constant. Rigidity is a severe state of hypertonia where muscle resistance occurs throughout the entire range of motion independent of velocity. Rigidity presents as simultaneous cocontraction of agonists and antagonists muscles, which results in an immediate resistance to a reversal of the direction of movement around a joint (Table 8.2) (Lundy-Eckman, 2018, p. 272)

In addition to the above muscle tone continuum, dystonia and ataxia are two other muscle tone disturbances that are often observed in children with neuromotor impairment.

- **Dystonia** or **fluctuating tone** is defined as a movement disorder in which involuntary sustained or intermittent muscle contractions cause twisting and repetitive movements, abnormal postures, or both (Sanger & Kukke, 2007). Dystonia is typically seen in children with neuromotor impairment of the basal ganglia such as athetoid cerebral palsy. These children present with large extraneous movement patterns that are involuntary, lacking control of motion in midranges. Children with fluctuation of tone are often influenced by primitive reflexive movements such as the asymmetrical tonic neck reflex (ATNR). Although this chapter is not dedicated to retention of primitive reflexes, it is important to note that the retention of primitive reflexes in children with neuromotor impairment are contributing factors to increased tone and decreased

variation of motion. NDT recognizes the influence of these reflexes and utilizes biomechanical principles of alignment as a means of dampening the involuntary influence on movement.
- **Ataxia** is a lack of muscle coordination during voluntary movements, resulting from an insult to the cerebellum.

Typically, children with neuromotor impairments exhibit abnormal postural muscle tone in their axial muscles impacting their ability to sustain their upright posture against gravity. These children develop compensatory movement patterns as a means of holding themselves up against gravity, such as scapula elevation, abduction and upward rotation, with lumbar extension and hip flexion instead of activating their deep postural back extensors, abdominals, hip extensor and abductors while standing or ambulating (Figure 8.5A).

In sitting many children resort to a W-sitting position as an inefficient stable base to free their hands for play. Long-term obligatory W-sitting puts the child at risk for hip abnormalities during their developing years (Figure 8.5B).

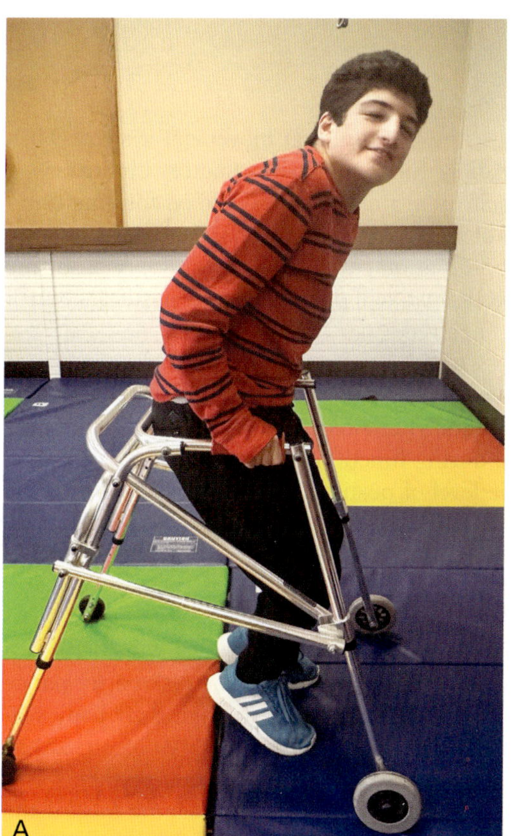

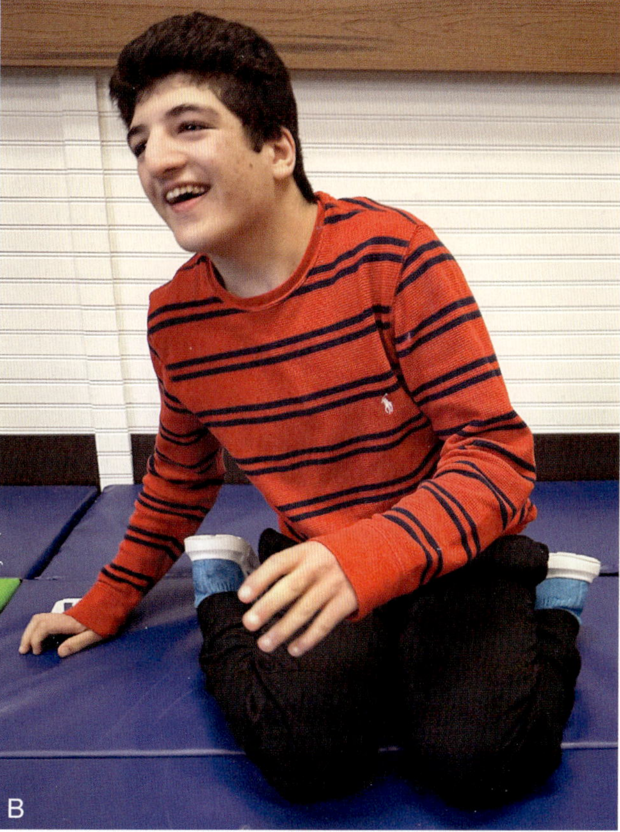

FIGURE 8.5 **A.** Boy with spastic diplegia cerebral palsy with crouched postural control in standing. Note the use of superficial postural muscles compensating for weak deep postural muscles, such as scapula elevation, humeral internal rotation, humeral extension, hip flexion, and lumbar extension. **B.** Boy with hypertonicity in W-sit. W-sit is a compensatory pattern allowing upright posture to free his arms for function.

Table 8.3 Function/Dysfunction Continuum: Postural Muscle Tone and Behavioral Indicators

Postural Muscle Tone	
Function	**Dysfunction**
Normal muscle tension at rest	Increased or decreased muscle tension at rest
Normal resistance to passive stretch	Hypo- or hyperresistance to passive stretch
Dissociation of body segments from and within each segment	Lack of dissociation or isolated control of body segments from and within each segment
Muscle tone responds to different postures	Muscle tone does not change with different postures

NDT views atypical muscle tone as a primary impairment of the neural system contributing to the impairments of posture and motor performance observed in children with neuromotor challenges (Barthel, 2020). Children with neuromotor pathology often present with mixed tone (Table 8.3).

Indicators of Postural Control

Motor control theories of neuroscience discuss how the postural and movement systems work together to achieve optimal motor efficiency for daily functional performance. Clinically, we define postural control as the ability to hold oneself up against gravity while performing functional tasks. As stated in the Assumptions section of this chapter, one of NDT's main principles is that impaired postural control and movement coordination patterns are the primary problems in clients with neuromotor impairments. In this section we will discuss what is postural control and how it impacts function or dysfunction when impaired.

Postural control involves controlling the body's position in space for the dual purposes of stability and orientation (Shumway-Cook & Woolcott, 2017). The primary role of the postural system is to provide the postural control needed to sustain and hold the body orientation through space, by providing dynamic stability and balance during functional activities. Postural control is essential for all upright functional activities. The level of postural control needed to maintain upright posture and move through gravity varies among individuals, tasks, and environments. Postural orientation and postural stability work together to establish postural control, enabling the maintenance and movement of the body within space (Figure 8.6).

Postural control relies on sensory input to determine the spatial position of the head and body, encompassing the ability to motorically manage this orientation, comprehend the necessary forces for movement, and consider the environmental constraints during the task performance (Howle, 2002). Postural orientation is defined as an individual's ability to align their body segments in relation to both their body and the task at hand (Shumway-Cook & Woolcott, 2012). For example, during a ball game, a child orients themselves to the ball, positioning themselves to either catch or throw the ball. Catching the ball may entail running and leaping toward the moving target, requiring a smaller BOS than when throwing the ball. In both scenarios, visual input contributes to the orientation of the ball. Additional sensory systems, such as the vestibular and proprioceptive systems, play roles in postural orientation by aligning the head to the body and the body to the surface, respectively. The discussion on the proprioceptive system will follow later in this chapter.

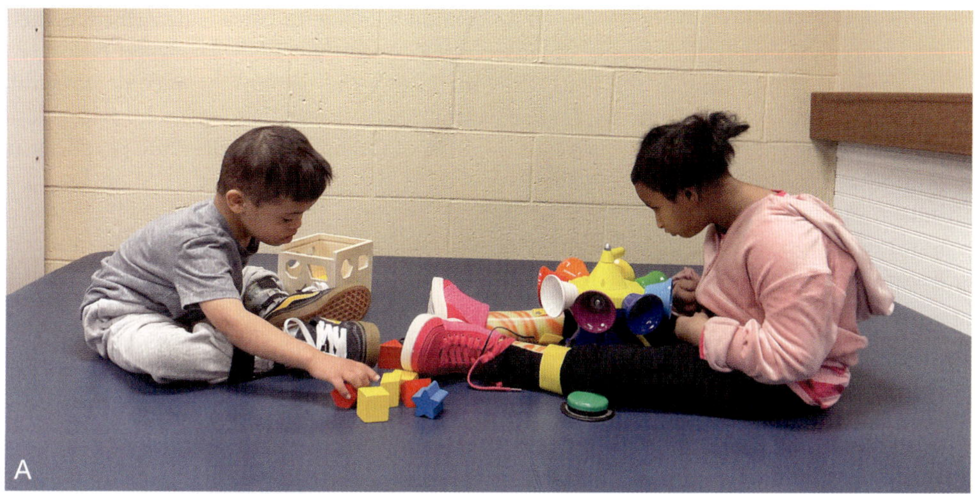

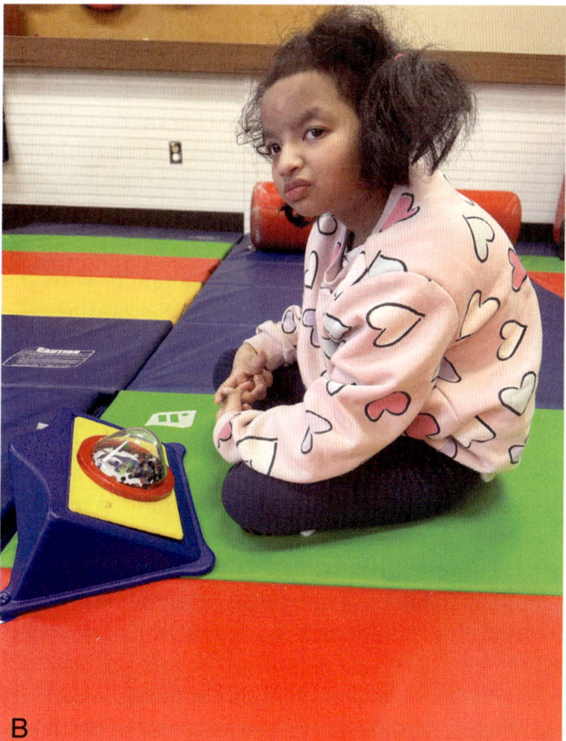

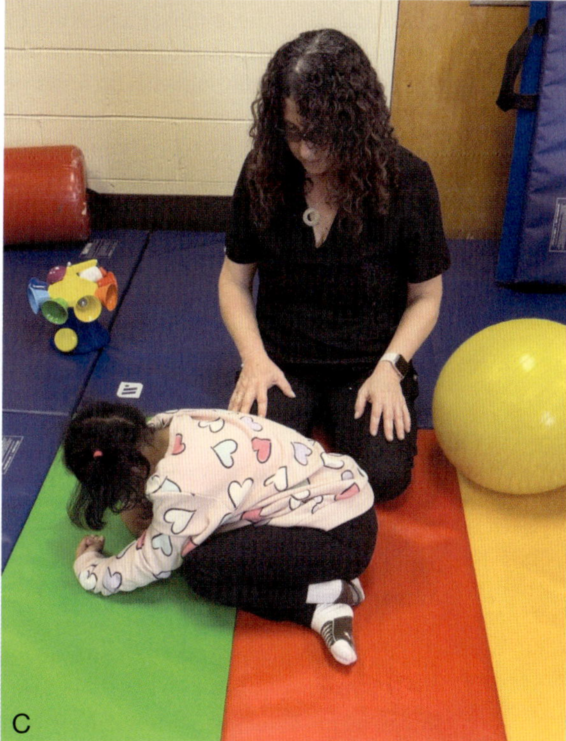

FIGURE 8.6 **A.** Two children with hypotonicity, demonstrating sacral sitting impacting postural spinal musculature, while engaged in play. **B.** Child with hypotonicity sits slumped forward. **C.** Child with hypotonicity is unable to maintain sitting posture.

Postural stability is another way of describing balance. Balance is described as the individual's ability to maintain their center of gravity (COG) over their BOS. The wider or larger the BOS, the easier it is to maintain the COG, thus increasing the person's balance or postural stability (Shumway-Cook & Woolcott, 2017). For example, when one first learns how to ride a bicycle, training wheels are provided to increase the BOS of the bicycle. As the child practices and learns how to maintain their COG over the two wheels, the training wheels are no longer required, indicating the child has developed the balance required for task efficiency. Postural control is required for most upright tasks, however postural orientation and postural stabilization vary according to the demands of each task (Shumway-Cook & Woolcott, 2017).

NDT assumes that normal movement requires integration of both the postural and movement systems allowing for the postural stability and mobility demands within variation of task and environment. Children with neuromotor pathology often have difficulty maintaining their balance in upright positions. Their postural muscles are often weak due to either low or high muscle tone and weakness. As a result, they often recruit inefficient movement muscles as a means of compensation. For example, children may posture their arms in a high guard position with scapula elevation, abduction and upward rotation, humeral internal rotation, elbow flexion for added stability. These movement components are muscles that primarily control the movement system, thus sacrificing functional mobility for inefficient stability. NDT intervention focuses on facilitation and handling with the intention of promoting postural control through experiences of weight bearing, weight shifting, and facilitation of movement through space (Figure 8.7). In tandem the practitioner provides muscle elongation and activation of those muscles in lengthened state during functional task performance.

In summary, postural stability and mobility serve as the foundation of functional movement. Dynamic stability or postural control is required for refined motions such as eye–hand coordination, manipulation, digital dexterity, and variation of motoric repertoires aligning with the individual's abilities and constraints, task, and environmental demands. Table 8.4 outlines the function/dysfunction continuum related to postural control.

Indicators of Range of Motion

Range of motion is described as the extent or distance a joint or a muscle can move and the direction in which it moves (Shumway-Cook & Woollacott, 2012, 2017). Range of motion includes active and passive and differs among individuals and across different joints. Normal, voluntary, active joint range of motion supports movement production. In the musculoskeletal system, muscles generate and transmit force through tendons to bones. To perform a specific task, a joint must be moveable into the "just right angle," considering factors such as amount of length, speed, and force produced by the muscle (Lieber, 2010).

Challenges related to flexibility, muscle length, and skeletal changes represent secondary impairments associate with range of motion in children with neuromotor dysfunction. Flexibility issues occur in joints, soft tissues, ligaments, tendons, and muscles. Joint mobility impairments include hypermobility or hypomobility. Hypermobility is observed in individuals who exhibit greater than normal range of motion in a given joint and increased ligamentous laxity. Children with hypotonia or muscle weakness around a joint often present with hypermobility or insufficient musculoskeletal support around their joints. Hypomobility, on the other hand, involves excessive stiffness or reduced range of motion in joints, contributing to maladaptive changes in joint alignment, deformities, and pain (Howle, 2002).

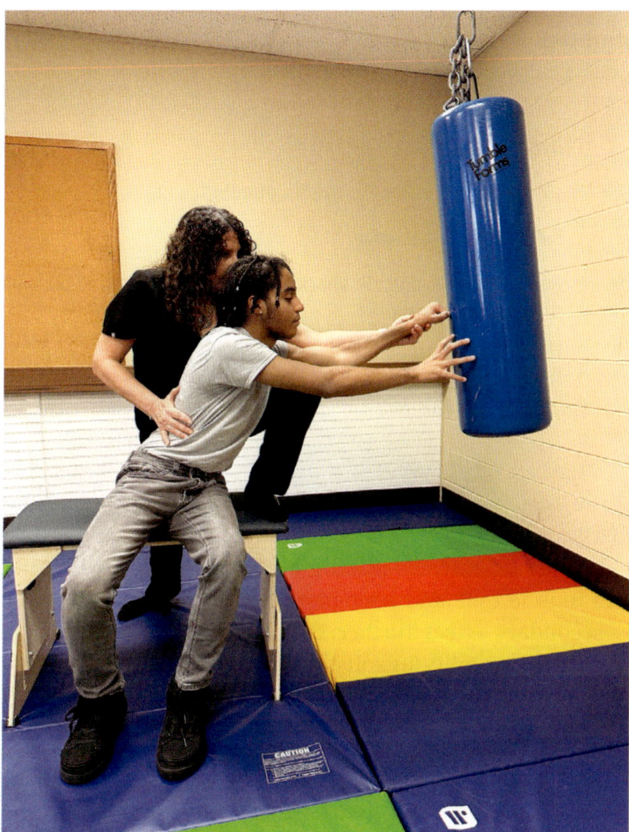

FIGURE 8.7 Range of the client's reach is beyond arm's length, therapist is facilitating a postural weight shift in his lower trunk and pelvis, to allow for reaching bilaterally toward the desired target.

Table 8.4 Function/Dysfunction Continuum: Postural Control and Its Behavior Indicators

Postural Control	
Function	**Dysfunction**
Ability to sustain the body in upright positions against gravity	Inability to sustain upright positions against gravity
Indicators of Function	**Indicators of Dysfunction**
Ability to maintain upright during functional tasks	Lacks postural control during functional tasks seeking external surfaces
Ability to weight shift over COG/BOS support during transitional movements	Loss of balance when COG is shifted over BOS during transitional movements
Ability to assume and maintain a variety of positions required for efficient task performance in a variety of environments.	Requires compensatory patterns of upper and lower extremities.

Table 8.5 Function/Dysfunction Continuum: Range of Motion and Its Behavioral Indicators

Range of Motion	
Function	**Dysfunction**
Full passive range of motion across all joints	Limited range of motion within affected joints
Indicators of Function	**Indicators of Dysfunction**
Full active and passive range of motion across all joints	Joint stiffness, muscle shortening resulting in limited passive or active range of motion
Ligamentous integrity for joint stabilization	Hypo- or hypermobility of joints Risk of developing joint contractures and musculoskeletal deformities, subluxations, or dislocation

Muscle length changes can occur due to atypical muscle tone, shortening of the viscoelastic properties of the muscle fibers, and excessive muscle recruitment or muscle spasms. Conversely, muscles may also become elongate excessively, leading to weakness and a diminished capacity to generate force. Changes in muscle tone and strength can also affect soft tissues, causing lose length and flexibility. This secondary effect further contributes to challenges in maintaining proper joint alignment. Promoting flexibility in soft tissue length and increasing muscle length are essential for preventing orthopedic impairments in later life (Howle, 2002). NDT intervention includes activating muscles in their elongated states while therapeutically increasing their length and range of motion. Activation is a central component in NDT intervention. Table 8.5 details function/dysfunction of range of motion.

Indicators of Musculoskeletal Alignment and Patterns of Weight Bearing and Weight Shifting

Biomechanical alignment of the musculoskeletal system refers to the arrangement of body segments in relation to each other, taking into account factors such as gravity, the BOS, and the nature of the task (Howle, 2002). The human body operates as a "linked system," where each segment biomechanically influences the others within the system. The alignment of body segments over the BOS determines the amount of effort required to support the body against gravity. Synergistic activation of muscle systems relies on these biomechanical relationships to produce accurate and efficient functional movement (Barthel, 2020).

Typically developing children practice movement in all planes of motion with symmetrical muscle forces around their joints. Through weight bearing and weight shifting during transitional movements, the child moves in all three planes of motion, ensuring symmetrical lines of pull in musculoskeletal development. However, children with neuromotor dysfunction, leading to asymmetrical tonal influences around their joint, are susceptible to vertebral column malalignment. The misalignment of the spinal column creates a biomechanical disadvantage for the deep intrinsic postural muscles, hindering their ability to engage effectively and resulting in weakened postural control. This compromised postural control affects the child's COG over their BOS, exacerbating issues related to posture, balance, and coordination. Children who struggle to maintain upright postural control face a heightened risk of developing spinal curvatures such as kyphosis, scoliosis, and lumbar lordosis.

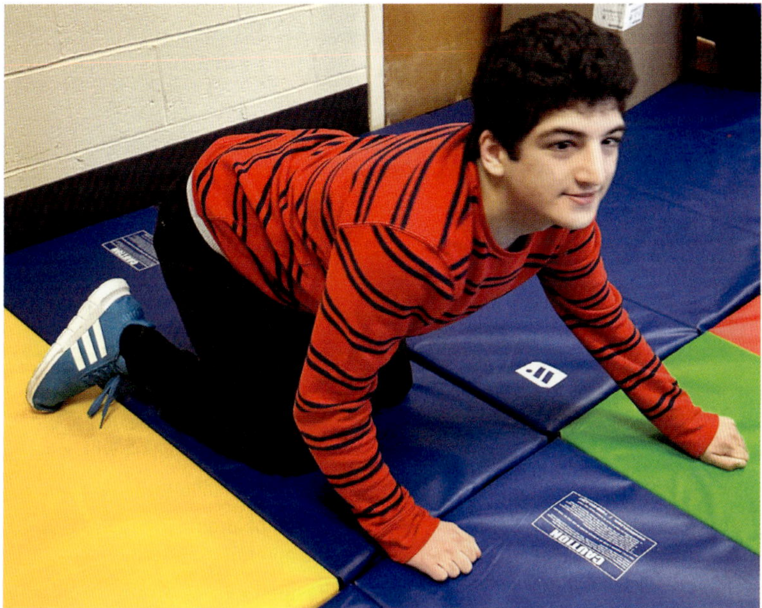

FIGURE 8.8 Boy is unable to generate sufficient force for weight shifting toward a new base of support.

Malalignment of the musculoskeletal system increases the likelihood of future orthopedic issues that may require surgical intervention for the child. Children with moderate-to-severe cerebral palsy often exhibit delayed skeletal maturation, low bone density, and diminished linear bone growth (Stamer, 2016). Atypical musculoskeletal changes typically manifest in the spine, lower extremities, and upper extremities. Notably, the wrist and hands are particularly at higher risk for muscle contractures due to their length and architecture.

Weight shifting is the ability to restore balance by moving the COG back over one's BOS, particularly during transitional movements or when moving in and out of positions. A child with neuromotor dysfunction who exhibits poor musculoskeletal alignment faces challenges in bearing weight and shifting it away from the loaded limb. For effective weight shifting from one BOS to the next, it is essential for the individual to establish efficient contact with the supporting surface (Figure 8.8). Children with atypical tone and alignment struggle to adapt their body to the supporting surface, resulting in an inefficient generation of forces necessary for shifting weight away from their supporting limb. This challenge can be observed during transitional movements like moving from sitting to standing, transitioning from quadruped to sitting, and during walking. Table 8.6 provides the indicators of function and dysfunction for musculoskeletal alignment and patterns of weight bearing and weight shifting.

Indicators of Dissociation of Movement

Dissociation is the ability to move specific body segments independently of others. It is linked to a neurologic insult to the lateral corticospinal tracts responsible for refined isolation of motion (Lundy-Ekman, 2018). Children with stereotypical patterns of movements have impaired dissociation of motion.

Table 8.6 Function/Dysfunction Continuum: Musculoskeletal Alignment and Patterns of Weight Bearing and Weight Shifting and Its Behavior Indicators

Musculoskeletal alignment and patterns of weight bearing and weight shifting	
Function	**Dysfunction**
Maintenance of upright postural musculoskeletal alignment in relationship to the base of support	Difficulty maintaining upright postural musculoskeletal alignment in relationship to the base of support Requires external support surfaces to sustain upright positioning
Indicators of Function	**Indicators of Dysfunction**
Postural musculoskeletal alignment in relation to body supporting movement in space	Poor postural alignment resulting in poor posture Atypical Postural Alignment in the Sagittal Plane: • Development of kyphosis (flexion of the thoracic spine) • Excessive posterior pelvic tilt with spinal flexion Atypical Postural Alignment in the Frontal Plane: • Development of lordosis (hyperextension of the lumbar spine) • Excessive anterior pelvic tilt with lumber extension Atypical Postural Alignment in the Horizontal/Transverse Plane • Asymmetrical postural alignment • Development of scoliosis (lateral asymmetrical curvature of the spine)
Ability to weight bear and push off of supporting surfaces to weight-shift body over weight-bearing limb during transitional positions and gait	Inability to weight bear and push off of supporting surfaces to weight-shift body over weight-bearing limb during transitional positions and gait

In the context of typical development, newborns are initially born in a state of physiologic flexion due to the confined space in utero, limiting their range of motion. As a child progresses in their development, they gradually engage in motion across all three planes—allowing diverse movements such as flexion, extension, medial and lateral motions, and rotation. As children develop increased control of rotation, they concurrently practice dissociation of movement both between (intralimb) and within (interlimb) body segments. An instance of intralimb dissociation occurs when a child supinates their right forearm while pronating their left forearm. Meanwhile, interlimb dissociation can be observed in actions like hip extension coupled with knee flexion. Furthermore, dissociation occurs in the spine as well, allowing individuals to, for example, turn their head to the right while keeping their lower trunk and pelvis oriented anteriorly.

As previously discussed, atypical development presents with atypical postural tone, compensatory stereotypical movements, with a limited movement repertoire available for task performance and environmental variables. In the context of atypical motoric development in children, there is a manifestation of stereotypical movement patterns that lack variation, indicating a lack of dissociation or the isolated control of body segments. Dissociation or fragmentation is the isolated control of movement in one joint without generating movement either between or within body segments in another joint (Shumway-Cook & Woolcott, 2017). The ability to flex your elbow and extend your wrist would be an example of intralimb dissociation. Children with stereotypical patterns of movements have impaired dissociation of motion.

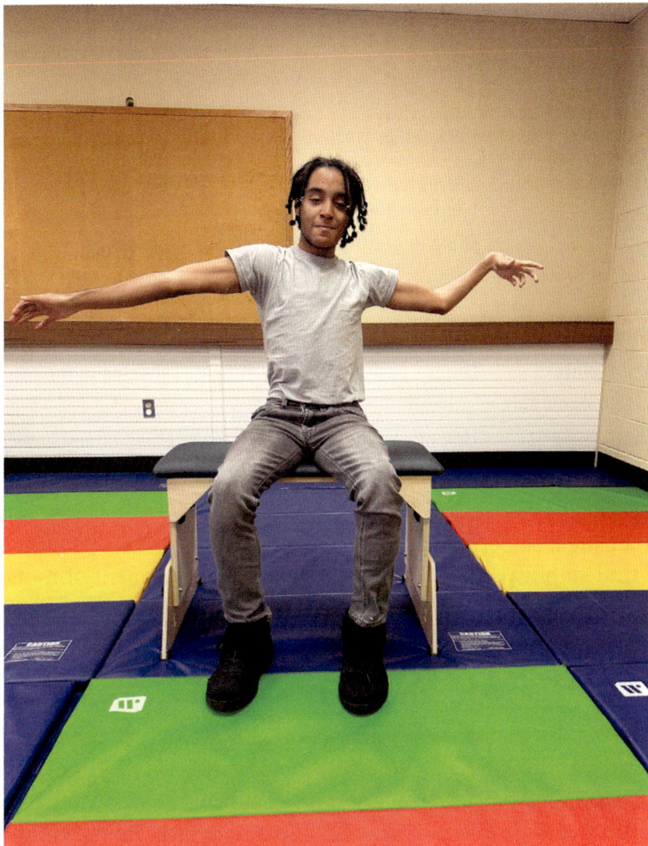

FIGURE 8.9 Boy shows a lack of interlimb dissociation impacting his active range of motion and reaching.

Children with hyper- or hypotonicity often exhibit a deficiency in dissociation and isolated movement productions (Figure 8.9). Those with hypertonicity face limited opportunities to elongate and activate muscles eccentrically in their lengthened state, hindering joint range of motion, and impeding the ability to perform dissociation and isolated movement productions. Children with hypotonicity experience joint instability stemming from postural weakness and ligamentous laxity. They tend to develop compensatory movement patterns that further impede dissociation of motion. Commonly, children displaying W-sit, log roll, a scissored gait pattern, commando crawls, or bunny hops often demonstrate a lack of dissociation. In the upper extremity, insufficient dissociation between the upper arm, forearm, wrist, and hand is observed, leading to compromised fine motor manipulation, digital isolation, and dexterity (Table 8.7).

Indicators of Motor Coordination and Efficiency

Occupational therapy practitioners assess motor coordination and efficiency as a crucial aspect of movement during functional activities. Evaluating motor coordination and efficiency involves a comprehensive analysis of temporal–spatial elements in task execution, considering factors like timing, velocity, and change of speed. It also involves observing the recruitment of isolated, dissociated motions for task efficiency. Motor coordination and efficiency relies on the integration of both

Table 8.7 Function/Dysfunction Continuum: Dissociation of Movement and Its Behavior Indicators

Dissociation of Movement	
Function	**Dysfunction**
Ability to perform isolated movements between or within body segments	Stereotypical movements Limited range of motion Muscle contractures and bony deformities
Indicators of Function	**Indicators of Dysfunction**
Ability to move joints in their full range of motion	Musculoskeletal contractures or deformities
Ability to activate muscles in their lengthened state (eccentric control) achieving full joint range of motion	Unable to eccentrically activate muscles in their fully lengthened state
Ability to use rotation during functional motions	Use of compensatory motions such as bunny hops, W-sits, commando-crawls, walks with scissored gait

gross and fine motor skill during task performance, with learning and practice. Motor coordination and efficiency reflect postural stability, emphasizing the minimal recruitment of motion necessary for accurate and timing task execution. Their foundation lies in the integration of the postural and movement systems, a critical element for skill acquisition across the lifespan. Throughout meaningful daily life occupations, the postural and movement systems work in refined synchrony, demonstrating the intricate interplay required for optimal motor coordination and efficiency.

In the typically developing child, coordination and efficiency develops as the child practices a variety of novel skills, through intrinsic self-correction and problem solving. Initially when a child learns a novel motor task, they recruit larger and more extraneous movements while paying increased attention to learning and problem solving for the motor task. As the child gains experience through practice and engages in self-correction, they recruit less extraneous motion and the task becomes more automatic in nature. The efficiency, trajectory, and response time of extremity movement hinge on the postural control, and the ability to dissociate movement based on the individual needs, the specific task, the variability of task demands, and environmental factors.

Conditions like compromised balance, reduced inter- and intralimb dissociation, limited ROM, and altered muscle tone collectively contribute to motor coordination and efficiency issues in children with atypically development. Those experiencing fluctuating tone or dystonia, such as those with athetosis, often demonstrated extraneous movement patterns, a lack of motion dissociation, and impaired response time, all of which contribute to dysfunction of motor coordination and efficiency.

Occupational therapy practitioners using an NDT framework create a safe environment, allowing the child to make mistakes, self-correct, and practice novel skills while providing the just right amount of handling to activate the postural control and movement needed for task performance. For example, when a child has difficulty sitting in their chair while using utensils, the practitioner may provide handling techniques to facilitate dynamic postural control and promote dissociation between and within both upper extremities (Table 8.8).

Indicators of Proprioception

The function of the proprioception in postural control is to provide the CNS with continuous and real-time sensory information about the position and movement of the body parts in space.

Table 8.8 Function/Dysfunction Continuum: Motor Coordination and Efficiency and Its Behavior Indicators

Motor Coordination and Efficiency	
Function	**Dysfunction**
Ability to perform motor tasks with fluid efficiency.	Inability to perform motor tasks with fluid efficiency. Task performance appears awkward, extraneous inefficient motions, decreased timing and accuracy.
Indicators of Function	**Indicators of Dysfunction**
The ability to maintain balance and coordination during complex motor tasks.	Inability to maintain balance and coordination required for complex tasks with variables of velocity, environmental demands such as uneven surfaces and reaction time.
Ability to grade reaction time to task demands such as response to a moving target, ball skills, driving, or use of scanning devices.	Inability to elicit reaction time in response to variation of velocity of moving targets. Inability to change direction of reach mid-stream toward a moving target.
Ability to move with speed and dexterity in response to task and environmental demands.	Inability to move with speed and dexterity in response to task and environmental demands.
Ability to dissociate and isolate inter- and intralimb body segments for refined dexterity and motor efficiency.	Inability to dissociate and isolate inter- and intralimb body segments resulting in stereotypical inefficient movement patterns for variation of task demands and environmental factors.

Proprioceptive receptors, located in muscles, tendons, and joints, detect changes in joint angles, muscle length, and tension. This information is crucial for the CNS to create an accurate and updated body schema, allowing for the coordination of muscle activity and adjustments in posture to maintain balance and stability during various movements and activities. Clinicians often emphasize the delivery of proprioceptive input through weight-bearing experiences. In the earlier section on postural control, we explored the significance of biomechanical joint alignment. In this section, we will delve into how proprioceptive information is received and underscore the importance of proper biomechanical joint alignment for the precision of proprioceptive data transmitted to the CNS. This precision is crucial for the CNS to formulate a detailed and accurate body schema image necessary for movement and error correction.

The functioning of the proprioceptive somatosensory system relies on the proper biomechanical and musculoskeletal alignment of joints, ensuring the accurate and precise reception of information by receptors regarding the body's spatial orientation. As mentioned earlier, a child with atypical muscle tone and musculoskeletal malalignment experiences asymmetrical or weak forces around their joints, impacting joint stability. When the child's joints lack proper alignment, they face a biomechanical disadvantage for both muscle firing and critical detection of muscle stretch essential for proprioceptive input to the spinal cord. Consequently, this poses challenges to the child's ability to perceive their body's position in space, affecting their postural control, postural adjustments, balance, coordination, and refined dexterity (Lundy–Ekman, 2018) (Table 8.9).

Table 8.9 Function/Dysfunction Continuum: Proprioception and Its Behavior Indicators

Proprioception	
Function	**Dysfunction**
Ability to detect where the body is in space with or without visual confirmation	Inability to detect where the body is in space with or without visual confirmation
Indicators of Function	**Indicators of Dysfunction**
Ability to self-correct body parts in motion	Inability to adjust body parts during weight-bearing activities in preparation for transitional movements
Ability to adapt motion in response to task and environmental demands	Inability to adapt postural control and movement in response to variable tasks and environmental demands

GUIDE FOR EVALUATION

The NDT problem-solving model serves as a guide for occupational therapy practitioners, leading them through goal setting, evaluation, and intervention implementation (Howle, 2002). An NDT evaluation is based on the theoretical assumptions section of this chapter. An understanding of typical motor development, biomechanics, kinesiology, and motor learning is crucial for navigating the complexity of neuromotor pathology and its impact on a child's development and occupational performance. The analysis includes observing the variability in the child's movement repertoire while recognizing stereotypical movement or repetition of compensatory movement patterns that interfere with motor learning, motor control, and ultimately, motor efficiency across the setting and throughout their lifespan. The evaluator focuses on the "quality" of task performance required for efficiency rather than merely the ability to use compensatory patterns for the skill. When using an NDT frame of reference, the practitioners direct their attention to areas of function and dysfunction previously highlighted, such as postural muscle tone, postural control, musculoskeletal alignment, weight bearing and weight shifting in and out of transitional positions, proprioceptive awareness, and motor coordination for developing task efficiency (Table 8.10).

Assessment of the Child

The assessment begins as soon as the child enters the room. The practitioner will observe how the child is brought into the room. For example, a parent carrying a child while supporting their head indicates that the child may have trouble with head control. In contrast, a child using an ambulatory assistive device, wheelchair mobility, or displaying independence in functional mobility presents a different scenario. The evaluator systematically examines the child's postural control during gross motor performance across various positions, assessing its impact on their ability to perform activities of daily living (ADLs) and play. Special attention is given to overall functional bimanual and upper extremity skills essential for daily life occupations. Throughout the evaluation process, the practitioner may also handle the child as a determinant of how the child receives and integrates sensorimotor information during therapeutic movement opportunities This encompasses an exploration of tone, posture, and balance, contributing to a comprehensive understanding of the child's capabilities and areas requiring therapeutic attention.

Table 8.10 Guideline for Neurodevelopmental Assessment

I. Examination of engagement in functional tasks and potential for change
  1. Gross and fine motor abilities/movements through space
  2. Gross and fine motor/task-directed functions
  3. Activities of daily living (ADLs) and Instrumental ADLs (IADLs)
  4. Communication
  5. Oral motor functions
  6. Social skills/behavior

II. Examination of posture and movement
  1. Biomechanical alignment
  2. Relationship of base of support and center of gravity
  3. Postural control and balance
     a. Anticipatory weight shift
     b. Steady-state balance
     c. Equilibrium
  4. Movement strategies and use of compensations
  5. Distribution and type of muscle and postural tone
  6. Symmetry/asymmetry
  7. Kinesiologic and biomechanical application of movement
  8. Coordination
  9. Description analysis of specific motor functions (handwriting, dressing, chewing)

III. Examination of system integrity and impairments
  1. Neuromuscular
     a. Muscle activation and execution including timing, initiating, sustaining, and terminating muscle activity
        i. Generation of force/tension
        ii. Coactivation/reciprocal patterns
        iii. Intra- and interlimb dynamics
        iv. Modulation and grading of forces
     b. Coordination of postural stability with movement
     c. Synergies
     d. Extraneous, fractionated, or dissociated movements
     e. Overall motor activity
  2. Musculoskeletal
     a. Range of motion; active and passive
     b. Muscle extensibility, functional range
     c. Muscle strength and endurance
     d. Skeletal abnormalities
  3. Sensory
     a. Vision
     b. Auditory
     c. Gustatory
     d. Olfactory
     e. Vestibular
     f. Somatosensory (tactile and proprioceptive)
     g. Interoception
     h. Sensory processing and modulation
  4. Regulatory
     a. Arousal
     b. State regulation
     c. Emotional regulation and control
  5. Perceptual/cognitive
     a. Cognitive capacity
     b. Attention
     c. Memory
     d. Adaptability
     e. Motor planning (gestalt of task, perception of position in space, and spatial relationships)
     f. Executive functions (goal setting, inhibiting impulsiveness, understanding consequences of actions)
  6. Other systems
     a. Integumentary
     b. Respiratory
     c. Cardiovascular
     d. Gastrointestinal
  7. Changes in performance and capacity based on response to facilitation, modification of task or environment

Adapted from Howle, J. M. (2002). *Neuro-Developmental treatment approach: Theoretical foundations and principles of clinical practice.* NDTA.

Within the NDT framework, ADLs represent specific domains of functional skills that often result from the integration of gross motor and upper extremity function. ADLs include participation in self-care such as feeding, and dressing, as well as the ability to explore, play, and interact with the environment (American Occupational Therapy Association [AOTA], 2020). In the context of NDT, the occupational therapy practitioner focuses on the impact of posture and movement dysfunction on the functional use of their upper extremities. This involves considerations of weight bearing and weight shifting during transitional movements, reach and grasp in space, hand manipulation required for dexterity in using tools, and independence in ADLs and instrumental ADLs (IADLs) across various settings. In addition, the practitioners assess factors such as cognition, motivation, arousal, vision, perception, sensory, and somatosensory processing, examining their relationship to motor control and task efficiency.

Occupational therapy practitioners analyze movement during task performance within the NDT framework. The specialized NDT lens enables practitioners to analyze and identify the primary movement components that impact the efficiency of a specific task within the context of the evaluation process. Importantly, the evaluation and analysis constitute a dynamic and continuous process, extending seamlessly throughout each treatment session.

Within the NDT framework, there is a recognition of the significant role that environmental factors play in anticipatory control of posture and movement. It is essential for practitioners to thoroughly assess the environmental demands associated with task performance and their impact on the child's postural and movement systems. Environment changes, such as seating or object placement can contribute to facilitating postural control (Figure 8.10). For instance, placing an object at a higher level can promote postural upright extension; and offering external support can facilitate optimal seating alignments. For detailed information on adaptive equipment that supports postural control for optimal task performance and efficiency, the

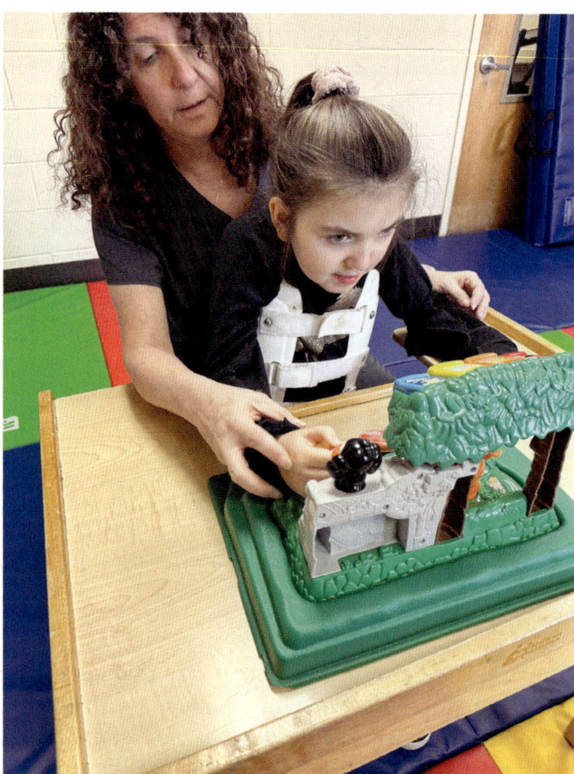

FIGURE 8.10 Child in thoracic-lumbar-sacral orthotic (TLSO) providing support of postural extension required for visual direction and manipulation. Play is essential for development and postural support allows for active participation in motor learning opportunities.

reader is encouraged to refer to Chapter 13, A Biomechanical Frame of Reference to Position Children for Function.

Evaluation of Posture and Movement

NDT places special emphasis on the assessment of posture and movement. A therapist assesses qualities along the function and dysfunction continua within this evaluation process. Attention is given to the quality of postural muscle tone, both at rest and the changes that occur during stable and mobile task demands. To facilitate a comprehensive assessment of posture and movement, a therapist observes postural alignment across all three planes of movements. In addition, the therapist evaluates the joint range of motion and postural control, specifically in relation to the BOS (Barthel, 2020).

To appreciate the importance of assessing posture and alignment, the author encourages the reader to engage in a practical exercise. Please long sit on the floor with a posterior pelvic tilt or sacral sitting. As you reach forward, observe that your humeri are biased toward scapula elevation, humeral internal rotation, biomechanically influencing the forearm toward pronation, accompanied by wrist flexion, ulnar deviation, and thumb adduction. Holding this position, bring your hands toward each other, noticing that the dorsum of your hands are facing each other. This restricted alignment limits visual inspection and digital manipulation. Now transition to an anterior pelvic tilt, where you are sitting on your ischial tuberosities with lumbar extension. Take note of the influence on your upper extremities. They are now in neutral alignment, offering full range of motion and dissociation at each joint needed for reach, grasp, and hand accommodation in space. This experiential exercise illustrates the significance of the quality of sit, which practitioners carefully examine. The practitioners aim to improve task efficiency and promote optimal musculoskeletal alignment by enhancing the fluency of motion through evaluating and adjusting the quality of body alignment in various positions such as sitting.

The assessment of interlimb and intralimb coupling are crucial for determining the degree of dissociation between different body parts. For example, many children with cerebral palsy experience restrictions in their hamstrings and hip flexors, demonstrating a "tightly linked" intralimb coupling relationship between the pelvis and the femur. In addition, children may demonstrate an intralimb relationship between wrist flexion and ulnar deviation, creating a tightly constrained that prevents "dissociation" of these joint segments. The relationship between body segments needs to be analyzed to assist in the planning of treatment implementation.

In the evaluation process, the therapist observes the child's postural control in various upright positions and during transitional movements. Central to this examination is the child's ability to maintain their COG over their BOS. When a child experiences dysfunction in this area, they may resort to using their upper extremities as a compensatory mechanism. This compensatory strategy, however, tends to impose further limitations on the child's upper extremity movement repertoire, particularly affecting their ability for refined fine motor manipulation.

Upon completion of the evaluation, the occupational therapy practitioner interprets the results by identifying consistent compensatory stereotypical patterns of movement that significantly impede the child's task performance across various contextual and environmental settings. The subsequent intervention and goal setting are determined based on the child's functional needs, current abilities, and expected performance within various environmental contexts. The objective is to design interventions that promote the generalization of motor learning and enhance task performance, aligning with the child's specific requirements and expectations.

POSTULATES REGARDING CHANGE

Postulates regarding change guide practitioners in developing strategies and methods of intervention that facilitate changes in functional performance. When the results of the evaluation indicate dysfunction, intervention focuses on the qualitative aspects of the movement that interfere with the child's ability to develop skills or functional abilities. Varying movement and postural problems may require different handling approaches. As previously emphasized, the primary technique of the NDT frame of reference is therapeutic handling provided by practitioners.

General Postulates Regarding Change

Therapeutic handling provides the opportunity for the child to develop variations of movements through active engagement in activities guided by therapists. By handling, while incorporating biomechanical alignment and guiding movement activation beyond their stereotypical ranges, the child will gain motor learning experiences that may be challenging for them to achieve independently.

Specific Postulates Regarding Change

1. If a practitioner uses graded sensory input during the guided movement, the child would more likely to dissociate body segments during movements and have typical motor responses to postural changes.
2. If a practitioner provides the opportunity to weight bear and weight shift through space while ensuring proper body alignment and offering therapeutic guidance, the child will be more likely to assume and maintain a variety of postures (postural control) required for effective task performance.
3. If a practitioner assists a child in moving through full range of motion, the child will reduce the possibility of joint contractures and musculoskeletal deformities, allowing them to more freely engage in activities.
4. If a practitioner provides aligned weight-bearing and weight-shifting experience with sensory inputs such as deep pressure and joint compression, a child will be more likely to perform cocontraction of musculature around a joint supporting movement in space and performing postural transitions.
5. If a practitioner provides handling to promote weight shifts and transitional movements while supporting proper alignment and the dissociation of coupled joint segments as the child moves in and out of positions, the child will be more likely to demonstrated reduced stiffness and less stereotypical patterns.
6. If a practitioner provides opportunities to promote graded reaction time, speed, and dexterity during complex motor tasks with therapeutic handling techniques, the child will be more likely to perform motor tasks with fluid efficiency.
7. If a practitioner provides deep pressure down toward the child's BOS when the body segments are aligned, a child will be able to initiate movements from the BOS by pushing against the BOS to aid in muscle activation.
8. If the practitioner provides stability and sensory input to proximal joints of the body, the child will become aware of their body in space and be able to adjust body parts in motion and in response to task and environmental demands.

APPLICATION TO PRACTICE

The NDT frame of reference emphasizes intervention strategies that require active initiation and participation from a child, often completed by the practitioner's manual guidance and direct handling. When evaluation results indicate movement dysfunction, practitioners target the primary components of movement that impede the child's occupational task performance within their age/stage developmental levels of functioning. The child's limited movement repertoire can result in motor inefficiency, potentially restricting play opportunities and environmental exploration. NDT places an emphasis on providing intervention to enable the child to effectively engage and participate in meaningful occupations. This is achieved through hands-on facilitation, focusing on typical movement components to increase motor efficiency for task performance.

The practitioner provides specific handling strategies to support the child's optimal biomechanical alignment, facilitating muscle activation within ranges that the child may struggle to assume or maintain independently, particularly in contexts crucial for their desired occupational task performance. NDT intervention strategies include preparatory strategies, coupled with precise therapeutic handling. The practitioner focuses on facilitating posture and movement while simultaneously inhibiting the child's atypical compensatory movement repertoires.

Preparation and Muscle Elongation

Children with neuromotor challenges often lack the capacity to independently select or activate the necessary motor patterns required for task performance. Frequently, the components of a movement sequence need to be prepared before a child can effectively integrate them into a functional sequence (Howle, 2002). Preparatory activities are those techniques that involve mobilizing or elongating tight structures and promoting proper alignment of body segments with respect to each other and in relationship to gravity (Figures 8.11 and 8.12). The purpose of preparation is

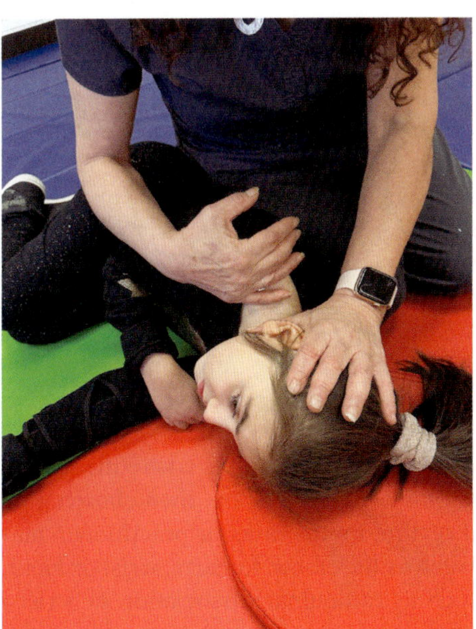

FIGURE 8.11 Passive cervical muscle elongation using gentle traction. Note that therapist's left hand is stabilizing while the right hand is providing gentle downward traction. This preparation allows for active muscle elongation in an activity.

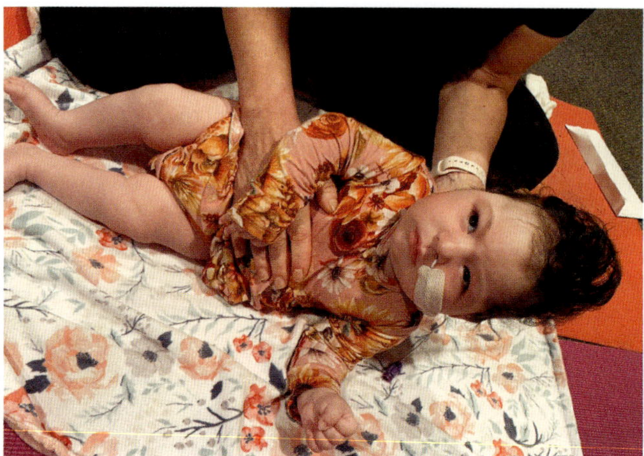

FIGURE 8.12 Facilitating active muscle elongation on the weight-bearing side provide preparation for transitional movements and head righting in supported side lying.

to establish a state of readiness, laying the foundation for the child's active initiation of posture and movement (Barthel, 2020).

Therapeutic Handling

The cornerstone of NDT intervention lies in therapeutic handling, which is grounded in contemporary knowledge of anatomy, neuroscience, biomechanics, and kinesiologic principles. The purpose of therapeutic handling is to facilitate active initiation and participation in a child's postural and movement systems, aiming to promote participation and independence in age/stage occupational performance. The selection of handling strategies is guided by the goal of optimizing motor efficiency while inhibiting neuromotor factors contributing to motor inefficiency and hinder skill acquisition. Using specific hand placement is one example of handling strategies. Practitioners purposefully place their hands to provide graded, directional, sensory cues with the intent to enhance the child's ability to "feel" and actively engage in new motor patterns within their optimized musculoskeletal alignment (Figure 8.13). Addressing muscle tone and range-of-motion limitations, practitioners may initiate their intervention with passive muscle elongation to increase range available motion. Through continuous movement analysis and clinical reasoning, practitioners adjust handling techniques by varying pressure, directions, forces, and the amount of sensory information provided. The overarching goal of therapeutic handling is to provide just enough support to enable activation in biomechanical alignment that the child cannot independently assume or maintain. The gradation of support is dynamically modified based on the specific task and environmental demands encountered during intervention.

"Key points of control" are the body segments that the practitioner uses to activate the motor components the child needs for task efficiency. Typically, proximal key points control refers to hand placement on the trunk, ribcage, shoulders or pelvis. In cases where the child demonstrates increased postural control or support, distal points of control are often chosen. For instance, to improve digital dexterity during bimanual or fine motor tasks, a practitioner may place their hands on the child's distal upper extremity, such as the elbow, forearm, wrist or hand, particularly when facilitating intralimb dissociation, such as radioulnar dissociation or wrist and forearm dissociation (Figure 8.14).

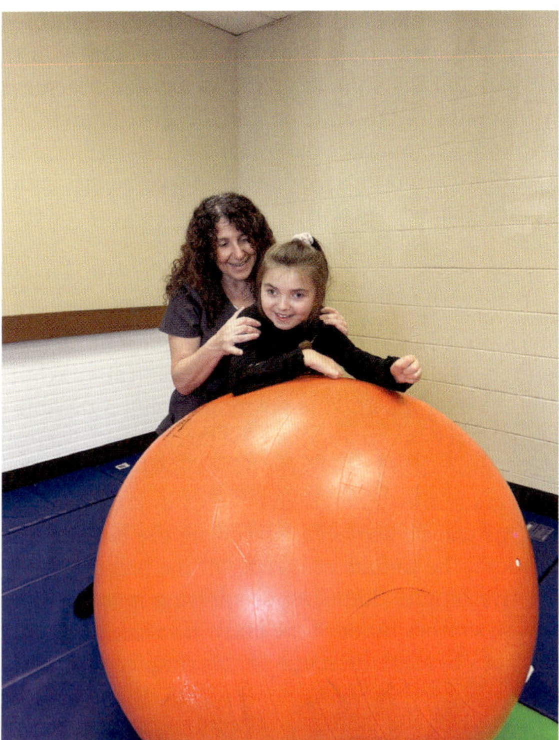

FIGURE 8.13 Handling on moveable surfaces allows the child to activate and sustain postural head, neck, and trunk alignment. The practitioner uses her body to promote postural extension in the child.

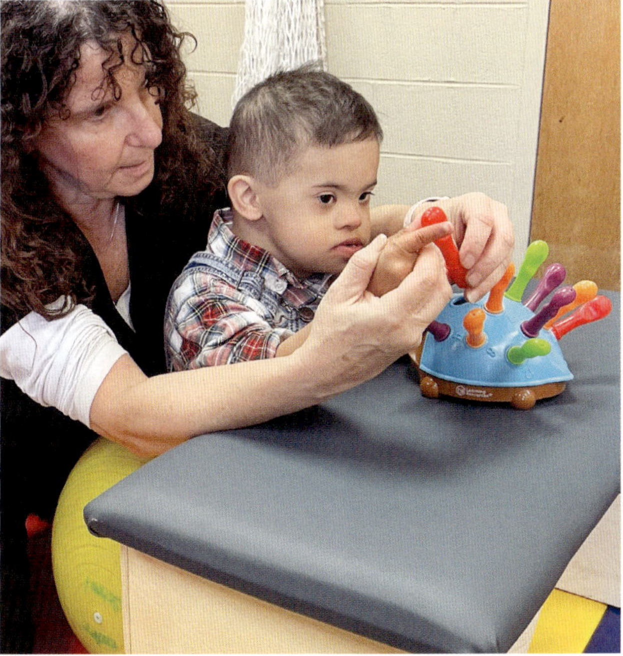

FIGURE 8.14 Facilitating isolated digital control in a child with hypotonicity. Therapist is providing deep touch into the palmar arch while stabilizing the ulnar side of the hand to support digital isolation for refined grasp.

Hand placement is dynamic and varies based on the neuromotor abilities of the child, the demands of the task, and environmental constructs. Therapeutic handling is a dynamic process that evolves throughout the treatment session, adjusting as the child achieves activation or requires additional support in line with the task demands and environmental factors. This process requires continuous observation, and analysis of movement/task by the practitioner. It is recognized that the child's level of arousal, emotions, and state of well-being significantly influence their optimal performance in each therapy session.

Use of Moveable Surfaces

Practitioners often use moveable surfaces, such as therapy balls and bolsters, as therapeutic tools during handling activities. These surfaces serve to facilitate postural activation while allowing for graded control of gravitational forces. When the child is positioned on a moveable surface, that surface becomes their BOS. The practitioner can manipulate the therapy ball, for example, inducing a postural response in the child to move their COG over the moveable BOS. The therapy ball offers the practitioner the ability to grade the gravitational forces in both gravity-assisted and gravity-resistive planes of motion. This can be achieved by moving the ball anteriorly or posteriorly to the line of gravity. Furthermore, the unique properties of the ball provide opportunities for linear vestibular and proprioceptive inputs. Bouncing or applying intermittent compression into the surface of the ball increase the sensory input of the body in space. It is important to note that skillful use of movable surfaces goes beyond the scope of this chapter (Figure 8.15). Readers

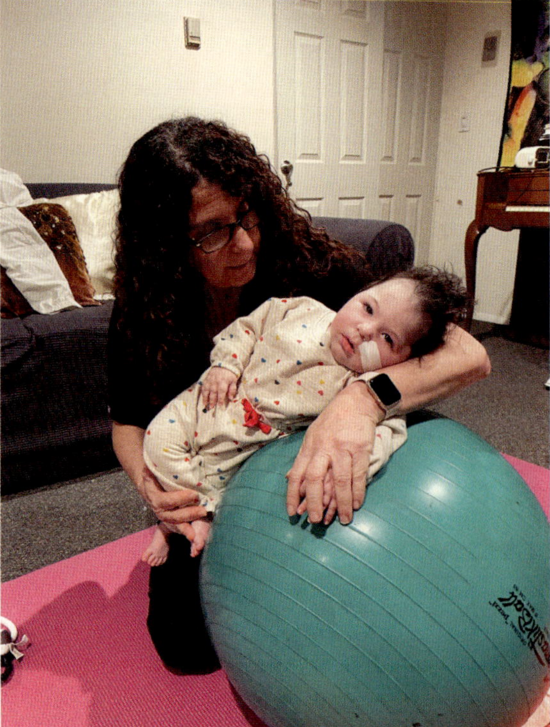

FIGURE 8.15 The use of a movable surface facilitates the activation of postural control in this baby.

are encouraged to expand their knowledge and techniques of using moveable surfaces through clinical supervisions and continuing education seminars.

Qualities of Touch

The touch provided by a practitioner during handling is direct, with the intensity varying depending on the specific sensory input required to elicit active movement or inhibit overactive movement patterns. To achieve optimal contact, a practitioner's hands are consistently molded and shaped to match the contours of the child's body. The degree of touch is graded according to the level of assistance the child requires for motor activation. Practitioners rely on their understanding of cutaneous and proprioceptive receptors to inform their clinical decision making when applying graded therapeutic touch. Both deep touch and proprioceptive input follow the same neural pathway to the CNS. In cases of neuromotor pathology, children often face challenges in receiving or integrating deep touch and proprioceptive input, hindering the facilitation of typical motor output (Lundy-Eckman, 2018).

Therapeutic handling often involves a combination of joint compression and traction or distraction. The application of joint compression is used specifically to provide proprioceptive input to the biomechanically aligned joint during facilitated active movement (Figures 8.16A,B). This is done with the intention of enhancing the proprioceptive information to the CNS while the child is

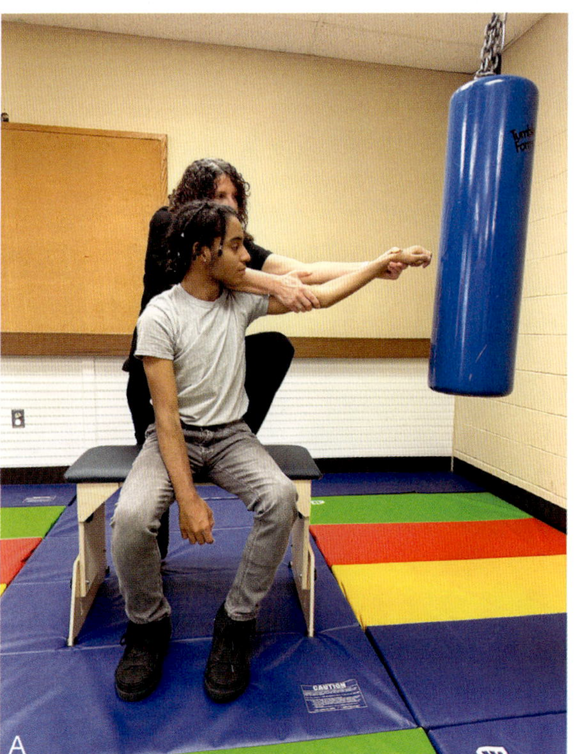

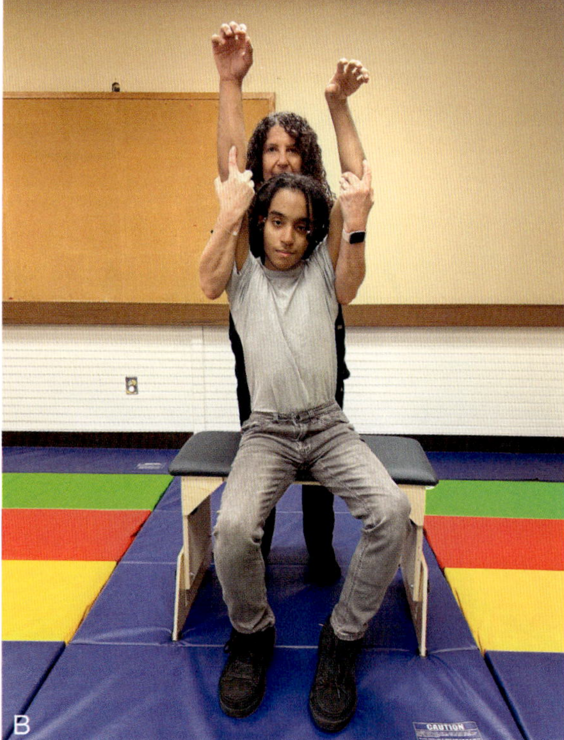

FIGURE 8.16 **A.** Intermittent compression is provided into affected upper extremity provided in preparation for extended arm reach. **B.** Intermittent compression is provided bilaterally into the boy's scapulae toward his base of support.

actively participating in novel therapeutic movement patterns. The primary source of proprioception information stems from the stretch receptors within the muscle spindle. Consequently, it is critical for the practitioner to determine the appropriate biomechanical alignment to ensure that the muscle is optimally aligned to initiate firing and generate an action potential.

Compression occurs when external pressure or weight is applied to body segments along the line of force, thereby decreasing the articular surface between the joints. Depending on the original state of targeted muscles, compression can be used as a strategy of relaxation or activation (Figure 8.17A,B).

Traction or distraction, is incorporated into therapeutic handling as a means of providing gentle stretch and elongate muscles and joints. Traction is used to facilitate elongation with activation, as a means of eliciting an active eccentric muscle contraction and facilitating desired movements. It is also used as a means for increasing ROM, reducing hypertonicity, and aiming for desired outcome of active facilitation. Traction occurs when a practitioner provides a pulling force to body segments in a distal direction. Slow sustained traction is particularly effective in elongating shortened muscles, releasing restricted fascia, and reducing the intensity of hypertonicity. This, in turn, allows for greater range of movement. Together, these dynamic forces applied to joints and muscles induce changes in body alignment and activation of muscle synergies, fostering functional improvements (Barthel, 2020).

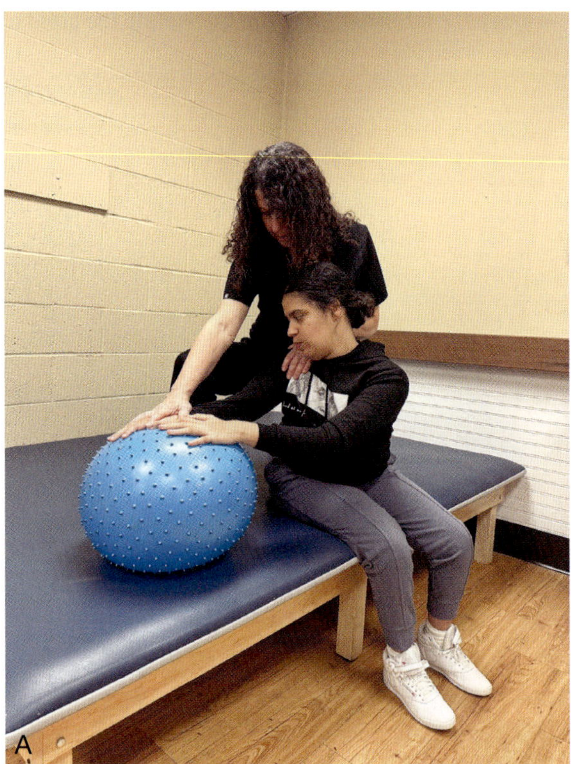

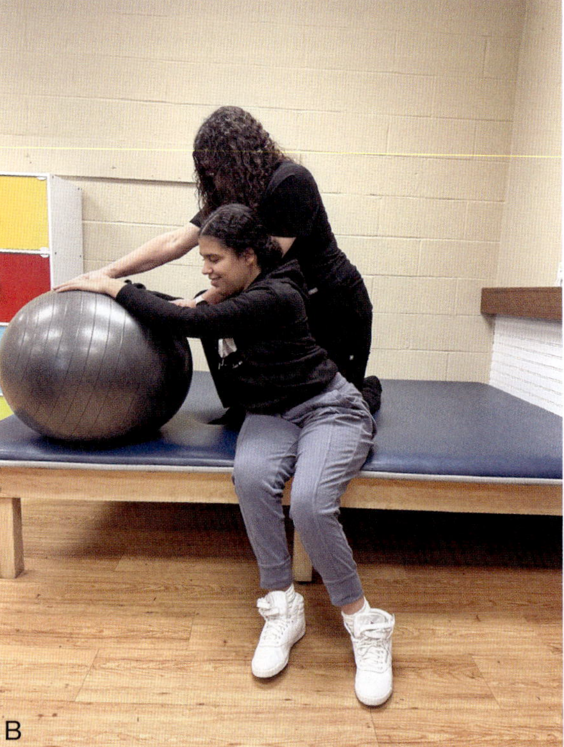

FIGURE 8.17 **A, B.** Both pictures demonstrate compression into the young woman's base of support. **A.** Tactile input and compression provided into weight-bearing surface of the young woman's right affected upper extremity. **B.** Compression provides proprioceptive input into base of support with trunk rotation, lower trunk, and pelvis weight shift in preparation for reaching.

Facilitation and Inhibition a Simultaneous Relationship in Therapeutic Handling

Facilitation or activation of motion is often provided in tandem with the inhibition of extraneous or overactive muscles that impede functional movement patterns. This facilitation or activation of motion is tailored to the child's atypical postural muscle tone and musculoskeletal constraint, which are identified during the initial NDT assessment and consistently reassessed throughout each treatment session. In this section, basic therapeutic principles will be introduced, aligning with children who exhibit weak postural control as a result of atypical muscle tone. It is crucial to note that neuromotor pathology presents as uniquely in each individual child. The information provided serves as a guideline for therapeutic handling within the NDT framework of treatment intervention.

Children with weak postural control often depend on a wide BOS as a compensatory strategy for their decreased trunk or postural control. When a child's BOS is narrowed, it imposes internal demands on the postural system to activate, in order to maintain balance by keeping their COG over their BOS. In essence, a wider BOS reduce the demands on the postural system, while a narrower BOS increases the demand for postural activation.

The initial step in activating or strengthening of postural muscles requires facilitation of biomechanical alignment of the muscle fibers to make them stretch sensitive for firing. When focusing on strengthening the postural muscles, the practitioner prioritizes providing activation in the following sequence:

1. **Isometric contractions** involve muscle contractions where the length of the muscle remains constant throughout the contraction. What does change, however, is the muscle tension. This type of contraction provides joint stabilization and ongoing muscle tension activation, enabling the sustenance and holding of postural muscles. This, in turn, allows individuals to maintain upright alignment, postural orientation, and stability. In the context of NDT handling, the facilitation of weak postural muscles includes working within their upright and shortened range, such as trunk extension and rotation. Activation within this shortened postural range is encouraged through small weight shifts over a weight-bearing limb (Stockmeyer, 2016).
2. **Eccentric contractions** occur during muscle lengthening. It is essential to facilitate eccentric control of the newly lengthened muscle, for readaptation and activation during mid-range functional activities. Eccentric contractions are facilitated once the postural muscle can sustain the isometric contraction for a long duration. Eccentric contractions are facilitated in mid-ranges, such as picking up an object from a table opposed to the floor.
3. **Concentric contractions** occur as postural muscles shorten to generate force. In cases of weak postural muscles, sustaining and holding in shortened range becomes challenging. Consequently, repetitive concentric contractions are introduced only when the child can sustain and hold in the shortened and or minimally lengthened range for an extended period. This duration is essential for the muscle to readapt and achieve the necessary length required for postural stability, crucial for maintaining the COG/BOS during upright functional daily activities.

Transitional Movement Patterns

Facilitating transitional movement patterns while incorporating the therapeutic handling principles discussed constitutes a dynamic process seamlessly woven into the NDT treatment session. Children experiencing atypical muscle tone often exhibit asymmetrical postures, increasing their

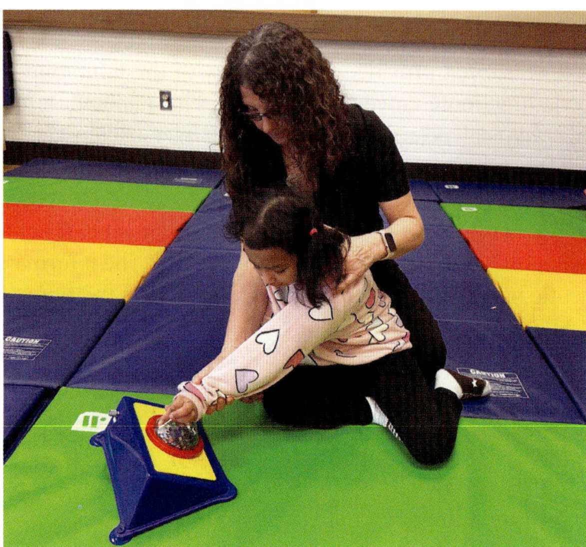

FIGURE 8.18 The practitioner is facilitating weight shifting in the child during adapted play experiences. The child is moving from side-sit toward kneel and back to sitting, within her small range of motor control.

susceptibility to conditions such as scoliosis and pelvic obliquities. These conditions can impede proper upright positioning and compromise postural control.

An occupational therapy practitioner following the NDT frame of reference focuses on activating postural control to enhance distal functioning in a single treatment session. The ongoing challenge lies in adeptly providing the just right amount of postural support required for the child to engage in purposeful play, learning, socialization, and ADLs (Figure 8.18). Through active engagement, repetition, and creation of a safe therapeutic environment for motor learning, the child can attain a sense of agency and mastery by successfully acquiring new skills. Practitioners utilizing an NDT frame of reference aim to enhance motor control and motor efficiency in the child's desired tasks, across various settings, and throughout their development.

CASE EXAMPLE

Background

Ari, a 7-year-old boy born prematurely at 32-week gestation who suffered a stroke in utero, resulting in left hemiparesis. He currently resides in an urban city center with his parents and younger sister, attending his local public school. Ari has an Individualized Education Plan (IEP) and is classified as a student with multiple disabilities. He is educated in a special education, self-contained classroom. Ari receives occupational, physical, and speech therapies to improve his functional mobility, bimanual coordination, and communication skills within the school environment. Ari ambulates independently, wears bilateral ankle foot orthotics (AFOs), a left functional hand orthotic and receives *Botox treatment* with serial casting to manage bilateral plantar flexion contractions caused by excessive lower extremity extensor tone and toe-walking gait pattern.

Ari sits in a typical classroom chair and desk. He lacks spontaneous use of his left upper extremity (LUE). There is minimal activation of elbow extension, resulting in a limited range of reach. In addition, there is no active forearm rotation, limiting his ability to orient his hand for manipulation. Ari also lacks activation of wrist extension, radial deviation, and digital isolation, severely impacting his ability to grasp, release, and manipulate objects within his hand. Despite these challenges, with verbal reminders, Ari will use his left hand as a functional stabilizer during tabletop activities. However, he demonstrates a compensatory behavior by "stuffing" an object in his left hand using his right hand, and he relies on his right hand to remove the object. This indicates a lack of active release in his left hand, highlighting the complexity of his motor difficulties.

Ari reports that he is interested in joining the robotics club, where participants construct robotics using Legos. However, Ari's parents are concerned about his fine motor limitations in his LUE, fearing that Ari might encounter frustrated, potentially leading to the development of poor self-esteem among his peers. Ari's parents advocate for focusing on ADLs, such as dressing and using a knife and fork to cut his food during mealtimes. Conversely, Ari does not share the same goal and is content to have his mother assist him with ADLs. This difference in perspective highlights a potential divergence in priorities between Ari and his parents regarding his developmental goals.

NDT Assessment and Goals

Upon quick stretch, Ari presents with spasticity in his LUE, including the biceps, forearm pronators, wrist flexors, ulnar deviators, extrinsic and intrinsic finger flexors, and digital adductors. This spasticity limits his ability to reach, grasp and manipulation of objects effectively. Ari demonstrates both passive and active range-of-motion limitations in his left upper and lower extremities. Physical examination reveals musculoskeletal issues including left-side trunk weakness, slight scoliosis, left scapula elevation, humeral internal rotation and adduction, elbow flexion, forearm pronation, wrist flexion with ulnar deviation, and flexed digits with thumb adduction. Notably, during challenging gross or fine motor activities and at increased velocities, the tone in Ari's LUE increases, leading to a more pronounced movement pattern described above. Sensory testing further indicates impairments in proprioception, deep touch, localization, and stereognosis (ability to identify an object within his hand with his vision occluded).

Ari presents with impairments in all bimanual tasks, such as keyboarding, constructional play activities, fastening buttons, zippering and using utensils for cutting his food. Ari uses only his right hand when engaging in the above tasks, tabletop activities and during gross motor tasks such as ball skills, riding an adapted bicycle and carrying his food tray in the cafeteria.

Ari's occupational therapist has developed the following goals using an NDT frame of reference to guide treatment planning and intervention.

- Spontaneously use LUE as a functional dominant assist, (with donned functional hand orthotic) to complete bimanual constructional tasks
- Grasp and release one-inch size Lego blocks with his LUE while constructing a 10-piece Lego design
- Independently carry his lunch tray in the cafeteria
- Independently use utensils during lunch and snack times

NDT Treatment Intervention

Using task analysis and environmental contexts to optimize motor learning and motor control opportunities, the following intervention plan is established.

Preparation: The occupational therapy practitioner assists Ari in initiating and sustaining musculoskeletal biomechanical alignment throughout the treatment session, optimizing desired muscle activation while inhibiting movements interfering with motor efficiency and proprioceptive input during weight bearing and weight shifting over his LUE through midranges of his transitional movement patterns. The occupational therapist (OT) uses manual handling to elongate his constricted muscles through muscle belly stretch, traction, and weight-bearing/shifting activities within mid-ranges.

Facilitation: Ari's occupational therapy sessions include motor opportunities on a variety of stationary and moveable surfaces focusing on facilitating trunk rotation, dissociation, and weight-bearing/weight-shifting experiences while reaching across midline for desired constructional play materials, such as Legos, play dough, building blocks, etc. The occupational therapy practitioner provides graded facilitation of the postural muscles within isometric ranges while encouraging reaching activities at Ari's end range of motor control. Proprioceptive input is provided through joint compression and active weight shifting of his trunk over his loaded upper extremity. All motor opportunities are facilitated bilaterally to promote symmetry of sensory input and motor output experiences.

Function: While Ari is engaged in constructional play activities with Legos, the OT continues to activate and assist in sustaining and holding the postural muscles while facilitating bimanual exploration of toy manipulation. The occupational therapy practitioner provides the proximal support needed to facilitate the intralimb dissociation within his LUE (e.g., scapula: humeral dissociation, humeral: forearm dissociation, forearm rotation, wrist: hand dissociation as well as radial-ulnar and digital: palm dissociation) required for digital dexterity and motor efficiency during bimanual constructional play activities.

The occupational therapy practitioner will collaborate with the school team members to optimize his carryover in the classroom and flexible therapeutic settings to generalize motor learning and align the task demands within various environmental settings. The occupational therapy practitioner may recommend that Ari use his functional hand splint during tabletop activities outside the OT clinical setting for optimal biomechanical carryover of his left forearm, wrist, and hand. Recommendations also include the team providing verbal reminders for Ari to position his LUE within his visual field to promote spontaneous use of his LUE as a functional dominant assist during bimanual fine motor tasks.

SUPPORTING EVIDENCE

Despite being widely used, there is limited evidence supporting effectiveness of NDT in addressing motoric deficits among children with neuromotor dysfunction (Butler & Darrah, 2001; teVelde et al., 2022). The existing evidence of NDT interventions often lacks consistency in demonstrating improved motor function and mobility. Moreover, the support for NDT is hindered by the scarcity of randomized control trials, and research is also often limited by the individualized nature of NDT interventions. In addition, alternative and activity-based approaches such as constraint-induced movement therapy (CIMT), conductive education, or task-oriented training, have shown promising efficacy in enabling children with neuromotor dysfunction to actively participate in their environments.

In an effort to evaluate the efficacy of NDT, several authors have conducted meta-analysis (teVelde et al., 2022) and systematic reviews (Butler & Darrah, 2001; Novak et al., 2013). According to an evidence report from the American Academy for Cerebral Palsy and Developmental Medicine (AACPDM), interventions using an NDT approach do not exhibit any advantage over alternative methods for addressing motor dysfunction (Butler & Darrah, 2001). Likewise, a systematic review by Novak et al. (2013) concluded that the use of NDT is ineffective in children with cerebral palsy. Specifically, their findings suggest that NDT lacks high-level evidence supporting improvement in contracture and tone compared to casting and pharmaceutical intervention. The study also reports weak evidence that the NDT improves function compared to goal-directed or context-focused therapy. Finally, a meta-analysis by teVelde et al. (2022) revealed that NDT is no more effective than activity-based or body structure- and function-related interventions in improving motor function. They also noted that the frequency of NDT intervention also had no impact on motoric outcomes.

In summary, the evidence supporting NDT as an effective treatment for children with neurologic dysfunction is lacking. There is limited higher-level study confirming the effectiveness of this treatment. The inherent challenge in establishing robust efficacy research lies in the individualized nature of the treatment protocol. Since each child presents unique characteristics, and the treatment is tailored to their specific needs, there is no standard protocol suitable in a clinical trial (Butler & Darrah, 2001). Adding complexity to the evaluation of NDT's efficacy, is the requirement for a high level of clinical skill, which currently lacks standardization. In addition, the measuring tools used to assess the intended changes resulting from NDT interventions may not be sufficiently sensitive to detect the differences. As the concepts of NDT are evolving, there is a need for more research exploring a combination of NDT with a context-focus and goal-directed approach (Barthel, 2020). To enhance inquiry into the efficacy of NDT, practitioners should consider developing fidelity models. In addition, the adoption of outcome measures such as goal attainment scaling could prove beneficial in assessing functionality while consideration of movement quality.

Summary

The NDT frame of reference traces its origins to the pioneering work of Dr. Karel and Berta Bobath in the mid-1940s. Functioning as a "living concept," NDT remains relevant by integrating contemporary principles of human development, neuroscience, biomechanics, and kinesiology with respect to dynamic system theories, neuronal selection, motor learning, motor control, and motor efficiency. The overarching goal is to maximize the child's development and participation in age/stage occupational performance through manual handling and facilitation of the postural and movement systems.

The hallmark of NDT intervention consists of hands-on therapeutic facilitation strategies implemented within the child's optimal biomechanical alignment, with the goal of activating primary movement components required for age/stage meaningful occupational participation and performance, while inhibiting atypical compensatory motions. NDT addresses quality of muscle tone through positioning and facilitation of active weight-bearing and weight-shifting experiences with emphasis on tactile and proprioceptive sensory input, with the desired outcome of enhancing the child's awareness of body schema in space.

Adaptive equipment and use of orthotics are often utilized to biomechanically support and carry over the optimal postural alignment with the goal of facilitating greater opportunity of initiation and activation of motor efficiency across settings. NDT intervention occurs during play and purposeful ADLs that are meaningful to the child, family, and environmental settings such as school, community, and home. NDT values the practice of skill with emphasis on quality of movement for motor efficiency and prevention of future musculoskeletal impairments related to stereotypical movements and atypical tonal asymmetries during growth and development. Application of NDT treatment intervention is a learned cognitive and motor skill that requires advanced additional training. The ultimate goal of NDT is to enhance the child's quality of motor efficiency in their desired occupational performance across settings and throughout their lifespan.

ACKNOWLEDGMENTS

The author wishes to thank Joan D. Mohr for sharing her knowledge as well as her unwavering mentorship throughout my clinical career and the many families and children who allowed their pictures to be used in the development of this work. The author acknowledges Kimberly Barthel for her previous edition of this chapter.

REFERENCES

American Occupational Therapy Association (AOTA). (2020). Occupational therapy practice framework: Domain and process (4th ed.). *American Journal of Occupational Therapy, 74*(Suppl 2), 7412410010. https://doi.org/10.5014/ajot.2020.74S2001

Barthel, K. (2020). A frame of reference for neuro-developmental treatment. In P. Kramer, J. Hinojosa & T. Howe (Eds.), *Frames of reference for pediatric occupational therapy* (4th ed., pp. 205–246). Wolters Kluwer.

Barthel, K. (2004). *Evidence and art: Merging forces in pediatric therapy*. Labyrinth Journeys.

Bierman, J. (2016). Neuro-developmental treatment practice and the ICF model. In J. Bierman, M. R. Franjoine, C. M. Hazzard, J. M. Howle & Stamer, M. (Eds.), *Neuro-developmental treatment: A guide to clinical practice* (pp. 308–324). Thieme Publishers.

Butler, C. & Darrah, J. (2001). Effects of neurodevelopmental treatment (NDT) for cerebral palsy: an AACPDM evidence report. *Developmental Medicine of Child Neurology*, 43(11), 778–790.

Darrah, J., & Bartlett, D. (1995). Dynamic systems theory and management of children with cerebral palsy: Unresolved issues. *Infants and Young Children, 8*(1), 52–59.

Edelman, G. M. (1987). *Neural Darwinism: The theory of neuronal group selection*. Basic Books.

Hadders-Algra, M. (2000). The neuronal group selection theory: Promising principles for understanding and treating developmental motor disorders. *Developmental Medicine and Child Neurology, 42*(10), 707–715. https://doi.org/10.1111/j.1469-8749.2000.tb00687.x

Howle, J. (2016). Motor control. In J. Bierman, M. R. Franjoine, C. M. Hazzard, J. M. Howle & M. Stamer (Eds.), *Neuro-developmental treatment: A guide to clinical practice* (pp. 308–324). Thieme Publishers.

Howle, J. M. (2002). *Neuro-Developmental treatment approach: Theoretical foundations and principles of clinical practice*. NDTA.

Ivanenko, Y., & Gurfinkel, V. S. (2018). Human postural control. *Frontiers in Neuroscience, 12,* 171. https://doi.org/10.3389/fnins.2018.00171

Kamm, K., Thelan, E., & Jensen, J. (1990). A dynamical systems approach to motor development. *Physical Therapy, 70*(12), 763–775. https://doi.org/10.1093/ptj/70.12.763

Lieber, R. (2010). *Skeletal muscle structure, function and plasticity*. Lippincott Williams & Wilkins.

Lundy-Ekman, L. (2018). *Neuroscience fundamentals for rehabilitation* (5th ed.). Saunders Elsevier.

Novak, I., Mcintyre, S., Morgan, C., Campbell, L., Dark, L., Morton, N., Stumbles, E., Wilson, S. A., Goldsmith, S. (2013). A systematic review of interventions for children with cerebral palsy: State of the evidence. *Developmental Medicine and Child Neurology, 55*(10), 885–910. https://doi.org/10.1111/dmcn.12246

O'Brien, J., Coker-Bolt, P., & Dimitropoulou, K. (2020). Application of motor control and motor learning, In J. Case Smith & H. Kuhaneck (Eds.), *Case Smith's occupational therapy for children and adolescents,* (8th ed., pp. 395–430). Elsevier, Inc.

Sanger, T. D., & Kukke, S. N. (2007). Abnormalities of tactile sensory function in children with dystonic and diplegic cerebral palsy. *Journal of Child Neurology, 22*(3), 289–293. https://doi.org/10.1177/0883073807300530

Schoen, S., & Anderson, J. (1999). NeuroDevelopmental treatment frame of reference. In P. Kramer & J. Hinojosa (Eds.), *Frames of reference for pediatric occupational therapy* (2nd ed., pp. 83–118). Lippincott Williams and Wilkins.

Shumway-Cook, A., & Woollacott, M. H. (2012). *Motor control: translating research into clinical practice* (4th ed.). Lippincott Williams & Wilkins.

Shumway-Cook, A., & Woollacott, M. H. (2017). *Motor control: Translating research into clinical practice* (5th ed.). Wolters Kluwer.

Smith, L., & Thelan, E. (1993). *A dynamic systems approach to development*. The MIT Press.

Stamer, M. (2016). Cerebral palsy. In J. Bierman, M. R. Franjoine, C. M. Hazzard, J. M. Howle & M. Stamer (Eds.), *Neuro-developmental treatment: A guide to clinical practice* (pp. 192–218). Thieme Publishers.

Stockmeyer, S. (2016). Application of a posture and movement model in practice. In J. Bierman, M. R. Franjoine, C. M. Hazzard, J. M. Howle & M. Stamer (Eds.), *Neuro-developmental treatment: A guide to clinical practice* (pp. 39–52). Thieme Publishers.

teVelde, A., Finch-Edmondson, M., McNamara, L., McNamara, M., Paton, M. C. B., Stanton, E., Webb, A., Badawi, N., & Novak, I. (2022). Neurodevelopmental therapy for cerebral palsy: A aeta-analysis. *Pediatrics, 149*(6):e2021055061

The Cognitive Orientation to Daily Occupational Performance Approach

Claire A. Sangster Jokić ■ Rose Martini ■ Helene J. Polatajko

Viewing the human as an occupational being is now a widely shared perspective among occupational therapists around the world. The viewpoint that enablement of human occupation is the core business of our profession is just as widely shared. However, that is where the global consensus seems to stop and opinions start to diverge. As is evident from the varied perspectives presented in this book, there are numerous ways of understanding human occupation. What is further evident is that each perspective invites differing approaches to working toward its enablement. This affords the potential for tremendous diversity in approaches to enabling human occupation, depending on the aspect of human occupation to be addressed (e.g., occupational engagement, occupational participation, occupational well-being, occupational justice) and at what level it is to be addressed (e.g., person, family, group, community, population). This chapter discusses one approach to enabling human occupation, the **Cognitive Orientation to daily Occupational Performance** (CO-OP) approach, or the trademarked **CO-OP Approach**.

CO-OP (Polatajko & Mandich, 2004) is not a perspective on human occupation; rather, it is a perspective on enablement that inherently holds a perspective on human occupation, more specifically on the performance of occupation. This chapter articulates both the CO-OP perspective on enablement and its inherent perspective on human occupational performance. However, CO-OP is concerned with more than simply the doing of an occupation or task (occupational performance), rather it is focused on addressing occupational performance goals that are set by the client and are therefore deemed important by the client and have relevance to their everyday living. Further, CO-OP is focused on the generalization and transfer of occupational goals addressed during intervention to the real world, thus ensuring that intervention outcomes have a meaningful impact on client's participation in everyday life situations. In this way, there are aspects of the Approach that supersede it and have relevance for our general understanding of participation in life through human occupation.

Historical Development of the CO-OP Approach

The CO-OP Approach was created in the 1990s out of frustration with the inability of traditional approaches to improve outcomes for children with motor-based learning problems (Polatajko &

Mandich, 2004). In particular, the CO-OP Approach was developed to enable children with developmental coordination disorder (DCD) to perform the typical skills of childhood. DCD is a neurodevelopmental disorder that affects motor performance (American Psychiatric Association, 2013). Children with DCD present with motor coordination problems that can interfere with the performance of daily occupations at home, school, and play. Although children with DCD can acquire many occupational skills, they require considerably more time and effort than their peers to do so and may experience inordinate difficulty in acquiring complex skills such as handwriting or bike riding. Traditional approaches to working with these children view their performance problems from a component, process-oriented perspective, or more specifically, from a neurodevelopmental or sensorimotor perspective. Interventions based in these perspectives focus on identifying underlying deficits and working to ameliorate them and promote the development of typical, neurosensorimotor processes. The reported failure of such approaches to demonstrate effectiveness in improving performance outcomes for children with DCD (Mandich et al., 2001a) and the need to enable children to succeed in the occupations of childhood led to the search for a new perspective on enabling goal-oriented performance, also known as occupational performance (Polatajko & Mandich, 2004).

After scrutinizing the results from a trial investigating the effectiveness of the process-oriented approach developed by Judith Laszlo and Phillip Bairstow (1985) that showed no improvement in goal-oriented performance (Polatajko et al., 1995), Polatajko noted that the children did demonstrate learning of the specific skill taught in the course of the component-based intervention. For Polatajko, these findings indicated that an approach situated in a learning paradigm warranted exploration. Polatajko had had considerable experience using a behavioral, learning approach to teaching children with severe intellectual impairments a number of basic occupational skills, and although antithetical to the thinking of the day, she reasoned that a learning approach may be useful in addressing the performance issues of children with motor-based learning problems. Given that the intelligence level of children with DCD is average or better, Polatajko further reasoned that a cognitive behavior modification approach may be more appropriate for this population. Accordingly, Polatajko and colleagues set out to create a cognitive-based intervention approach to address the performance needs of children with motor-based performance problems. Work on this new approach, initially called Verbal Self-Guidance (Wilcox & Polatajko, 1994), eventually led to the creation of the CO-OP Approach presented in this chapter.

The Cognitive Orientation to Daily Occupational Performance Approach

"CO-OP is a client-centered, performance-based, problem-solving approach that enables skill acquisition through a process of strategy use and guided discovery." (Polatajko & Mandich, 2004, p. 2)

The CO-OP Approach is a complex intervention designed to enable occupational performance, also known as **goal-oriented performance.** CO-OP has four specific objectives: (1) skill acquisition, (2) strategy use, (3) generalization, and (4) transfer. The ultimate objective of the CO-OP Approach is to enable individuals who have activity limitations as a result of occupational performance issues to acquire the necessary skills and strategies to enable optimal participation in the everyday activities of living. The accumulating evidence indicates that the CO-OP Approach is successful in enabling individuals with a number of different diagnoses and performance issues to reach their occupational performance goals and participate in everyday life (Scammels et al., 2016).

The CO-OP Approach is composed of seven key features: (1) client-chosen goals, (2) dynamic performance analysis (DPA), (3) cognitive strategy use, (4) guided discovery, (5) enabling principles, (6) parent or significant other involvement, and (7) session structure and format (Polatajko & Mandich, 2004). These features are described in detail in the book *Cognitive Orientation to daily Occupational Performance in Occupational Therapy: Using the CO-OP Approach™ to Enable Participation Across the Lifespan* (Dawson et al., 2017). The first five key features are considered essential elements of the intervention, that is, they must be present for the intervention to be considered consistent with the CO-OP Approach (Skidmore et al., 2017). The key features of DPA, cognitive strategy use, and guided discovery are referred to as the CO-OP "trifecta." They happen simultaneously and iteratively to advance skill acquisition, while the enabling principles underly these three key features. The last two key features (parent or significant other and session structure) are considered to be structural elements. These are elements that determine the structure and context of the intervention and that can vary according to the client's or clinical practice situation (Skidmore et al., 2017). The seven key features, further discussed later in this chapter, each play an important role in the CO-OP intervention process.

The CO-OP intervention process is client centered and relies on the skills of therapists to engage clients in actively enabling the client to solve performance problems using cognitive strategies and verbal self-guidance. The process starts with having the client determine the performance goals that will be the focus of the intervention. The therapist then establishes the baseline performance of each and teaches the client a global problem-solving strategy. From this point, the therapist guides the client in the use of that strategy to uncover performance problems and discover effective domain-specific strategies to improve performance and enable skill acquisition and goal attainment. The Approach is goal focused and operates entirely at the task performance level; it does not involve any direct intervention at the level of performance components.

THEORETICAL BASE

The CO-OP Approach is a complex approach whose development and implementation are informed by diverse theoretical and empirical perspectives and foundations derived from disciplines of occupational therapy, movement science and psychology. These foundations will be discussed briefly here in relation to three key characteristics of the Approach: client-centeredness, performance-based or task-oriented, and a learning (problem-solving) paradigm.

Client-Centeredness

"Client-centred practice refers to collaborative approaches aimed at enabling occupation with clients who may be individuals, groups, agencies, governments, corporations or others. Occupational therapists demonstrate respect for clients, involve clients in decision making, advocate with and for clients in meeting clients' needs, and otherwise recognize clients' experience and knowledge." (Canadian Association of Occupational Therapists, 1997, p. 49)

The term **client-centeredness** describes an orientation to practice, rather than a specific theory or approach. It is predicated on the belief that the client is the expert with respect to their own occupations and the contexts in which they are performed. Being a client-centered therapist means working in a collaborative partnership with the client starting at goal setting and continuing through all aspects of the interaction. Client-centeredness should pervade all aspects of the interaction and should involve the active and informed participation of the client throughout. Interactions should be structured to promote autonomy, empowerment, choice, and control for clients (Sumsion, 1999).

Client-centered enablement is evident in all aspects of the CO-OP Approach from the initial identification of the performance goals that will be the focus of the intervention through the iterative process of noticing performance problems, proposing performance solutions, trying them out, and checking to see if they were effective in achieving the desired goal and whether it would be of use in the client's real-world context.

Performance Based

The term **performance based,** when used to describe an intervention, indicates that the intervention is focused on goal-oriented performance, rather than on underlying processes. These processes, as defined by the Canadian Model of Occupational Performance and Engagement (Townsend & Polatajko, 2013), can be cognitive, affective, or physical. In occupational therapy, there are two broad perspectives on intervention approaches designed to address occupational performance issues that are physical (i.e., sensorimotor) in nature (as is the case in DCD). The more long-standing perspective is to focus on the foundational components of performance, often referred to as a process-oriented or "**bottom-up**" approach. The newer perspective, and the one underlying CO-OP, is to focus directly on performance, often referred to as a task-oriented or "**top-down**" approach (Polatajko et al., 2013). The two approaches stand in direct contrast to each other: bottom-up approaches work on ameliorating deficits that underlie performance issues, putting foundational skills in the foreground and holding goal-oriented performance in the background, whereas top-down approaches work to put performance in the foreground and hold foundational skills in the background.

Top-down approaches emphasize the importance of working on goal-oriented performance directly. They are based on the premise that performance is learned, that the performance requirements for any task are specific to that task, and that learning is best achieved through task-specific training. Top-down approaches, by definition, are learning approaches where learning is defined "as an enduring change in behavior or in capacity to behave in a given fashion, which results from practice or other forms of experience" (Shuell, 1986). Learning is considered to be an active process of acquiring, remembering, and using knowledge that occurs through unobservable cognitive processes such as memory and attention. Learning theorists emphasize the important role that the mental organization of knowledge, including problem solving, reasoning, and thinking, plays in the acquisition and performance of behaviors or skills (Schunk, 2000).

Top-down approaches, as applied to motor-based performance, emerged jointly with the shift in the movement science literature from deficit-driven models to learning models—that is, from traditional hierarchical models to contemporary systems models (Mathiowetz & Bass Haugen, 1994). Based in contemporary systems theory, these models showed that as motor behavior emerges, it is self-organized and arises from a heterarchical, dynamic interaction of multiple subsystems of the individual (sensory, motor, perceptual, cognitive, attentional, and anatomical systems) and that task and environmental factors also play a key role (Thelen, 2005; Thelen, 1995). Motor learning theories indicate that the early stages of motor learning are cognitively driven (Fitts & Posner, 1967; Gentile, 1992), or rather require conscious cognitive effort to plan, execute, and adjust the movements necessary to perform a goal-oriented task.

In keeping with a movement science framework, top-down approaches look at the performance as a whole, attending to the interaction between the person, task (activity/occupation), and environment in producing performance (Polatajko & Mandich, 2004). From a top-down perspective, a child experiencing the difficulties learning to ride a bicycle discussed previously would first be observed attempting to ride a bike, during which the aspects of bike riding observed to be problematic for the child would be noted. Having ascertained these performance breakdowns, therapy would focus on having the child learn the missing aspects in context (e.g., getting feet on the pedal, steering). No attempt would be made to assess foundational components such as balance or eye–hand coordination nor work specifically on improving them; rather, intervention would focus on learning the missing aspects of bike riding and would end when the child could successfully ride a bike. Evidence from both the pediatric (Novak et al., 2013; Polatajko et al., 2004) and adult (McEwen et al., 2009) literature supports the use of top-down approaches. With respect to bicycle riding, there is evidence from CO-OP studies in which children with cerebral palsy (Cameron et al., 2010, 2016), DCD (Polatajko et al., 2001a), developmental disabilities (Halayko et al., 2016), and dystonia (Gimeno, 2015) and adults with chronic stroke (McEwen et al., 2009) all learned to ride bikes.

Emerging neuroscience also supports performance-based/task-specific approaches. As Hebbian theory postulates, learning, which is synonymous with neural plastic changes, occurs at the level of the synapse as a result of the presynaptic cell's repeated and persistent stimulation of the same postsynaptic cell (Hebb, 1949, as cited in Doidge, 2007). This is succinctly captured in the catchphrase coined by Shatz in 1992: "Cells that fire together, wire together" (as cited in Doidge, 2007, p. 63).

Carey et al. (2012) reviewed the neuroscience evidence to understand how best to support the proper presynaptic/postsynaptic connections needed to prompt neuroplastic changes intrinsic to learning. They noted that the evidence from animal studies and studies of humans after stroke demonstrated that experience and training are critical ingredients for such neuroplastic changes to occur. However, it would seem that not just any experience or any training suffices, rather, a specific, targeted approach is required. Carey and colleagues concluded that the neuroscience evidence suggests that for training to support the neuroplastic changes in the brain associated with improved outcomes, it must be:

- Explicit, task specific, and goal driven;
- A task with real-world relevance;
- Active in problem solving;
- Responsive to environmental demands; and
- Able to provide opportunities for variation and practice.

In the CO-OP Approach, being performance based means that the intervention meets these prerequisites. Specifically, it is explicit, task specific, and goal driven:

> "CO-OP is performance based. A major objective of CO-OP is skill acquisition, in particular, the acquisition of those skills the child wants to, needs to, or is expected to perform. By using instruments that emanate from a client-centered philosophy, the therapist enables the identification of goals that are meaningful." (Polatajko & Mandich, 2004, p. 25)

Explicit task performance is central to and pervades the CO-OP Approach. Every CO-OP session is focused on improving performance of the occupational goals specified by the client at the outset of the intervention. "Performance based" requires that the client specifies meaningful and relevant performance goals from an unlimited number of potential occupational performance goals. Furthermore, the CO-OP Approach is a learning approach that applies a problem-solving paradigm and offers varied practice of skills under varied conditions and environments. It is imperative that the client is motivated to address the goals and that the goals have real-world relevance for the client. The real-world relevance of the skills learned is what ensures generalization, as will be seen in the cases of Morris, Marcus, and Roger in examples presented later in this chapter.

A Learning Perspective

"Understanding effective performance requires understanding the psychology of strategies; promoting human effectiveness at a task requires understanding of the strategies that can accomplish the task and how to develop such strategies among learners" (Pressley & Harris, 2006, p. 265).

This quote by Michael Pressley and Karen Harris (2006) captures the specific perspective on occupational performance inherent in the CO-OP Approach. As previously stated, the approach is a complex one concerned with improving occupational, or goal-oriented, performance. First and foremost, it is a cognitive learning approach based on the premise that human occupational performance is learned. It is derived from a number of distinct theoretical perspectives drawn from disciplines concerned with human performance, especially from psychology and its perspectives on behavior, learning, and cognition and from human movement science and its perspectives on motor learning and motor control. Taken together, these perspectives suggest that all goal-oriented performance, and even motor-based occupational performance such as riding a bike or writing your name, is learned; that learning is, at least in its' early stages, dependent on cognition; and that cognitive strategies can be used to support performance learning. The evidence from CO-OP studies bears this out.

Further, the psychology and human movement science literatures suggest that performance is influenced by the task to be performed and the context of the performance—in other words, performance is the result of the interaction of the person with the task and the environment. This perspective is in keeping with many of the models of human occupational performance, including Person–Environment–Occupation Model, Person–Environment–Occupation–Performance Model, and Ecological Model of Occupation. It has a particularly good fit with the Canadian Model of Occupational Performance and Engagement (Townsend & Polatajko, 2013). The Canadian Model of Occupational Performance and Engagement identifies occupational performance as the interaction between person, occupation, and environment and specifically identifies cognition as a component of the person that contributes to performance. This perspective is also inherent in the more contemporary theories of motor learning, such as the dynamic systems theory (Thelen, 2005) and internal models of motor learning (Imamizu et al., 2000; Thoroughman & Shadmehr, 2000).

The unique perspective on occupational performance inherent in the CO-OP is that the person's individual cognitive process has primacy in occupational performance. That is, although occupational performance results from the interaction of person, occupation, and environment, it all starts with the person. From a CO-OP perspective, all understanding of occupational performance, and its enablement, needs to start with an understanding of the role the person, and most especially the role cognition, plays in performance. In contrast, the CO-OP is embedded in a learning paradigm in which the perspective of cognition, and cognitive strategies specifically, drives the interaction and is the catalyst that supports the transformation of ability into performance (Pressley & Harris, 2006). Accordingly, the CO-OP perspective places the person at the center of occupational performance and emphasizes the importance of cognition in performance. From a CO-OP perspective, the person is at the forefront of and central to any and all understanding of human occupation; therefore, engaging the individual's cognition should be at the forefront of intervention.

Problem Solving and Strategy Use

Problem-solve, verb: "to use cognitive processing to find a solution to a difficult question or situation; to use deep thought to solve a problem." (Problem-solve, n.d.)

Problem solving is the ability to combine previously learned knowledge in a new way to solve a new problem. From a CO-OP perspective, occupational performance issues are viewed as a problem to be solved. This applies to all manner of performance problems including motor-based performance issues, such as riding a bicycle, as discussed earlier. Viewing motor-based performance issues from a problem-solving perspective is in line with a movement science framework, where it is understood that problem-solving processes naturally occur during motor learning (Swinnen et al., 1990). As has been suggested by Gentile (1992), movement issues are problems to be solved, and the therapist working within a movement science framework must become an active problem solver using a broad knowledge base to generate ways to help achieve a specific performance goal.

Problem solving is a higher-order process and is considered the most complex of all functions. It is generally held that all people can become more effective problem solvers through the use of problem-solving strategies. A problem-solving strategy refers to the steps that one would use to identify and resolve the problems that pose barriers to achieving one's own goal (Bransford & Stein, 1993). Generally speaking, strategies are tools or plans of action used for accomplishing a task or achieving a purpose; they are always goal directed (Toglia et al., 2012). **Cognitive strategies** are goal-directed, cognitive operations put into place to help learn, memorize, and problem solve and are over and above those that are inherent to the task itself. These operations are involved in all activities that require thinking, planning, and decision making. They are used to acquire new skills and to make task performance easier, quicker, or more efficient across different tasks and domains (Toglia et al., 2012).

In the CO-OP, problem solving and strategy use go together because problem solving is promoted through strategy use. **Strategy use** involves the employment of consciously controlled cognitive processes to achieve a goal and is essential to skill acquisition in the CO-OP Approach. Namely, strategies are used to help develop internal procedures that promote skilled performance; to bridge the gap between ability and performance; and to support skill acquisition, generalization, and transfer.

Many strategies are available to guide problem solving, but the strategy used in the CO-OP Approach comes from the cognitive behavior modification approach developed by Donald Meichenbaum (1977), which used verbal self-instruction and the global (metacognitive) problem-solving strategy GOAL-PLAN-DO-CHECK to change behavior. GOAL-PLAN-DO-CHECK is a problem-solving strategy that draws on metacognitive ability and encourages the individual to monitor, reflect upon, and evaluate progress toward a goal, to develop a plan for achieving that goal and to adjust the plan as necessary. This metacognitive strategy involves determining what specific skills or strategies a performance requires and then monitoring those skills and strategies to achieve the goal.

The CO-OP Approach, initially called Verbal Self-Guidance (Wilcox & Polatajko, 1994), departed from Meichenbaum's intervention by incorporating client-centered principles from occupational therapy and actively engaging the child throughout the intervention. Rather than providing the child with the goal to be addressed and using modeling both to demonstrate the use of GOAL-PLAN-DO-CHECK and to identify self-instructions for improved performance, therapists using Verbal Self-Guidance enable the child to set their own goals. Verbal Self-Guidance also guides the child to notice their own performance problems and identify performance solutions through a process of guided discovery. The intervention was renamed CO-OP to highlight the importance of cognition in skill acquisition, the focus on goal-oriented performance, and the cooperative nature of the practitioner–client interaction (Polatajko, 2010).

In addition to the global problem-solving strategy, the CO-OP Approach also makes use of domain-specific strategies (Polatajko & Mandich, 2004). These are strategies that are specific to a person, situation, and task or part of a task. They are introduced to solve specific performance issues as they arise and are often used only for a short time. In contrast, global strategies such as GOAL-PLAN-DO-CHECK, also referred to as metacognitive or executive strategies, are higher-order strategies that are used to control and coordinate other strategies (Pressley et al., 1987) and to ensure that the goal has been achieved (Flavell, 1981). In this way, they serve to guide the problem-solving process. Conscious and explicit use of a metacognitive strategy, like GOAL-PLAN-DO-CHECK, enables the learner to become more aware of the learning process and the factors (including specific strategies) that contribute to learning and successful skill acquisition, which in turn allows for more effective monitoring and evaluation of one's own learning (Bjorklund & Causey, 2018). Once learned, a problem-solving strategy can also be applied to other situations to solve new problems and promote further learning. In this way, strategies, like GOAL-PLAN-DO-CHECK, become key to facilitating the generalization and transfer of outcomes beyond the intervention context.

DESCRIBING FUNCTION AND DYSFUNCTION

In line with the client-centered, performance-based, and learning paradigms that make up the theoretical base underlying the CO-OP Approach, individual function or dysfunction is considered in terms of the child's performance of a meaningful task or occupation. From a learning perspective, function might be argued to represent the acquisition of knowledge and skills necessary to successfully reach a functional goal, or in this case to perform a task or occupation. From this perspective, "function" implies that something has been learned and can be performed. Conversely, dysfunction arises when knowledge and skills have not yet been learned and therefore the child experiences difficulties performing the task or occupation. From the perspective underlying CO-OP, this learned versus not-yet-learned distinction can be further considered with respect to the person performing the occupation (performance components), the occupation itself, and the environment in which the occupation is performed (Table 9.1).

In CO-OP, several tools support the evaluation of the child's function in performing meaningful tasks or occupations, and the person, occupation, and environment factors that influence learning and performance. These tools are described in the following section.

GUIDE FOR EVALUATION

The originators of the CO-OP Approach have specified numerous tools to support the focus on performance. First, the CO-OP intervention is initiated with the identification by the client of (usually) three occupational performance goals using the Canadian Occupational Performance Measure (Law et al., 2014), which is a measure designed to identify performance issues that are

Table 9.1 Describing Function and Dysfunction From a Learning Perspective

Domain	Function (learned)	Dysfunction (not-yet-learned)
Occupational Performance	The child successfully performs daily occupations they want, need, or are expected to do.	The child experiences problem(s) during performance of daily occupations (performance breakdown).
Person	The child possesses sufficient motivation/interest, task knowledge, and skill to perform the occupation.	The child lacks motivation, knowledge, and/or skill for performing the occupation.
Occupation	The demands of the occupation/task are in line with the child's skill level.	The demands of the occupation/task are not in line with the child's skill level.
Environment	The environment in which the occupation is performed supports performance (offers appropriate supports and resources).	The environment in which the occupation is performed constrains or interferes with performance (inadequate or inappropriate supports and resources).

important to the client and have real-world relevance. It is also used to measure the client's perceived level of performance and satisfaction with the identified goals. Once goals are identified, the baseline performance of the client-chosen target skills is established. Both the client and the therapist rate the performance before intervention; the client uses the Canadian Occupational Performance Measure, and the therapist uses the Performance Quality Rating Scale (Polatajko & Mandich, 2004).[1] The **Performance Quality Rating Scale,** designed specifically for the CO-OP Approach, is an observational tool used to rate performance on a scale of 1 to 10. When rating performance, the therapist considers observed (or reported) performance relative to the desired (e.g., "I want to be able to julienne vegetables"), required (e.g., "I want to write legibly"), or typical (e.g., "I want to ride my bike") performance, where 1 indicates the performance is not at all competent and 10 indicates the performance is very competent. To establish the baseline performance level, the client is asked to perform the skills in question (or report on their performance if performing that skill in the therapy session is not practical or possible). Then, using the Performance Quality Rating Scale, the therapist rates the observed performance on a 10-point scale. At the same time, the therapist conducts the first **DPA,** a dynamic process of analyzing actual performance to identify performance problems or performance breakdown (Dawson et al., 2017; Polatajko & Mandich, 2004; Polatajko et al., 2000).

Carrying out a DPA involves direct observation (when possible) or reported observations of all aspects of the performance. DPA is akin to activity analysis, but in contrast to activity analysis, it is a dynamic process that cannot be done in isolation of the actual performance; it is focused on analyzing the idiosyncrasies of performance by a specific person in a specific context. In the DPA process, careful attention is paid to the various aspects of the performance, including the movements performed relative to the skills required and the fit (perfect match of therapeutic goals and client's needs) with occupational and environmental demands. To assist in the DPA process, the originators of CO-OP created the DPA decision tree (Polatajko et al., 2000). This decision tree (Figure 9.1) poses a series of questions that serve to establish the client's motivation for the task

[1]Polatajko and Mandich (2004) describe the manner in which the Performance Quality Rating Scale is used in practice. The application and psychometric properties of the PQRS have been examined in more detail in other work (Gimeno et al., 2021; Martini et al., 2014).

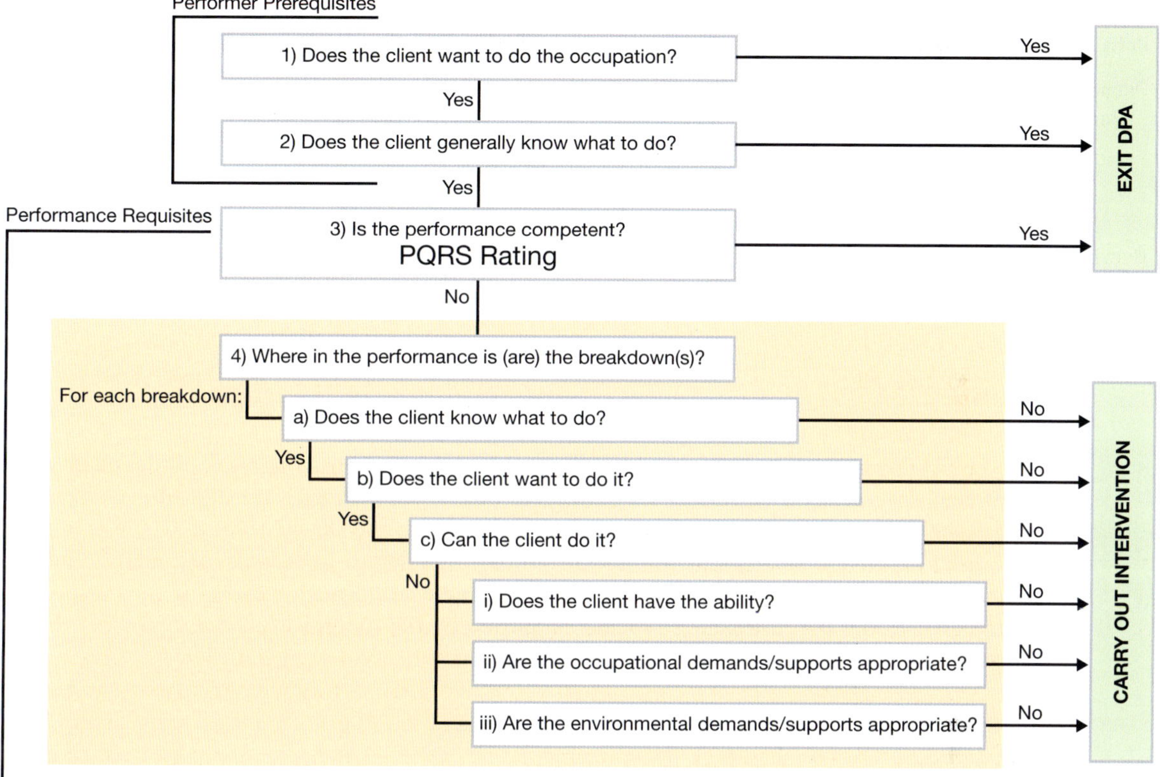

FIGURE 9.1 Dynamic performance analysis (DPA) decision tree. (Adapted from Polatajko, H. J., Mandich, A. D., & Martini, R. [2000]. Dynamic performance analysis: A framework for understanding occupational performance. *American Journal of Occupational Therapy*, *54*[1], 65–72. https://doi.org/10.5014/ajot.54.1.65. Copyright retained by author.)

at hand, their knowledge of the task demands, and the competency of the performance of each aspect of the task. The DPA process also prompts consideration of the various person, task, and environment factors influencing performance and performance breakdown. Although created for the therapist's use, there is good evidence that the client, through participation in the CO-OP, learns to independently carry out DPA (Hyland & Polatajko, 2012). In the CO-OP Approach, DPA becomes a tool for the continuous identification, evaluation, monitoring, and resolution of occupational performance problems for the therapist and ultimately, through the systematic application of (meta)cognitive strategies during problem solving, for the client.

In the CO-OP, the DPA process is an iterative one. In as much as CO-OP is performance based, once the baseline has been established, all remaining sessions of CO-OP involve using DPA repeatedly. Throughout each session, each time the target skill is performed, be that in part or as a whole, both the therapist and the client (with therapist guidance) carry out a DPA to identify and analyze performance breakdowns. The DPA process is embedded in the global problem-solving strategy that frames the approach, a feature of CO-OP that will be discussed in more detail later in this chapter.

POSTULATES REGARDING CHANGE

As an approach grounded in a learning paradigm, CO-OP applies several key features aimed at promoting learning and skills acquisition as a means to support change or, more accurately, to enable successful performance of meaningful tasks or occupations. These features are informed by the theoretical foundations of learning discussed previously. From a neuropsychological perspective, learning is considered as a process of neurologic change and adaptation through repeated and sustained activation or *neuroplasticity*. This notion was first captured by Donald Hebb in 1949:

Hebb's General Postulate: Constant activation of a target (postsynaptic) neuron by a presynaptic neuron results in a rise in synapse effectiveness (Hebb, 1949, 2002).

According to Hebb's postulate, the learning process can be considered as one in which neurons and neuronal connectivity change in response to new information. To promote the connectivity needed to prompt neuroplastic changes essential to learning, the learning process must be one that affords sustained activation of neural pathways through active, purposeful, variable, and repeated learning and practice opportunities (Carey et al., 2012).

In CO-OP, promoting learning and skill acquisition is achieved using three key features of the approach, specifically: DPA (discussed in the previous section), strategy use and guided discovery. Together, DPA, strategy use, and guided discovery make up the CO-OP *trifecta,* which is applied and used iteratively throughout the CO-OP process and serves to identify and analyze performance problems (DPA) and discover, apply, and evaluate strategies for resolving these problems (strategy use) through a learning process supported by the therapist (guided discovery). These elements and the way they function together as the trifecta are described next.

Strategy Use

The CO-OP Approach starts with the client being taught to use the GOAL-PLAN-DO-CHECK problem-solving strategy to structure the process of solving the performance problems that their self-selected goals present. This strategy subsequently focuses and frames all interactions between the client and the therapist. Each component of the strategy represents a cognitive operation inherent in the problem-solving process: identifying a clear GOAL, determining a PLAN or strategy for how the goal will be achieved, applying or DOing the plan to determine whether it is effective for achieving the goal and CHECKing whether the goal has been achieved or the problem resolved. Once the strategy has been taught to the client, it is used throughout the CO-OP intervention, where the therapist and client are continuously engaged in an iterative exchange regarding the goal, the plan for achieving that goal, implementation of the plan, and checking the results of the implementation of the plan. In essence, the GOAL-PLAN-DO-CHECK strategy is a metacognitive strategy that structures and supports the problem-solving process by prompting the learner (client) to engage in self-monitoring, self-reflection, and self-evaluation processes critical for effective and efficient learning.

As previously indicated, there are two types of cognitive strategies used in the CO-OP Approach—global and domain-specific (Polatajko & Mandich, 2004). While the global strategy used in CO-OP (GOAL-PLAN-DO-CHECK) is explicitly taught to the client at the outset of the intervention, domain-specific strategies are not taught. Rather, they are discovered during the DPA process through a process of guided discovery; hence, the CO-OP trifecta.

More specifically, problem-solving and cognitive strategy use (one pillar of the trifecta) is supported by two major tools that are also the remaining two pillars of the trifecta—DPA and guided discovery. DPA, described earlier, is embedded in the GOAL-PLAN-DO-CHECK framework; it is used each time a performance is discussed either in the PLAN phase or in the CHECK phase of the problem-solving framework. Guided discovery, which is described next, ensures that the client is actively engaged in problem solving and the identification of domain-specific strategies, becomes skilled at engaging in this process, and that the developed strategies are relevant to the client in their real-world context. This, in turn, ensures that the client feels ownership of the discovered solutions to performance problems, attributes success to strategy use, and is therefore more likely to apply these solutions outside of the therapy setting, thus achieving generalization and transfer (Pressley & Harris, 2006).

Guided Discovery

> *"Can it be, Ischomachus, that asking questions is teaching? I am just beginning to see what is behind all your questions. You lead me on by means of things I know, point to things that resemble them, and persuade me that I know things that I thought I had no knowledge of"* (Socrates, n.d.).

Guided discovery is a method of instruction designed to facilitate active learning. Guiding discovery elicits the learner's active involvement in the discovery of new learning. In guided discovery, the learner is led to discover answers to problems rather than being given the answers outright. On an instructional continuum, it sits in the middle between didactic learning, or direct teaching, where the learner is specifically taught the answer, and pure discovery learning, where the learner is left to discover the answers on their own with little or no guidance (Figure 9.2). Guided discovery has been shown to be more effective than discovery learning in supporting skill acquisition and transfer (Mayer, 2004).

The basic premise of guided discovery is that meaningful learning occurs when the learner strives to make sense of the presented material by selecting the relevant information to attend to, organizing it into a coherent structure, and then integrating it with previous knowledge to form new knowledge (Mayer, 2004). Using guided discovery ensures that the learner identifies the solutions that make sense, fit with existing knowledge, and have relevance to real-world context. The defining characteristic of

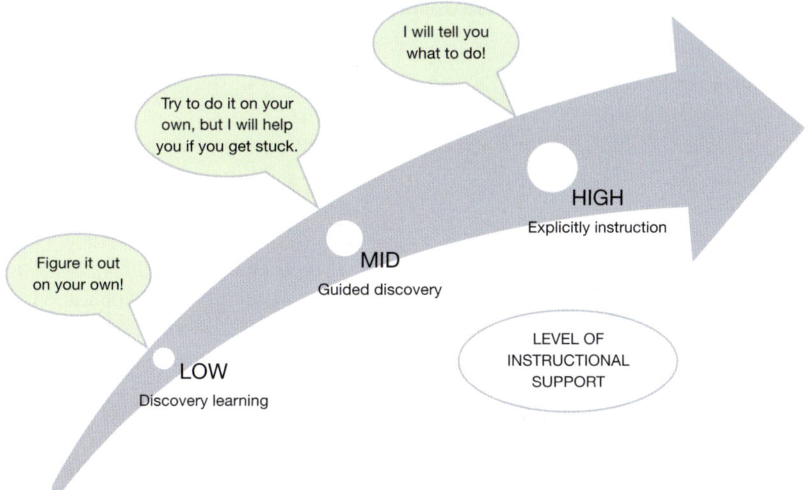

FIGURE 9.2 Instructional continuum. (Adapted from McEwen, S. E., Wolf, T., Baum, C. M., & Polatajko, H. J. [2014]. *Combined task-specific and cognitive strategy training in subacute stroke: A phase II randomized controlled trial.* Paper presented at the International Stroke Conference, San Diego, CA. Copyright retained by author.)

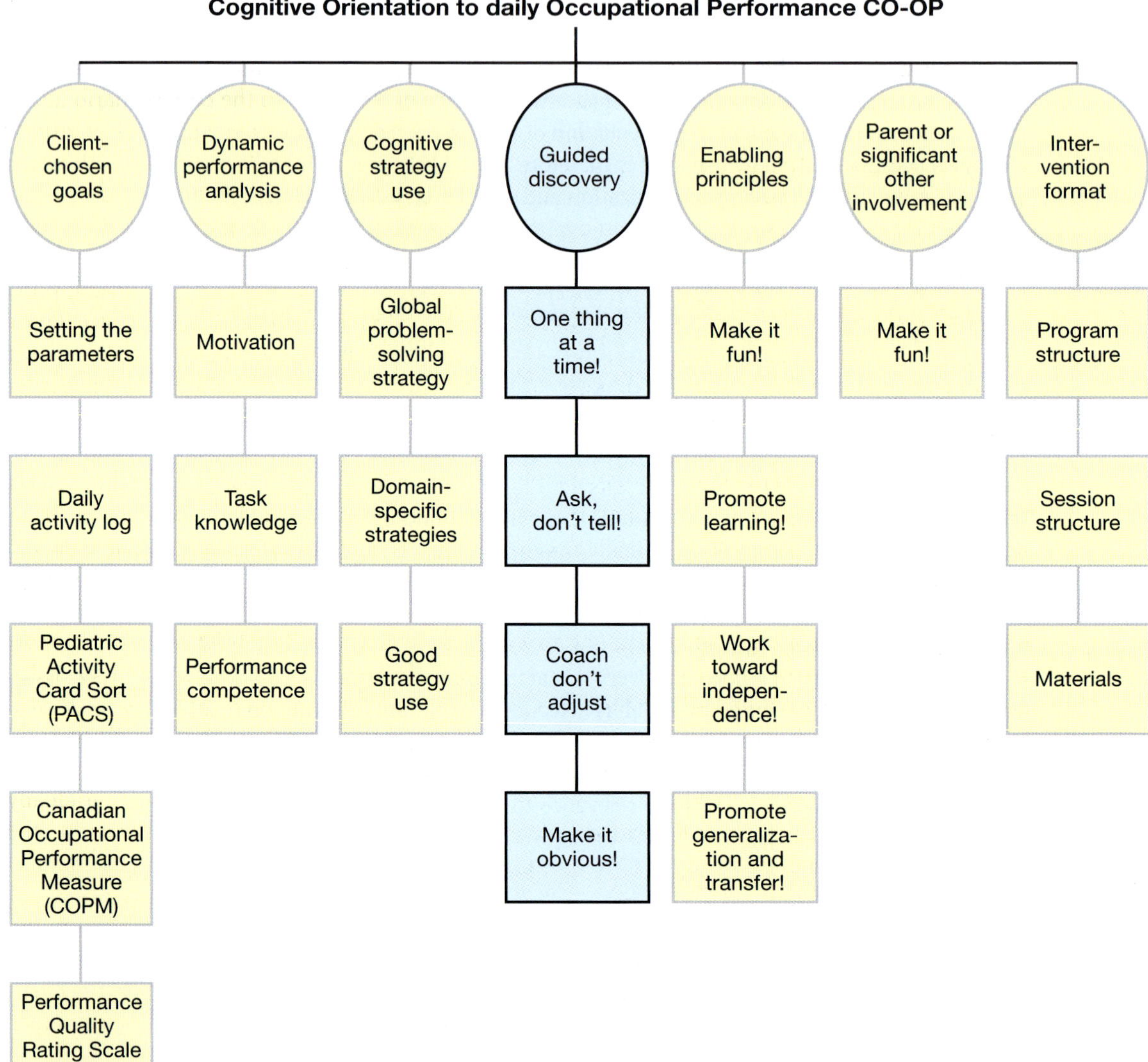

FIGURE 9.3 Guided discovery keys. (Adapted from Polatajko, H. J., & Mandich, A. [2004]. *Enabling occupation in children: The Cognitive Orientation to daily Occupational Performance (CO-OP) Approach*. CAOT Publications ACE. Copyright retained by author.)

guided discovery is the logical and sequential use of a series of questions or techniques that lead the learner to discover a concept, principle, relationship, rule, or action that was previously unknown.

In the CO-OP, the process of guided discovery is captured in five keys that are used by the therapist to "unlock" the learning and skill acquisition process (Figure 9.3). Each key is written in the form of imperatives to emphasize its importance to the approach: *One thing at a time! Ask, don't tell! Coach, don't adjust! Stay in sync!* and *Name that strategy!* Each key is designed to support active problem solving and learning.

Together, these five keys firmly establish CO-OP as a learning approach. For example, "One thing at a time!" points to the importance of focus and attention to learning, recognizing that learning is done best when only one thing is presented and practiced. Although the therapist may identify that there are many issues with the performance of a skill, as in the case scenario at the end of this chapter, the therapist guides the client to focus on only one element of a skill at a time. The remaining guided discovery keys are designed to help the therapist focus the client's attention on specific aspects of performance that require adjusting and guide the client toward possible strategies that offer a solution. For example, the therapist may do this by using "Ask don't tell!" This imperative reminds the therapist to pose a question to draw attention to a performance issue rather than directly identifying the performance issue. Or the therapist can use "Coach, don't adjust!" This imperative reminds the therapist to pose a question or make a comment to draw attention to a performance issue, rather than simply making unobtrusive adjustments to support performance success. The therapist supports discovery and application of strategies by encouraging the child to "Name that strategy!", giving an explicit label to the discovered domain-specific strategy and recognizing it as a tool for resolving problems and achieving goals. Naming the strategy increases the likelihood that the child will remember and apply the strategy during task performance and recognize its role in improving performance. Finally, the therapist must endeavor to "Stay in sync!" with the child's current level of knowledge and skill by responding to observed performance, behavior, verbalizations, and emotional responses with the appropriate level of support and guidance for supporting task practice, global strategy use, and domain-specific strategy discovery. For example, the therapist might apply the "hourglass" method (Figure 9.4) to support strategy discovery by posing questions that are in sync with the child's current level of knowledge and skill—posing broad, general questions when the child possesses a larger repertoire of knowledge about the task and more specific questions when the child is in an earlier phase of skill acquisition and therefore would benefit from provision of more directed and knowledge-rich questions to successfully identify performance problems and potential strategies. As the child gradually acquires knowledge and skill and discovers strategies appropriate for advancing performance, the therapist "stays in sync" with the child's learning by moving between broad and specific questions.

Guided discovery is congruent with client-centeredness; in fact, it is essentially a form of client-centeredness. Guided discovery provides a structure to foster a spirit of collaboration and mutual respect and empowers the client to address problems and identify their own solutions. Using guided discovery ensures that the client works on problems that are important to the client and identifies the solutions that make sense, fit with existing understanding, and have relevance to the real-world context.

As mentioned previously, using guided discovery enables the client to be actively involved in noticing performance problems and proposing performance solutions (strategies), which in turn ensures that the client is fully engaged in the process. This can be seen in the following exchange between Markus (pseudonym), a young boy with Asperger syndrome, and the therapist when discussing strategies regarding his handwriting. In this excerpt, Markus was in the midst of trying out his strategy for letter formation and positioning:

Therapist (observing Markus writing slowly): You know I really also like how you are taking your time when you make the letters.

Marcus: Yes, but in school, sometimes there isn't as much time and then my mind says "rush-rush-rush, rush-rush-rush, rush-rush-rush."

Therapist: What can you tell your mind when it does that; what can you say?

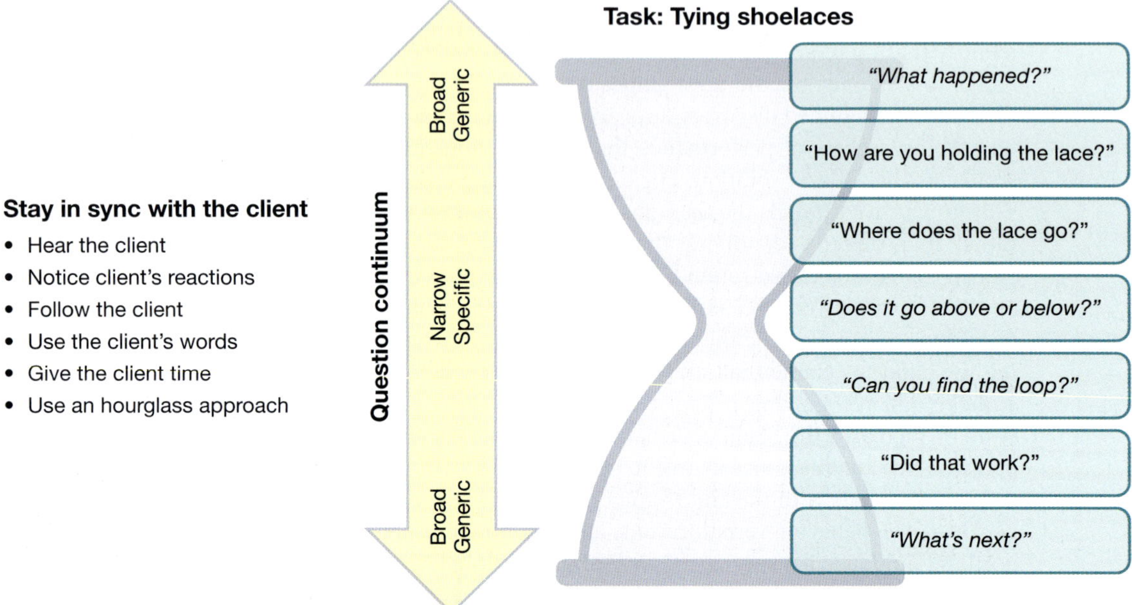

FIGURE 9.4 Hourglass approach to guided discovery. (Adapted from CO-OP Workshop. [2022]. International Cognitive Approaches Network (ICAN). Copyright retained by author.)

Marcus: But it is also, like, what the school does (pausing to think); but I'll try, I'll try to … (thoughtful pause) I don't know!

Therapist: What can you say? What can you say to yourself? Can you say maybe, can you say (hesitating) m-a-y-b-e "I am going to slow down"? Can you say that?

Marcus: OK! (thoughtful pause; then with excitement) I know a better idea—I'm going to try to take my t-i-m-e!

Here, all three elements of the CO-OP trifecta can be observed, where Marcus is prompted to analyze his handwriting problems and identify the problem (DPA) through questions and prompts from the therapist (guided discovery), which in turn leads to the identification of a domain-specific strategy or PLAN for achieving a specified performance GOAL (strategy use).

Conducting the intervention in a collaborative, client-centered manner using guided discovery enhances the client's feelings of ownership of the solutions and the strategies identified, as can be seen when Markus proudly declares his strategy to the therapist in the previous excerpt. In turn, this collaboration enhances the client's sense of self-efficacy as they begin to attribute performance success to strategy use, and not innate ability. This, in turn, supports performance learning and generalization and transfer. This is vividly described in the following quote from a client's father after his son, Roger, learned to ride his bike during CO-OP intervention:

> "There is no doubt about it, that for Roger, bike riding has been a lifeline, a lifeline into the social community, and a lifeline so far as his self-esteem, it has definitely grown. It sort of was a rite of passage, a real marker for him" (Mandich & Polatajko, 2003, p. 588).

Enabling Principles

Enabling occupation refers to "processes of facilitating, guiding, coaching, educating, prompting, listening, reflecting, encouraging, or otherwise collaborating with people so that individuals, groups, agencies, and organizations have the means and opportunity to be involved in solving their own problems" (CAOT, 1997, 2002, p. 180).

As previously mentioned, the CO-OP Approach is grounded within a client-centered philosophy and a learning paradigm in which the focus is on enabling people to perform and participate in meaningful occupations by supporting skill acquisition, strategy use, generalization, and transfer. The **enabling principles**, another key feature of CO-OP, represent a collection of key concepts, theories, and ideas underlying this process of enablement. Drawn from theoretical, clinical, and empirical knowledge regarding learning and cognition, they are used to facilitate strategy use, guide skill acquisition, and promote generalization and transfer by ensuring client motivation and engagement throughout the CO-OP process. Similar to guided discovery, the enabling principles are captured within four building blocks: *Make it fun!* or *Actively engage the client!*; *Promote learning!*; *Work towards independence!*; and *Promote generalization and transfer!* (Figure 9.5).

While guided discovery represents a technique the therapist performs during the CO-OP process as a means to support DPA, strategy use and skill acquisition on the part of the client, the enabling principles represent a collection of postulates that guide the therapist's actions with the aim to promote learning. As building blocks, they represent the 'foundations' upon which the techniques and tools in other key features are applied. This includes techniques such as creating the 'just right challenge' to encourage effort and perseverance and active participation in the CO-OP process; nurturing positive self-efficacy by encouraging the client to actively engage in the problem-solving process, embrace challenges and reframe failures as opportunities for learning; and applying principles and techniques based in learning theory to structure task practice and provide appropriate and timely feedback, with the ultimate aim of improving performance and gaining independence. Working toward independence (i.e., when guided practice of the task becomes automatic performance) involves the scaffolded provision (and eventual removal) of various forms of support from the therapist, with the ultimate goal of generalization and transfer.

Together, the fundamental elements of the CO-OP Approach described thus far are used to achieve the main objectives of CO-OP: to promote strategy use, skill acquisition, and the generalization and transfer of acquired skills to other contexts and tasks. Grounded in Hebb's general postulate for learning and within a learning paradigm more generally, these features can be summarized under four **postulates regarding change** that capture the actions applied by the therapist to promote learning within the CO-OP Approach. While they do not represent general postulates representing incontestable truths (such as *Hebb's postulate*), these propositions represent assumptions about the underlying mechanisms through which the CO-OP Approach promotes change and learning based on current evidence supporting the approach (presented later in this chapter). The CO-OP postulates regarding change are:

1. The use of the global cognitive (GOAL-PLAN-DO-CHECK) strategy enables the identification and analysis of performance problems (DPA) and the discovery of solutions (domain-specific strategies) for successful performance of self-selected goals.
2. The use of the guided discovery keys during the CO-OP process supports the adoption of a cognitive, problem-solving approach to skill acquisition and goal (task) performance.

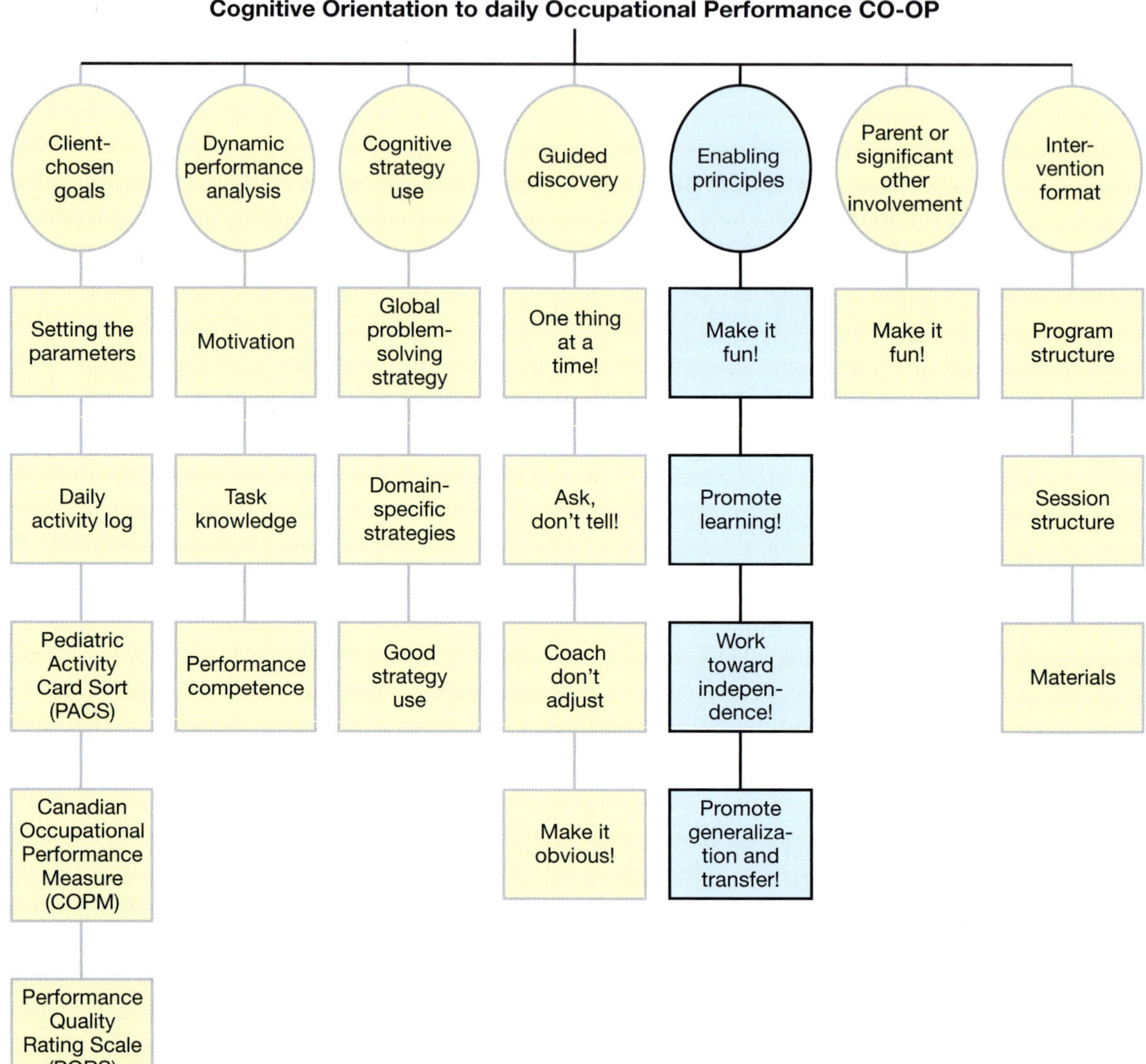

FIGURE 9.5 Enabling principles building blocks. (Adapted from Polatajko, H. J., & Mandich, A. [2004]. *Enabling occupation in children: The Cognitive Orientation to daily Occupational Performance (CO-OP) Approach*. CAOT Publications ACE. Copyright retained by author.)

3. The enabling principles enhance motivation and readiness for active engagement in the learning process and therefore support learning.
4. The combination of DPA, guided discovery, strategy use, and enabling principles promotes the generalization and transfer of learning.

The following section will describe in more detail how the many elements intrinsic in the CO-OP Approach are applied together during the intervention process to promote strategy use, enable skill acquisition, and achieve generalization and transfer of both the skills acquired for achieving performance goals and the strategies used to support problem solving and successful performance.

APPLICATION TO PRACTICE

Current evidence, discussed below, indicates that CO-OP is an effective approach for achieving occupational goals and thus enabling performance and participation among a diverse range of client populations with varied performance problems. However, before implementing the CO-OP Approach in practice, a few prerequisites should be established. Namely, due to the highly interactive nature of the Approach and the expectation that the client actively collaborates and participates in all aspects of goal-setting, performance analysis, and strategy discovery, it is imperative that both the therapist and client are ready and able to engage in such a process. For the therapist, this means that they possess a client-centered philosophy, a thorough understanding of disability and learning theory, and skills in communication and behavior management. For a client to benefit from the CO-OP Approach, they must be able to identify their own occupational goal(s) with the support of the therapist and/or significant other and demonstrate sufficient communication skills, behavioral responsiveness, and cognitive ability to learn, understand and engage in the problem-solving process that is inherent to the CO-OP Approach.

The CO-OP Process

Implementing the CO-OP Approach with a client involves a process consisting of five steps. It typically begins with a preintervention phase, in which the Approach is introduced to the client, client-centered and occupation-based goals are identified, and baseline performance level is established. This is followed by a series of intervention sessions (typically 10) focused on the advancement of skill performance (i.e., resolving performance problems and achieving identified goals) using the CO-OP trifecta. Finally, a postintervention session is conducted to re-evaluate performance and measure change.

In the CO-OP Approach, client-centered occupation-based goal setting is completed using the Canadian Occupational Performance Measure (Law et al., 2014), which therapists use to enable the client to identify their occupational performance issues and initiate the process of setting the client-centered occupational performance goals to be addressed. This ensures the goals are meaningful to the client and have relevance to the client's life and that the client is motivated to work on acquiring the relevant skills in therapy and will use the newly acquired skills in their everyday life. To quote a client's mother in a follow-up interview after her son, Morris, completed the CO-OP intervention:

> "I didn't think that learning to be a goalie was a good goal for therapy. I thought writing was the important thing. Well I have to tell you that he learned to be a good goalie with you, and then he made the school floor hockey team. They went to the championships and won. He is living his dream!" (Mandich et al., 2003, p. 584)

Once the client, together with the therapist, has identified occupation-based goals, the next step in the process is establishing baseline performance level for each identified goal. To do so, the therapist uses two previously described tools: the Canadian Occupational Performance Measure (Law et al., 2014) is used to collect client's self-ratings of current performance and their level of satisfaction with that performance, while the Performance Quality Rating Scale

(Polatajko & Mandich, 2004) is used by the therapist to evaluate observed performance directly.

Following this preintervention phase, the CO-OP process continues with the intervention sessions themselves, where the global GOAL-PLAN-DO-CHECK strategy is used collaboratively by the therapist and client in a continuous and iterative fashion to set performance goals (identify performance problems), to make and implement plans (domain-specific strategies) for achieving goals and to evaluate outcomes. This process instigates the CO-OP trifecta: identifying problems and setting plans using DPA, discovering and applying domain-specific strategies to resolve problems and ensuring active engagement of the client in all aspects of this process using guided discovery. The iterative and interactive nature of these key features of CO-OP and the way they all come together during practice of the client's goals is illustrated in Figure 9.6.

Specifically, guided discovery is combined with strategy use and the DPA process to enable clients to themselves discover the strategies that will solve their performance problems. In particular, guided discovery is entwined with the global problem-solving strategy; it is used iteratively to elucidate the PLAN, identify the domain-specific strategies, and carry out the CHECK. Although it is possible to use strategies without using guided discovery—for example, Donald Meichenbaum (1972) used modeling and direct instruction—combining them enables the learner to achieve a sense of ownership of the strategies used to resolve performance problems and more deeply understand the role of these strategies in achieving goals, which in turn means that they are more likely to apply such strategies to resolve future performance problems. To quote Jean Piaget (1970), "Remember also that each time one prematurely teaches a child something that he could have discovered himself, that child is kept from inventing it and consequently from understanding it completely" (p. 715).

Alongside the iterative and collaborative application of the GOAL-PLAN-DO-CHECK strategy, DPA and guided discovery, two additional features of the CO-OP Approach serve to advance the client's performance on their chosen goals. First, the client is assigned homework at the end of each CO-OP session, usually in the form of a brief task to be carried out at home prior to the next

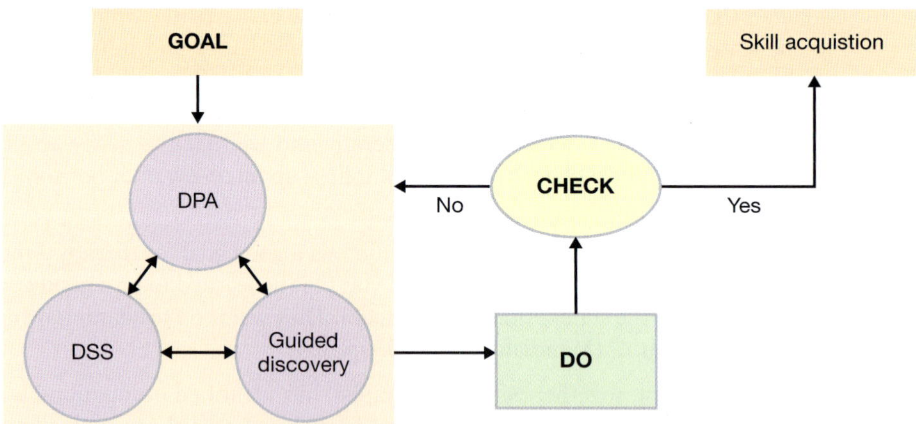

FIGURE 9.6 Global strategy flow chart showing the trifecta. (Adapted from Polatajko, H. J., & Mandich, A. [2004]. *Enabling occupation in children: The Cognitive Orientation to daily Occupational Performance (CO-OP) Approach*. CAOT Publications ACE. Copyright retained by author.)

session. Second, the involvement of a significant other throughout the CO-OP process (most often a parent or caregiver in the case of a child client) is considered key to the Approach's success. This involvement can be in the form of active participation in initial goal setting and baseline measurement, learning the basics of the CO-OP Approach (and the GPDC strategy in particular), attending CO-OP therapy sessions and supporting the client's completion of homework activities between sessions. Both homework and involvement of a significant other are considered crucial for the generalization and transfer of strategies and learned skills.

Upon completion of the intervention sessions, the CO-OP process concludes with a post intervention session aimed at re-evaluating the client's performance on their chosen goals and measuring change. This is achieved using the same tools used in the preintervention session: the Canadian Occupational Performance Measure (Law et al., 2014) and the Performance Quality Rating Scale (Polatajko & Mandich, 2004). Using these measures, observational and self-ratings of the client's performance are collected and subsequently compared to the ratings from pretest to determine the degree of change. In this way, the CO-OP process possesses a mechanism for clearly determining and demonstrating performance-based outcomes of the intervention and thus gathering evidence for one's own practice.

CASE EXAMPLE

Matthew: A Young Child With Developmental Coordination Disorder*

Matthew is a 6-year-old boy who was referred to therapy by his family physician. He attends first grade at a local school. Matthew's parents and his teacher observed him having significant difficulty with fine motor skills. He could not do up his zipper, and tying his shoes was extremely difficult. Matthew's mother had bought him Velcro shoes, but he really wanted a pair of Nike running shoes for Christmas. Mathew met the criteria for DCD but had not been given a formal diagnosis. Psychological assessment revealed that Matthew also had a nonverbal learning disability. Children with DCD exhibit significant difficulty acquiring new motor skills and are often restricted from participating in the typical activities of childhood. They are referred to occupational therapy for a variety of performance issues when they perform poorly in school-related motor-based activities, in particular, handwriting problems (Mandich & Polatajko, 2003).

In Preparation

On referral to the clinic, Matthew's parents were very frustrated and felt that they wanted to intervene early. Accessing therapy service had been a struggle for the family. Matthew's parents were very concerned about the effect his difficulties were having on his self-confidence and felt that early intervention would facilitate Matthew's optimal functioning in the classroom.

---

*Adapted from Polatajko, H. J., & Mandich, A. (2004). *Enabling occupation in children: The Cognitive Orientation to daily Occupational Performance (CO-OP) Approach*. CAOT Publications ACE. Adapted with permission.

Developmentally, Matthew's milestones were all within normal limits. At the time of referral, he was having difficulty printing his letters. He was also having difficulty at mealtime and often spilled his food. He really wanted to use a knife but could not manage to coordinate the movements. He could not do up the buttons or the zipper on his coat or snowsuit, and this often interfered with his ability to go out for recess on time with his friends.

Results of standardized testing on the Movement Assessment Battery for Children (Henderson et al., 2007) placed Matthew in the 1st percentile for his age; on the Test of Visual Perceptual Skills (Martin, 2017), he was in the 60th percentile; and on the Beery Developmental Test of Visual Motor Integration (Beery et al., 2010), he was in the 20th percentile. A parent questionnaire identified functional problems in the areas of self-care, and school and leisure activities. Matthew began CO-OP intervention.

Because younger children sometimes have difficulty using the 10-point rating scale of the Canadian Occupational Performance Measure (Law et al., 2014), it was decided that Matthew and his mom would complete the measure together. Matthew and his mom identified three GOALs (Box 9.1) that were important to both Matthew and his mom. The Canadian Occupational Performance Measure scores given by Matthew and his mother both indicated that Matthew had difficulty with these skills. The therapist observed Matthew perform these skills. The therapist's Performance Quality Rating Scale scores concurred with the results of the Canadian Occupational Performance Measure (Table 9.2).

The therapist used the DPA decision tree to analyze Matthew's performance and identified points of performance breakdown, presented in Box 9.1.

The Intervention

Matthew chose to start by working on tying his shoes. The therapist modeled how to tie a shoelace and verbalized the steps. She described the steps in the process to Matthew and then encouraged him to try. She broke the skill into steps. Starting with crossing the laces and making the first knot, the therapist prompted Matthew to describe each step, ensuring that she did not talk while Matthew was concentrating on performing the task. Matthew commented that when he crossed his laces it looked like an "X." Matthew was able to

Box 9.1 Case Example: Matthew's Performance Goals and Breakdown Points

GOAL	Performance Breakdown Points
Tying his shoes	He does not know how to start and do the first knot. He does not know how to form the loops. He does not know how to tie the final knot.
Cutting his food	He does not hold the fork or knife in the proper position. He holds his elbows way up in the air when cutting. He tries to tear the food instead of cutting it.
Printing	His letters are too large. His words are too close together and some letters overlap. He does not hold his pencil with a functional grasp. He sits on the edge of the chair.

Table 9.2 Case Example: Matthew's Strategies and PLAN Development

Domain-Specific Strategy Type	Specific Strategy	Bridging of Strategy
Body position	Helper-hand-doer-hand	From cutting food to throwing and catching a baseball, eating a bowl of soup
Body position	READY position	Computer, eating at the table, doing homework at the desk, hitting a baseball
Body position	Chicken arms down	Eating, cutting with scissors
Attention to task	Make an "X" Glue my loop to the shoe	Tying his hockey skates and soccer shoes
Motor mnemonic	Make a bunny ear	Tying his hockey skates and soccer shoes
Task specification/ modification	Use of a pencil grip	Provided a grip for school and home

Parents were informed of the strategies and encouraged to have Matthew use these strategies at home and school.

form the loop, but it was far too big and far too high off the shoe. Through prompting and questioning Matthew was made to realize that he had to "glue the loop to the shoe." The following dialogue during shoe tying practice illustrates this process:

Therapist: Okay. So what we're doing now is tying shoes, right? What's our PLAN for tying shoes? Do you remember? What's the first part of the PLAN?

Matthew: Hold them here and make an "X." (demonstrating)

Therapist: Umhmm.

Matthew: And go through here. And then pull.

Therapist: Wow!

Matthew: Yup. Then make a loop with the tail, then come around, then there's a hole. You go through the hole and then you've got a tie.

Therapist: Yup. And you know, you have the right word, and you're doing the right thing, but there's one little thing I noticed that made a difference.

Matthew: It went through this loop instead?

Therapist: That's right, and how long should our tail be?

Matthew: About that long. (showing therapist)

Therapist: Yeah. So let's try it that way.

Matthew: Make a loop with this hand, and come around.

Therapist: Okay, stop for a second. Hold that still. Now you've got the loop, and that is a great loop. But you know what? I noticed something about that loop.

Matthew: What?

Therapist: And I bet Commander GOAL-PLAN-DO-CHECK[1] would notice this too. (brings over puppet) It's floating in space. Look, it's way up here! It's like a hot air

---

[1]Please note that Commander GOAL-PLAN-DO-CHECK is a character puppet sometimes used to introduce the global strategy to children and help them remember and apply the strategy during task practice.

balloon launching. But do you know what? I think it should be in a different spot. What do you think? You try to finish it and see if that will work now.

Matthew: (ties shoes)

Therapist: What do you think? (looking at Matthew) What do you think, Commander? (looks at puppet)

Matthew: One loop's bigger than the other.

Therapist: It is.

Therapist: Okay, so we've got a loop bigger than the other, that's one problem, but watch when I do it. Okay, let's see. You can be the detective here. You've already done this part for me (therapist ties the shoelaces to the point of making the loop), so the next thing you told me to do was ....

Matthew: Make a loop.

Therapist: Okay, so where should I grab the loop? Is it close to the shoe, or up here? (makes a very small loop at the top of the lace)

Matthew: Close to the shoe.

Therapist: Okay. So I grab the loop close to the shoe; now what do I do here?

Matthew: Come around the loop, and then make a hole.

Therapist: Okay. I've made a hole.

Matthew: And make it go in it, but not ... only halfway in.

Therapist: Okay, halfway in.

Matthew: And then you have a loop.

Therapist: Okay, and now what do you do?

Matthew: I don't know. What?

Therapist: What comes next? What do I do with the loops?

Matthew: Pull them.

Therapist: Pull them. Tada. Now what was different about what you did and what I did?

Matthew: I don't know.

Therapist: Okay, you start from the beginning again. Okay, so first thing is ...

Matthew: Come around; make the next one come around.

Therapist: Umhmm.

Matthew: Then pull. (pulls tightly, finishes tying) Tada!

Therapist: Tada. That's excellent. What do you think about that?

Matthew: I'm good!

Matthew's second GOAL was printing. The therapist began by working on letter size. Through questioning, comparison, and exaggeration, Matthew came to realize that not all letters are the same size. He discovered that the letters have to stay on the line (he called this the racing track) and that the letters cannot cross into the next track (line), either the track above or the track below. His small letters sat on the track and took up half of the space and the tall letters touched the top of the racing track. Using the same analogy, the therapist led Matthew to discover that cars should not bump into each other, nor should the letters. Each letter had its own space.

Matthew held the pencil with an awkward grasp, so the therapist next targeted correcting his pencil grasp. Although the therapist had planned to address pencil grasp before letter size, Matthew did not want to change his grasp and became frustrated with the therapist when she suggested doing so. As such the therapist put this breakdown point aside for the time. After several sessions, Matthew was able to increase his success with printing and was then willing to work on his pencil grasp. The therapist tried a variety of pencil grips to keep his fingers in the correct position. The therapist used questioning to help Matthew come up with a strategy for an appropriate body position and pencil grasp. He called it his "READY" position. The therapist talked about how racing car drivers have a ready position at the starting gate just as Matthew has a ready position for writing.

Matthew had difficulty forming some letters correctly. The therapist addressed those letters directly and guided Matthew to come up with his own PLANs. For example, Matthew was having difficulty with letters that required diagonal lines and he would make his "V's" using vertical lines. He identified the verbal mnemonic "leaning tower" for the letter V and the mnemonic "roof" to remind him to curve the top of the "r."

Matthew also discovered strategies to help him cut his food and was able to bridge his READY position from writing to cutting his food. Matthew tended to elevate his elbows when he was cutting his food and so he came up with the strategy of "chicken arms down." He learned to "saw" his food instead of tearing it and to hold his fork with the handle "hidden in his hand" (not pointing straight up).

These domain-specific strategies and PLANs were developed and reinforced using a strategy summary sheet was created for Matthew, which he took home to support generalization. He was encouraged to use his strategies at school. The PLANs and strategies that he developed and the situations to which the strategies were bridged are summarized in Table 9.3.

At the End of the Intervention

After the 10 acquisition sessions, the therapist:

- Readministered the Canadian Occupational Performance Measure.
- Readministered baseline, using Performance Quality Rating Scale.

Table 9.3 Matthew's Canadian Occupational Performance Measure (COPM) and Performance Quality Rating Scale (PQRS) Scores Before and After CO-OP Intervention

	COPM													
	Importance				Performance				Satisfaction					
	Pretest		Posttest		Pretest		Posttest		Pretest		Posttest		PQRS	
GOAL	P	C	P	C	P	C	P	C	P	C	P	C	Pretest	Posttest
Tying his shoes	9	10	9	10	1	5	9	10	2	5	10	10	1	9
Cutting his food	9	10	9	10	2	5	8	10	2	5	9	10	3	9
Printing	10	5	10	5	3	5	9	10	2	5	9	10	3	8

All scores are made on a 10-point scale.
P, parent; C, child.

- Probed the child for generalization and transfer of Global (GOAL-PLAN-DO-CHECK) and Domain-Specific Strategies.
- Reviewed and reinforced CO-OP Approach and cognitive strategy use with parents and caregivers.

In the final meeting, the therapist repeated the Canadian Occupational Performance Measure and the Performance Quality Rating Scale, and both sets of scores showed significant improvement on all occupational goals (Table 9.1). Matthew and his mom were very pleased with the results.

SUPPORTING EVIDENCE

In addition to being an intervention that allows therapists to demonstrate the effect of CO-OP in their own practice, significant evidence has accumulated over the past 25 years to demonstrate the effectiveness of the Approach for improving performance and achieving client goals.

The new approach developed by Polatajko in the 1990s, initially called Verbal Self Guidance (Wilcox & Polatajko, 1994) was first tested with children with DCD using a series of 10 single-case experimental studies (Wilcox & Polatajko, 1994). This study demonstrated that the approach could help children with DCD improve performance in a wide variety of occupations and meet their occupational goals. The approach was further tested with additional children with DCD in a series of four systematic replications (Martini & Polatajko, 1998). These findings again demonstrated that the approach could help children improve performance in a variety of occupations and meet their goals. It was further demonstrated that the results were reproducible with a different therapist and that the outcomes were maintained over time.

Careful analysis of these early studies helped to refine the approach and identify its key features, especially the importance of focusing on an occupation of importance to the child (client-chosen goals), of analyzing the performance of that activity (key feature: DPA), and of the client-centered engagement of the child in the identification of performance problems and the discovery of solutions (key feature: guided discovery) (Polatajko et al., 2001b). The analyses of the intervention videos also revealed that, in addition to the global strategy, children discovered a number of domain-specific strategies and used them to improve performance to meet a variety of goals (Mandich et al., 2001b). Accordingly, the identification of domain-specific strategies was added to the process (key feature: cognitive strategy use). These analyses indicated that although verbal self-guidance was an important component of the approach, it did not capture the essence of the approach; broader cognitive strategy use and a focus on goal-oriented performance did. Therefore, to highlight the importance of cognition in skill acquisition, the focus on goal-oriented/occupational performance, and the cooperative nature of the interaction between therapist and client in the approach, it was renamed the CO-OP.

Subsequent studies of the CO-OP Approach with children with DCD not only demonstrated that the original findings were reproducible across children and therapists but also that gains in occupational performance were maintained, generalized, and transferred (Capistran & Martini, 2016; Chan, 2007; Green et al., 2008; Polatajko et al., 2001b; Yasunaga et al., 2023). Furthermore, the results from the CO-OP intervention have been shown to be superior to results of traditional approaches in improving outcomes for children with DCD (Miller et al., 2001), even when carried out in a group setting (Anderson et al., 2018; Thornton et al., 2016). Studies of CO-OP with other populations have also yielded similar results, showing it to be effective with a broad range of other diagnostic groups, both children and adults. These populations included children with acquired brain injury (Lebrault et al., 2023; Missiuna et al., 2010), autism spectrum disorder (Phelan et al., 2009; Rodger & Brandenburg, 2009; Rodger et al., 2008; Rodger & Vishram, 2010), cerebral palsy (Cameron et al., 2016; Jackman et al., 2018), ADHD (Gharebaghy et al., 2015), developmental disabilities (Halayko et al., 2016), and dystonia (Gimeno, 2015; Gimeno et al., 2019). CO-OP has also been shown to be effective with adults with a variety of conditions including adults with acute stroke (Linkewich et al., 2019; McEwen et al., 2015; McEwen et al., 2014; Song et al., 2019), chronic stroke (Henshaw et al., 2011; McEwen et al., 2009; McEwen et al., 2010; Polatajko et al., 2012), cerebral palsy or spina bifida (Öhrvall et al., 2020), and traumatic brain injury (Dawson et al., 2007; Dawson et al., 2009; Ng et al., 2011); as well as older adults with self-reported cognitive difficulties (Dawson et al., 2014) and following a hip fracture (Appleton et al., 2023). The application of the CO-OP intervention continues to be explored with different populations. For example, Davies et al. (2023) described a study protocol evaluating the efficacy and feasibility of CO-OP with adults with Parkinson disease.

In addition to growing evidence to support the use of the CO-OP Approach with increasingly diverse populations, research has also indicated that is not only an effective intervention for enabling performance of the motor-based tasks examined in the original research with children with DCD (e.g., riding a bicycle, handwriting, tying shoelaces), but also for tasks and skills in different occupational domains, including social, participation, and organizational goals among children with autistic spectrum disorder (Rodger et al., 2008; Rodger & Vishram, 2010) and adults with executive dysfunction following brain injury (Dawson et al., 2009). More recently, studies have also suggested that delivery of CO-OP intervention via telehealth may be a feasible and effective approach for improving performance on task-oriented goals (functional, performance-based goals) (Beit Yosef et al., 2019; Shiozu & Kurasawa, 2023).

While a considerable amount of evidence has accumulated for the effectiveness of CO-OP at addressing performance-based goals for diverse tasks and occupations among a range of client populations, the evidence for the mechanisms through which these changes are achieved is currently less well understood. However, existing research does suggest that learning is central to the success of the CO-OP Approach. Specifically, the adoption of a systematic, problem-solving approach to discover and apply strategies enables the client to identify and resolve performance problems and transfer this learning to everyday situations. This was first evident in early studies examining the effect of CO-OP with children with DCD, which demonstrated that children with DCD participating in CO-OP, along with improved performance of occupational goals, exhibited more frequent and more effective cognitive strategy use (Sangster et al., 2005) and engaged in more frequent and more complex DPA (Hyland & Polatajko, 2012) following intervention than those following other intervention approaches. Importantly, research has also indicated that the use of the global and domain-specific strategies is individual to both the child and goal (Rodger & Liu, 2008). Other studies have suggested that such changes in strategy use indicate that children participating in CO-OP adopt a more strategic approach to task learning and skill acquisition by learning to apply metacognitive skills for identifying problems, discovering domain-specific strategies, and monitoring and evaluating performance that, in turn, enables them to be more self-regulated in their approach to skill acquisition (Hyland & Polatajko, 2012; Sangster et al., 2013). This change has also been linked to improved self-efficacy following CO-OP (e.g., Roy et al., 2017), where developing a metacognitive awareness of the role of strategies in addressing performance problems prompts a move from a fixed mindset that affirms that success is determined by innate ability (or lack thereof) toward a growth mindset and belief that success can be achieved by discovering and applying the appropriate strategy. While this research provides support for the cognitive, learning paradigm framing the CO-OP Approach, it should be noted that research examining the mechanisms of change underlying the success of the Approach in resolving problems in performance of task-oriented goals remains in the earlier stages and further investigation is necessary to more fully explore the hypothesized mechanisms for change across different client groups.

Most recently, neuroimaging studies have begun to explore the effects of CO-OP at the neurologic level. In a recent MRI study (Izadi-Najafabadi et al., 2022), children with DCD demonstrated increased functional connectivity in networks associated with self-, emotional-, and attention-regulation alongside functional gains in motor and task performance and goal achievement following CO-OP intervention. On the basis of their results, the authors argue that the CO-OP Approach is an effective intervention that induces changes at both brain and behavioral levels. These results are consistent with the literature on the neuroscience of learning discussed earlier in this chapter, which argues that neuroplastic changes associated with learning are best supported through training situations that are task specific and goal driven, and that require active problem solving in a real-world context that provides opportunities for variation and practice.

Finally, there is evidence indicating that the gains achieved during the CO-OP intervention are generalized to real-life situations and transferred to tasks not directly addressed during intervention for clients from various populations, including children with cerebral palsy and spina bifida (Öhrvall et al., 2023), adults with traumatic brain injury (Dawson et al., 2009) and stroke (McEwen et al., 2010). A scoping review confirmed that transfer following CO-OP intervention was reported on at least one, and in many cases several, outcome variables in all of the 25 studies included in the review (Houldin et al., 2018). Such generalization and transfer, a gold-standard outcome for any therapeutic intervention, suggest that the outcomes of the CO-OP Approach have a relevant and meaningful effect on the performance of occupations the client wants, needs, or is expected to do in their daily life.

Taken together, the cumulative evidence indicates that the CO-OP Approach enables various populations with a variety of occupational performance issues, including motor-based performance issues, to use cognitive strategies to attain their occupational performance goals. Moreover, the skills acquired can be generalized to real-world situations and transferred to novel tasks. The observation that adopting a cognitive orientation to the enablement of occupational performance is successful across a variety of diagnostic groups with varied occupational performance issues and occupational goals has important implications for current understanding of occupational performance and its enablement.

CONCLUSIONS

The CO-OP Approach is a learning-based approach to the enablement of human occupational performance, and although it is an approach to intervention, it is based on an inherent, if not explicit, perspective on occupational performance. The primary characteristics of the Approach—client-centeredness, performance-based, and problem solving—together with the primary active ingredients of the approach—strategy use and guided discovery—point to the inherent perspective, with each characteristic and ingredient articulating an aspect of the perspective of the CO-OP Approach. This perspective, embedded in a learning paradigm, views goal-based performance as learned behavior, and that the learning of the behavior is driven by cognition and supported by cognitive strategies. The CO-OP perspective on occupational performance is in keeping with the models of occupational performance that view it as the interaction of person, occupation, and environment, but the CO-OP perspective gives the person, and most especially cognition, primacy in occupational performance. Accordingly, our understanding of human occupational performance must start with the person and their cognitions. The evidence presented in this chapter demonstrating that the CO-OP Approach is effective at enabling occupational performance through application of a cognitive, problem-solving intervention supports this perspective.

REFERENCES

American Psychiatric Association. (2013). *Diagnosis and Statistical Manual of Mental Disorders* (5th ed., text revision). Author.

Anderson, L., Wilson, J., & Carmichael, K. (2018). Implementing the Cognitive Orientation to daily Occupational Performance (CO-OP) approach in a group format with children living with motor coordination difficulties. *Australian Occupational Therapy Journal, 65*(4), 295–305. https://doi.org/10.1111/1440-1630.12479

Appleton, E., Maeir, T., Kaufman, Y., Karni, S., & Gilboa, Y. (2023). Cognitive Orientation to daily Occupational Performance (CO-OP) for older adults after a hip fracture: A pilot study. *American Journal of Occupational Therapy, 77*(1), 7701205130. https://doi.org/10.5014/ajot.2023.050073

Beery, K. E., Buktenica, N. A., & Beery, N. A. (2010). *Beery-Buktenica Developmental Test of Visual-Motor Integration* (6th ed.). Psychological Corp.

Beit Yosef A., Jacogs, J. M., Shenkar, S., Shames, J. Schwartz, I., Doryon, Y., Naveh, Y., Khalailh, F., Berrous, S., & Gilboa, Y. (2019). Activity performance, participation and quality of life among adults in the chronic stage after acquired brain injury: The feasibility of an occupation-based telerehabilitation intervention. *Frontiers in Neurology, 10,* 1247. https://doi.org/10.3389/fneur:2019.01247

Bjorklund, D. F., & Causey, K. B. (2018). Learning to think on their own: executive function, strategies and problem-solving. In *Children s Thinking: Cognitive Development and Individual Differences*. Sage Publications Inc.

Bransford, J., & Stein, B. (1993). *The Ideal Problem Solver*. W. H. Freeman.

Cameron, D., Craig, T., Edwards, B., Missiuna, C., Schwellnus, H., & Polatajko, H. J. (2016). Cognitive Orientation to daily Occupational Performance (CO-OP): A new approach for children with cerebral palsy. *Physical & Occupational Therapy in Pediatrics*, *37*(2), 183–198. https://doi.org/10.1080/01942638.2016.11855000

Cameron, D., Polatajko, H., Schwellnus, H., Missiuna, M., Roy, R., & Craig, T. (2010). Cognitive Orientation to Occupational Performance (CO-OP): A new approach for children with cerebral palsy. Poster presented at the World Federation of Occupational Therapist Congress, Santiago, Chile.

Canadian Association of Occupational Therapists. (1997). *Enabling Occupation: An Occupational Therapy Perspective.* CAOT Publications.

Capistran, J., & Martini, R. (2016). Exploring inter-task transfer following a CO-OP approach with four children with DCD: A single subject multiple baseline design. *Human Movement Science*, *49*, 277–290. https://doi.org/10.1016/j.humov.2016.07.004

Carey, L. M., Polatajko, H. J., Tabor Connor, L., & Baum, C. M. (2012). Stroke rehabilitation: A learning perspective. In L. M. Carey (Ed.), *Stroke Rehabilitation: Insights from Neuroscience and Imaging*. Oxford University Press.

Chan, D. Y. K. (2007). The application of Cognitive Orientation to daily Occupational Performance (CO-OP) in children with developmental coordination disorder (developmental coordination disorder) in Hong Kong: A pilot study. *Hong Kong Journal of Occupational Therapy, 17,* 39–44. https://doi.org/10.1016/S1569-1861(08)70002-0

Davies, S. J., Gullo, H. L., & Doig, E. (2023). Efficacy and feasibility of the CO-OP approach in Parkinson's disease: RCT study protocol. *Canadian Journal of Occupational Therapy, 90*(4),363–373. https://doi.org/10.1177/00084174231156287

Dawson, D. R., McEwen, S. M., & Polatajko, H. J. (Eds.) (2017). *Cognitive Orientation to daily Occupational Performance in Occupational Therapy: Using the CO-OP Approach™ to Enable Participation Across the Lifespan.* AOTA Press.

Dawson, D. R., Gaya, A., Hunt, A., Levine, B., Lemsky, C., & Polatajko, H. J. (2009). Using the Cognitive Orientation to Occupational Performance (CO-OP) with adults with executive dysfunction following traumatic brain injury. *Canadian Journal of Occupational Therapy/Revue Canadienne D'Ergotherapie, 76,* 115–127. https://doi.org/10.1177/000841740907600209

Dawson, D., Polatajko, H., & Levine, B. (2007). Naturalistic rehabilitation for executive dysfunction. *Journal of the International Neuropsychological Society, 13*(1 Suppl 1), 120.

Dawson, D., Richardson, J., Troyer, A., Binns, M., Clark, A., Polatajko, H., Winocur, G., Hunt, A., & Bar, Y. (2014). An occupation-based strategy training approach to managing age-related executive changes: A pilot randomized controlled trial. *Clinical Rehabilitation, 28,* 118–127. https://doi.org/10.1177/0269215513492541

Dictionary.com (n.d.) Problem-solve. In Dictionary.com. Retrieved from http://dictionary.reference.com/browse/problem-solve

Doidge, N. (2007). The brain that changes itself: Stories of personal triumph from the frontiers of brain science. Penguin Life.

Fitts, P. M., & Posner, M. I. (1967). Human performance. Brooks/Cole.

Flavell, J. H. (1981). Cognitive monitoring. In W. P. Dickens (Ed.), *Children's Oral Communication Skills* (pp. 35–60). Academic Press.

Gentile, A. M. (1992). The nature of skill acquisition: Therapeutic implications for children with movement disorders. In H. Forssberg & H. Hirschfeld (Eds.), Movement Disorders in Children. *Medicine and Sport Science* (Vol. 36, pp. 31–40). Karger.

Gharebaghy S., Rassafiani, M., & Cameron, D. (2015). Effect of cognitive intervention on children with ADHD. *Physical & Occupational Therapy in Pediatrics, 35*(1), 13–23. https://doi.org/10.3109/01942638.2014.957428

Gimeno, H. (2015, May). *Scales and outcomes for managing dystonia in childhood: What have we learned from previous studies?* Paper presented at the Satellite DBS symposium, European Paediatric Neurology Society Congress, Vienna, Austria.

Gimeno, H., Brown, R. G., Lin, J.-P., Cornelius, V., & Polatajko, H. J. (2019). Cognitive approach to rehabilitation in children with hyperkinetic movement disorders post-DBS. *Neurology*, 92(11), e1212–e1224. https://doi.org/10.1212/WNL.0000000000007092

Gimeno, H., Farber, J., Thornton, J., & Polatajko, H. (2021). The Relative merits of an individualized versus a generic approach to rating functional performance in childhood dystonia. *Children, 8,* 7, https://dx.doi.org/10.3390/children8010007

Green, D., Chambers, M. E., & Sugden, D. A. (2008). Does subtype of developmental coordination disorder count: Is there a differential effect on outcome following intervention? *Human Movement Science, 27,* 363–382. https://doi.org/10.1016/j.humov.2008.02.009

Halayko, J., Magill-Evans, J., Smith, V., & Polatajko, H. (2016). Enabling two-wheeled cycling for youth with Down syndrome. *Pediatric Physical Therapy, 28*(2), 224–230. https://doi.org/10.1097/PEP.0000000000000240

Hebb, D. O. (1949). *The organization of behaviour: A neuropsychological theory*. John Wiley and Sons, Inc.

Hebb, D.O. (2002). *The organization of behavior: A neuropsychological theory*. Taylor Francis. https://doi.org/10.4324/9781410612403

Henderson, S. E., Sugden, D. A., & Barnett, A. L. (2007). *Movement assessment battery for children-2 second edition (Movement ABC-2)*. The Psychological Corporation.

Henshaw, E., Polatajko, H. J., McEwen, S. E., Ryan, J. D., & Baum, C. (2011). A cognitive approach to improve participation after stroke: Two case studies. *American Journal of Occupational Therapy, 65*(1), 55–63. https://doi.org/10.5014/ajot.2011.09010

Houldin, A., McEwen, S. E., Howell, M. W., & Polatajko, H. J. (2018). The Cognitive Orientation to daily Occupational Performance approach and transfer: A scoping review. *OTJR: Occupation, Participation and Health, 38*(3), 157–172. https://doi.org/10.1177/1539449217736059

Hyland, M., & Polatajko, H. J. (2012). Enabling children with developmental coordination disorder to self-regulate through the use of dynamic performance analysis: Evidence from the CO-OP approach. *Human Movement Science, 31*(4), 987–998. https://doi.org/10.1016/j.humov.2011.09.003

Imamizu, H., Miyauchi, S., Tamada, T., Sasaki, Y., Takino, R., PuÈtz, B., Yoshioka, T., & Kawato, M. (2000). Human cerebellar activity reflecting an acquired internal model of a new tool. *Nature, 403*(6766), 192–195. https://doi.org/10.1038/35003194

Izadi-Najafabadi, S., Kamaldeep, K. G., & Zwicker, J. G. (2020). Training-induced neuroplasticity in children with developmental coordination disorder. *Current Developmental Disorders Reports, 7,* 48–58. https://doi.org/10.1007/s40474-020-00191-0

Izadi-Najafabadi, S., Gunton, C., Dureno, Z., Zwicker, JG. (2022). Effectiveness of cognitive orientation to occupational performance intervention in improving motor skills of children with developmental coordination disorder: A randomized waitlist-control trial. *Clinical Rehabilitation*, 36(6), 776–788. doi: 10.1177/02692155221086188

Jackman, M., Novak, I., Lannin, N., Froude, E., Miller, L., & Galea, C. (2018). Effectiveness of Cognitive Orientation to daily Occupational Performance over and above functional hand splints for children with cerebral palsy or brain injury: A randomized controlled trial. *BMC Pediatrics, 18*(1), 248. https://doi.org/10.1186/s12887-018-1213-9

Law, M., Baptiste, S., Carswell, A., McColl, M. A., Polatajko, H., & Pollock, N. (2014). *Canadian Occupational Performance Measure* (5th ed.). CAOT Publications ACE.

Lebrault, H., Martini, R., Manalov, R., Chavanne, C., Krasny-Pacini, A., & Chevignard, M. (2023). Cognitive orientation to daily occupational performance to improve occupational performance, goals for children with executive function deficits after acquired brain injury. *Developmental Medicine and Child Neurology*, *66*(4). 501–513. https://doi.org/10.1111/dmcn.15759

Linkewich, E., Avery, L., Rios, J., & McEwen, S. (2019). Minimally clinically important differences in functional independence after a knowledge translation intervention in stroke rehabilitation. *Archives of Physical Medicine and Rehabilitation*, *2020*(101), 587–591. https://doi.org/10.1016/jp.apmr.2019.10.185

Mandich, A., & Polatajko, H. (2003). Developmental coordination disorder: Mechanisms measurement management. *Human Movement Science, 22,* 406–411.

Mandich, A., Polatajko, H. J., Macnab, J. J., & Miller, L. T. (2001a). Treatment of children with developmental coordination disorder: What is the evidence? *Physical and Occupational Therapy in Pediatrics, 20*(2/3), 51–68. https://doi.org/10.1080/J006v20n02_04

Mandich, A., Polatajko, H. J., Missiuna, C., & Miller, L. (2001b). Cognitive strategies and motor performance in children with developmental coordination disorder. *Physical and Occupational Therapy in Pediatrics, 20*(2/3), 125–144. https://doi.org/10.1080/J006v20n02_08

Mandich, A., Polatajko, H., & Rodger S. (2003). Rites of passage: Understanding participation of children with developmental coordination disorder. *Human Movement Science, 22,* 583–595. https://doi.org/10.1016/j.humov.2003.09.011

Martin, N. A. (2017). *Test of visual perceptual skills* (4th ed.). Academic Therapy Publications.

Martini, R., & Polatajko, H. J. (1998). Verbal self-guidance as a treatment approach for children with developmental coordination disorder: A systematic replication study. *OTJR: Occupation, Participation and Health, 18*(4), 157–181. https://doi.org/10.1177/153944929801800403

Martini, R., Rios, J., Polatajko, H., Wolf, T., & McEwen, S. E. (2014). The Performance Quality Rating Scale (PQRS): Reliability, convergent validity, and internal responsiveness for two scoring systems. *Disability and Rehabilitation, 29*(6), 526–536. https://doi.org/10.3109/09638288.2014.913702

Mathiowetz, V., & Bass Haugen, J. (1994). Motor behavior research: Implications for therapeutic approaches to central nervous system dysfunction. *American Journal of Occupational Therapy, 48,* 733–745. https://doi.org/10.5014/ajot.48.8.733

Mayer, R. E. (2004). Should there be a three-strikes rule against pure discovery learning? The case for guided methods of instruction. *American Psychologist, 59*(10), 14–19. https://doi.org/10.1037/0003-066X.59.1.14

McEwen, S. E., Huijbregts, M., Ryan, J., & Polatajko, H. (2009). Cognitive strategy use in motor skill acquisition post stroke: A critical review. *Brain Injury, 23*(4), 263–277. https://doi.org/10.1080/02699050902788493

McEwen, S. E., Polatajko, H. J., Baum, C., Rios, J., Cirone, D., Doherty, M., & Wolf, T. (2015). Combined cognitive-strategy and task-specific training improves transfer to untrained activities in sub-acute stroke: An exploratory randomized controlled trial. *Neurorehabilitation and Neural Repair, 29*(6), 526–536. https://doi.org/10.1177/1545968314558602

McEwen, S. E., Polatajko, H. J., Huijbregts, M. P. J., & Ryan, J. D. (2010). Inter-task transfer of meaningful, functional skills following a cognitive-based treatment: Results of three multiple baseline design experiments in adults with chronic stroke. *Neuropsychological Rehabilitation, 20,* 541–561. https://doi.org/10.1080/09602011003638194

McEwen, S. E., Polatajko, H. J., Huijbregts, M. P., & Ryan, J. D. (2009). Exploring a cognitive-based treatment approach to improve motor-based skill performance in chronic stroke: Results of three single case experiments. *Brain Injury, 23,* 1041–1053. https://doi.org/10.3109/02699050903421107

McEwen, S., Wolf, T., Baum, C., & Polatajko, H. (2014, February 12). *Combined task-specific and cognitive strategy training in subacute stroke: A Phase II randomized controlled trial.* American Heart Association; International Stroke Conference 2014, San Diego, California.

Meichenbaum, D. (1972). Cognitive modification of test anxious college students. *Journal of Consulting and Clinical Psychology, 39*(3), 370–380. https://doi.org/10.1037/h0033896

Meichenbaum, D. (1977). *Cognitive-behaviour modification*. Plenum Press.

Miller, L. T., Polatajko, H. J., Missiuna, C., Mandich, A. D., & Macnab, J. J. (2001). A pilot trial of a cognitive treatment for children with developmental coordination disorder. *Human Movement Science, 20*(1/2), 183–210. https://doi.org/10.1016/S0167-9457(01)00034-3

Missiuna, C., DeMatteo, C., Hanna, S., Mandich, A., Law, M., Mahoney, W., & Scott, L. (2010). Exploring the use of cognitive intervention for children with acquired brain injury. *Physical & Occupational Therapy in Pediatrics,* 30, 205–219. https://doi.org/10.3109/01942631003761554

Ng, E., Polatajko, H., & Dawson, D. (2011). Addressing dysfunction after brain injury: A pilot tele-rehabilitation study. *Archives of Physical Medicine and Rehabilitation, 92,* 1690–1722. https://doi.org/10.1016/j.apmr.2011.07.003

Novak, I., McIntyre, S., Morgan, C., Campbell, L., Dark, L., Morton, N., Stumbles, E., Wilson, S., & Goldsmith. S. (2013). A systematic review of interventions for children with cerebral palsy: State of the evidence. *Developmental Medicine and Child Neurology, 55*(10), 885–910. https://doi.org/10.1111/dmcn.12246

Öhrvall, A. Hofgren, C., Lindquist, B., Bergqvist, B., Himmelmann, K., Opheim, A. Sjöwall, D., Brock, K., & Peny-Dahlstrand, M. (2023) Intervention with the CO-OP approach leads to a transfer effect over time to untrained goals for children with cerebral palsy or spina bifida, *Disability and Rehabilitation*. https://doi.org/10.1080/09638288.2023.2225875

Öhrvall, A. M., Bergqvist, L., Hofgren, C., & Peny-Dahlstrand, M. (2020). "With CO-OP I'm the boss"—experiences of the Cognitive Orientation to daily Occupational Performance approach as reported by young adults with cerebral palsy or spina bifida. *Disability and Rehabilitation*, *42*(25), 3645–3652. https://doi.org/10.1080/09638288.2019.1607911

Phelan, S., Steinke, L., & Mandich, A. (2009). Exploring a cognitive intervention for children with pervasive developmental disorder. *Canadian Journal of Occupational Therapy, 76,* 23–28. https://doi.org/10.1177/000841740907600107

Piaget, J. (1970). Piaget's theory. In P. H. Mussen (Ed.), Carmichael's *Manual* of Child Psychology (3rd ed., Vol. 1, pp. 703–732). Wiley.

Polatajko, H. J. (2010). The CO-OP twist. *Physical & Occupational Therapy in Pediatrics, 30*(4), 277–279. https://doi.org/10.3109/01942638.2010.510381

Polatajko, H. J., & Mandich, A. (2004). *Enabling occupation in children: The Cognitive Orientation to daily Occupational Performance (CO-OP) Approach*. CAOT Publications ACE.

Polatajko, H. J., Cantin, N., Amoroso, B., McKee, P., Rivard, A., Kirsh, B., & Lin, N. (2013). Occupation-based enablement: A practice mosaic. In E. A. Townsend & H. J. Polatajko (Eds.), *Enabling occupation II: Advancing an occupational therapy vision for health, well-being and justice through occupation* (2nd ed., pp. 177–201). CAOT Publications ACE.

Polatajko, H. J., Macnab, J., Anstett, B., Malloy-Miller, T., Murphy, K., & Noh, S. (1995). A clinical trial of the process-oriented treatment approach for children with developmental co-ordination disorder. *Developmental Medicine and Child Neurology, 37,* 310–319. https://doi.org/10.1111/j.1469-8749.1995.tb12009.x

Polatajko, H. J., Mandich, A. D., & Martini, R. (2000). Dynamic performance analysis: A framework for understanding occupational performance. *American Journal of Occupational Therapy, 54*(1), 65–72. https://doi.org/10.5014/ajot.54.1.65

Polatajko, H. J., Mandich, A. D., Miller, L., & Macnab, J. (2001a). Cognitive Orientation to daily Occupational Performance: Part II—the evidence. *Physical and Occupational Therapy in Paediatrics, 20*(2/3), 83–106. https://doi.org/10.1080/J006v20n02_06

Polatajko, H. J., Mandich, A. D., Missiuna, C., Miller, L., Macnab, J., Malloy-Miller, T., & Kinsella, E. A. (2001b). Cognitive Orientation to daily Occupational Performance (CO-OP): Part III—the protocol in brief. *Physical and Occupational Therapy in Pediatrics, 20*(2/3), 107–123. https://doi.org/10.1300/J006v20n02_07

Polatajko, H. J., McEwen, S. E., Ryan, J. D., & Baum, C. M. (2012). Brief report: A pilot randomized controlled trial investigating cognitive strategy use to improve goal performance post stroke. *American Journal of Occupational Therapy, 66*(1), 104–109. https://doi.org/10.5014/ajot.2012.001784

Polatajko, H. J., Rodger, S., Dhillon, A., & Hirji, F. (2004). Approaches to the management of children with motor problems. In D. Dewey & D. E. Tupper (Eds.), *Developmental Motor Disorders: A Neuropsychological Perspective* (pp. 461–486). Guilford Press.

Pressley, M., & Harris, K. R. (2006). Cognitive strategies instruction: From basic research to classroom instruction. In E. Anderman, P. H. Winne, P. A. Alexander, & L. Corno (Eds.), *Handbook of Educational Psychology* (2nd ed., pp. 265–286). Lawrence Erlbaum.

Pressley, M., Borkowski, J. G., & Schneider, W. (1987). Cognitive strategies: Good strategy users coordinate metacognition and knowledge. In R. Vasta (Ed.), *Annals of Child Development* (Vol. 4, pp. 89–129). JAI Press.

Rodger, S., & Brandenburg, J. (2009). Cognitive Orientation to (daily) Occupational Performance (CO-OP) with children with Asperger's syndrome who have motor-based occupational performance goals. *Australian Occupational Therapy Journal, 56,* 41–50. https://doi.org/10.1111/j.1440-1630.2008.00739.x

Rodger, S., & Liu, S. (2008). Cognitive Orientation to (daily) Occupational Performance: Changes in strategy and session time use over the course of intervention. *OTJR: Occupation, Participation and Health, 28*(4), 168–179. https://doi.org/10.3928/15394492-20080901-03

Rodger, S., & Vishram, A. (2010). Mastering social and organization goals: Strategy use by two children with Asperger syndrome during Cognitive Orientation to daily Occupational Performance. *Physical and Occupational Therapy in Pediatrics, 30,* 264–276. https://doi.org/10.3109/01942638.2010.500893

Rodger, S., Ireland, S., & Vun, M. (2008). Can Cognitive Orientation to daily Occupational Performance (CO-OP) help children with Asperger's syndrome to master social and organisational goals? *British Journal of Occupational Therapy, 71*(1), 23–32. https://doi.org/10.1177/030802260807100105

Roy, A., Mann, S., Polatajko H., & Gimeno, H. (2017). Participation and goal-oriented metacognitive intervention and self-efficacy in children and youth with dystonia and other hyperkinetic movement disorders. *Developmental Medicine & Child Neurology, 59,* 101–101. https://doi.org/10.1111/dmcn.37_13512

Sangster Jokic, C., Polatajko, H., & Whitebread, D. (2013). Self-regulation as a mediator in motor learning: the effect of the Cognitive Orientation to Occupational Performance approach on children with DCD. *Adapted Physical Activity Quarterly, 30*(2), 103–126. https://doi.org/10.1123/apaq.30.2.103

Sangster, C. A., Beninger, C., Polatajko, H. J., & Mandich, A. (2005). Cognitive strategy generation in children with developmental coordination disorder. *Canadian Journal of Occupational Therapy, Revue Canadienne D'ergotherapie, 72*(2), 67–77. https://doi.org/10.1177/000841740507200201

Scammels, E. M., Bates, S. V., Houldin, A., & Polatajko, H. J. (2016). The Cognitive Orientation to daily Occupational Performance: A scoping review. *Canadian Journal of Occupational Therapy, Revue Canadienne D'ergotherapie,* 83(3), 1–10. https://doi.org/10.1177/0008417416651277

Schunk, D. (2000). *Learning theories*. Merrill.

Shiozu, H., & Kurasawa, S. (2023). Cognitive Orientation to daily Occupational Performance (CO-OP) approach as telehealth for a child with developmental coordination disorder: A case report. *Frontiers in Rehabilitation Science, 14*. https://doi.org/10.3389/fresc.2023.1241981

Shuell, T. J. (1986). Cognitive conceptions of learning. *Review of Educational Research, 56,* 411–436. https://doi.org/10.3102/00346543056004411

Skidmore E. R., McEwen S. E., Green D., van de Houten J., Dawson D. R., & Polatajko H. J. (2017). Essential elements and key features of the CO-OP approach. In Dawson D. R., McEwen S. E., Polatajko H. J. (Eds.), *Cognitive Orientation to daily Occupational Performance in occupational therapy: Using the CO-OP Approach™ to enable participation across the lifespan* (pp. 11–20). American Occupational Therapy Association Press.

Song, C.-S., Lee, O.-N., & Woo, H.-S. (2019). Cognitive strategy on upper extremity function for stroke: A randomized controlled trials. *Restorative Neurology and Neuroscience, 37*(2019), 61–70. https://doi.org/10.3233/RNN-18053

Sumsion, T. (1999). The client-centred approach. In T. Sumsion (Ed.), *Client-centred practice in occupational therapy* (pp. 15–20). Harcourt Brace.

Swinnen, S., Schmidt, R. A., Nicholson, D. E., & Shapiro, D. C. (1990). Information feedback for skill acquisition: Instantaneous knowledge of results degrades learning. *Journal of Experimental Psychology: Learning, Memory, and Cognition, 16,* 706–716. https://doi.org/10.1037/0278-7393.16.4.706

Thelen, E. (1995). Motor development: A new synthesis. *American Psychologist, 50*(2), 79–95. https://doi.org/10.1037//0003-066x.50.2.79

Thelen, E. (2005). Dynamic systems theory and the complexity of change. *Psychoanalytic Dialogues, 15*(2), 255–283. https://doi.org/10.1080/10481881509348831

Thornton, A., Licari, M., Reid, S., Armstrong, J., Fallows, R., & Elliott, C. (2016). Cognitive Orientation to (daily) Occupational Performance intervention leads to improvements in impairments, activity and participation in children with developmental coordination disorder. *Disability and Rehabilitation, 38,* 979–986. https://doi.org/10.3109/09638288.2015.1070298

Thoroughman, K. A., & Shadmehr, R. (2000). Learning of action through adaptive combination of motor primitives. *Nature, 407,* 742–747. https://doi.org/10.1038/35037588

Toglia, J. P., Rodger, S. A., & Polatajko, H. J. (2012). Anatomy of cognitive strategies: A therapist's primer for enabling occupational performance. *Canadian Journal of Occupational Therapy, 79,* 225–236. https://doi.org/10.2182/cjot.2012.79.4.4

Townsend, E. A., & Polatajko, H. J. (2013). *Enabling Occupation II: Advancing an occupational therapy vision for health, well-being and justice through occupation* (2nd ed). CAOT Publications ACE.

Wilcox, A., & Polatajko, H. J. (1994). The impact of verbal self-guidance on children with developmental coordination disorder. *11th International Congress of the World Federation of Occupational Therapists Congress Summaries, 3,* 1518–1519.

Yasunaga, M., Miyaguchi, H., Ishizuki, C., Kita, Y., & Nakai, A. (2023). Cognitive Orientation to daily Occupational Performance: a randomized controlled trial examining intervention effects on children with developmental coordination disorder traits. *Brain sciences, 13*(5), 721. https://doi.org/10.3390/brainsci13050721

A Frame of Reference for Teaching–Learning: The Four-Quadrant Model of Facilitated Learning (4QM)

Craig Greber ■ Jenny Ziviani

Occupational therapy practitioners draw on skills and knowledge in teaching and learning when they facilitate task proficiency as a component of an occupational therapy service. In doing so, they do not reproduce the wide and varied roles of professional teachers. Rather, they use effective teaching–learning strategies in ways that enable goal attainment for those with whom they work. This chapter explores the ways occupational therapy practitioners can use teaching–learning to enable their clients to attain task proficiency integral to occupational performance. Tasks can be viewed as subcomponents of activities, which are themselves components of occupations. In this chapter, the term "learners" refers to children accessing occupational therapy services, and "facilitator" refers to the practitioners, parent, or others working directly with children to enable learning.

Facilitating learning is a complex behavior that includes what we do, as well as how we do it. The Four-Quadrant Model of Facilitated Learning (4QM) (Greber et al., 2011) has been advanced as one way of informing the selection of effective learning strategies based on the changing needs of learners when learning a task. Grouped into four broad clusters, these strategies provide a scaffold for identifying and attending to children's various learning needs throughout task learning. In this chapter, the theoretical base of the 4QM will be outlined, the concepts contained in the model defined, characteristics of function and dysfunction identified, and evaluation procedures will be linked to indicators of function and dysfunction. To establish the relationship between theory and practice, a practice scenario will illustrate how the 4QM can be used as a frame of reference to guide teaching–learning interventions in occupational therapy.

THEORETICAL BASE

This section presents the underlying theoretical base of the 4QM. The model focuses primarily on the intrinsic process of learning that results in changes to tasks the child is able to perform in pursuit of agreed goal occupations. In this section, the assumptions that validate teaching–learning as a useful intervention in occupational therapy will be reviewed, and the theoretical postulates that illustrate the relationship between essential concepts embedded in the 4QM will be described.

Occupational therapy practitioners use teaching–learning as an approach to service delivery when proficiency in the performance of fundamental tasks is viewed as an important step in occupational goal attainment. Occupational performance barriers are often addressed by either building a child's personal physical, cognitive, and/or psychosocial capacities required for performance, or modification of the occupation or environment to better align with the child's existing capacities. Teaching–learning approaches instead make the important assumption that the child has the underlying capacities to perform the occupation, yet needs to acquire proficiency in the key tasks underpinning it. Teaching–learning approaches can also be used in combination with compensatory ones when occupational form is adapted or simplified and proficiency is attained in the key tasks relevant to that adapted form. For example, when fitting a shoe is problematic, the use of a shoehorn can simplify the process; however, proficiency in grasping and manipulating the shoehorn is a necessary prerequisite. Alternatively, when the entire activity is too difficult for the child, a compensatory approach can be used to find an easier alternative (e.g., a child who is unable to tie shoelaces might perform more autonomously when using Velcro straps). In both these cases, repeated practice, embedded in daily routines, can be used to enhance the proficiency with which key tasks are performed. The defining assumption in teaching–learning approaches, then, is that the child's occupational goals can be attained through acquiring proficiency in the tasks comprising the occupation, regardless of whether that performance occurs in its original or adapted form.

Occupational therapy practitioners routinely utilize teaching–learning as a prominent method of intervention in pediatric practice to enhance self-care, productivity, and leisure occupations (Rodger et al., 2005). It is therefore essential that practitioners have a fundamental understanding of the theoretical base underpinning teaching and learning. They should become familiar with the characteristics of a range of strategies used to facilitate learning, and embrace the factors that determine the most appropriate strategies for an individual on a given task at various stages of the learning process.

In his seminal work, developmental psychologist Lev Vygotsky (1978) proposed a process by which children with superficial competencies could develop advanced competence through guidance from a facilitator. Vygotsky identified a principle of learning called the Zone of Proximal Development (Vygotsky, 1978), which represented a stage of learning where a learner required support to perform a task successfully. In Vygotsky's theory, progress toward autonomy was made possible through systematic facilitator's supports called scaffolds. As the learner became increasingly competent, Vygotsky observed the initiation of scaffolding to move from the facilitator to the child. Similarly, the use of prompts transitioned from being overt to covert. Vygotsky's person-centered approach to learning provides an appropriate theoretical framework that is well aligned philosophically with principles of enablement guiding occupational therapy practice.

Direct instruction teaching methods have been contrasted with more indirect inductive approaches in conceptualizations of the teaching–learning process (e.g., Joyce et al., 2009; Woolfolk, 2015). Mosston and Ashworth (2008) positioned a range of teaching styles on a continuum from "command style" at one extreme to "self-teaching" at the other, based on the cognitive focus of the style. Direct instruction is based on behaviorist approaches to learning that reinforce specific patterns of response (Joyce et al., 2009). Indirect strategies are seen to engage the learner to a greater extent in the decision-making process, drawing on a cognitivist approach to learning (Joyce et al., 2009). More direct styles inform the learner of key elements of the task or the response required, while indirect styles facilitate the learner to arrive at those solutions with support.

The Four-Quadrant Model of Facilitated Learning

When practitioners choose teaching–learning as an intervention strategy, they take on the role of a facilitator, with the child as a learner. The 4QM not only provides a means of understanding, planning, and coordinating the use of learning strategies in occupational therapy but also lends itself to multidisciplinary use by others involved with the child, such as teachers, teaching assistants, and parents (Greber et al., 2007a).

The 4QM groups together the various cognitive, physical, and language-based learning strategies useful in leading children to perform tasks more autonomously. As Mosston and Ashworth (2008) theorized, some learning strategies are more direct and overt than others. For instance, learning can be based on telling the child what to do and how to do it. These direct strategies serve the need for knowledge, and they provide information about the characteristics of the task or the response required. Less direct strategies (such as provision of feedback) engage the learner to a greater extent in the decision-making process. These strategies encourage the learner to be more active in planning, executing, and evaluating performance. Direct strategies can be viewed as being at one extreme of a continuum of teaching–learning styles, with indirect strategies at the other end.

Approaches to teaching and learning vary not only in their directness but also on the basis of the person initiating the strategy. Some learning strategies are initiated by the person facilitating the learning (in this case, the practitioner), whereas others employ the learner as a source of initiation. The source of initiation of learning strategies can be viewed as a progression in the relationship between facilitator-initiated strategies and learner-initiated strategies.

When the continua representing directness and source of facilitation are integrated, the 4QM is created. Four distinct clusters of learning strategies become apparent, each serving a different learner need (see Figure 10.1). Those strategies that are direct and initiated by a facilitator (Quadrant 1) specify the characteristics of the task and/or the performance required. Other strategies that are indirect in nature, yet still facilitator-initiated, fall into Quadrant 2. These are useful in supporting decision making by the learner. Quadrant 3 groups those overt self-prompting strategies initiated by the learner that help them to recall key points essential to task performance. A range of self-regulatory strategies that are not obvious to observers underpins autonomy, and these strategies are grouped in Quadrant 4. The 4QM helps a practitioner to plan and coordinate the learning strategies used to promote task autonomy by providing a structure that allows the practitioner to respond to learner needs as task learning proceeds. Specific learning strategies can be articulated within each quadrant. When these are documented, the complete 4QM becomes a useful frame of reference to guide therapists in implementing teaching–learning during service delivery.

Assumptions

In many professions, practitioners use forms of teaching–learning during their practice. Occupational therapy practitioners use teaching–learning in ways that are at once both similar to and different from how they are used in other professions. The relationship between teaching–learning and the overarching theoretical principles of occupational therapy is central to the 4QM. This relationship is based on the assumption that targeted occupational performance can be enhanced by more autonomously enabling proficiency in essential tasks and activities. By enabling a child to enhance competence in occupation-relevant tasks, occupational performance is enhanced by improving the congruence between the person, occupation, and environment.

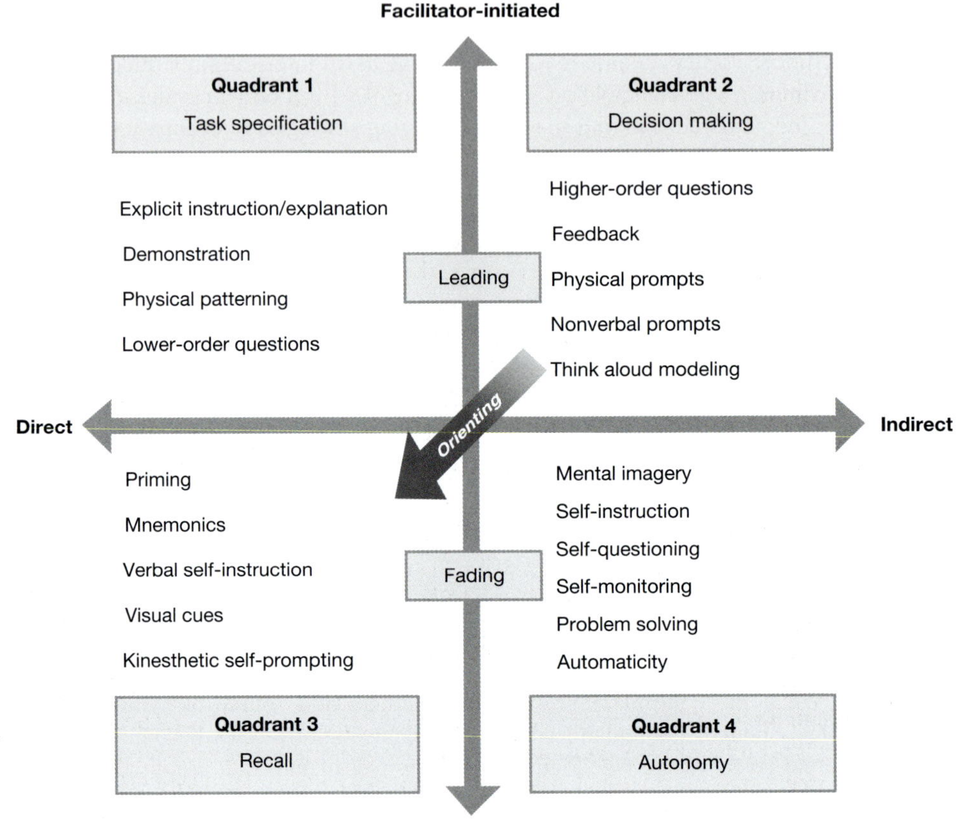

FIGURE 10.1 The Four-Quadrant Model of Facilitated Learning. (Reprinted with permission from Greber, C. (2011). *The Four-Quadrant Model of Facilitated Learning: Development and clinical utility* (Ph.D. thesis). School of Health & Rehabilitation Sciences, The University of Queensland.)

Acquiring proficiency in key tasks fundamental to the target occupation can be facilitated by either structuring practice routines to optimize acquisition, altering the activity to simplify its performance, or invoking specific teaching–learning strategies to facilitate learning of the tasks essential to occupational performance. Although these three options are sometimes combined, it is the use of specific teaching–learning strategies with which the 4QM is specifically concerned.

Assumptions about the development of autonomy are important to the 4QM.

- Proficiency in key tasks is only the first step in improving occupational performance and attaining occupational goals.
- Enhancing occupational performance involves more than learning the tasks necessary for performance. It also requires the ability to adapt and perform tasks in the unique contextual features of the target occupation.
- Autonomy therefore includes mastery of key tasks, competence in using the decision-making procedures that enable generalization, and contextual competence in incorporating learned tasks into occupational performance.

Delimitation

This frame of reference can be employed only when the child is judged to have the necessary performance components (e.g., strength, dexterity, bilateral coordination) to complete the task in its current or an agreed, adapted form.

Foundational Concepts and Definitions

Teaching–learning is the basis of intervention in this frame of reference. Occupational therapy service delivery consists of activity analysis, the teaching learning encounter, and generalizations and transfer. Activity analysis helps identify relevant tasks and unpack core skills and abilities necessary for their completion. While the ability to perform key tasks is a central part of this process, teaching–learning as an approach to therapy looks beyond autonomy in specific tasks and toward improved performance in the target occupation. The focus of the service is occupational performance.

Activity analysis assists in identifying barriers to occupational performance, including allowing the practitioner to understand the occupations of the child and how the child creates meaning through purposeful engagement. Activity analysis is useful in establishing priorities for service provision when constraints are based on either task performance, or a more fundamental breakdown of performance components, such as strength, dexterity, and/or sensory processing. This helps to distinguish the need for services related to learning a new task from those focused on capacity development.

When selecting teaching–learning approaches, practitioners typically address barriers to occupational performance created by the lack of proficiency in specific tasks. By enabling the child to learn the necessary tasks, personal capacities are not enhanced through other therapeutic means. Rather, through teaching–learning, proficiency in the essential tasks and activities for attaining occupational goals is acquired. For example, when reviewing a child's mealtime occupations, the use of knife and fork might be a central activity. Activity analysis helps the practitioner to identify the child's ability to perform specific tasks (such as holding the fork steady or making the sawing action with the knife) that are potential barriers to performing the activity and hence limits performance of the child's mealtime occupations. The teaching–learning approach has the appeal of directness. It requires a thorough understanding of the occupation, the activities that comprise it, and the tasks that facilitate performance. In this approach, emphasis is not placed on performance components, such as strength, dexterity, or bilateral coordination that might be targeted when using other frames of reference.

To assist a child to attain occupational goals, it is first necessary to identify the components of the occupation. Activity analysis is a means through which this can occur and is a core skill in occupational therapy. Activity analysis should provide the practitioner with a thorough understanding of the activity, its place in occupational performance, and the tasks fundamental to its performance. Activity analysis, therefore, forms an important basis for clinical reasoning when using teaching–learning approaches.

The teaching–learning encounter involves an interaction between the practitioner and the child. The practitioner can set about designing services that will support learning, after key tasks that are barriers to performance have been identified. The teaching–learning encounter is a complex aspect of practice that requires the practitioner to be responsive to the changing needs of the learner and adapt the strategies employed in response to those needs. Within this context, a range of child and practitioner characteristics, such as preferred learning style, communication mode and interpersonal factors should be considered. These factors are discussed more explicitly below.

For the learning of tasks to occur, the learner needs to understand the task and the performance requirements, engage effective decision making to modify performance in response to errors, recall the key elements of successful performance, and monitor performance through both concurrent and reflective analyses. Once a task is able to be performed, these processes might become automatic, but during the learning phase, strategies that support these processes need to be developed. This is the scaffolding Vygotsky (1978) described as essential to supporting learning.

The strategies employed by a practitioner during intervention must therefore match not only the characteristics of the learner, task, and environment but also the learning needs of the child at any point in time. Each child has unique learning requirements that change as task learning proceeds, so their needs cannot always be predicted. Therein lies a challenge for practitioners. They are faced with the task of developing an intervention that depends on high levels of teaching skill and in-depth knowledge about the teaching–learning process. In this sense, knowledge of effective teaching–learning strategies, and the ability to match them with a learner's needs, is paramount to the outcomes for the child. The 4QM supports the practitioner's reasoning in this process.

Generalization and transfer of learned tasks to enable occupational performance is a key component of occupational therapy. Teaching performance within a real-life context minimizes the adaptation a child needs to make to the contextual features of their occupational performance. For example, teaching a child to use a knife and fork during mealtime enables the child to generalize those tasks to other mealtime environments more easily. This is preferable to teaching knife and fork use when cutting playdough in a play-based setting. Autonomy in occupational performance is attained when a child has the necessary knowledge of the task, decides on an appropriate course of action, and is able to independently enact, monitor, and mediate performance in such varied contexts as the occupation might entail.

To illustrate the point, consider a child who has a goal to brush their teeth before going to bed. The practitioner might facilitate learning of the fundamental tasks of toothbrushing—putting toothpaste on the brush, grasping and manipulating the brush, rinsing, and so on. The child then develops performance autonomy—competence in the tasks required to brush their teeth. In order to engage in toothbrushing; however, the child must orient to other features of performance, such as locating the toothbrush, judging the amount of paste and the temperature of rinsing water, and completing the task in an appropriate amount of time. Making decisions about these variables engages the child in procedural autonomy—autonomy in transfer of learned tasks to the real-life context. The closer the learning context is to that of the goal occupation, the fewer adaptations needed. Intervention that takes place in the child's own bathroom, for example, minimizes the degree of transfer needed.

Becoming "able" is an important stage in developing occupational autonomy; however, if the child expects to be reminded to brush their teeth (as often develops when a child has become reliant on help from others), complete autonomy has not yet been attained. Implementing strategies that encourage the child to recognize the appropriate time to brush teeth and to engage in the occupation without prompting can help to develop autonomy. Only when the child initiates task performance in ways that respond to changing contexts can they become truly autonomous in the goal occupation.

Concepts and Definitions

The 4QM builds upon the integration of "directness" and "source of initiation" continua by detailing the various learning strategies that can be used to address learner needs in each of the four quadrants. The complete 4QM is illustrated in Figure 10.1. For a child to become proficient in a task, they must understand the task, decide on a plan of action, recall the important features of performance, and monitor the outcomes of each effort. When a child finds particular parts of this process troublesome, the 4QM can assist the practitioner to identify strategies relevant to the child's unique needs. Each of these strategies conceptualizes a mode of scaffolding that can be used to attain successful performance of the target task. In the various theories that have been used to inform the development of the 4QM, these concepts have sometimes been given different names in the many bodies of knowledge that refer to the same phenomena. The labels used in the 4QM represent a consolidation of these many names into terms that are best understood by occupational therapy practitioners.

In order to establish each of the learning strategies in the 4QM as separate and discrete entities, it is necessary to define and exemplify each. This enables distinctions to be made between the strategies available to the practitioner and supports the practitioner to select the most facilitatory approach for a learner at a given time and on a given task, and to effectively link or combine those strategies used throughout the learning process.

Quadrant 1: Direct, Facilitator-Initiated Strategies

Quadrant 1 strategies use direct instruction methods to communicate information from the facilitator to the learner to inform the learner of the goal of the task, the task requirements, and/or the nature of performance. Practitioners can use explicit instruction and explanation, demonstration, physical patterning, and/or lower-order questions to provide this information. Each of these strategies involves the facilitator providing the learner with direct prompts, which provide task-specific information in a way that encourages the learner to reproduce or build on previously learned responses. They inform or remind the learner what to do in order to complete the task successfully.

Explicit instruction and explanation provide the learner with descriptions of various characteristics of the task itself and/or the expected response. Such strategies can be used to inform the learner of the requirements of the task ("Do this") or key features of performance ("Do it this way"). Verbal, print, and technology-based forms of instruction may all provide the same type of information if their purpose is specifically to impart information. A practitioner is using explicit instruction and explanation when they say:

- "You need to hold the food still with your fork while you cut to stop it sliding around."
- "Push your arm through the sleeve."
- "Turn the paper with your left hand, and open and close the scissors with your right hand."

Explicit instruction and explanation are frequently used in conjunction with demonstration to provide the learner with a clear understanding of what is required (Figure 10.2).

Demonstration occurs when a practitioner provides an example of the expected response or performance. It can be used to highlight specific aspects of the technique, clarify ambiguity in verbal instructions, and/or provide a reference of correctness for the learner's efforts. Demonstration usually employs visual modalities, but it can also be used to model appropriate verbal responses (e.g., in social interaction). Demonstration can occur when:

- the practitioner shows the learner how to perform the task
- the learner views a video of the task being performed
- a cartoon or simulated performance is used as an example of the expected response
- the facilitator models a verbal response appropriate to a social interaction.

Physical patterning (Greber et al., 2007b) has been used to identify a specific element of physical manipulation of the learner's body. The terms "physical assistance," "physical guidance," and "manual guidance" have variously been used in the literature to describe a range of physical

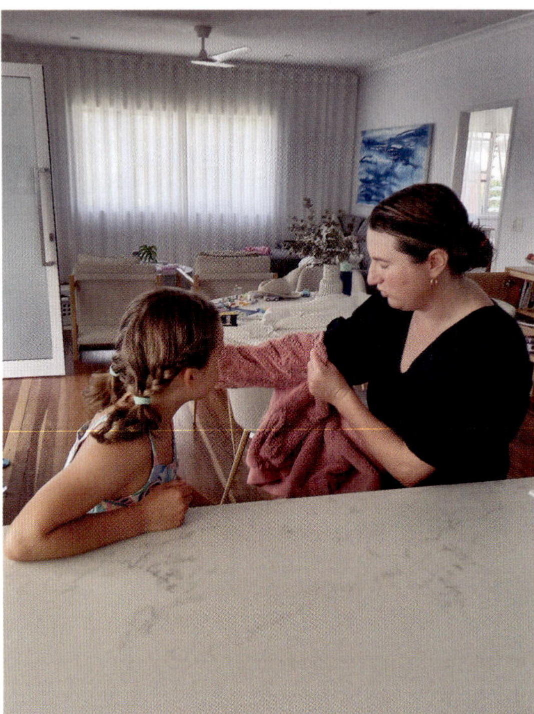

FIGURE 10.2 The therapist uses demonstration and explanation to facilitate dressing.

facilitations, from partial prompts to complete patterning (Carr & Shepherd, 2010; Chen et al., 2001; Libby et al., 2008; Schmidt & Wrisberg, 2008). In understanding how these strategies might be employed in task learning, it is useful to draw a distinction between those strategies that manipulate the child's body through the entire movement (*physical patterning*), those that direct but do not control the movement (*physical guidance*), and intermittent strategies that use tactile and kinesthetic prompts to support motor planning (*physical prompts*). Each of these strategies involves the learner to varying degrees in planning and executing the movement, and consequently supports different outcomes. These three labels have been used in the 4QM to identify particular learning strategies based on physical input by the facilitator.

In physical patterning, the learner does not contribute to the movement but allows the practitioner to passively manipulate the body part. Physical patterning might be used to establish the general form or the spatial characteristics of the movement. This might occur when:

- the practitioner manipulates the learner's limbs to provide an example of the appropriate performance of the task;
- the practitioner works hand over hand with the learner to perform a task, while the learner remains passive; and
- the practitioner moves the learner's limb through the range of motion required to perform the task to provide a general feel for the movement (Figure 10.3).

The use of questioning has received considerable attention in many bodies of the literature. One way of distinguishing the various types of questions a practitioner might ask a child is to use a hierarchical system that distinguishes the cognitive skills involved, such as Bloom's taxonomy

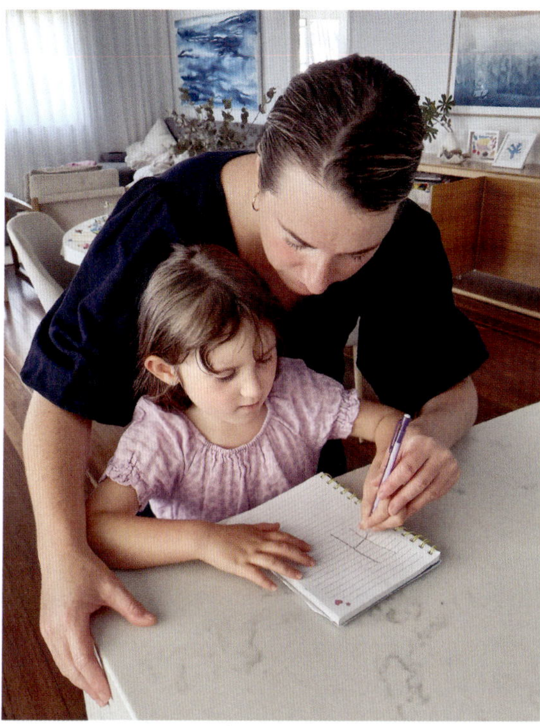

FIGURE 10.3 The therapist uses physical patterning to facilitate letter formation.

(Anderson et al., 2013; Bloom et al., 1956). Several authors have used this taxonomy to discriminate questions that evoke lower-level processes, such as recalling and understanding, from those that stimulate higher-order productive cognitions (e.g., Bissell & Lemons, 2006; Erdogan & Campbell, 2008; Walsh & Sattes, 2017). The use of this taxonomy in the 4QM has distinguished between the labels *lower-order questions* (Quadrant 1) and *higher-order questions* (Quadrant 2).

Lower-order questions is a term that describes questions used to promote the learner's performance by facilitating recall of information with which the learner has previously been provided. This type of questioning ensures that the learner's interpretation of the task is accurate. It can also be used to focus the learner's attention on key aspects of performance by challenging them to recall previously learned material. Examples of lower-order questions include:

- "What do you do next?"
- "Where should you look?"
- "How should you be standing?"

Quadrant 2: Indirect, Facilitator-Initiated Strategies

When the learner understands the task requirements but is unable to generate an effective plan for performing the task, different learning tools are necessary. Strategies that engage the learner in decision making have different features to those that specify the task. Although they remain facilitator-initiated, they are less direct in nature. These strategies are represented in Quadrant 2. They encourage problem solving and decision making rather than providing specific instructions. Strategies such as higher-order questions, feedback, physical prompts, nonverbal prompts, and think aloud modeling all serve this purpose. Each of these approaches encourages the learner to make appropriate decisions about their own performance.

Higher-order questions are used to provoke thoughts and draw the learner's attention to elements of the task that need to be considered. This type of question requires the application of knowledge to engage the learner in analysis, problem solving, judgment, reasoning, and/or evaluation. Questions that facilitate the use of higher-order cognitive processes stimulate the production of new cognitions rather than the recall of old ones. For example:

- "What might be the problem here?"
- "How could you do it differently?"
- "Why do you think that happened?"
- "How does that look?"

Statements such as "I wonder why that happened," though not phrased as a question, still imply one. They function to engage the learner in analysis, problem solving, and critical evaluation. For that reason, statements such as these can be considered higher-order questions.

Feedback (Schmidt & Lee, 2014) can be intrinsic, but it can also be provided by others observing performance to support the learner by orienting them to the use of self-regulatory procedures. Feedback therefore reports the practitioner's observations to the learner but does not instruct the learner in what to do or what to change (which would be akin to *explicit instruction*). For example, a practitioner might comment:

- "Uh-Oh, I think there's a problem."
- "You're leaning a little to the left."
- "Your book is sliding around while you write."

Symbolic representations that record or evaluate performance, such as checklists, can also provide useful feedback to learners in a visual form.

Physical prompts (Libby et al., 2008; Thompson et al., 2004) involve touch that reminds the child to use a body part, or promotes the initiation of movement. Such strategies support the learner to make successful efforts, without detracting from their ability to plan and execute a response. Physical prompts can include tapping or pushing a limb in response to delayed movement initiation. With complex activities, it may be necessary to provide physical prompts on various subtasks rather than just at the commencement of movement. For example, separate physical prompts may be used sequentially to initiate grasping the spoon, loading it, transporting food to the mouth, and then replacing the spoon in the bowl. Physical prompts challenge the learner to plan, monitor, and execute movements in ways that physical facilitation (Quadrant 1) does not do (Figure 10.4).

Nonverbal prompts are facial expression, eye gaze, and gestures used by the practitioner. Learner performance can be initiated, modified, and/or terminated by an array of nonverbal inputs from the facilitator. For example, a practitioner might:

- Give a quizzical look to indicate a need to reassess performance.
- Point at a potential hazard.
- Direct eye gaze at key objects involved in a task.
- Point to a body part that needs to be used in the performance (Figure 10.5)

Think aloud modeling (Polatajko & Mandich, 2004) is the verbalization of physical performance and modeling of the use of cognitive strategies. In this strategy, the practitioner audibly describes the decision-making processes that are occurring as they perform the task. While

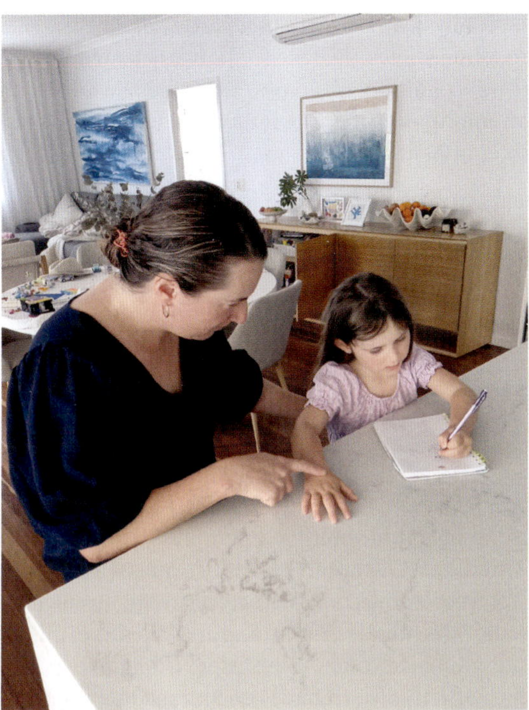

FIGURE 10.4 The therapist uses a physical prompt to facilitate pencil–paper tasks.

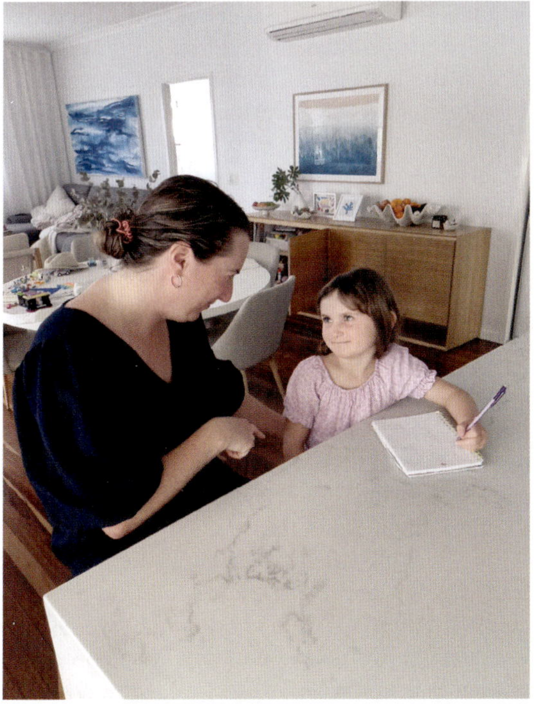

FIGURE 10.5 The therapist uses nonverbal prompting to facilitate pencil–paper tasks.

demonstration (from Quadrant 1) of physical performance provides the learner with task-specific information, think aloud modeling shows the learner how to engage in higher cognitive processes. The dialog can model the recognition of errors, describe the problem-solving and decision-making processes, and/or exemplify self-monitoring procedures. While performing the task themselves, a practitioner might comment:

- "That doesn't seem right. What went wrong there? Maybe if I concentrate on keeping my hand a bit steadier."
- "What happens if I put it on there? Oh no, it fell off. Where else could I put it? Maybe over here."

Performance of the task while describing the associated cognitions aloud combines the use of two strategies: demonstration (from Quadrant 1) and think aloud modeling (from Quadrant 2). The visual representation of the response is considered demonstration, while the verbalization is think aloud modeling.

Quadrant 3: Direct, Learner-Initiated Strategies

Strategies that involve learners reminding or prompting themselves using strategies that are observable to others are grouped in Quadrant 3. Learners might use any of a number of strategies to recall key points about the task for successful performance. Priming strategies, mnemonics, verbal self-instruction, visual cues, and kinesthetic self-prompting all serve this purpose. It is noteworthy that the terms "verbal self-guidance" and "rote script" (Polatajko & Mandich, 2004) have been used to distinguish two types of self-talk strategies encouraged by occupational therapy practitioners working with children. Because both procedures serve the same purpose of talking oneself through a difficult task, they are described collectively in the 4QM as *verbal self-instruction*.

Priming (Greber et al., 2007b) is a learner-initiated strategy that involves verbal or physical rehearsal. Priming differs from practice strategies that involve repeating with the objective of improving the quality of performance in the long term. Priming strategies bring together the various skills involved in a performance as a rehearsal of previously learned procedures to ensure that the intended response is the correct one. An example of priming is when the child verbally rehearses what they will say to a cashier while waiting in line or do a "dry run" of a task before performing it. The goal of priming, then, is to prepare for performance rather than improve it, and this distinguishes it from "practice." Priming strategies can use various modalities to organize general response schemas in order to meet the temporal and contextual demands of the imminent performance. The key element here is the *intention* of priming. If the goal is to prepare and optimize the response, rather than to provide an avenue for improving performance, the strategy can be considered to be a priming one. Practice is instead an opportunity to implement previously acquired strategies to refine and improve specific task performance (Schmidt & Wrisberg, 2008).

Mnemonics (Joyce et al., 2009) are a type of associative learning that enables learners to increase their capacity to store and retrieve information. Mnemonics aid the recall of key features, processes, facts, and procedural steps. They include the use of link words, acronyms, nonsense phrases, and rhymes. Although a facilitator might aid in the development of a mnemonic, its use becomes the responsibility of the learner, making it a learner-initiated strategy. For instance, a learner might use the nonsense phrase "Every Good Boy Deserves Fun" to prompt the recall of the notes E, G, B, D, F in musical notation. Alternatively, a child might say, "Nose over toes and up she goes" to focus on body position during transition to standing. Mnemonics use simple and/or symbolic language to focus on key elements of the task.

Verbal self-instruction (Greber et al., 2007b; Martini & Polatajko, 1998) is when a child uses verbal strategies to engage in the problem-solving process or to recall the steps involved in performance. Complex tasks are not easily reduced to a few key points represented in a mnemonic. Sometimes, a child might find it more valuable to think out loud, describing the task and the decisions necessary for its performance. On occasion, a formal rote script might be recited to guide the child through the task. The use of verbal self-instruction, and tools such as a formal script, supports both cognitive (e.g., memory) and metacognitive (e.g., self-monitoring) processes. These strategies have also been shown to enhance sustained attention to task in some contexts (Bairami et al., 2016).

Some examples of verbal self-instruction include a child saying to themselves:

- "I hold it like this and tip it in like that"
- "What happens if I put it on there. Oh no, it fell off. Where else could I put it?"
- "Put my feet on here. Put my hands on here. Ready to push. Go. Whoops, I have to try to stay balanced."

Visual cues (Frey & Fisher, 2010; Greber et al., 2007b) that prompt the learner to recall steps in a task or prompt action can include picture cues, checklists, computer-generated visual prompts, real-object cues, mind maps, graphic organizers, visual displays, and computer-assisted instruction. Mirrors and video recordings can also be useful visual prompts to enhance performance. Simple examples of visual cues include picture charts that remind the learner to engage in particular behaviors, or a sequence of pictures that guide the learner through the steps of a task (Figure 10.6).

1. Cow horns
2. Over
3. Under
4. Pull
5. Make a loop
6. Around and through
7. Pull

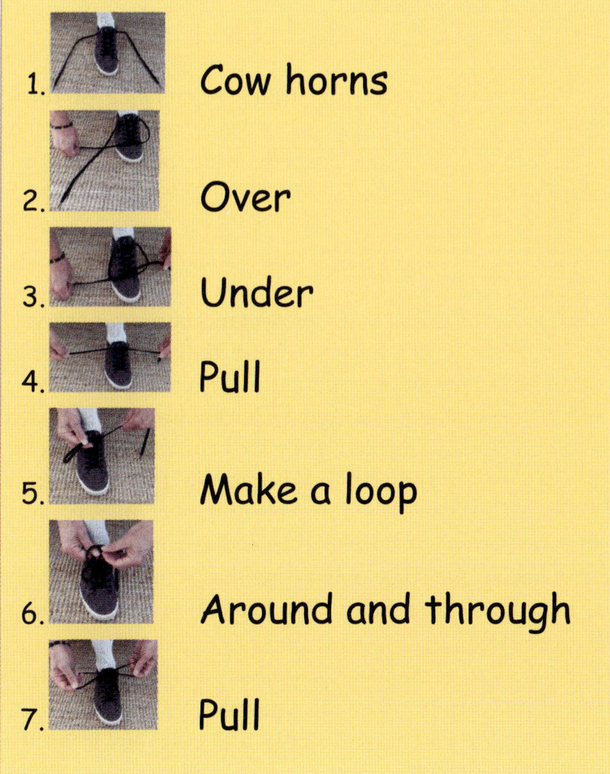

FIGURE 10.6 A visual prompt is developed to support recall of steps for shoelace tying.

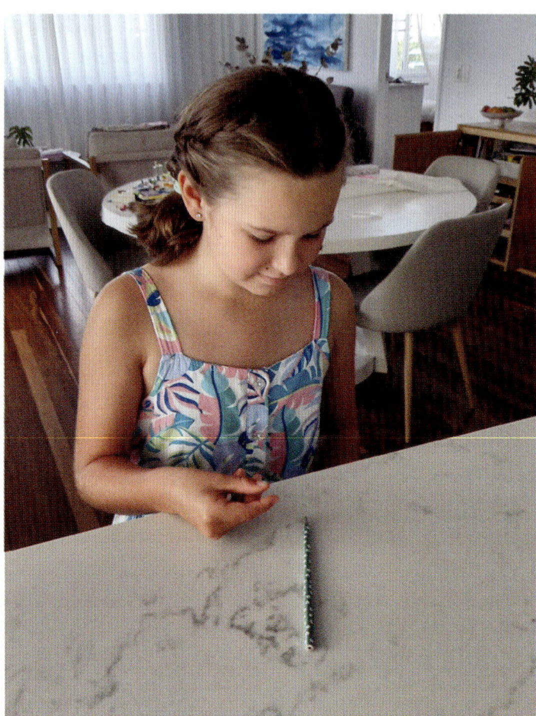

FIGURE 10.7 The child uses kinesthetic self-prompting to facilitate pencil grasp.

Kinesthetic self-prompting (Greber et al., 2007b) strategies enhance or direct the child's attention to a particular action or body part during learning. When a child taps their fingers and thumb together to remind themselves to use a tripod grasp on the pencil, they are using kinesthetic self-prompting (Figure 10.7).

Quadrant 4: Indirect, Learner-Initiated Strategies

Internalized strategies for monitoring and evaluating performance are not observable to onlookers but are necessary for autonomous performance. Because they are not overtly observable, these strategies can be deemed indirect in nature. Such strategies and processes are assessable only by learner self-reports, making the content of strategies in Quadrant 4 somewhat speculative. Zimmerman and Schunk (2011) provided a thorough review of cognitive and metacognitive factors that can lead to self-regulated learning and performance across a range of learning contexts. Additionally, Schmidt and Wrisberg (2008) described the role of *mental imagery* and *problem solving* as aids in the preparation for performance, as well as in overcoming barriers. *Automaticity* is a term that has been used to describe a final stage of learning that is independent of the cognitive processes that mark earlier periods of learning (Schmidt & Lee, 2014). These processes have each been reflected in Quadrant 4 of the 4QM.

Mental imagery (Schmidt & Wrisberg, 2008) can support decision making, planning, and other cognitive strategies. Mental imagery is a process that occurs entirely within the learner's mind, making it unobservable to onlookers. It is a higher-order process and is often a useful strategy to recall the visual cues used in Quadrant 3.

Self-instruction (Theodorakis et al., 2010), the use of inner speech to direct the learner's actions, is symbolic of the internalization of verbal self-instruction strategies. Whereas verbal self-instruction is an observable learning strategy, self-instruction provides no observable signs. Self-instruction helps to identify and direct the use of problem-solving strategies. It is particularly useful in recalling procedural steps involved in a performance or attending to specific cues.

Self-questioning (Steele, 2005) utilizes internal dialog to analyze information and regulate the use of cognitive strategies through reflective thinking. The distinction between self-instruction and self-questioning is a redundant one because neither process is obvious to the observer. Reports from the learner can be used to identify the characteristics of internal dialog if this is likely to be helpful to the learning process, and if the learner has sufficient insight to distinguish the strategies used. As with self-instruction, inner speech can be used to engage in silent reviews of performance, development and critique of plans of action, and clarification of goals.

Self-monitoring (Richards & Farrell, 2005; Sinha & Sharma, 2001) supports the evaluation of specific strategies, analyses their effectiveness, critiques performance, and assesses the need for modification. Self-monitoring enables the child to assess the extent to which their performance matches the anticipated response. Once again, this is an internal process and not observable.

Problem solving (Sternberg & Frensch, 2014) includes various cognitive processes that are employed to plan, judge, and reason. Individually, each of these processes can be used in either observable or unobservable ways to overcome difficulties in performance. Collectively, the synthesis of these processes in deciding on a course of action is a covert process termed problem solving. To the practitioner, it becomes obvious that problem solving is occurring when a child overcomes barriers to performance independently.

Automaticity (Schmidt & Lee, 2014) is the innate ability to perform a task spontaneously and independently. It is the ultimate outcome where performance is not attention demanding and is unregulated by cognitive or metacognitive activity. As automaticity develops, processing occurs without the forms of internalized self-prompting that mediated earlier autonomous stages. Responses become routine, consistent, and predictable and occur in the absence of conscious planning.

Intermediate Strategies Through Quadrants

Strategies exhibiting characteristics of adjoining quadrants can be considered *intermediate strategies*. They might perform dual functions, or link the content of one quadrant to that of another. Three forms of intermediate strategies are discernable: *leading strategies* (bridging Quadrant 1 and Quadrant 2), *orienting strategies* (linking Quadrant 2 and Quadrant 3), and *fading strategies* (used to move from Quadrant 3 to Quadrant 4) (see Figure 10.1).

Leading strategies are forms of questions, incomplete statements, and physical guidance that reflect characteristics of both task specification (Quadrant 1), and facilitation of problem-solving processes (Quadrant 2). These strategies might provide effective links between information giving strategies of Quadrant 1 and the cognitive scaffolds of Quadrant 2. Examples of leading strategies include:

- "cloze" (incomplete statements) such as "Do this. Now, you need to ...(pause)"
- Stabilizing a child's elbow to enable them to brush hair (physical guidance) (Figure 10.8)
- Questions that stimulate both higher- and lower-order cognitive processes (e.g., "What part of your body should you use to overcome that problem?")
- Partial demonstration of the expected response.

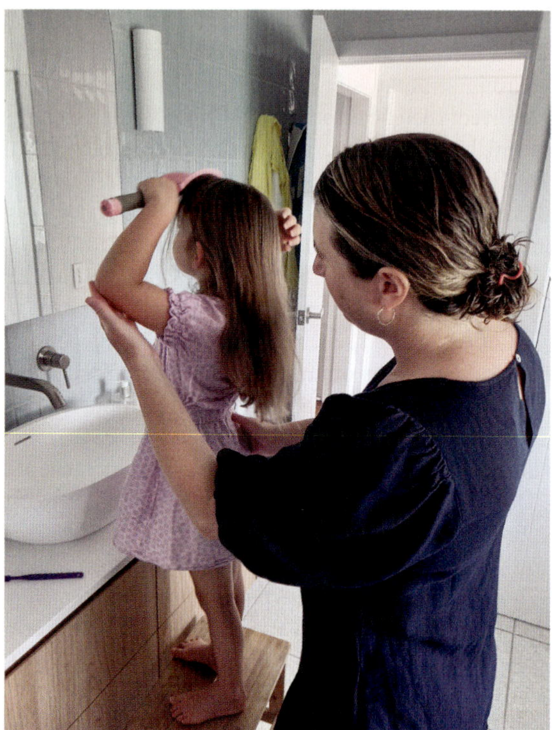

FIGURE 10.8 The therapist uses physical guidance to facilitate hair brushing.

Orienting strategies include verbal and nonverbal strategies that provide no information to the child apart from a reminder to use learner-facilitated procedures. These strategies share the characteristics of Quadrant 2 (engaging the learner in decision-making processes) and Quadrant 3 (recalling the key features of performance) and help orientate learners to the need for self-regulated instruction. For instance, a practitioner might orient a child to the use of verbal self-instruction strategies by asking, "What could you say to remind yourself what to do next?" or directing the child to a visual cue by pointing to the child's picture prompt card.

Fading is a gradual process involving internalization of the overt self-regulatory strategies of Quadrant 3. Some forms of self-prompting can become less obvious to observers yet are not representative of the covert self-instruction of Quadrant 4. Strategies such as subvocalization (whispering) are on the margin of both quadrants. Similarly, when a child begins to orient to only a few of the steps in a picture sequence, it is clear they are internalizing some of the procedures but are not yet able to do without the visual prompt. In these cases, fading of overt self-prompting strategies is occurring.

Theoretical Postulates

The 4QM embeds Vygotsky's notion of the Zone of Proximal Development as a stage during development of task proficiency, wherein learning and performance can be scaffolded by self and others. The relationship between quadrants enables scaffolds to be systematically reduced as the learner proceeds toward greater proficiency. At the same time, throughout the learning process, the facilitator may increase or decrease scaffolding as the learner's needs demand at any point in time. As Vygotsky (1978) theorized, learning and performance can be enabled by the provision of appropriate learning supports.

In the 4QM, these supports are specific learning strategies that are appropriate to the learner's needs at a given point in time:

- In earlier stages, the learner's efforts are shaped by information from the facilitator (Quadrant 1).
- Stimuli are used to prompt appropriate decisions about performance (Quadrant 2).
- Later stages of task proficiency are characterized by the gradual internalization of self-mediated prompts (Quadrant 3 and Quadrant 4).
- Intermediate strategies are used to move the child from one quadrant to another and from facilitator initiated to learner initiated.
- A facilitator of learning needs to respond to the child's needs in ways that are fluid and adaptable.
- Implementation should include the need to move between quadrants in a bidirectional manner depending on the learner's needs at the time.

Within the 4QM, specific learning strategies are grouped together based on the learner needs they support. At the same time, strategies in one quadrant are closely related to those in other quadrants. For example, physical patterning in Quadrant 1 is aligned with physical prompts in Quadrant 2 and kinesthetic self-prompting in Quadrant 3. Similarly, explicit instruction and explanation (Quadrant 1) has similarities to think aloud modeling in Quadrant 2 and verbal self-instruction in Quadrant 3. In this way, learning strategies used in different parts of the learning process can be well coordinated by using consistent learning modalities.

FUNCTION/DYSFUNCTION CONTINUUM

As a child develops proficiency in the key tasks that underpin occupational performance, the types of scaffolding required to enable performance change. Four broad types of scaffolding have been described earlier: task specification, decision making, recall, and autonomy. Each of these corresponds to a different quadrant in the 4QM and illustrates varied degrees of function and dysfunction on the task. These indicators are discussed below. It is important to note that the learner can enter the learning encounter exhibiting the need for any or all of these scaffolds. Although they might generally be expected to move through the quadrants sequentially, in practice this might not be the case. The learner might move quickly toward autonomous performance after the task has been explained. Alternatively, some learners might require varied levels of scaffolding within a single learning encounter or even on a single trial. For some children, performance will always be marked by a need for facilitator support or overt self-mediation. Such children may never develop independence on the task in its current form and might require development of an alternative occupational form.

The 4QM has four function–dysfunction continua, describing performance of the child as they move through the four quadrants toward autonomous task performance. The first continuum describes the child's abilities to respond to direct, facilitator-initiated strategies (Table 10.1). The second continuum is indirect facilitator-initiated strategies, where the child requires less input on the part of the facilitator to begin a task and carry it out (Table 10.2). The third continuum indicates occasions where the child is able to initiate tasks independently, without direct or indirect facilitation from the practitioner (Table 10.3). The fourth and final continuum is when the child is able to perform a task successfully and autonomously, without direct or indirect

Table 10.1 Indicators of Function and Dysfunction for Quadrant 1: Direct, Facilitator-Initiated Strategies

Quadrant 1	
Function	**Dysfunction**
Responds to direct instructor-facilitated strategies	Difficulty responding to direct instructor-facilitated strategies
Indicators of Function	**Indicators of Dysfunction**
Responds to specific instructions from the practitioner and others	The child is not able to respond to specific instructions from the practitioner and others
Responds to the practitioner's specific explanations about the task	Not able to respond to the practitioner's specific explanations about the task
Responds to the practitioner's direct prompts	Does not respond to the practitioner's direct prompts
Responds to the practitioner's demonstration of the task	Not able to follow the practitioner's demonstration of the task
Responds to physical patterning, such as hand over hand, by the practitioner to assist in the performance of the task	Does not respond to physical patterning, such as hand over hand, by the practitioner to assist in the performance of the task

facilitation from the practitioner, and without reliance on any overt self-prompting (Table 10.4). There is a difference (as the child's learning shifts from one quadrant to another) between the need for external facilitation to stimulate successful performance and the ability to use overt self-mediating strategies for successful performance. In the 4QM, the continuum is not truly linear, as a child moves from dysfunction to function; the path is more like a Z, as illustrated in Figure 10.9. In some instances, the child might move directly from Quadrant 1 or Quadrant 2 to Quadrant 4 (autonomy) without requiring facilitator- or learner-initiated prompting in other

Table 10.2 Indicators of Function and Dysfunction for Quadrant 2: Indirect, Facilitator-Initiated Strategies

Quadrant 2	
Function	**Dysfunction**
Is able to develop an effective plan for performing the task	Is not able to develop an effective plan for performing the task
Indicators of Function	**Indicators of Dysfunction**
Responds to higher-order questions that facilitate the use of higher cognitive skills	Not able to respond to higher-order questions
Responds to feedback from others	Not able to respond to feedback from others
Responds to physical prompts	Does not respond to physical prompts
Responds to nonverbal prompts	Does not respond to nonverbal prompts
Responds to "think aloud modeling"	Does not respond to "think aloud modeling"

Table 10.3 Indicators of Function and Dysfunction for Quadrant 3: Direct, Learner-Initiated Strategies

Quadrant 3	
Function	**Dysfunction**
Able to perform the task using learner-initiated strategies	Not able to use learner-initiated strategies to perform the task
Indicators of Function	**Indicators of Dysfunction**
Uses priming to perform the task	Cannot use priming to support performance
Responds to the use of mnemonics as a memory aid	Does not respond to the use of mnemonics as a memory aid
Uses verbal self-instruction to complete the task	Not able to use verbal self-instruction to complete the task
Responds to visual cues to perform the task	Does not respond to visual cues to perform the task
Uses kinesthetic self-prompting to perform the task	Unable to use kinesthetic self-prompting to perform the task

quadrants. Hence, the path from dysfunction to function might form a direct line, a right angle, or a Z shape depending on the way the child responds. It is also important to note that the child's learning needs might also change from one occasion to another as the shift toward autonomy becomes consolidated.

Within these continua, four groups of behaviors indicate the characteristics of function and dysfunction, based on the discussion above. These characteristics can be used as the basis for the evaluation of autonomy in tasks and activities relevant to occupational performance.

A child may not demonstrate all behaviors in a quadrant.

Table 10.4 Function and Dysfunction Indicators for Quadrant 4: Indirect, Learner-Initiated Strategies

Quadrant 4	
Function	**Dysfunction**
Able to use internalized learner-initiated strategies for effective task performance	Has not internalized learner-initiated strategies for effective task performance
Indicators of Function	**Indicators of Dysfunction**
Uses self-imagery as part of cognitive strategies to perform tasks	Not able to use self-imagery as part of cognitive strategies to perform tasks
Uses internal self-instruction to perform tasks	Cannot use internal self-instruction to perform tasks
Uses self-questioning to analyze information for reflective thinking and to develop cognitive strategies	Does not engage in self-questioning to analyze information for reflective thinking and to develop cognitive strategies
Uses self-monitoring to evaluate and engage in task performance	Cannot use self-monitoring to evaluate and engage in task performance
Uses problem solving skills to evaluate and engage in task performance	Does not use problem solving skills to evaluate and engage in task performance
Performs the task automatically	Cannot perform the task automatically

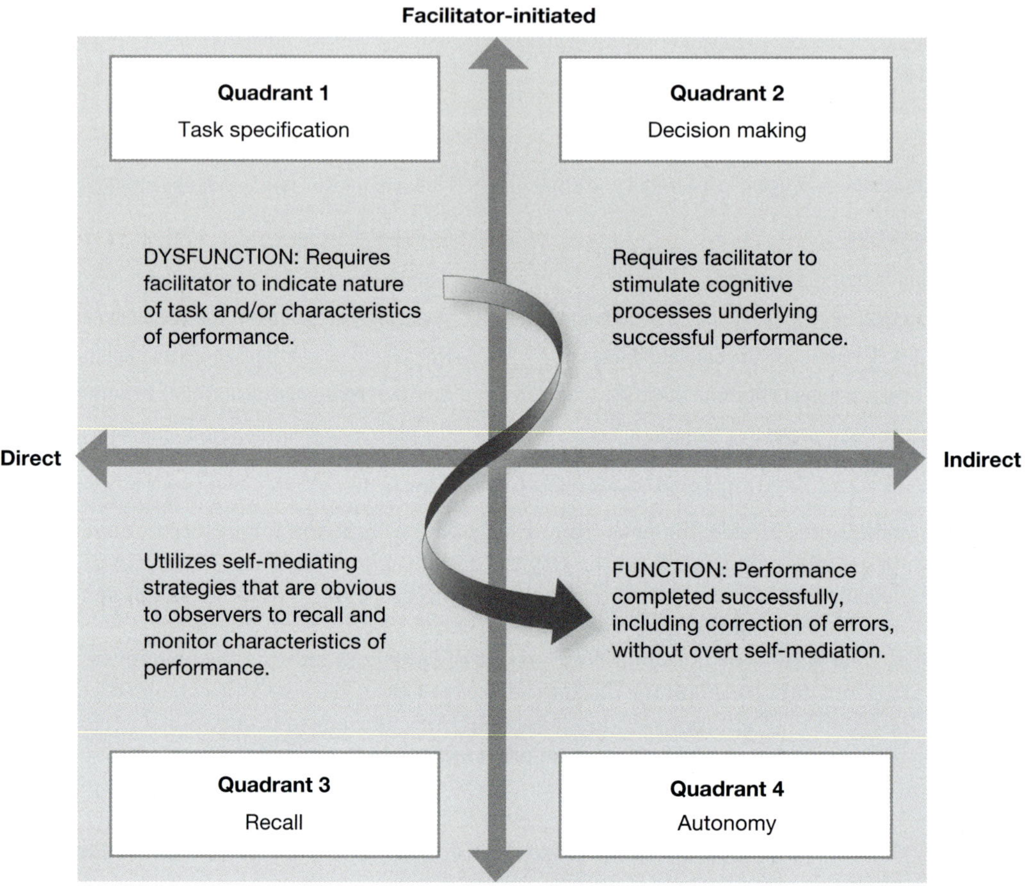

FIGURE 10.9 Features of Function and Dysfunction on the Four-Quadrant Model of Facilitated Learning.

GUIDE FOR EVALUATION

Activity analysis can be useful both in identifying the core tasks that need to be mastered to enhance occupational performance, and also in establishing the characteristics of the individual's current performance. Notably, an individual's performance can change not only from one occasion to the next, but even during sustained performance of the same task (such as when maintaining balance while transferring from the toilet). Through the process of activity analysis, the therapist needs to ascertain that the child has the necessary performance capacities, such as strength, dexterity, cognition, or emotional resilience, to successfully complete the task.

In establishing the learning strategies that are likely to be most appropriate for a child, the therapist must maintain a fluid view of the child's learning needs, systematically guiding them through various stages of the learning process. Understanding the characteristics of performance that indicate the learner's needs leads the therapist to select learning strategies most likely to enable successful performance. This dynamic approach to the use of activity analysis leads to

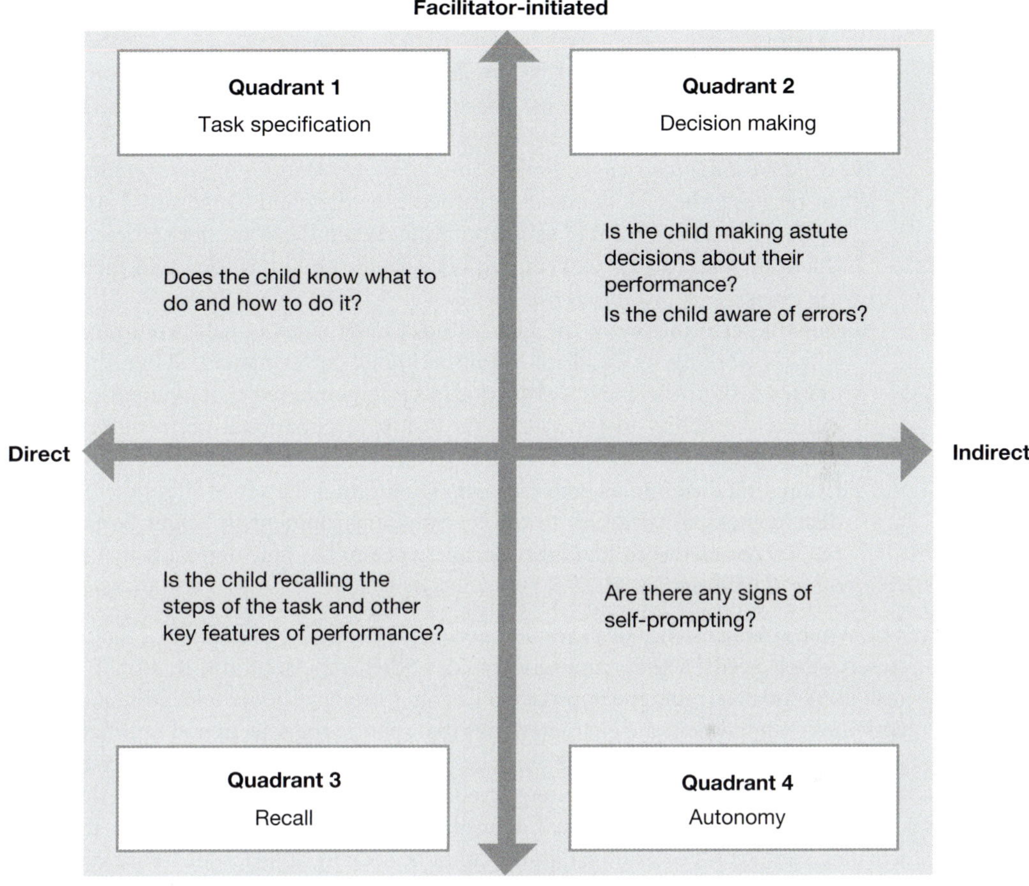

FIGURE 10.10 Guidelines for Evaluating Learning Needs.

the coordinated adoption of learning strategies, which is essential in developing autonomy. A therapist might consider specific questions when evaluating a child's learning needs, as described in Figure 10.10. The answer to each question helps to establish the child's learning needs, and consequently the quadrant from which appropriate learning strategies might be drawn. Repeated use of these questions throughout the learning encounter ensures the child's learning needs are met, and task performance is optimized.

"Does the child know what to do and how to do it?"

On most occasions, task learning must commence with an understanding of the task at hand. During formative stages of learning, the child would not have an understanding of the task. This directs the therapist to use Quadrant 1 strategies in the first instance to establish knowledge of the desired response. Once that has occurred; however, the child would usually be expected to retain this knowledge, and so the use of Quadrant 1 strategies becomes redundant unless the child has difficulties remembering those requirements. Re-evaluation of the child's learning needs should then ensue through asking subsequent evaluation questions.

Is the child solving problems and making astute decisions about their performance? Is the child aware of errors?

Quadrant 2 strategies should be employed if problem solving, decision making, and error recognition are not apparent. These strategies support the learner to engage in cognitive processes that lead to successful performance.

"Is the child recalling the steps of the task and other key features of performance?"

When recalling the task demands is difficult for the child, Quadrant 3 strategies can be used by the learner as a form of self-prompting. When these are not sufficient to generate recall, Quadrant 1 strategies are required because the child has forgotten the task demands.

"Are there any signs of self-prompting?"

Successful performance of the task without overt signs of self-prompting indicates that the child is working in Quadrant 4 (autonomous performance). While this suggests progress toward task proficiency, it should also be remembered that occupational goal attainment reflects the ability to generalize the task to occupational performance, including performance in other contexts and/or performing consistently within the same context over time. Evaluating the child as performing in Quadrant 4 therefore offers the opportunity to introduce contextual variables to the learning environment. It might be necessary to support the learner as the child adapts performance to the new demands by using strategies from other quadrants.

While characteristics of the child's performance can be indicative of the quadrant most likely to serve their needs, activity analysis provides other important information. Characteristics of the task itself can determine the approach a learning strategy should take. Motor, cognitive, and social activities each have unique characteristics that require the selection of optimal learning strategies. For example, while physical tasks lend themselves to demonstration and physical facilitation, cognitive and verbal tasks may be better served by higher-order questioning and think aloud modeling.

In various cases, the physical environment may or may not support the use of particular learning strategies. For example, it might not be socially appropriate to use verbal self-instruction strategies if the environment is an inherently quiet one. Similarly, visual prompts, such as picture sequences, might not be able to be used in environments that do not have a location for affixing them. Consideration of the environment in which the occupation takes place enables the therapist to select strategies that are socially valid.

A synthesis of these factors provides the therapist with the basis for selecting and using learning strategies that are appropriate to the needs of the learner, the characteristics of the environment, and the target occupation. Greber et al. (2012) provided a detailed account of how these considerations might be framed with reference to the 4QM.

Greber et al. (2012) described a simple acronym that can be used to assist identification of relevant teaching and learning strategies. The ALERT acronym stops short of prescribing ways of deciding upon appropriate learning strategies. Instead, it identifies five factors that therapists should be "alert" to when selecting the most appropriate learning strategy within any of the four quadrants. These are factors relating to the:

- **Activity** itself
- **Learner** characteristics
- **Environment** in which the task is performed
- **Relationship** between the practitioner, therapist, and child
- **Therapist**'s own skills in facilitating learning.

In this way, while specific strategies might be selected from the 4QM, the way they are implemented should be informed in a nuanced manner by considering each of those factors.

POSTULATES REGARDING CHANGE

At the center of the 4QM frame of reference are two general postulates regarding change:

1. Learning can be enhanced by appropriately scaffolding performance so that the learner achieves a successful outcome. In this way, the social environment can be manipulated to enhance performance and learning, as proposed by Vygotsky (1978).
2. In order to enable a child to progress through the stages of task learning and hence advance through the quadrants, it is useful to employ intermediate strategies that straddle two quadrants.

Directional Postulates

There are two directional postulates regarding change for this frame of reference.

1. When a practitioner dually seeks to facilitate task proficiency and maximize self-mediation, they will be most effective by moving from those strategies that are facilitator initiated and involve the child in reproductive cognitions (Quadrant 1), toward those that are covert, learner initiated and internalized (Quadrant 4).
2. The intervention would begin at the proficiency of the child in whichever quadrant that proficiency falls, and move through the subsequent quadrants as necessary. Because proficiency might be variable across time, it might be necessary to draw on different quadrants at different times. The rule of thumb should always be to offer only as much prompting as is necessary to enable performance.

Specific Postulates Regarding Change

The various learning strategies in the 4QM have been described and defined earlier. In order to enact the general postulates above, they must be linked to provide a pathway toward autonomy, while at the same time maintaining the flexibility to respond to individual learning needs on a temporal and contextual basis. This can be achieved by using the concepts in the 4QM in a well-directed and coordinated fashion. Accepting the general postulates regarding change to be true, a number of specific postulates regarding change enable the 4QM to be implemented.

1. If the practitioner employs facilitator-initiated methods such as explicit instruction and explanation, physical patterning, and lower-order questions, then the child will be able to understand the task requirement and complete the task.
2. If the practitioner employs additional facilitator-initiated strategies, such as higher-order questionings, verbal feedback, and/or physical prompts/gesture, then the child will be able to develop an effective plan for task performance.
3. If the practitioner provides opportunities to allow the child to recall key points about the tasks, then the child will be able to engage in self-initiated strategies to complete a task.
4. If the practitioner encourages the child to use indirect, learner-initiated strategies, then the child will be able to internalize these strategies for effective task performance, which can lead to a stage of automaticity.

APPLICATION TO PRACTICE

This frame of reference can be employed only when the child is judged to have the necessary performance capacities (e.g., strength, dexterity, bilateral coordination) to complete the task in its current form. Each strategy in the 4QM reflects a body of knowledge about the way that learning occurs and has been validated as an effective method of facilitating learning. These are grouped into various quadrants based on shared characteristics.

In order to provide only as much scaffolding as necessary on any attempt at completing a task, it is recommended that the practitioner work backward to determine where to begin the intervention. A practitioner should first provide sufficient time for a child to perform the task autonomously (with or without overt self-prompting), and if that is not possible, use orienting strategies to remind the child of the self-prompting strategies in Quadrant 3. If the child still does not embrace Quadrant 3 strategies, the practitioner should utilize indirect (Quadrant 2) prompts, employing more direct (Quadrant 1) prompts only if necessary. This process eliminates the likelihood of dependent behaviors that can develop when practitioner anticipate failure, assume the need for guidance, and/or provide scaffolds that are not required.

When the 4QM frame of reference is used, the practitioner integrates knowledge of the task, child, environment, and their own clinical skills, to develop specific learning strategies that will result in enhanced occupational performance for the child. One way of approaching the development of specific strategies for a child is to begin by identifying the features of autonomous performance. Using knowledge of the child's characteristics, and those of the environment and task itself, the practitioner can then work backward through the model to identify effective strategies in earlier quadrants that will be useful in establishing autonomy.

It is helpful to use a "what if...?" questioning route to inform the development of teaching–learning strategies. By working backward from Quadrant 4 to Quadrant 1, the practitioner is able to identify where the child is experiencing difficulties with the task. For example, with a child learning to tie shoelaces (Quadrant 4), the practitioner might ask, "What could the child do to remind themselves if they forget the sequence of movements?" (Quadrant 3). Next, the practitioner might ask, "What would the child do if they were internalizing their self-prompting strategies?" (Fading). After that, the practitioner could ask, "What could I say or do if the child forgets their prompts?" (Orienting). Subsequently, they might ask, "What will I do to help the child to decide what to do if they don't use self-prompting?" (Quadrant 2), and then, "What will I do if the child forget what they should do and can't figure it out?" (Quadrant 1). Finally, the practitioner might ask, "What could I do if the child is reluctant to attempt the task without direct prompting?" (Leading). Armed with these questions, the practitioner can construct an individualized set of strategies using the 4QM in a coordinated and sequential way.

CASE EXAMPLE

To understand how the 4QM might be implemented in practice, it is useful to consider its application in the following situation:

Implementing the 4QM: Ishaan

Ishaan's family migrated from India shortly after he was born and they strive to maintain links with their traditional culture. He is 5 years old and has recently transitioned to formal schooling. Ishaan previously attended early childhood education in an inclusive setting where his individual needs arising from a moderate developmental delay were well addressed.

Ishaan's parents take responsibility for many of his self-care needs, assisting him with dressing and bathing and supporting him closely with toileting and grooming. They see this as an important way of fulfilling their parenting roles in line with their cultural beliefs. Indian mealtime practices do not traditionally involve the use of cutlery, and Ishaan has not been introduced to the use of a knife, fork, or spoon. Ishaan's teacher has reported to his parents that Ishaan has become socially isolated at mealtimes because other children have noticed him using his hands to eat foods for which his peers would use cutlery. The teacher is aware of Ishaan's developmental delays and assumes he does not have the fine motor skills to use cutlery effectively. They recommend the family access occupational therapy services.

When the occupational therapy practitioner meets with the family, Ishaan's parents do not share the teacher's concerns and do not appear to understand the importance of establishing proficiency in cutlery use during mealtimes, as this would not normally be of concern in India. It is only when Ishaan and his parents meet with the teacher and therapy practitioner to negotiate therapy goals that collaborative goal setting occurs. Ishaan says he has friends at school, but reports they sometimes tease him when he uses his hands to eat. While cutlery use is not important within the home, Ishaan's parents begin to recognize the importance of peer relationships and agree it would be valuable for Ishaan to adopt mealtime practices like those of his peers when in the school environment. They also recognize they have limited knowledge of how to teach the relevant tasks due to their ambivalence in using cutlery during their own mealtimes. Ishaan and his parents collaborate in setting occupational goals relating to school mealtimes and seek guidance from the occupational therapy practitioner.

The occupational therapy practitioner begins by analyzing the occupation. Ishaan is beginning to enjoy and find meaning in becoming autonomous in a range of occupations at school and home. During mealtimes at school, there are many occasions where spoons might be used, but relatively few where knife and fork might be required. However, Ishaan and his parents would like to address both tasks so that Ishaan becomes well prepared for future mealtime experiences. Ishaan has indicated keenness to master these skills. The family acknowledge that the way knife and fork are used differs across countries, and they decide they will follow traditional British usage because of their extended family ties to that country.

Further analysis confirms that Ishaan is able to perform many activities relevant to mealtimes: he can pour from a jug, drink without spilling, open containers, and accurately bring food to his mouth. On occasions where a spoon is required at home, Ishaan's mother feeds him with the spoon rather than letting him feed himself. When presented with knife and fork, Ishaan is unable to orientate the implements, or grasp and use them effectively.

Given Ishaan's developmental delay, the practitioner investigates Ishaan's fine motor and cognitive skills. While there are some minor delays, the practitioner is satisfies that Ishaan has the requisite motor capacities to effectively use cutlery and the cognitive skills to learn those tasks. Most importantly, he is able to form appropriate grasp patterns, including isolating his index finger as he will need to do when using knife and fork. The practitioner decides to use teaching–learning as a primary focus during service delivery.

The occupational therapy practitioner also considers several complementary aspects of service delivery. Simplification of the occupation by grading the texture and firmness of food would make the tasks easier to learn, and careful positioning of plates, bowls and cutlery would also support learning. Cutlery with built up handles would be easier for Ishaan to grasp; however this would require further adaptation for Ishaan in the future as he progresses to regular cutlery. The practitioner considers the use of lipped bowls and plates but decides this might encourage Ishaan to rely unnecessarily on those supports. In the end, the practitioner decides to use teaching–learning to master the tasks in their most conventional form without the use of adaptive cutlery or crockery. However, the practitioner also chooses to grade characteristics of food and to arrange the equipment in ways that facilitate success, and these factors become important parts of the teaching–learning process.

To approach this scenario, the practitioner identifies three key observations:

1. That Ishaan is not proficient in some of the tasks required to feed himself using cutlery.
2. That his motor and cognitive skills are sufficient to acquire proficiency in cutlery use.
3. That with appropriate use of teaching–learning strategies, Ishaan will develop proficiency in the tasks required for mealtimes and generalize his performance to the school and home environments as required.

The practitioner focuses specifically on three tasks perceived as barriers to occupational performance: loading the spoon when eating from a bowl, stabbing food with a fork, and cutting food using a knife and fork. Sequenced learning strategies will be required as Ishaan develops proficiency in these tasks. This leads the therapist to use the 4QM as a frame of reference to guide teaching–learning.

The practitioner uses a series of questions to determine Ishaan's learning needs:

- Does he know what is required to hold the various implements?
- Is he aware when he is holding or using the implements inefficiently?
- Is he choosing appropriate tactics for grasping and manipulating the implements?
- Can he recall the steps involved in using each tool, or does he omit/repeat some steps?
- Is he using any obvious strategies to remember how to use the cutlery effectively?
- Are there any signs that he requires self-prompting to perform the tasks?

Additionally, the practitioner uses the ALERT acronym to guide the selection of appropriate strategies in each quadrant of the 4QM:

- What type of **activity** is this? (e.g., physical, verbal, cognitive)
- What are the characteristics and capacities of the **learner**? (e.g., physical, cognitive, psychosocial)?
- Are there **environmental** features that make it difficult to use particular strategies? (e.g., space, noise, distractibility)
- What **relationship** factors between therapist–client, teacher–student, and parent–child need to be considered? (e.g., learned helplessness, engagement, support, risk-taking behaviors)
- What are the limits of the **therapist's** own skills and knowledge in this area? (e.g., professional experience, cultural awareness, skills in teaching–learning)

The occupational therapy service available to Ishaan allows therapy to take place in the school environment. Although it is not always possible to time the sessions to correspond with mealtimes, embedding services in the school context will help to minimize the transfer of skills necessary to the target occupation. Services in the home are not possible; however Ishaan's mother is able to attend sessions at school, and has decided to implement similar learning opportunities in the home environment. This will help to minimize the transfer of skills necessary to the target occupation in each context. Features of the environment in which learning takes place will therefore be consistent with those inherent in performance of the occupation. Ishaan's mother has requested guidance in the use of supportive teaching–learning strategies in the home.

With these factors in mind, the practitioner develops a series of coordinated learning strategies and records them in each quadrant of the 4QM. They do so by working backward through the model beginning in Quadrant 4, linking each of the learning strategies directly with the target tasks (Figure 10.11).

Quadrant 4 represents autonomous performance. The practitioner begins by identifying the features of autonomous performance to serve as a reference point for the development of teaching and learning strategies. As a physical activity, it will be easy to observe when Ishaan's performance uses only covert self-prompting. Working in the school will allow the practitioner to identify any relevant features of that context. The occupational therapy practitioner will also support Ishaan's mother to use strategies to optimize Ishaan's performance in the home environment.

The practitioner works together with Ishaan to consider the tasks and make initial attempts. To engage in autonomous performance, Ishaan will need to have a clear understanding of task requirements and covertly instruct and monitor his own performance. The practitioner will observe Ishaan's performance and note the way Ishaan responds to any difficulties. By identifying what autonomous performance will look like, the practitioner is then able to identify the key features of the performance that need to be addressed (see Figure 10.11, Quadrant 4).

Quadrant 3 strategies are useful in helping the learner recall the key features of performance. In developing appropriate strategies for Quadrant 3, the practitioner considers Ishaan's strength in verbal recall, and his enthusiasm for action rhymes and songs. This suggests he will be able to use kinesthetic self-prompts and simple mnemonics to recall key aspects of the target tasks. Firstly, the practitioner encourages Ishaan to isolate and point his index fingers and tap the tips of them only the desk. This acts as a kinesthetic self-prompt to remind him of the importance of pointed fingers when grasping the knife and fork. Then the practitioner collaborates with Ishaan to develop simple phrases he could use to remind himself of how to use the cutlery. Ishaan will say aloud, "scoop and in" when using the spoon, and, "hold and cut" when using knife and fork. For knife and fork use, it is also important that Ishaan uses the correct hand for each implement. The occupational therapy practitioner notices a prominent freckle on the back of Ishaan's left hand and suggests he could that to help him orient himself. Ishaan agrees to use alliteration—"F for freckle, F for fork"—to help himself. This is essentially a visual prompt but is supported by the use of a mnemonic. These self-prompting strategies together will enable Ishaan to recall all the key points of the task identified in Quadrant 4. As Ishaan moves from the overt self-prompting strategies of Quadrant 3 to the covert ones of Quadrant 4, he may naturally choose to whisper the mnemonic rather than say it aloud (Fading). The use of mnemonics could prove intrusive (and even embarrassing) in the school environment, so while they will be used during therapy, it is important they are faded as quickly as possible. If Ishaan does not spontaneously use his mnemonics or kinesthetic self-prompts, the facilitator might use an orienting prompt such as, "What could you say or do to help you remember?". Quadrant 3, Orienting and Fading strategies are all detailed in Figure 10.11.

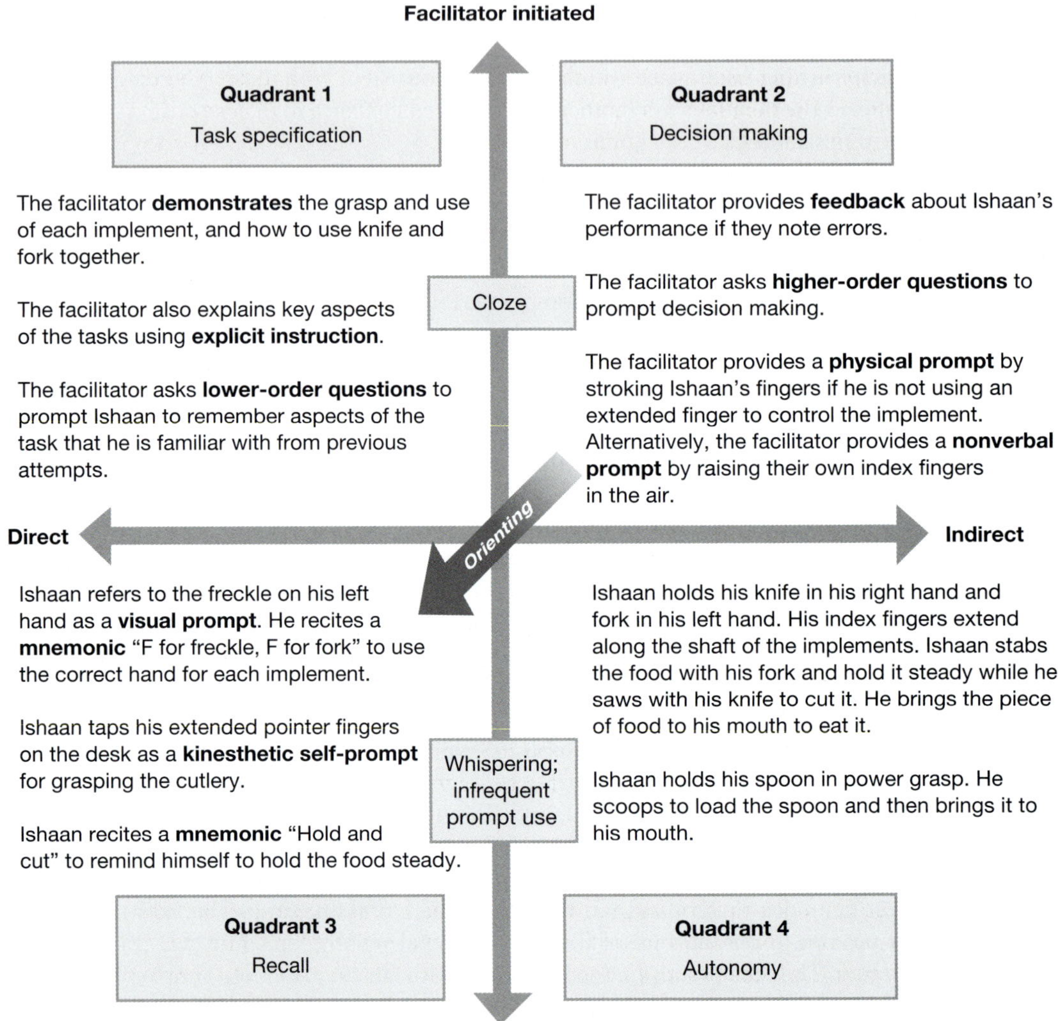

FIGURE 10.11 Ishaan's Four-Quadrant Model of Facilitated Learning for using cutlery.

Whereas Quadrant 3 strategies are initiated by the child, Quadrant 2 strategies involve the facilitator (in this case the occupational therapy practitioner, teacher, or parent) providing the impetus for learning. Strategies in this quadrant should be congruent with those in Quadrant 3, so that they naturally lead the child to become more self-directed. Quadrant 2 strategies engage the child in decision making, fostering the cognitive skills necessary to select, organize, and monitor a course of action. Although the tasks involved in using cutlery are physical ones, the practitioner observes that Ishaan's difficulties are often the result of not understanding what to do, rather than not having the physical competencies to perform the task. The practitioner works with Ishaan to select a number of strategies to support him to learn the procedures for using a spoon, knife, and fork. First, they agree that the facilitator will use feedback to alert Ishaan if he needs to try another way of performing the task. For example, if Ishaan is not securing the food in place while using the knife, the facilitator will say, "Uh-oh—the food is moving around." If required, the facilitator will prompt further using higher-order questions such as, "What could you do to hold the food steady?" The facilitator will also ask, "Why do you think that happened?" if an error occurs. The other strategies used in Quadrant 2 will be the use of nonverbal prompts. The facilitator will either raise their index fingers or stroke Ishaan's index fingers (if he is not watching the facilitator) to prompt Ishaan to alter his grasp to a more appropriate one. These strategies are summarized in Figure 10.11, Quadrant 2. The development of a supportive and nonjudgmental relationship will be important in encouraging Ishaan to problem solve, even when he is uncertain of the best response.

Strategies in Quadrant 1 provide information about either the task itself or the anticipated response. During the initial stages of learning, Quadrant 1 strategies are used so that Ishaan understands what he needs to do. As learning progresses, Quadrant 1 strategies are only used when Ishaan is unsuccessful in implementing strategies from other quadrants. The practitioner establishes a series of strategies to clarify the characteristics of the task. The practitioner works with Ishaan to identify the best strategies to specify the task. Ishaan prefers to observe demonstration of knife, fork, and spoon use. He has a positive relationship with his mother and teacher and will accept guidance from them. The practitioner recognizes Ishaan's strength in verbal communications and decides to use explicit instruction alongside those demonstrations. Once Ishaan has been shown how to use the implements, a lower-order question such as, "How should you hold your spoon?" might be appropriate. Only if Ishaan continues to have difficulty will hand-over-hand physical patterning be used. Once Quadrant 1 strategies are established, the practitioner develops leading strategies that bridge Quadrant 1 and Quadrant 2. A cloze sentence like, "Hold and ... (pause)" is selected. Ishaan will consider the task and identify the next step when the facilitator pauses. Quadrant 1 and leading strategies are identified in Figure 10.11, Quadrant 1.

The occupational therapy practitioner has now developed a complete 4QM that will guide them in delivering services. Service delivery takes place in the school environment in the presence of Ishaan's mother, and she receives a copy of the complete 4QM to inform her support for Ishaan's learning in the home environment. The practitioner begins by establishing Ishaan's knowledge of the task. Ishaan is observed attempting to use cutlery and asked about his performance (e.g., "What should you do first?"), technique (e.g., "What do you think is the best way to hold the spoon?"), and outcome (e.g., "Why do you need to hold the food steady when we cut?"). This gives an indication of Ishaan's orientation to the task. The answers to these questions indicate that although Ishaan understands the task at a general level, he has not acquired an appreciation of the key features of the task that determine success, such as the importance of stabbing food with the fork, or the various grasp patterns required.

The practitioner uses demonstration and explicit instruction to draw Ishaan's attention to the need to grasp and use utensils in particular ways. Answers to lower-order questions indicate that Ishaan is able to recall those key features when prompted. The practitioner then begins to use incomplete instructions (cloze) during their demonstrations, and Ishaan is able to complete the sentence.

The practitioner then focuses on the decision-making process, rather than the critical physical skills, by asking higher-order questions. Prompting becomes less direct and encourages Ishaan to engage in problem solving when he has having difficulty with the task. After some practice, Ishaan is mostly able to perform the target tasks without ongoing support from the facilitator but continues to have difficulty recalling some specific characteristics of the task. Over the course of a few sessions, he becomes able to use learner-initiated (Quadrant 3) strategies to prompt himself on grasp and use of cutlery. Sometimes, he forgets to use these strategies, so the practitioner uses an orienting prompt to remind Ishaan to engage them. Less frequently, he cannot recall his self-prompting strategies and so the practitioner re-engages Quadrant 2 strategies to support Ishaan's learning. Over time, Ishaan begins to whisper self-prompting verbalizations to himself, and relies less on kinesthetic self-prompts. He eventually becomes able to use knife, fork, and spoon independently on eating tasks at home and school. Ishaan's mother and teacher are present during therapy sessions and implement the same strategies during eating occurring outside of therapy time. They refer to the documented 4QM strategies when deciding how best to enable Ishaan at any point in the learning process, depending on his identified learning needs.

At this point, Ishaan demonstrates autonomy in performing some key tasks when eating. However, when rushed to complete the activity, as occurs during time-limited lunch breaks, this performance sometimes breaks down. Similarly, he sometimes has difficulty recognizing when to use a spoon and when to use knife and fork. Using the strategies detailed in the 4QM, Ishaan's teacher and parents take on the role of facilitator, using consistent learning strategies to promote the acquisition of skills. The use of Quadrant 3 (self-prompting) strategies and exposure to feedback, nonverbal prompts, and higher-order questions (Quadrant 2) enable Ishaan to make astute decisions about the contextual demands of the occupation. When the task becomes difficult due to time restrictions, or eating in an unfamiliar context, Ishaan's facilitator uses orienting strategies to encourage Ishaan to employ the self-mediating strategies of Quadrant 3 to think and talk his way through difficult situations. This develops his ability to initiate processes in flexible ways that will enable occupational performance across varied contexts.

As the result of a carefully thought-through teaching–learning process, Ishaan has been able to attain proficiency in the tasks necessary to eat meals using cutlery. Through attention to the many factors that influence development of proficiency in key tasks and generalizing them to occupational performance, his therapist has used the 4QM as a frame of reference in enabling Ishaan to develop occupational autonomy.

SUPPORTING EVIDENCE

Development of the 4QM began as an action research project that sought to understand and improve the way that teaching–learning was utilized as a therapeutic approach in the first author's practice (Greber et al., 2007c). Early incarnations of the model were the outcomes of successive cycles of reflecting, planning, acting, and observing when the model was used to guide teaching–learning interventions. Action research has been championed as an important way for occupational therapy practitioners to improve their practice (Gilbert-Hunt, 2017). A version of this process was subsequently undertaken by Pullen (2011) to investigate the teaching–learning practices of teaching assistants in New Zealand, using the 4QM as a reference point. This form of practice-based investigation is an important feature of the evidence driving the 4QM. The postulates derived from conscious experience and theory were subsequently formalized in the 4QM as a way of guiding occupational therapy practitioners in the use of teaching–learning approaches, where the proficiency in particular tasks is deemed pivotal in client goal attainment. This clinically focused approach to gathering evidence has continued to characterize the 4QM as a frame of reference that directly informs practice.

Throughout its development, anecdotal reports from practitioners employing the 4QM in their practice have suggested applicability of the model in informing teaching–learning interventions across a wide range of child and adult practice areas. This has subsequently been supported by other researchers. Juntorn et al (2017) have demonstrated the effectiveness of combining two formal frameworks—the Perceive, Recall, Plan, Perform System of Task Analysis (Chapparo & Ranka, 1997) and the 4QM. The Perceive, Recall, Plan, Perform System of Task Analysis system offers a standardized, criterion-referenced way of assessing occupational performance, and the 4QM provides a supporting conceptual framework for organizing teaching–learning interventions. The authors demonstrated the effectiveness of combining these two frameworks in improving learning outcomes in academic activity in Thai children with learning difficulties.

Another example of where the 4QM has been used in conjunction with other approaches is reported by Pijarnvanit & Scriphetcharawut (2023). In their study of the implementation of Occupational Performance Coaching (OPC) (Graham et al., 2021) with parents of children with attention deficit hyperactivity disorder, those authors found that the strategies captured in the 4QM provided parents with learning opportunities when supporting the executive functioning of their children. This intervention was delivered by telehealth, an expanding approach to service delivery, and hence offers some insights into future intervention approaches which could incorporate the 4QM.

In another area of practice, Breeden (2014) used the 4QM to inform development of visual strategies to enhance adult home safety. Furthermore, Steed (2014) presented a client-centered model for designing psychoeducational content based on theoretical elements from the 4QM, combined with Cronjé's Integrative Design Model (2006). This created a hybrid client-centered instructional design model intended to guide occupational therapists in the creation of psychoeducational content for clients with emotional regulation deficits. Borges Da Costa (2014) also cited the 4QM in proposing ways of engaging clients in learning tasks related to physical leisure activities that promoted general well-being. Interestingly, the 4QM has also been discussed as a way of informing classroom teachers about effective ways to enhance executive skills in the classroom (Cooper-Kahn & Foster, 2013). These authors proposed the use of the 4QM as a framework for teachers to engage cognitive strategies in supporting and optimizing student learning in school settings.

Each of these authors has used the 4QM based on perceived applicability to particular practice areas, and in many cases employed it alongside other intervention strategies. The value of the 4QM as a framework for supporting novice practitioners and students to become more proficient in the use of teaching–learning approaches has been evident both anecdotally and also by its use in occupational therapy education programs. DeCleene et al. (2013) have argued that, while occupational therapy practitioners routinely use teaching–learning as an element of their practice, formal education in learning theory is often limited. These authors agreed that the 4QM presents occupational therapy students with one way of conceptualizing the learning process and the actions that support learning and encouraged occupational therapy educators to support students to develop appropriate teaching–learning skills as part of their training. They found that students were able to benefit from additional knowledge about teaching and learning theory by becoming more able to integrate it into their practice. This tenet is supported by research that has shown that training in the 4QM enhanced the clinical reasoning of early career therapists utilizing teaching–learning approaches by (1) enhancing the range of teaching–learning strategies they consider, (2) providing a structure for planning teaching–learning interventions, and (3) engaging in more organized clinical reasoning that parallels contemporary pedagogic theories. It also illustrated, however, that other factors, such as previous experiences, practice in the use of the model, and stage of professional development, also influence the impact of the training process (Greber, 2011). This research provided preliminary evidence that the nature of clinical reasoning itself was enriched when the 4QM was used as a framework for planning teaching–learning interventions.

Given that teaching–learning approaches are identified as being a part of almost every occupational therapy intervention (Greber et al., 2011), it is hardly surprising that other researchers have suggested that practitioners implement the 4QM in combination with other frames of reference to "create their own way" of working with particular clients. For example, Nelson et al. (2009) noted that practitioners indicated they frequently used approaches in combination, creating a "multi-model" approach in order to best meet the needs of their clients. More importantly, they reported that practitioners were able to articulate the complex and multifaceted clinical reasoning behind their choices.

Opportunities exist to advance our understanding of the applications of the 4QM by gathering evidence of the effects of use of the model on client goal attainment in a range of contexts and when used in combination with other treatment approaches. In an unpublished Honors thesis, Wilson (2014) undertook preliminary work toward this goal by surveying the perceptions of final year students trained in the 4QM regarding its contribution to client goal attainment. There was general agreement from participants that 4QM training placed the students in a better position to plan teaching–learning interventions, and participants perceived that these well-planned interventions led to faster and more complete task mastery in pediatric clients. To date, no studies have directly evaluated the effect of 4QM training on task learning in children, nor compared it with other pedagogic frameworks.

REFERENCES

Anderson, L. W., Krathwohl, D. R., Airasian, P. W., Cruikshank, K. A., Mayer, R. E., Pintrich, R. J., & Wittrock, M. C. (2013). *A taxonomy for learning, teaching, and assessing: A revision of bloom's taxonomy of educational objectives, Abridged edition*. Pearson Education.

Bairami, F., Adibi, K., & Mohammadi, I. (2016). The effectiveness of verbal self-instruction on sustained attention (based on continuous performance test) among students with mathematics learning disabilities. *International Journal of Humanities and Cultural Studies, 2*(4), 1286–1296. http://www.ijhcs.com/index.php/ijhcs/index

Bissell, A. N., & Lemons, P. P. (2006). A new method for assessing critical thinking in the classroom. *BioScience, 56*(1), 66–72. https://doi.org/10.1641/0006-3568(2006)056[0066:ANMFAC]2.0.CO;2

Bloom, B., Englehart, M. B., Furst, E. J., Hill, W. H., & Krathwohl, O. R. (1956). *Taxonomy of educational objectives: The classification of educational goals. Handbook 1: The cognitive domain*. Longman.

Borges Da Costa, A. L. (2014). *An investigation into circle dance as a medium to promote occupational well-being* (Ph.D. thesis). University of Bolton.

Breeden, L. E. (2014). *Exploring older adult home safety with photo elicitation via telehealth* (PhD thesis). Ball State University.

Carr, J. H., & Shepherd, R. B. (2010). *Neurological rehabilitation: Optimizing motor performance* (2nd ed.). Churchill Livingstone.

Chapparo, C., & Ranka, J. (1997). The PRPP system of task analysis. In Chapparo, C., & Ranka, J. (Eds.), *Occupational performance model (Australia). Monograph 1* (pp. 189–198). Occupational Performance Network, School of Occupational Therapy, The University of Sydney.

Chen, S., Zhang, J., Lange, E. Miko, P., & Joseph, D. (2001). Progressive time delay procedure for teaching motor skills to adults with severe mental retardation. *Adapted Physical Activity Quarterly, 18*(1), 35–48.

Cooper-Kahn, J., & Foster, M. (2013). *Boosting executive skills in the classroom: A practical guide for educators*. John Wiley & Sons.

Cronjé, J. (2006). Paradigms regained: Toward integrating objectivism and constructivism in instructional design and the learning sciences. *Educational Technology Research & Development, 54*(4), 387–416. https://doi.org/10.1007/s11423-006-9605-1

DeCleene, K. E., Ridgway, A. J., Bednarski, J., Breeden, L., Mosier, G. G., Sachs, D., & Stephenson, D. (2013). Therapists as educators: The importance of client education in occupational therapy. *The Open Journal of Occupational Therapy, 1*(4), Article 5. https://doi.org/10.15453/2168-6408.1050

Erdogan, I., & Campbell, T. (2008). Teacher questioning and interaction patterns in classrooms facilitated with differing levels of constructivist teaching practices. *International Journal of Science Education, 30*(14), 1891–1914. https://dx.doi.org/10.1080/09500690701587028

Frey, N., & Fisher, D. (2010). Identifying instructional moves during guided learning. *The Reading Teacher, 64*(2), 84–95. https://doi.org/10.1598/RT.64.2.1

Gilbert-Hunt, S. (2017), Sylvia Rodger's contribution to a dynamic and diverse curriculum and education evidence base. *Australian Occupational Therapy Journal, 64*, 45–48. https://doi.org/10.1111/1440-1630.12404

Graham, F., Kennedy-Behr, A., & Ziviani, J. (2021). *Occupational Performance Coaching: A manual for practitioners and researchers.* Routledge.

Greber, C. (2011). *The Four-Quadrant Model of Facilitated Learning: Development and clinical utility* (Ph.D. thesis). School of Health & Rehabilitation Sciences, The University of Queensland.

Greber, C., Hinojosa, J., & Ziviani, J. (2012). Achieving success: Facilitating skill acquisition and enabling participation. In Ziviani, J., Poulsen, A., & Cuskelly, M. (Eds.). *The art and science of motivation: A therapist's guide to working with children* (pp. 123–158) Jessica Kingsley.

Greber, C., Ziviani, J., & Rodger, S. (2007a). The Four-Quadrant Model of Facilitated Learning (part 1): Using teaching-learning approaches in occupational therapy. *Australian Occupational Therapy Journal, 54*(s1), S31–S39. https://doi.org/10.1111/j.1440-1630.2007.00662.x

Greber, C., Ziviani, J., & Rodger, S. (2007b). The Four-Quadrant Model of Facilitated Learning (part 2): Strategies and applications. *Australian Occupational Therapy Journal, 54* (s1), S40–S48. https://doi.org/10.1111/j.1440-1630.2007.00663.x

Greber, C., Ziviani, J., & Rodger, S. (2007c). The Four-Quadrant Model of Facilitated Learning: A clinically-based action research project. *Australian Occupational Therapy Journal, 54*, 149–152, https://doi.org/101111/j.1440-1630.2006.00558.x

Greber, C., Ziviani, J., & Rodger, S. (2011). Clinical utility of the Four-Quadrant Model of Facilitated Learning: Perspectives of experienced therapists. *Australian Occupational Therapy Journal, 58*, 187–194. https://doi.org/10.1111/j.1440-1630.2010.00901x

Joyce, B. R., Calhoun, E., & Hopkins, D. (2009). *Models of learning: Tools for teaching* (3rd ed.). Open University.

Juntorn, S., Sriphetcharawut, S., & Munkhetvit, P. (2017). Effectiveness of information processing strategy training on academic task performance in children with learning disabilities: A pilot study. *Occupational Therapy International*, 2017, Article ID 6237689. https://doi.org/10.1155/2017/6237689

Libby, M. E., Weiss, J. S., Bancroft, S., & Ahearn, W. H. (2008). A comparison of most-to-least and least-to-most prompting on the acquisition of solitary play skills. *Behavioral Analysis in Practice, 1*(1), 37–43. https://doi.org/10.1007/BF03391719

Martini, R., & Polatajko, H. J. (1998). Verbal self-guidance as a treatment approach for children with developmental coordination disorder: A systematic replication study. *Occupational Therapy Journal of Research, 18*(4), 157–181. https://doi.org/10.1177/153944929801800403

Mosston, M., & Ashworth, S. (2008). *Teaching physical education* (1st online edition). Spectrum Institute for Teaching and Learning. www.spectrumofteachingstyles.org

Nelson, A., Copley, J., Flanigan, K., & Underwood, K. (2009). Occupational therapists prefer combining multiple intervention approaches for children with learning difficulties. *Australian Occupational Therapy Journal, 56*, 51–62. https://doi.org/10.1111/j.1440-1630.2007.00712.x

Pijarnvanit, P., & Scriphetcharawut, S. (2023). The effects of telehealth parent coaching on occupational performance and executive function of children with attention-deficit/hyperactivity disorders, and parent self-efficacy: A preliminary study. *Occupational Therapy in Health Care, 38*(3), 783–799. https://doi.org/10.1080/07380577.2023.2169976

Polatajko, H. J., & Mandich, A. (2004). *Enabling occupation in children: The Cognitive Orientation to daily Occupational Performance (CO-OP) Approach*. Canadian Association of Occupational Therapists.

Pullen, R. (2011). Research and reflection: Promoting independence in the classroom through mixed methods: A trainee's perspective. *OT Insight, 32*(7), 1–2, 4.

Richards, J. C., & Farrell, T. S. C. (2005). *Professional development for language teachers: Strategies for teacher learning*. Cambridge University Press.

Rodger, S., Brown, G. T., & Brown, A. (2005). Profile of paediatric occupational therapy practice in Australia. *Australian Occupational Therapy Journal, 52*, 311–325. https://doi.org/10.1111/j.1440-1630.2005.00487.x

Schmidt, R. A., & Lee, T. D. (2014). *Motor learning and control: From principles to applications* (5th ed.). Human Kinetics.

Schmidt, R. A., & Wrisberg, C. A. (2008). *Motor learning and performance: A situation-based learning approach*. Human Kinetics.

Sinha, S. P., & Sharma, A. (2001). Cognitive strategy instruction approach of problem solving for learning disabled children. *Journal of Indian Psychology, 19*(1–2), 33–38.

Steed, R. (2014). A client-centered model of instructional design for psychoeducation interventions in occupational therapy. *Occupational Therapy in Mental Health, 30*(2), 126–143. https://doi.org/10.1080/0164212X.2014.878536

Steele, M. M. (2005). Teaching students with learning disabilities: Constructivism or behaviorism. *Current Issues in Education [Online], 8*(10). http://cie.asu.edu/volume8/number10/

Sternberg, R. J., & Frensch, P. A. (2014). *Complex problem solving: Principles and mechanisms*. Psychology Press.

Theodorakis, Y., Hatzigeorgiadis, A., & Zourbanos, N. (2010). Cognitions: Self talk and performance. In Murphy, S. M. (Ed.), *The Oxford handbook of sport and performance psychology* (pp. 191–212). Oxford University Press.

Thompson, R. H., McKerchar, P. M., Paige, M., & Dancho, K. A. (2004). The effects of delayed physical prompts and reinforcement on infant sign language acquisition. *Journal of Applied Behavior Analysis, 37*(3), 379–383. doi:10.1901/jaba.2004.37-379

Vygotsky, L. S. (1978). Mind in society: The development of higher psychological processes. Translated by Cole, M., Scribner, S., John-Steiner, V., & Souberman, E. In: Reiber, R. W., & Robinson, D. K. (Eds.), *The essential Vygotsky* (pp. 345–400). Kluwer Academic.

Walsh, J. A., & Sattes, B. D. (2017). *Quality questioning: Research-based practice to engage every learner* (2nd ed.). Sage.

Wilson, N. (2014). *Final year occupational therapy students' perceptions of client goal attainment following training in the Four-Quadrant Model of Facilitated Learning (Unpublished Honours thesis)*. University of the Sunshine Coast.

Woolfolk, A. E. (2015). *Educational psychology* (13th ed.). Pearson.

Zimmerman, B. J., & Schunk, D. H. (2011). *Handbook of self-regulation of learning and performance*. Routledge.

Motor Skill Acquisition Frame of Reference

Katherine Dimitropoulou

11

Motor skills are the abilities that allow individuals to perform intentional, variable, goal-directed, motor actions in the context of functional activities. Motor skills support children and adolescents to explore their worlds, implement plans and decisions, and interact with others. The development of motor skills occurs through intense practice and interactions in the context of daily tasks and activities. Throughout the life span these skills continue to adapt and develop across activities, and occupations, in different environments.

Movements are the building blocks of motor skills that under the agency and intent of the individual, allow for variability, increasing complexity, flexibility, and adaptability in functional behavior. Infants engage and constantly expand in the development of motor skills through exploratory movements of reaching, touching, grasping, rolling, sitting, crawling, etc., gaining awareness of their bodies, the objects around them, and their environments. Toddlers, new to walking, average thousands of steps (and falls) per hour, constantly moving toward their favorite persons, toys, or intriguing new spaces. Experienced walkers spend 8 to 10 hours a day moving, navigating, reaching, grasping, throwing, catching, and engaging in complex coordinated motor actions. Children and adolescents spend most of their days practicing, learning, developing, and performing skillful movements as they engage in occupations, express their thoughts, and interact with others.

Motor skill acquisition is a multidimensional process that expands children's and adolescents' existing abilities and builds their functional, cognitive, and psychosocial skills, empowering them to engage in meaningful occupations. Neurodevelopmental problems (e.g., cerebral palsy, autism, developmental coordination disorder [DCD], etc.), trauma (e.g., traumatic brain injury, etc.), and psychosocial problems (e.g., obsessive compulsive disorder, etc.) can impact motor skill acquisition and hinder the development of functional abilities and occupational engagement in infants, children, and adolescents. The scope of this chapter is to examine the functional use of existing motor abilities, and how practitioners can further support their learning, practice, development, and adaptation. The goal is to provide occupational therapy practitioners with tools to assess and identify children's existing motor skills and the tools to facilitate the development of new ones.

THEORETICAL BASE

This frame of reference utilizes current theoretical work and scientific evidence in the fields of functional ability, motor development, motor control, and motor learning in pediatrics. The theoretical framework suggests that motor skill acquisition in pediatrics should always be considered in the context of development to support functionality. Functionality is the ability of individuals to carry out daily tasks that are meaningful to them (Beard et al., 2016). Motor development is a multidimensional dynamic process underlying an individuals' ability to: (a) gain and maintain control of their bodies; (b) plan and execute goal directed actions; and (c) anticipate the consequences of these actions (Von Hofsten, 2004). Motor control explains how neural/musculoskeletal and behavioral processes guide motor skill acquisition and function (Wolpert & Landy, 2012) while considering the possible roles of the task and environment may play. Finally, *motor learning* describes processes of learning that are developmentally appropriate and can enhance and expand individuals' functional abilities in natural environments (Magill & Anderson, 2010). This frame of reference aligns conceptually with the principles of the Occupational Therapy Practice Framework, 4th Edition (OTPF-4) (American Occupational Therapy Association [AOTA], 2020) and the International Classification of Function (ICF) system (World Health Organization, 2021).

Assumptions

The motor skill acquisition frame of reference accepts three assumptions:

1. Occupational therapy practitioners prioritize and expand functional abilities (not disabilities) and motor skills to enable function and participation in occupations, taking under consideration the children's and adolescents' developmental level.
2. Motor skill acquisition prioritizes strategies that acknowledge and respect children's agency, and enable prospectivity, flexibility, and adaptation so that skills can be used to carry out daily activities.
3. Occupational therapy practitioners adopt the role of facilitator when guiding children's and adolescents' motor skill acquisition.

Motor Development and Motor Skill Acquisition

In pediatrics, we consider motor skill acquisition to be nested in motor development (Adolph et al., 2012; Adolph & Robinson, 2015; Eccleston, 2015). Motor development is a complex process of overall growth, change, and neuromaturation (Adolph & Robinson, 2015; Eccleston, 2015; Von Hofsten, 2004). It is guided by general principles of skill progression and follows a highly individualized pattern among children (Adolph et al., 2018; Adolph & Robinson, 2015).

Motor skill acquisition is a multilevel process. A useful way to scaffold the taxonomy of complex components of motor skills is to first conceptualize *movements* as the building blocks for all motor skills. *Movements* (or primitive movements) are simple, fundamental, goal-directed motor patterns (Schambra et al., 2019). For example, when eating a meal, movements involve basic actions, such as: grasp the fork, transfer of the food, etc. Movement combinations support the completion of specific *tasks*. A *task* is a subcomponent of a functional activity. Using the same activity example, reaching to grasp the spoon is a task, etc. *Combining/sequencing tasks* support the completion of an activity. In the eating example, reaching and grasping the fork, stabbing the food, transferring the food in the mouth to bite it, etc., comprise the eating activity. Following this scaffolded taxonomy in clinical practice may be a useful tool for practitioners to characterize motor skill acquisition and children's abilities more accurately.

Principles guiding motor development include the following concepts:

1. Motor skills do not follow a successive/linear progression. Often, children skip motor development "milestones" and/or present at the same time behaviors that are a "mix" or overlap

among "milestones." For example, some infants never crawl but instead transition directly from sitting to standing and walking. Some infants begin walking for a few days and revert to crawling for months before starting to walk again.

2. The maturation of many systems (not just motor processes) contributes to motor skill development. Motor skills are dependent on the maturation and integration of sensory systems to detect information on the consequences of motor actions. In fact, sensorimotor systems share common neural processes that cannot be distinguished (in sensory and motor) when examining children's functional motor abilities. In addition, increase in memory capacity and cognitive organization systems (executive function) open new possibilities for interactions with the world and lead to more complex motor skills.
3. Learning is embedded in development. Motor skills can be learned if they are in concert with the child's developmental level. For example, children are "ready" to reach beyond their arms' length if their postural control and balance in sitting allows them to move their bodies forward without falling. New walkers must focus on their steps and have a hard time carrying their toys while walking, and experienced walkers can carry two or three toys with little effort. Likewise, kindergarteners spend much of their effort to formulate each letter rather than think of how to write entire words or sentences. Mastery of letter formation allows for thought and formation of full words and sentences as children mature developmentally.
4. New motor skills and abilities facilitate a cascade of real-time events that can foster further learning and development. When infants take their first steps, parents are excited and provide opportunities for their infants to repeat this behavior. Infants respond to these social cues and further expand and adapt their steps developing walking skills.
5. Variability is at the core of motor skills practiced in the real world. For neurotypically developing children this variability supports skill refinement and adaptation.
6. Contexts (i.e., social, cultural) and experiences matter. Motor development does not occur with the mere passage of time. Chronologic age is not synonymous with developmental level. Opportunities for exploration, exposure to meaningful activities, practice, feedback, and interactions enrich children's skills and can support or hinder development.

Motor Control and Functional Ability

Motor skills are behavioral indicators of the child's motor control. *Motor control* is the ability to organize movements in response to task/activity demands toward accomplishing goal-directed actions in natural contexts (Gordon et al., 2021; Michalski et al., 2020; Thura et al., 2022). This ability is dependent on children's experiences, and it entails the organization of various underlying processes (person factors) related to the capacity of neural systems (i.e., sensorimotor, memory, cognitive control, and behavioral systems), and musculoskeletal systems (i.e., bone, joint, and muscle health). This ability is also relevant to the nature of the task and the environment. Analysis of person, task, and environment factors can provide insights on the nature and the magnitude of the difficulties and inform clinical interventions.

Person Factors

Motor skills acquisition is affected by a multitude of systems. Development and maturation as well as specific neurodevelopmental problems, or trauma impact the response and integration of these systems to support functional behavior.

The following systems impact the acquisition of motor skills:

1. The specific body structures (i.e., joint range of motion) and functions (i.e., spasticity, dystonia, ataxia, etc.), related to sensorimotor systems.
2. Planning and error detection related to processing of motor actions.
3. Cognitive control of motor actions (i.e., inhibitory control, ability to alter the strategies and/or plans).
4. Behavioral processes affect motor actions (i.e., performance stress, emotional state, self-efficacy).

Contemporary theories of motor control such as the ecologic theory (Adolph & Kretch, 2015; Gibson, 1992; Pezzulo & Cisek, 2016) suggest that neural and musculoskeletal factors are not enough to explain functional ability. The premise is that functional behavior is organized by additional psychological processes. Specifically, the ecologic theory suggests that children organize motor responses based on what they perceive the task affords for them to do specific to the context in which it is to be executed (Gibson, 1992). Inherent in this process is their perceived ability and how this ability matches the task demands. As children develop more complex motor skills, they discover new opportunities for movement and new strategies to explore and implement. Success in utilizing new motor skills leads to an increase in their perceived ability, leading to more possibilities for task engagement.

Four psychological processes guide the ability to translate underlying neural and musculoskeletal processes into function. These processes are agency, prospectivity, flexibility, and adaptability (Adolph & Hoch, 2019; Adolph & Kretch, 2015; Adolph & Robinson, 2015; Reddy et al., 2013). Persistent lack of agency, prospectivity, flexibility, and adaptability results in motor dysfunction.

Agency is the ability to use motor skills to control an object (e.g., grasp a spoon, etc.), aspects of a task, an activity or a set of activities. Agency is important in motor skill acquisition and can be explicit or implicit. The implicit process refers to the sequences of actions that are habitually carried out without requiring children's attention. Explicit processes refer to the awareness of the steps required to problem solve and complete a motor task. It empowers children to make decisions, to test, refine, and revise their motor skills to accomplish their goals and impact their environments. Thus, agency leads to self-efficacy. Agency is present in the first months of life. Infants discover that when moving their arms/hands in a specific rhythmic pattern they can swipe a mobile hanging over them and can create a series of pleasant sounds. The initial random movements get organized in a rhythmic pattern (agency) and accomplish a desired goal (self-efficacy) (D'Souza et al., 2017; Haggard, 2017).

Studies in children with neurodevelopmental problems demonstrate that lack of agency can impact motor skills acquisition in various ways. For example, children with autism spectrum disorders, demonstrate lack of agency in motor skills, that is lack of intention in their movements, lack of action selection, or the motivation to achieve the goal resulting in errors, and /or loss of interest and frustration (Zalla & Sperduti, 2015). Studies in children with DCD reveal that an altered sense of agency is evident when children use their motor skills to carry out functional tasks. For example, children with DCD appear unable to detect the consequences of their actions and do not update internal models and strategies for future action selection. Their motor skills appear "stuck" to specific strategies even if these strategies do not work (Nobusako et al., 2020).

Prospectivity is the ability to plan motor actions anticipating task and environmental demands and consequences of the behavior (Adolph & Kretch, 2015). Prospectivity is heavily dependent on practice and experience. For example, children learn to assume effective trunk and arm postures to effectively engage in ball games. With experience they are able to succeed in increasingly more complex task scenarios that require high levels of accuracy and speed (e.g., playing soccer, or tennis, etc.) (Bäckström et al., 2021; Donath et al., 2015). They can relate to accuracy and/or timing of movements in response to task demands, and usually characterize the efficiency of motor actions. When children have difficulty with prospectivity it can lead to frustration and potentially hinder motor skill acquisition.

Flexibility is the ability to recognize and address errors in motor actions and update actions and strategies for better performance (Adolph & Hoch, 2019). It is associated with the ability to learn from failed attempts and strategies. Detection and exploration of the errors leads to movement modification to match the task demands. Given the variable nature of daily activities this ability is essential for functional behavior. As an example, children with Down syndrome may engage in several attempts to button and unbutton a coat using the same strategies without success. Although they recognize that they are not successful, lack of manipulation ability and cognitive control may hinder their ability to address the problem (Alesi & Battaglia, 2019).

Adaptability is the ability to use strategies learned in a specific task, to problem solve a novel task in the same or new environments (transferring of skills). Children with problems in adaptability can successfully perform a specific task in a specific environment but cannot use their motor actions to perform similar tasks or the same task in different environments (Delgado-Lobete et al., 2022).

Task Factors

To better promote motor skill acquisition from a developmental perspective, tasks and activities should be selected to pose "the just right challenge" (Novak & Honan, 2019) between the current skill level and the next anticipated more mature or complex skill. This is important for engagement and learning. However, this process is not easy and requires constant adaptation of the task demands as children progress. Task complexity is taken under consideration to grade task demands and is understood from three dimensions: (1) motor demands, (2) dual demands, and (3) psychosocial demands.

1. Motor demands refer to the coordination and postural processes required for task execution. These include:
   a. unimanual versus bimanual;
   b. stationary (e.g., hold your arm/hand up) versus dynamic (e.g., climbing stairs);
   c. low coordination and precision (e.g., touch a target) versus high level of coordination and precision (e.g., pour water from a pitcher to a cup) (Dimitropoulou et al., 2025).
2. Dual demands refer to tasks that have motor and cognitive demands:
   a. motor tasks that have complex rules (e.g., playing a game of mini-golf);
   b. motor tasks that require concurrent thinking and creative processes (i.e., handwriting an essay)
   c. multitasking (e.g., walking and talking to a friend) (McIsaac et al., 2015)
3. Psychosocial demands refer to performance stress carrying out:
   a. novel tasks;
   b. tasks performed for an audience;
   c. difficult (for the person) tasks (Engel-Yeger & Hanna Kasis, 2010; Gasser-Haas et al., 2020)

Environment

According to the OTPF-4 (AOTA, 2020) occupational therapy practitioners examine the physical, social, cultural, temporal, virtual, and personal contexts in which motor skill and motor skill acquisition occur. Physical parameters such as light, sound, etc. can influence a child's motor performance and the process of motor skill acquisition (Mansini et al., 2020; Williams et al., 2019). The social environment can function as support, or as an obstacle for motor performance. For example, a child may be able to form letters in the intervention session (one-to-one conditions) but is unable to write in the classroom (classroom noise and sounds, performance anxiety). Cultural habits and expectations may influence motor actions and motor skill acquisition. Temporal aspects refer to the child's developmental stage and are always a consideration when assessing motor skills. Virtual contexts may include motor interactions with a computer screen. For example, children may practice their motor skills using a virtual reality (VR) system and a virtual environment.

Motor Learning

Motor learning is a process that describes a change in current motor skills that results in better motor performance (Krakauer et al., 2019). Motor learning is related to children's overall learning processes. It is embedded in their development and maturation process (Babik et al., 2022; Risen et al., 2015).

Levels and Stages of Motor Skill Acquisition

Learning and motor learning share similar neural networks and processes. Explicit (cognitive use of steps to carry out a task) and implicit processes (habitually used actions not needing cognitive awareness) are frequently observed to overlap in the process of motor learning and motor skill acquisition. For example, in the activity of brushing teeth, all sequences and actions the child completes to rhythmically brush their teeth are implicit because they are not occupying the child's attention, but they are still refined as the child continues to engage in the activity. In the same example, we may now introduce instructions about the use of a new toothpaste that requires specific application to be effective. Explicit control engages the child's attention systems to pay attention to instructions and learn a new method.

Motor skill acquisition is accomplished in two stages: early stages of learning and late stages of learning (Gentile, 1998). In early stages of learning, children learn movements with the goal to develop accurate movement strategies to match the task demand. Children focus on the nature of the movements, the consequences of their motor actions, their movements are slow and there are frequent errors in execution of the movement. Past experiences with similar motor tasks are retrieved from memory to serve as initial strategies that are then refined through practice. Practice conditions have little variability and errors of performance are either avoided (errorless learning) if the child has poor memory skills or they are clearly indicated to facilitate accuracy (Maxwell et al., 2017). This process has significant motor and cognitive demands. Tasks are constrained to a specific context. Strategies related to learning such as practice programs, feedback, and task adaptation are utilized in this stage.

In the later stages of learning, children frequently develop more than one strategy when executing a motor action. They are working on speed and accuracy at the same time need to practice under variable task conditions or may develop strategies to transfer the acquired motor skills in other similar tasks or contexts.

To better understand the processes underlying these stages of learning concepts of dynamic systems theory are incorporated into the theory of motor learning. According to dynamic systems theory, movement is multidimensional and is shaped by experience and practice tasks embedded in natural and meaningful contexts (Thelen, 2005). Like ecologic theory, dynamic systems theory suggests that motor skill acquisition is dependent on nonlinear and transactive person factors, task characteristics, and environments (Thelen, 2005). Initially, in early stages of learning, learners focus on the control parameters of movements that is the coordination, and constraint of the shape and nature of the movement. For example, children are asked to recognize and get used to the overall shape of the movement, that is, a reaching movement or a grasping movement. It also entails utilizing the necessary systems (i.e., postural control and dynamic coordination of the upper limb and trunk) in preparation and support of the movement. In later stages of learning, children focus on the regulatory parameters of movements (e.g., speed, force, acceleration, etc.) that are usually acquired and modified as children refine and recalibrate their task interactions.

Therefore, motor skill acquisition can be optimized by utilizing specific strategies and conditions (Wulf & Lewthwaite, 2016). According to the optimal theory of motor learning, motor skill acquisition can be facilitated utilizing tasks that are intrinsically motivating to children and capture their attention toward goals that are important to them. In early stages of learning, a key factor is to enhance children's expectations (boost their confidence) for future performance to support their stamina through intense practice, repetitions, and possibly frustration. Giving children choices (promoting autonomy and agency) within the given tasks motivates engagement and activity participation.

Intense Physical and Mental Practice

Intense practice is a well-established principle in motor skill acquisition. Although specific practice regimes are not established, general principles are clearly outlined to guide occupational therapy interventions. Specific strategies further enhance the effectiveness of practice:

1) Expand on children's abilities, using their problem-solving skills (error-based learning) in the context of tasks. Start by simplifying the task to provide the "just right challenge" in order to be close to the child's current level of abilities. Then introduce challenges requiring problem-solving strategies that improve memorization and retention of motor skills (Chien & Chen, 2018; Polatajko et al., 2001). For example, instead of providing hand-over-hand assistance or detailed verbal instructions, practitioners can better support motor skill acquisition if they simplify the task to the level that the child can problem solve their movements and strategies with limited external assistance. In Figure 11.1, the therapist has set up the task so that the child starts stacking the single hole shapes, then moves to the more complex hole shapes. After the child problem solves through the first easier versions of the task, they can then proceed to more complex shapes (matching the holes of the square shapes).

   Following this facilitatory process, children can learn motor skills in a meaningful and engaging manner expanding on their abilities. In this picture when the child starts with the single hole shape, they learn the control parameters of movement, that is how to position their body away from the structure, use their fingers to reach grasp, hold, and manipulate shapes, and align the hole on the shape to the stacking pole. After a few repetitions with the single-hole shape, they learn the regulatory parameters of the task. The child learns to use adequate timing and force to make the shape go through. They have

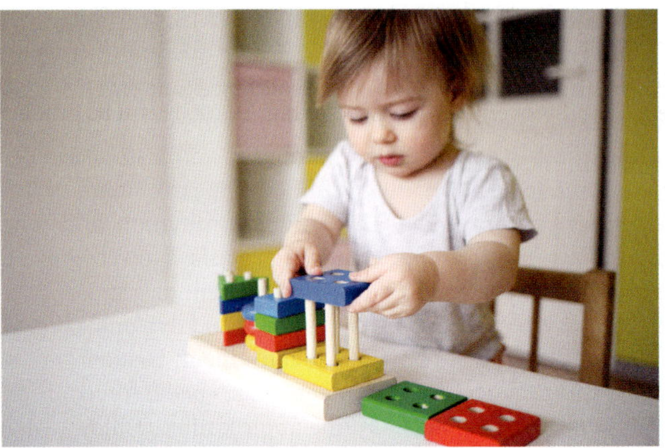

FIGURE 11.1 Child problem solves through the task. Note: Task progresses from east to difficult providing intrinsic feedback. Credit: Natalia Bodrova iStock photo ID:1254783988.

the opportunity to self-correct increasing their agency and autonomy with the task with high probability of developing, planning (prospectivity), and flexibility skills as the task progresses to higher levels of difficulty.

2) Repetitive practice alone does not enhance motor skill acquisition. Repetitive practice can support movements but does not translate in motor skill acquisition and functionality. Using repetitive movements to increase range of motion or improve strength can support motor skill acquisition if it is accompanied by practice and training of motor skill in the context of natural tasks and activities.

3) Practice should be embedded in activities that resemble daily life situations. However, these activities can be complex and may require multiple movements, multiple tasks, and several motor skills. If this process is too complex for the child, the therapist needs to structure practice relative to the tasks and movements the specific child needs to learn. Whole/part-activity practice is very important to translate movement to motor skill acquisition and functional ability (de Camargo Barros et al., 2017). See case study for examples/pictures of whole/part practice.

   a. Whole-activity practice: Even in the early stages of learning, engaging in whole-activity practice provides children with a goal that is real and meaningful, exposes them to the nature of the entire problem they need to solve, and has them engage in practice using multiple systems. Whole-activity practice is interspersed between part-task/activity practice to assist with transfer of skills. Children are motivated and learn more effectively when the whole activity is embedded in their practice. Typically developing children and children with neurodevelopmental problems alike practice more, perform better, and acquire motor skills, when they engage in whole-activity practice. Engaging in the whole activity requires children to process stimuli and respond to changes within and between systems (i.e., person, task, environment). The ability to respond in variable ways is a hallmark of goal-directed functional movement. Typically developing children, for example, use multiple motor strategies when moving, as opposed to children with DCD, who have been found to exhibit limited variability and adaptability in their movement. Therefore, one goal of occupational therapy intervention geared toward improvement in motor control, is to promote variability and flexibility in movements through whole training.

b. Part-task/activity practice: Part-task practice aims to build motor capacity (i.e., improve joint alignment, planning, precision) by reducing complex activity into smaller component steps. Tasks are still part of the overall activity, but they receive increased attention and repetition. Parts of the task and movement that need to be developed can be practiced separately and within the activity. The best way to integrate part-task practice to the whole activity is through the process of backward chaining. In this process, the child practices the last steps of the activity first (faster access to the rewarding result of the activity). From there the child works backward toward gradually completing the entire activity. This process not only supports learning of specific movements (i.e., thumb opposition when holding a spoon) and learning of parts of the activity that may be hard for the child (i.e., bring the spoon to the mouth without spillage) but it also is the best way to teach motor plans for sequential tasks.

4) Early stages of learning and difficult motor patterns require blocked practice (presenting the same activity repeatedly) with little variability to support memorization of motor patterns and movement sequences that are complex and difficult for the child. Later stages of learning require gradual transition to random and distributed practice (changing sequence and activities), with rest between practice regimes to allow for memory consolidation (Gill et al., 2018).

5) Mental practice refers to the ability to mentally rehearse a skill without any physical execution. Typically developing children as young as 8 years of age can engage successfully in mental practice. It is an effective method for practicing motor skills as it requires little effort and can be applied in different environments. It has strong evidence for supporting motor skill acquisition and transfer of skills from one activity to another and from one context to the other (Hall, 1985).

Feedback

Feedback is an important strategy to enhance motor skill acquisition. There are two types of feedback. *Extrinsic feedback* is verbal, visual, and haptic (hand over hand) feedback provided by the practitioner and *intrinsic feedback* is feedback provided from the interaction with the activity itself. Early stages of learning require extrinsic and intrinsic feedback to better understand the activity, tasks, and movements involved (Bishop et al., 2018). Later stages of learning mostly focus on intrinsic feedback to promote autonomy and sustain motor performance. A well-known form of extrinsic feedback is *knowledge of performance*. This is feedback that provides cues helpful to improve movement quality, task sequencing and completion, and supports the establishment of basic motor performance. *Knowledge of results* is another type of feedback that focuses on the motor skill outcomes. It communicates the goals and can be used as a means of motivation to support achievements as children accomplish tasks (parts of an activity).

Variability

Variability is the hallmark of daily function and participation. It poses a significant challenge in the process of motor skill acquisition, as it can introduce confusion and hinder the process of learning if children are exposed to it too early in the learning process. However, without variability motor skill flexibility and adaptability is not possible (Adolph et al., 2018). Variability can be introduced gradually within the context of one activity in one environment and based on the child's performance increase to multiple activities in multiple environments.

Transfer of Skills

Transfer of skills refers to generalization of skills from one activity and situation to novel activities and alternative situations. Children need to work toward this level of motor skill acquisition prior to discharge. For example, excellent handwriting skills in the context of the therapy session does not accomplish the functional goal of improving handwriting in the classroom. Some children can transfer skills partially or entirely and others need practice in new environments to be able to perform learned skills within novel contexts. Transfer of skills training should not be the last aspect of the intervention. It is better accomplished if children are exposed to natural environment conditions as part of the motor skill acquisition training process (Jarus & Gutman, 2001).

FUNCTION/DYSFUNCTION CONTINUA

The motor skill acquisition frame of reference has two continua that define the child's ability to perform specific tasks based on indicators of functional ability and indicators of motor skills. The function/dysfunction continua of the motor skill acquisition frame of reference begin with acknowledging that motor skills support functional activities that are meaningful for the child. Functional abilities are examined in natural environments taking into consideration children's developmental level. Practitioners examine children's agency, prospectivity, flexibility, and adaptability when addressing motor skills in the context of daily activities (Table 11.1).

Practitioners must also consider function/dysfunction as related to a child's developmental level, their motor control, and in the context of motor learning. Therapists evaluate underlying person factors (sensorimotor, cognitive, psychosocial skills) and musculoskeletal factors (bone, joint, muscle health, and function). Task complexity is assessed using knowledge of tasks analysis and skilled behavior required in the contexts in which children are required to perform their functional activities. Often, neurodevelopmental problems or trauma interfere with the expected developmental level of motor skills associated with the child's chronologic age. Therefore, as with all assessment, the developmental level of current motor skills always needs to be considered. It is also recommended that therapists evaluate two to three contexts in which the activities are performed to measure the impact of context on motor skill acquisition (Table 11.2).

Practitioners can identify function/dysfunction continua for any task that is necessary for the child to perform in their environment. When applying the motor skill acquisition frame of reference, practitioners need to always consider the environment and should analyze each environment in which the child is expected to perform those tasks.

GUIDE FOR EVALUATION

Occupational therapists use their knowledge of human development, motor control, and learning to assess children's abilities in the context of functional tasks. The evaluation process starts with the formation of an occupational profile that establishes children's occupations, interests, and priorities. Families and school systems, as the supportive systems for motor skill acquisition, collaborate in the development of the occupational profile. Interviews and checklists are used to gather this information. Then utilizing the function and disfunction continua, therapists are able to determine the child's skill level and appropriate goals areas.

Therapists evaluate functional abilities (agency, prospectivity, flexibility, and adaptability) as well as underlying person factors (sensorimotor, cognitive, psychosocial skills) and musculoskeletal

Table 11.1 Function/Dysfunction Continua: Indicators of Functional Ability

Agency	
Function	**Dysfunction**
Chooses own goals, practices motor skills, engages or self-initiates in decisions, positive affect	Does not set goals, does not practice motor skills, disinterested in making decisions, flat or negative affect
Indicators of Function	**Indicators of Dysfunction**
Chooses own goals	Does not set goals
Practices motor skills	Does not practice motor skills
Engages or self-initiates in decisions	Is not interested in making decisions
Demonstrates positive affect	Demonstrates flat or negative affect
Prospectivity	
Function	**Dysfunction**
Plans and anticipates the consequences of motor actions	Does not plan or anticipate the consequences of motor actions
Indicators of Function	**Indicators of Dysfunction**
Plans motor actions	Unable to plan or poorly plans motor actions
Accurately anticipates the consequences of motor actions	Does not anticipate the consequences of motor actions or makes inaccurate estimates
Flexibility	
Function	**Dysfunction**
Able to detect errors in motor actions and shift the behavior to alter the outcome	Unable to detect errors, unable to shift behavior to alter the motor outcomes
Indicators of Function	**Indicators of Dysfunction**
Error detection	Unable to detect errors
Change strategies to improve motor outcomes	Unable to change strategies to improve movement outcomes
Adaptability	
Function	**Dysfunction**
Able to use learned strategies in novel tasks and contexts	Unable to use learned strategies in novel tasks and contexts
Indicators of Function	**Indicators of Dysfunction**
Detects and uses learned strategies in novel tasks	Unable to detect and use learned strategies in novel tasks
Detects and uses learned strategies to accomplish tasks in novel contexts	Unable to detect and use learned strategies in novel contexts

Table 11.2 Function/Dysfunction Continua: Motor Control & Motor Learning

Function	Dysfunction
Person factors: sensorimotor, cognitive, psychosocial, and musculoskeletal systems are functional	One or more person factors: sensorimotor, cognitive, psychosocial, and musculoskeletal systems are not fully functional
Indicators of Function	**Indicators of Dysfunction**
Specific body structures and functions support motor skill	Specific body structures and functions do not support motor skill
Planning and error detection is evident in motor actions	Planning and/or error detection are not evident in motor actions
Cognitive control of motor actions is present	Cognitive control of motor actions is not present
Behavioral processes support motor actions	Behavioral processes hinder motor actions
Motor learning	
Function	**Dysfunction**
Implicit learning is present	Implicit learning is not present
Explicit learning is present	Explicit learning is not present
Indicators of Function	**Indicators of Dysfunction**
Able to problem solve task	Has difficulty or is unable to problem solve task
Able to detect intrinsic feedback	Has difficulty or is unable to detect intrinsic feedback
Able to engage in intense practice	Has difficulty or is unable to engage in intense practice
Able to engage in whole-activity, part-task practice	Has difficulty or is unable to engage in whole-activity, part-task practice
Able to engage in mental practice	Has difficulty or is unable to engage in mental practice
Able to understand and use explicit feedback	Has difficulty or is unable to understand and use explicit feedback
Able to transfer learned skills in novel tasks and environments	Has difficulty or is unable to transfer learned skills in novel tasks and environments

factors (bone, joint, muscle health, and function) when assessing motor control (see Tables 11.1 and 11.2). Therapists need to consider task complexity using knowledge of tasks analysis and skilled behavior in the contexts in which children are required to perform their functional activities when evaluating the ability to perform motor tasks within their daily occupations. It is recommended that therapists evaluate several contexts in which the activities are performed to measure the impact of context on motor skill acquisition.

POSTULATES REGARDING CHANGE

General Postulates Regarding Change

Motor skill acquisition is a gradual process that starts with learning of the control parameters (nature and shape) of movements that are necessary to accomplish tasks and activities (early stages of learning) and progresses to learning regulatory aspects of movements (i.e., speed, timing, force) as movements become more automated and integrated in tasks and activities (later stages of learning). Early stages of learning benefit from intense part-task practice, more blocked practice, and the use of explicit feedback. Later stages of learning benefit from using whole-task practice, intrinsic feedback, and variability.

Directional Postulates Regarding Change

Based on the theoretical base the following general directional principles apply for motor skill acquisition:

1. Children's motor skills will improve if practiced within daily activities that are interesting and meaningful to them.
2. Children's motor skills will improve if children are presented with activities that present the "just right challenge."
3. Children's motor skills will improve if the therapist provides activities that follow motor control and learning principles taking into consideration the child's developmental level.
4. Children's motor skills will improve if they are practiced within the context of natural activities in the child's natural environment.

Specific Postulates Regarding Change

1. If the therapist provides the child with tasks that encourage the use of movements the child needs to learn and develop, within tasks that are meaningful and simplified to the child's level of "just right challenge," the child's motor skill performance will improve.
2. If the therapist provides intense blocked and randomized practice of movements and tasks the child needs to develop, the child's motor skill performance will improve.
3. If the therapist provides opportunities for practicing part-task movements and tasks to improve the child's motor capacity, as well as whole-activity practice, the child's motor skill performance will improve.
4. If the therapist provides explicit feedback (knowledge of performance, knowledge of results) in early stages of learning and gradually replaces this feedback with intrinsic feedback embedded in the tasks and activities, the child's motor skill performance will improve.
5. If the therapist provides opportunities for problem solving (error-based learning) during learning to enhance memory of strategies, the child's motor skill performance will improve.
6. If the therapist provides problem solving with immediate feedback (errorless learning) when the child has significant problems with memory and processing skills, the child's motor skill performance will improve.
7. If the therapist provides opportunities for variable practice of movements, tasks, and activities in a variety of environments, the child's motor skill performance will improve.

APPLICATION TO PRACTICE

The intervention process begins with the practitioner examining the functional goals and priorities for the child and their families. The level of functional abilities is determined, and it is clearly communicated that the focus of the intervention is to expand on these functional abilities. The child's agency, that is the active engagement, choice demonstration, and initiation of tasks pertaining to the functional activities, is examined. Providing choices supports learning and increases self-esteem. Children and adolescents are likely to practice motor skills that are important to them in order to expand their functional abilities. The practitioner functions as a facilitator; tasks, activities, and challenges are discussed and agreed in common.

As children/adolescents engage in the intervention process the practitioner observes prospective control of motor actions. Is the child able to plan ahead? Do they have expectations of specific outcomes for their actions? If not, is the activity too complex? How can it be simplified? Are the children able to problem solve through the activity or are they fully dependent on external assistance and feedback? At this stage, practitioners utilize evaluation findings related to person factors (sensorimotor system, cognition, psychosocial abilities) to modify task complexity and the environment with the goal to create "the just right challenge" conditions in order for the child to problem solve, receive and use intrinsic feedback, and accomplish the task.

Early stages of learning are marked with slow, elaborate movements that are practiced constantly to perceive the shape and goal of the movement. Feedback, such as knowledge of performance and knowledge of results helps to improve precision and success. Practice is usually blocked with low to no variability so that movements can be shaped. Part tasks occupy the majority of the session with whole-activity practice serving as a reminder of the functional goal. As children/adolescents feel more comfortable they will demonstrate variability in their strategies to complete the tasks, practice regulatory task components (i.e., speed, timing, force), and are able to vary their motor responses and still succeed in the task. Later stages of learning involve whole-activity practice with increased variability. Movements, tasks, or whole activities are practiced in more than one context and feedback is mostly intrinsic (the child is able to receive it directly from the task).

It is important to note that although functional activities (i.e., dressing, writing, etc.) are specific and the ultimate goal of the intervention process, tasks, and movements can be broader and shared across functional activities. For example, the functional ability to get dressed (wearing a button-down shirt) is specific and during intervention practice will entail engaging in buttoning a shirt. However, the process of buttoning involves smaller tasks that practice movements using the pincer grasp, manipulating garments and small objects, finger isolation, planning, and sequencing motor patterns. These skills can be practiced using a variety of other tasks. For example, building structures with small Lego blocks, using tweezers or tongs to pick up small objects, etc. These alternative tasks introduce some variability and make the sessions engaging while still working on the specific motor skill acquisition and functional goals. Children and adolescents should be encouraged to think of these alternative tasks and problem solve through them with the therapist. This process supports agency and facilitates the client's ability to think of ways to practice their skills outside the session.

CASE EXAMPLE

Mark

Mark is a 5.5-year-old body diagnosed with cerebral palsy, spastic hemiplegia. He lives in a three-bedroom apartment with his two sisters and his parents. He attends a local public school for most of the day and has physical and occupational therapy sessions right after school. He receives some therapy services at school as well. Mark is ambulatory with some safety concerns when using the stairs (Gross Motor Function Classification System Level II). At school he attends an inclusive classroom and has a paraprofessional assigned to him for safety.

Occupational Therapy Evaluation

Mark's interests are drawing and creating superhero posters, engaging in play with peers at school and at home, and being able to dress independently so that he does not need to find his paraprofessional when going to the bathroom at school. His parents are concerned with his ability to remain seated during class work and lessons. He frequently gets tired and slides off his chair after 10 minutes of seat work. They also want him to improve his graphomotor and scissor cutting skills to keep up with first-grade expectations for reading and writing.

During the evaluation process, Mark was very motivated to engage in graphomotor tasks such as drawing and writing letters as well as using scissors. He was able to stop the activities and indicate where he was having specific difficulties. For example, he mentioned that he is bothered that his lines in his drawings are very curvy, and they interfere with the drawing outcome. He voiced his frustration with the scissors as he has difficulty placing the scissors and cutting within the lines. His letters had significant issues with alignment and spacing making his writing product illegible. He is aware of his performance and gets frustrated, stops working on the task and says that he is "stuck." Clinical observation on how he performs these activities indicates problems with prospective control of his actions (cannot organize more than two steps and does not anticipate the outcome of his work). He presents with a lack of flexibility in the strategies used, even when he is aware they are not working for him.

Assessments were utilized to better understand his functional activity performance in dressing (ABILHAND-Kids, Arnould et al., 2004), writing (Minnesota Handwriting Assessment, Reisman, 1999), and drawing as these were all noted to be areas of high priority for him. The therapist also assessed scissor cutting skills as this was a parental priority for Mark. Two developmental assessments were used to capture Mark's developmental level. A motor skill assessment (the Peabody Developmental Motor Scales-3, Folio & Fewell, 2023) and visual motor assessment (the Beery-Buktenica Developmental Test of Visual-Motor Integration [VMI], 6th Edition) (Beery & Beery, 2010). The Quality of Upper Extremity Skills Test (QUEST, DeMatteo et al., 1992) was also used to analyze movement patterns for unilateral and bilateral skills. The assessments revealed variable levels of abilities across different domains. Mark has strong visual perceptual skills and uses these to learn and organize his actions. His trunk and upper extremity on the left side are weak but functional. He can engage in bilateral tasks but when strength, precision, or stability are required his left side is not able to support the task. This particularly interfered with tasks that require coordination and precision such dressing, use of scissors, and writing.

Goals for the Occupational Therapy Intervention

Mark and his parents agreed to the following goals that address the functional abilities of using scissors, getting dressed, and writing drawing. His goals are as follows:

Goal 1: Mark will be able to use scissors to cut curved lines with 1/8 of an inch precision without assistance 80% of the time within 1 year.

Objective: Mark will be able to cut a straight line with 1/8 inch precision without assistance and with no need for supports (table).

Objective: Mark will be able to cut a semicircle with 1/8 inch precision without assistance and with no need for supports (table).

Goal 2: Mark will be able to dress independently using a button-down shirt with ¼ inch buttons, and pants with a zipper and a belt 80% of the times within 1 year.

Objective: Mark will be able manipulate buttons ½–¼ width with no assistance.

Objective: Mark will be able fasten and fasten a belt in a timely fashion with no assistance.

Objective: Mark will be able to zip and unzip zippers that require strength with no assistance.

Goal 3: Mark will be able to print legible letters and complete schoolwork at home using lined paper without assistance 80% of the times within 1 year.

Objective: Mark will be able to print two lines of legible letters without needing assistance to stabilize the paper or using breaks.

Objective: Mark will be able to a page of legible letters and short words without needing assistance to stabilize the paper or using breaks.

Intervention

Intervention began at home with the plan to practice and integrate the skills at school once he had developed some consistency in his desired motor skills. The first goal was to improve scissor skills. According to the motor skill acquisition frame of reference and the general postulate regarding change, Mark should be able to improve his scissor skills if we introduce a gradual process of learning. The first step was to analyze his motor patterns in the tasks or the entire activity. We observe (Figure 11.2) that the overall posture of his movement needs to shift. Mark needs to learn the control parameters of the movement, that is the nature and the shape of his movement and his ability to orient the scissors. We also observe that the task is too complex for him, as it poses challenges for him to concurrently stabilize the paper, plan his movements, and orient his scissors. Learning of the new motor skills begins with a task modification (Figure 11.3) to learn the shape of the movement and practice motor skills that relate to cutting through specific tasks: aligning the scissors to the paper for cutting, holding the paper with the assisting hand, snipping, and cutting parts of the line with the scissors. Practice within the session and in-home activities with his sisters was set to learn these tasks and the associated movements.

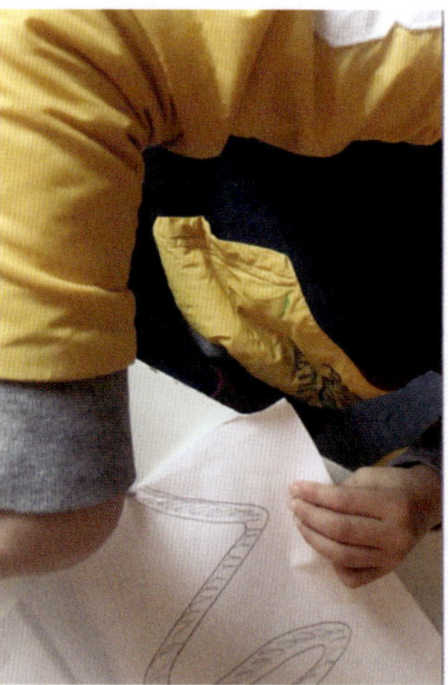

FIGURE 11.2 Child's posture and movement planning is inadequate for the task. Note: Task is too complex for the child to problem solve and learn.

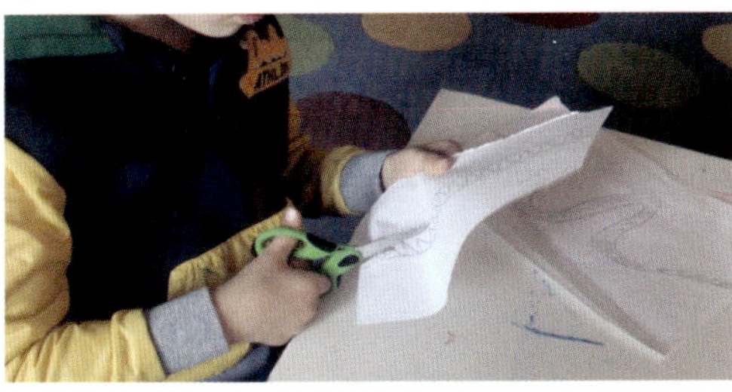

FIGURE 11.3 Task provides opportunities for problem solving and success ("Just right challenge"). Note: Child is able to learn new movements and practice them.

Similar to the paper cutting activity, cutting playdough for his younger sister, etc. helped him learn the shape of the movements and the motor plans. Eventually, he was able to shift the force he applied to the scissors and the paper, increase his speed, and the timing of his overall activity completion improved significantly. Communication with his teachers expanded this practice regime to school arts and crafts projects. Mark felt very proud and often said "I am the master of cutting straight lines." Mark progressed gradually from straight lines to slightly curved lines. Explicit feedback was provided to draw his attention to the assisting hand. While the shape and the pressure as well as the flexibility in the primary (dominant hand) were evident, the curved lines posed a need for the assisting hand to develop flexible motor patterns or turning the paper to accommodate cutting. Similarly, he slowed down to learn the shape of the new movements and the coordination between the two hands. Practice was somewhat variable between cutting straight lines and slightly curved lines. The occupational therapy sessions also included simple bilateral tasks where each arm/hand were given a different role (opening containers, bottles, etc.). Mark was challenged by these activities but persisted. Mark continued to practice at school and at home. He was now able to cut complex curved lines without any assistance but needed to improve his strength and coordination (Figure 11.4) to meet his functional goal. Variable practice was embedded in his free time activities of creating superhero posters. His hand and arm got stronger and this process facilitated improvement of his pencil grasp and increase in his stamina for both cutting and writing activities.

The second goal was for Mark to learn how to use buttons and zippers to be able to dress independently. For this goal, along with the general postulate regarding change, we used the specific postulate regarding change that if the therapist provides opportunities

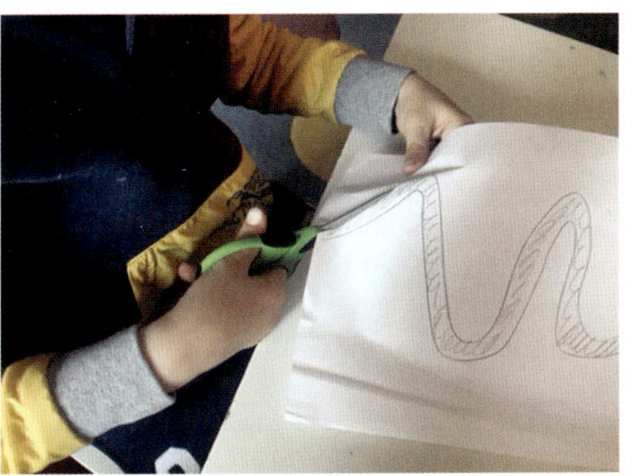

FIGURE 11.4 Task complexity can increase as the child acquires new motor skills. Note: The child practices speed, timing, forces needed for this complex activity.

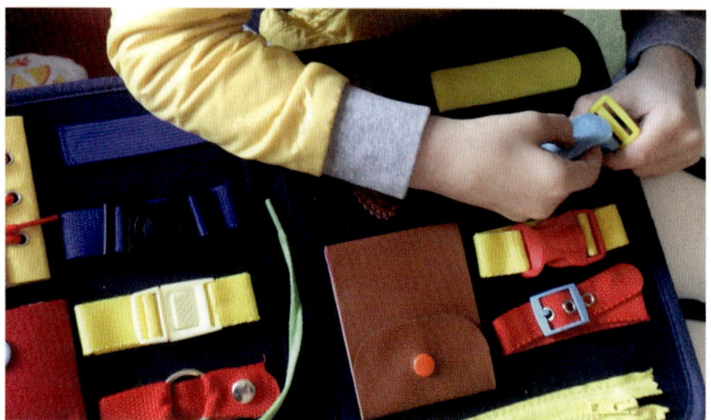

FIGURE 11.5 Part-task practice. Note: The child practices the steps and movements to learn how to use a belt.

for practicing part-task movements and whole activities the child will improve their motor capacity. To accomplish part task practice we introduced a fasteners activity board. The board had all types of fasteners for Mark (Figure 11.5). He was able to practice breaking the steps down even further and learn to plan his movements, the coordination of both sides of the body, and the shape of his grasp (early stages of learning).

Eventually, he was able to increase the speed, applied the correct pressure, sequenced his movements, and was able to zip/unzip, button/unbutton, and fasten/unfasten the belt on the board. As part of his whole-activity practice, he practiced putting on and button/unbutton a shirt with large buttons, using the mirror for feedback. The practitioner also provided explicit feedback of knowledge of performance (i.e., "remember your three steps," "slow down and look at your fingers"). Other activities (i.e., small Lego construction, chalkboard drawing) that practiced manipulation skills, sequencing of movements, and visual motor skills were used in the session to keep Mark engaged. Mark was able to put on his pants without help within 6 months, became independent in donning/doffing his coat, and continued to challenge himself with button down shirts.

Last, for handwriting and drawing, we built upon the manipulation skills (from work in dressing activities), and the grasp strength skills (via scissor skills) he had developed. Mark also needed to work on his core and shoulder strength and stability, as well as his wrist/finger flexibility as writing and drawing tasks required more stamina and precision than the other two tasks. Using environmental modification by providing a vertical board helped lower the task expectation and to build both core and shoulder strength. Parallel to learning motor skills in the context of the actual activity, exercises for developing core strength were introduced. Mark's letters were more legible at the end of 6 months. We introduced a slanted board at home and at school for his writing activities. We also introduced a visual cue for him to monitor his posture (while he continues to build his skills). When he felt he was sliding on his chair or his body was moving away from his hand he would "stop" and "sit up tall." We introduced this strategy in the context of the game where he won points every time he remembered to stop and sit up for a prize. Mark got used to this process and was able to readjust his body on the chair about 50% of the time.

SUPPORTING EVIDENCE

There are several motor skill acquisition guidelines in pediatrics (Araneda et al., 2020; Friel et al., 2016; Izadi-Najafabadi et al., 2015; Yu et al., 2018; Molinaro et al., 2022). Most of them focus on children with specific diagnosis and aim to improve motor patterns and address underlying person, task, and environmental factors. One such example is the Hand-Arm Bimanual Intensive Therapy (HABIT) protocol. The HABIT protocol (Friel et al., 2016) suggests task simplification for children to learn new motor tasks, supports part-task practice of movements needed for the performance of complex activities, as well as working on whole-task learning for functional ability development. Systematic studies suggest that there should be at least 60 hours of intensive practice with the HABIT protocol for changes in behavior and for neuroplasticity to occur. In a recent study, Friel et al., 2016, tested the effects of HABIT on manual skills and motor cortex plasticity in children with unilateral spastic cerebral palsy. The researchers compared structured skill training using HABIT with unstructured hand use activities (controls). Each group received 90 hours of intervention across 3 weeks. The groups were tested before, immediately after, and 6 months after the intervention using as a primary outcome the Jebsen-Taylor Test of Hand Function. Both groups showed significant improvements in bimanual hand use and hand dexterity. However, only the HABIT group showed increases in the size of the affected hand's motor cortical region.

For most of these interventions functional ability is a secondary outcome. However, in the motor skill acquisition guidelines, functionality is the starting point for the evaluation and intervention process. The premise here is that working to facilitate improvement in children's/adolescents' motor skills is not enough to promote function. Activity-based interventions that are meaningful, promote agency, autonomy, flexibility of strategies and adaptability are necessary components in the acquisition of motor skills.

REFERENCES

Adolph, K. E., & Hoch, J. E. (2019). Motor development: Embodied, embedded, enculturated, and enabling. *Annual Review of Psychology*, *70*, 141–164. https://doi.org/10.1146/annurev-psych-010418-102836

Adolph, K. E., & Kretch, K. S. (2015). Gibson's theory of perceptual learning. *International Encyclopedia of the Social and Behavioral Sciences*, *10*, 127–134. https://doi.org/10.1016/b978-0-08-097086-8.23096-1

Adolph, K. E., & Robinson, S. R. (2015). Motor development. *Handbook of Child Psychology and Developmental Science*, 1–45. https://doi.org/10.1002/9781118963418.childpsy204

Adolph, K. E., Cole, W. G., Komati, M., Garciaguirre, J. S., Badaly, D., Lingeman, J. M., Chan, G. L. Y., & Sotsky, R. B. (2012). How do you learn to walk? Thousands of steps and dozens of falls per day. *Psychological Science*, *23*(11), 1387–1394. https://doi.org/10.1177/0956797612446346

Adolph, K. E., Hoch, J. E., & Cole, W. G. (2018). Development (of walking): 15 suggestions. *Trends in Cognitive Sciences*, *22*(8), 699–711. https://doi.org/10.1016/j.tics.2018.05.010

Alesi, M., & Battaglia, G. (2019). Motor development and Down syndrome. In: *International Review of Research in Developmental Disabilities* (Vol. 56, pp. 169–211). Academic Press. https://doi.org/10.1016/bs.irrdd.2019.06.007

American Occupational Therapy Association. (2020). Occupational therapy practice framework: Domain and process-fourth edition. (2020). *The American Journal of Occupational Therapy*, *74*(Supplement_2), 7412410010p1–7412410010p87. https://doi.org/10.5014/ajot.2020.74S2001

Araneda, R., Sizonenko, S. V., Newman, C. J., Dinomais, M., Le Gal, G., Ebner-Karestinos, D., Paradis, J., Klöcker, A., Saussez, G., Demas, J., Bailly, R., Bouvier, S., Nowak, E., Guzzetta, A., Riquelme, I., Brochard, S., & Bleyenheuft, Y. (2020). Protocol of changes induced by early Hand-Arm Bimanual Intensive Therapy Including Lower Extremities (e-HABIT-ILE) in pre-school children with bilateral cerebral palsy: A multisite randomized controlled trial. *BMC Neurology*, *20*(1), 1–10. https://doi.org/10.1186/s12883-020-01820-2

Arnould, C., Renders, A., Penta, M., & Thonnard J-L. (2004). ABILHAND-Kids. A measure of manual ability in children with cerebral palsy. *Neurology*, *63*, 1045–1052.

Babik, I., Galloway, J. C., & Lobo, M. A. (2022). Early exploration of one's own body, exploration of objects, and motor, language, and cognitive development relate dynamically across the first two years of life. *Developmental Psychology*, *58*(2), 222–235. https://doi.org/10.1037/dev0001289

Bäckström, A., Johansson, A. M., Rudolfsson, T., Rönnqvist, L., von Hofsten, C., Rosander, K., & Domellöf, E. (2021). Motor planning and movement execution during goal-directed sequential manual movements in 6-year-old children with autism spectrum disorder: A kinematic analysis. *Research in Developmental Disabilities*, *115*, 104014. https://doi.org/10.1016/j.ridd.2021.104014

Beard, J. R., Officer, A., De Carvalho, I. A., Sadana, R., Pot, A.M., Michel, J. P., Lloyd-Sherlock, P., Epping-Jordan, J. E., Peeters, G., Mahanani, W. R., Thiyagarajan, J. A., Chatterji, S. (2016). The World report on ageing and health: a policy framework for healthy ageing. *The Lancet*, *387*(10033), 2145–2154. https://doi.org/10.1016/s0140-6736(15)00516-4

Beery, K. E., & Beery, N. A. (2010). *The Beery-Buktenica developmental test of visual-motor integration: Administration, scoring, and teaching manual* (6th ed.). NCS Pearson.

Bishop, J. C., Kelly, L. K., & Hull, M. (2018). Knowledge of performance feedback among boys with ADHD. *Research in Developmental Disabilities*, *74*, 31–40. https://doi.org/10.1016/j.ridd.2017.12.003

Chien, K. P., & Chen, S. (2018). The influence of guided error-based learning on motor skills self-efficacy and achievement. *Journal of Motor Behavior*, *50*(3), 275–284.

D'Souza, H., Cowie, D., Karmiloff-Smith, A., & Bremner, A. J. (2017). Specialization of the motor system in infancy: From broad tuning to selectively specialized purposeful actions. *Developmental Science*, *20*(4), e12409. https://doi.org/10.1111/desc.12409

de Camargo Barros, J. A., Tani, G., & Corrêa, U. C. (2017). Effects of practice schedule and task specificity on the adaptive process of motor learning. *Human Movement Science*, *55*, 196–210.

Delgado-Lobete, L., Montes-Montes, R., Pértega-Díaz, S., Santos-Del-Riego, S., Hartman, E., & Schoemaker, M. M. (2022). Motor performance and daily participation in children with and without probable developmental coordination disorder. *Developmental Medicine & Child Neurology*, *64*(2), 220–227. https://doi.org/10.1111/dmcn.15036

DeMatteo, C., Law, M., Russell, D., Pollock, N., Rosenbaum, P., & Walter, S. (1992). *QUEST: Quality of upper extremity skills test*. McMaster University, CanChild Centre for Childhood Disability Research.

Dimitropoulou, K., O'Brien, J., & Coker-Bolt, P. (In press). Application of motor control and learning. In *Case-Smith's occupational therapy for children and adolescents*.

Donath, L., Faude, O., Hagmann, S., Roth, R., & Zahner, L. (2015). Fundamental movement skills in preschoolers: A randomized controlled trial targeting object control proficiency. *Child: Care, Health and Development*, *41*(6), 1179–1187. https://doi.org/10.1111/cch.12232

Eccleston, C. (2015). Embodied and embedded. *Embodied*, 251–260. https://doi.org/10.1093/acprof:oso/9780198727903.003.0012

Engel-Yeger, B., & Hanna Kasis, A. (2010). The relationship between developmental co-ordination disorders, child's perceived self-efficacy and preference to participate in daily activities. *Child: Care, Health and Development*, *36*(5), 670–677. https://doi.org/10.1111/j.1365-2214.2010.01073.x

Folio, M. R., & Fewell, R. R. (2023). *Peabody developmental motor scales, third edition (PDMS-3)*. Pro-Ed Inc.

Friel, K. M., Kuo, H. C., Fuller, J., Ferre, C. L., Brandão, M., Carmel, J. B., Bleyenheuft, Y., Gowatsky, J. L., Stanford, A. D., Rowny, S. B., Luber, B., Bassi, B., Murphy, D. L. K., Lisanby, S. H., & Gordon, A. M. (2016). Skilled bimanual training drives motor cortex plasticity in children with unilateral cerebral palsy. *Neurorehabilitation and Neural Repair*, *30*(9), 834–844 https://doi.org/10.1177/1545968315625838

Gasser-Haas, O., Sticca, F., & Wustmann Seiler, C. (2020). Poor motor performance–do peers matter? Examining the role of peer relations in the context of the environmental stress hypothesis. *Frontiers in Psychology*, *11*, 498. https://doi.org/10.2378/peu2022.art10d

Gentile, A. M. (1998). Movement science: Implicit and explicit processes during acquisition of functional skills. *Scandinavian Journal of Occupational Therapy*, *5*(1), 7–16. https://doi.org/10.3109/11038129809035723

Gibson, E. J. (1992). How to think about perceptual learning: Twenty-five years later. In H. L. Pick, P. W. van den Broek, & D. C. Knill (Eds.), *Cognition: Conceptual and methodological issues* (pp. 215–237). American Psychological Association. https://doi.org/10.1037/10564-009

Gill, S. V., Pu, X., Woo, N., & Kim, D. (2018). The effects of practice schedules on the process of motor adaptation. *Journal of Musculoskeletal and Neuronal Interactions*, *18*(4), 419–426.

Gordon, J., Maselli, A., Lancia, G. L., Thiery, T., Cisek, P., & Pezzulo, G. (2021). The road towards understanding embodied decisions. *Neuroscience & Biobehavioral Reviews*, *131*, 722–736. https://doi.org/10.1016/j.neubiorev.2021.09.034

Haggard, P. (2017). Sense of agency in the human brain. *Nature Reviews Neuroscience*, *18*(4), 196–207. https://doi.org/10.1038/nrn.2017.14

Hall, C. R. (1985). Individual differences in mental practice and imagery of motor skill performance. *Canadian Journal of Applied Sport Science*, *10*, 17S–21S.

Izadi-Najafabadi, S., Mirzakhani-Araghi, N., Miri-Lavasani, N., Nejati, V., & Pashazadeh-Azari, Z. (2015). Implicit and explicit motor learning: Application to children with Autism Spectrum Disorder (ASD). *Research in Developmental Disabilities*, *47*, 284–296. https://doi.org/10.1016/j.ridd.2015.09.020

Jarus, T., & Gutman, T. (2001). Effects of cognitive processes and task complexity on acquisition, retention, and transfer of motor skills. *Canadian Journal of Occupational Therapy*, *68*(5), 280–289. https://doi.org/10.1177/000841740106800504

Krakauer, J. W., Hadjiosif, A. M., Xu, J., Wong, A. L., & Haith, A. M. (2019). Motor learning. *Comprehensive Physiology*, *9*(2), 613–663. https://doi.org/10.1002/cphy.c170043

Magill, R. A., & Anderson, D. I. (2010). *Motor learning and control*. McGraw-Hill Publishing.

Masini, A., Marini, S., Leoni, E., Lorusso, G., Toselli, S., Tessari, A., Ceciliani, A., & Dallolio, L. (2020). Active breaks: A pilot and feasibility study to evaluate the effectiveness of physical activity levels in a school-based intervention in an Italian primary school. *International Journal of Environmental Research and Public Health*, *17*(12), 4351. https://doi.org/10.3390/ijerph17124351

Maxwell, J. P., Capio, C. M., & Masters, R. S. (2017). Interaction between motor ability and skill learning in children: Application of implicit and explicit approaches. *European Journal of Sport Science*, *17*(4), 407–416. https://doi.org/10.1080/17461391.2016.1268211

McIsaac, T. L., Lamberg, E. M., & Muratori, L. M. (2015). Building a framework for a dual task taxonomy. *BioMed Research International*, 2015. https://doi.org/10.1155/2015/591475

Michalski, J., Green, A. M., & Cisek, P. (2020). Reaching decisions during ongoing movements. *Journal of Neurophysiology*, *123*(3), 1090–1102. https://doi.org/10.1152/jn.00613.2019

Molinaro, A., Micheletti, S., Pagani, F., Garofalo, G., Galli, J., Rossi, A., Fazzi, E., & Buccino, G. (2022). Action Observation Treatment in a tele-rehabilitation setting: A pilot study in children with cerebral palsy. *Disability and Rehabilitation*, *44*(7), 1107–1112.

Nobusako, S., Osumi, M., Hayashida, K., Furukawa, E., Nakai, A., Maeda, T., & Morioka, S. (2020). Altered sense of agency in children with developmental coordination disorder. *Research in Developmental Disabilities*, *107*, 103794. https://doi.org/10.1016/j.ridd.2020.103794

Novak, I., & Honan, I. (2019). Effectiveness of paediatric occupational therapy for children with disabilities: A systematic review. *Australian Occupational Therapy Journal*, *66*(3), 258–273. https://doi.org/10.1111/1440-1630.12573

Pezzulo, G., & Cisek, P. (2016). Navigating the affordance landscape: feedback control as a process model of behavior and cognition. *Trends in Cognitive Sciences*, *20*(6), 414–424. https://doi.org/10.1016/j.tics.2016.03.013

Polatajko, H., Mandich, A.D., Miller, L.T. (2001). Cognitive Orientation to daily Occupational Performance (CO-OP): Part II—the evidence. *Physical & Occupational Therapy in Pediatrics*, *20*, 83–106. https://doi.org/10.1080/j006v20n02_06

Reddy, V., Markova, G., & Wallot, S. (2013). Anticipatory adjustments to being picked up in infancy. *PloS one*, *8*(6), e65289. https://doi.org/10.1371/journal.pone.0065289

Reisman, J. (1999). *Minnesota Handwriting Assessment*. Harcourt Assessment.

Risen, S. R., Barber, A. D., Mostofsky, S. H., & Suskauer, S. J. (2015). Altered functional connectivity in children with mild to moderate TBI relates to motor control. *Journal of Pediatric Rehabilitation Medicine*, *8*(4), 309–319. https://doi.org/10.3233/prm-150349

Schambra, H. M., Parnandi, A., Pandit, N. G., Uddin, J., Wirtanen, A., & Nilsen, D. M. (2019). A taxonomy of functional upper extremity motion. *Frontiers in Neurology*, *10*, 857. https://doi.org/10.3389/fneur.2019.00857

Thelen, E. (2005). Dynamic systems theory and the complexity of change. *Psychoanalytic Dialogues*, *15*(2), 255–283.

Thura, D., Cabana, J. F., Feghaly, A., & Cisek, P. (2022). Integrated neural dynamics of sensorimotor decisions and actions. *PLoS Biology*, *20*(12), e3001861. https://doi.org/10.1371/journal.pbio.3001861

Von Hofsten, C. (2004). An action perspective on motor development. *Trends in Cognitive Sciences*, *8*(6), 266–272. https://doi.org/10.1016/j.tics.2004.04.002

Williams, U., Law, M., Hanna, S., & Gorter, J. W. (2019). Personal, environmental, and family factors of participation among young children. *Child: Care, Health and Development*, *45*(3), 448-456. https://doi.org/10.1111/cch.12651

Wolpert, D. M., & Landy, M. S. (2012). Motor control is decision-making. *Current Opinion in Neurobiology*, *22*(6), 996–1003. https://doi.org/10.1016/j.conb.2012.05.003

World Health Organization. (2021). International classification of functioning, disability and health (ICF). https://doi.org/10.1037/t76403-000

Wulf, G., & Lewthwaite, R. (2016). Optimizing performance through intrinsic motivation and attention for learning: The OPTIMAL theory of motor learning. *Psychonomic Bulletin & Review*, *23*, 1382–1414. https://doi.org/10.3758/s13423-015-0999-9

Yu, J. J., Burnett, A. F., & Sit, C. H. (2018). Motor skill interventions in children with developmental coordination disorder: A systematic review and meta-analysis. *Archives of Physical Medicine and Rehabilitation*, *99*(10), 2076–2099. https://doi.org/10.1016/j.apmr.2017.12.009

Zalla, T., & Sperduti, M. (2015). The sense of agency in autism spectrum disorders: a dissociation between prospective and retrospective mechanisms?. *Frontiers in Psychology*, *6*, 1278. https://doi.org/10.3389/fpsyg.2015.01278

SECTION III

Section III

Frames of Reference With Specific Scope

Introduction to Section III

The frames of reference presented in this section focus on a specific area of practice or the development of specific skills. These frames of reference are often used in conjunction with other frames of reference. We believe that it is easier to learn a frame of reference in isolation, however in the real world frames of reference are rarely used alone. Given the complexity of children, it is unusual when one frame of reference can meet all of the clients' needs. Learning frames of reference one at a time allows the student or new practitioner to become fluent with the theories and understand its translation into application. Constructing an effective plan of intervention for a child with multiple areas of concern often requires more than one frame of reference (Mosey, 1986; Howe et al., 2020). The practitioner may use multiple frames of reference together sequentially, in parallel, or by combining them.

FRAMES OF REFERENCE IN SEQUENCE

This approach requires the practitioner to use one primary frame of reference to address the main areas of concern and then use another frame of reference for a more discrete problem that may not be covered with the first frame of reference. Alternatively, this approach may be used, when the first frame of reference really prepares the child for the use of the second frame of reference. In this case, the theoretical bases may not use the same approach to the change process. Each frame of reference would address different performance components and therefore does not necessarily need to be theoretically congruent. An example of this would be the use of Ayres Sensory Integration Frame of Reference (Chapter 6) to prepare an adolescent's sensory system for self-regulation and then implementing the use of the social participation frame of reference (Chapter 14) for peer-to-peer interaction in a group.

FRAMES OF REFERENCE IN PARALLEL

This approach has the practitioner use two frames of reference at the same time. These frames of reference are approaching similar problems from different perspectives. They are not combined but used separately, during the intervention process. While they are using different approaches, they are often addressing similar problems. Two frames of reference that work well in parallel and are often used this way are the neurodevelopment treatment approach (Chapter 8) and the biomechanical approach (Chapter 13). While neurodevelopment treatment uses handling as a tool for application, the biomechanical approach uses external positioning as a means of application. The biomechanical approach can help maintain the preferred position for an extended period of time, after a child receives physical input from handling. This is an oversimplification of these frames of reference, but it is meant to give an example of how two frames of reference can be used in parallel.

COMBINING FRAMES OF REFERENCE

This approach requires experience, skill, and a thorough understanding of the application of the theoretical components of a variety of frames of reference and is not recommended for novice practitioners. It is important for the practitioner to ensure the theoretical orientation of the two frames of reference are compatible. Combining two frames of references requires the approach used for the change process to be congruent as well, as in they are both developmentally oriented or both focusing an acquisitional orientation. An example of frames of reference that work well together are motor skill acquisition (Chapter 11) and handwriting (Chapter 12) as they both build upon congruent theoretical concepts and intervention techniques of how a child develops motor skills.

REFERENCES

Howe, T. H., Hinojosa, J., & Kramer, P. (2020). Frames of reference in the real world. In P. Kramer, J. Hinojosa, & T. H. Howe (Eds.), *Frames of reference for pediatric occupational therapy* (4th ed., pp. 557–569). Wolters-Kluwer.

Mosey, A. C. (1986). *Psychosocial components of occupational therapy*. Raven Press.

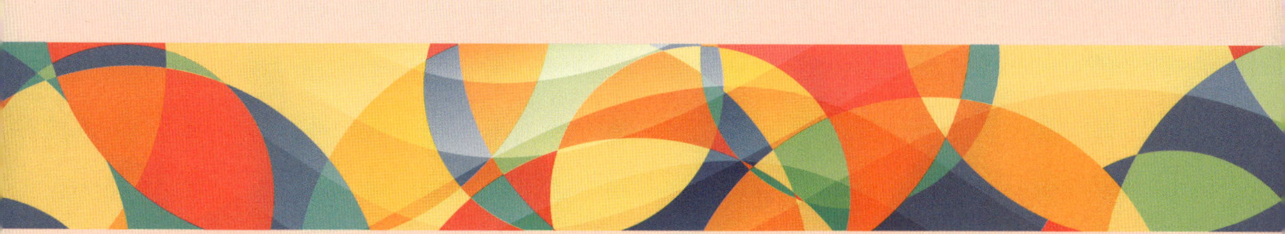

A Frame of Reference for Developing Handwriting Skills

Mindy Garfinkel

One of the primary occupations in which children engage, as identified in the *Occupational Therapy Practice Framework, 4th Edition* is education (American Occupational Therapy Association [AOTA], 2020). Handwriting remains a critically necessary skill for school-aged children, despite the increased time being used keyboarding, in and out of the school setting (Denton et al., 2006; Feder & Majnemer, 2007; Schneider et al., 2023; Schwellnus et al., 2013). It impacts academic participation, academic progress, and subsequently, inclusion of students in environments with same-aged peers (Denton et al., 2006; Feder & Majnemer, 2007; Graham et al., 2008). In a typical school day, students are required to copy from the board or books for assignments, transcribe class notes, complete worksheets, math problems, and write in journals. Handwriting and other literacy-based occupations take up approximately 30% to 60% of a student's school day (McHale & Cermack, 1992; Ritty et al., 1993); yet nearly 30% of typically developing children exhibit handwriting difficulties during their school career (Bonneton-Botte et al., 2023; Cermak & Bissell, 2014; Döhla & Heim, 2016; Karlsdottir & Stefansson, 2022). As such, the World Health Organization includes handwriting difficulties as one of the barriers to school participation (Jiménez, 2017). Further, handwriting difficulties are listed in the *Diagnostic and Statistical Manual of Mental Disorders* (5th ed.; American Psychiatric Association, 2013), coded under specific learning disorder, with impairment in written expression or developmental expressive writing disorder.

Handwriting, a complex process, and important occupation that a child performs as part of their role of being a student, requires the integration of several skills and systems. It involves language, cognitive, perceptual, sensory, and motor skills (Benbow, 2006; Donica et al., 2013; Lust & Donica, 2011). Additionally, psychosocial factors, postural control (Pade et al., 2018), visual–motor integration (Tse et al., 2019), bilateral integration, and writing tool use play significant roles in a student's success in mastering handwriting skills (Vico et al., 2023).

Poor handwriting performance has been linked to a child's overall emotional and physical well-being (Case-Smith et al., 2014; Graham et al., 2008). The literature suggests that children with poor handwriting skills may exhibit hand discomfort/pain, anxiety, lowered self-esteem, frustration, and fatigue (Feder & Majnemer, 2007; McHale & Cermak, 1992). Further, children who have difficulty with handwriting frequently use more energy and effort during handwriting tasks than their same-aged peers, leading to the need to focus on the mechanics of handwriting rather than the content of their message (Tseng & Cermak, 1993). Though these references are somewhat older, handwriting is still one of the primary reasons for occupational therapy referrals.

Further, evidence supports academic success is positively correlated to legible handwritten work that is completed in a timely manner. Graham et al. (2000) noted that students who were proficient in taking written notes in class demonstrated an increased ability to retain information presented in the classroom and produced schoolwork that was more grade appropriate and completed in a timelier manner, as compared to students exhibiting handwriting difficulties. Perceptual and perceptual-motor skills are critical predictors of academic performance and success during literacy-based tasks (Carlson et al., 2013; Pienaar et al., 2013; Schneck, 2020). The legibility of transcribed classwork is critical to a student's success in school (Laszlo & Broderick, 1991; Sudsawad et al., 2002; Weintraub & Graham, 1998). Further, higher grades are more frequently given to students producing legible work, which has been linked to the student's ability to advance to the next grade in school (Hammerschmidt & Sudsawad, 2004; Weintraub & Graham, 1998).

The frame of reference for developing handwriting skills targets elementary, middle, and high school-aged children and adolescents who exhibit difficulty communicating via written means, using a writing implement and paper. This frame of reference focuses on acquiring, developing, and/or remediating students' handwriting skills so that students may express themselves more effectively and efficiently (Graham et al., 2006; Howe et al., 2013; Santangelo & Graham, 2016).

It should be noted that the use of assistive technology, such as a laptop computer, may help a student to compensate for handwriting difficulties. However, there are many situations in life where handwriting is necessary. The use of assistive technology is not included in this frame of reference, as it does not address the acquisition, development, and/or remediation of handwriting skills.

THEORETICAL BASE

The theoretical base for this frame of reference for developing handwriting skills comes from theories of human development (Bronfenbrenner, 1986; Piaget, 1954), motor acquisition (Schmidt, 1975), visual perception, and sensory integration and processing (Ayres, 2005). Each of these theories are aligned with the tenets of occupational therapy as they consider the individual (person), the context (environment), and the task (occupation) (AOTA, 2020).

Human Development

Motor Development

Fine motor skills are the movements we make with our hands and fingers, including coordination of small muscle groups, and they allow us to perform our daily occupations. Children develop fine motor skills beginning at birth. Below are fine motor developmental milestones that must be mastered for a child to be successful in handwriting:

- 0 to 6 months of age: grasping
- 6 to 12 months: pinching objects between the thumb and other finger(s) and transferring objects from one hand to the other (crossing midline and bilateral coordination)
- 1 to 2 years: feeding self with a utensil; turning pages in a book (Figure 12.1)
- 2 to 3 years: turning a single page in a book; holding a crayon with the thumb and first two fingers
- 3 to 4 years: drawing copies of circles; using nondominant hand to assist and stabilize objects while using them

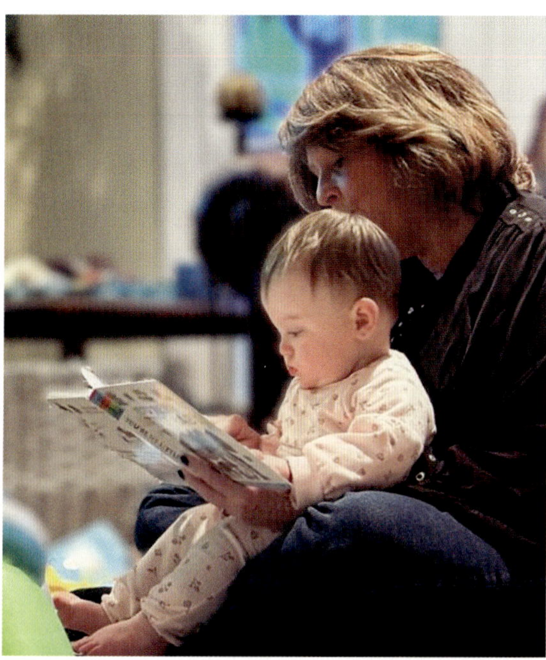

FIGURE 12.1 Child is turning pages in a book.

- 4 to 5 years: printing your name and the numbers 1 through 5
- 5 to 6 years: coloring within the lines; using a three-fingered grasp of a pencil
- 6 to 7 years: writing consistently on lines; writing most numbers and letters correctly (Cleveland Clinic, n.d.).

From a biomechanical perspective, the refined and precise fine motor skills required for handwriting are also contingent upon a stable base of support. Therefore, stability of the trunk, shoulder girdle, elbow, forearm, and wrist must be considered to support the child as they learn and develop their handwriting skills. Please see Chapter 13, A Biomechanical Frame of Reference to Position Children for Function for more information related to biomechanical theory and intervention guidelines.

Cognitive Development

Just as a certain level of physical maturation is necessary for a child to be able engage in handwriting tasks, so is a certain level of cognitive maturation. Jean Piaget saw cognitive development in children as resulting from the dynamic relationship between the child's abilities and the environment. Piaget is best known for identifying four stages of cognitive development in children (Piaget, 1954). He emphasized that child maturation and their interaction with the environment are two critical influences in child cognitive development, and that they occur in each of the four stages.

- The first stage is the *sensorimotor stage.* During this stage, young children aged birth to 2 years get to know the world through their senses and movements. Tactile, oral, kinesthetic, and visual systems are learning about the environment as the child masters motor milestones.

- The second stage of development is the *preoperational stage* and it occurs at approximately 2 to 7 years of age. During this stage, the child develops language and begins to use symbolic play. This stage is crucial for the development of handwriting skills, as handwriting is a form of language expression. Further, the concept of symbolism is critical to a child's ability to recognize that the letters of the alphabet, especially when used in words, represent things and concepts other than randomly configured lines on paper.
- The third and fourth stages of cognitive development *concrete operations* (ages 7 to 11), and *formal operations* (ages 12 through adulthood), respectively, are stages wherein the emergence of logical thought, the ability to reason deductively, and abstract thought become more developed. These skills are necessary for writing composition, a higher-level writing occupation.

Bronfenbrenner's Ecological Systems Theory (EST) of human development is a dynamic systems theory that considers the interplay of biologic, psychological, and social sciences, and how all the systems impact one another and the individual (Bronfenbrenner, 1986) (Figure 12.2). Five systems are identified as they relate to one another, and the child over time: the microsystem, mesosystem, exosystem, macrosystem, and the chronosystem. A description of each system with a school-based example is provided below.

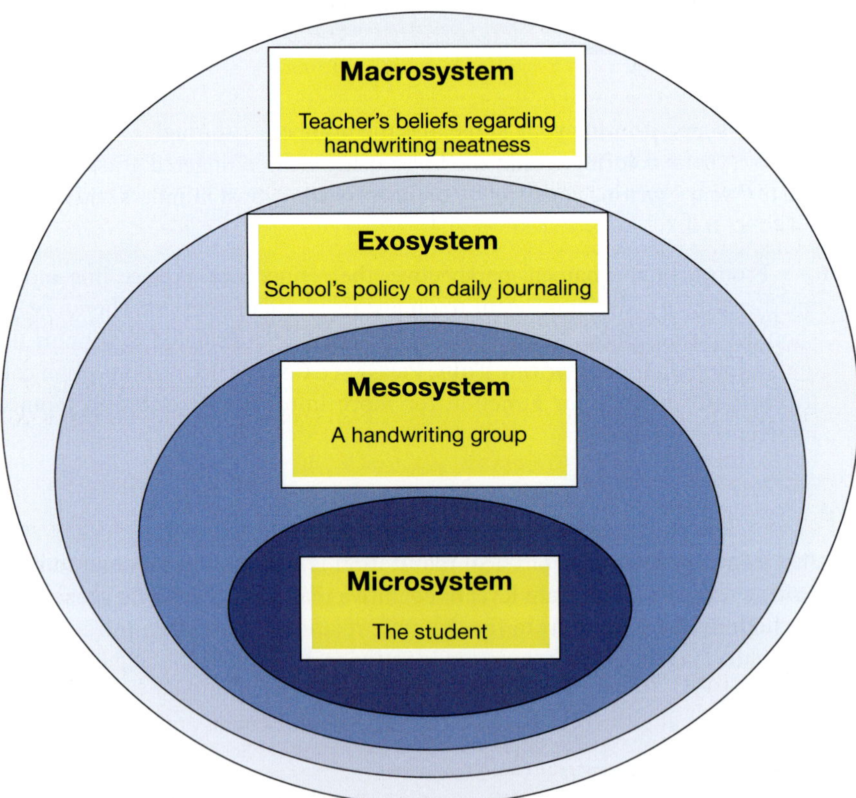

FIGURE 12.2 Bronfenbrenner's ecological systems theory as it relates to handwriting. (Adapted from Santrock, J. W. (2021). *Essentials of life-span development* (7th ed.). McGraw Hill Higher Education.)

The *microsystem* includes the child's personality, beliefs, and temperament, as well as individuals with whom a child has daily, face-to-face contact. This may include family members and educators (Bronfenbrenner, 1986). An example of a microsystem that impacts handwriting is a child's emotional state. Consider May, a 7-year-old whose father left on a long business trip over the weekend. When asked to write about how she spent her weekend, May sits in her seat and quietly cries, refusing to write in her journal.

The *mesosystem* is made up of links between multiple microsystems in a child's life (Bronfenbrenner, 1986). The classroom, classmates, and educators create a microsystem for an individual student. The school, broader student body, and the school staff comprise a mesosystem for the student (Bronfenbrenner, 1986). If we use the case of 7-year-old, May, an example of a mesosystem that impacts her handwriting in the classroom is her writing group. The small group discusses ideas in preparation for writing, and the students encourage one another to "do a good job."

The *exosystem* is like the mesosystem; however, at least one of the microsystems do not contain the student at the center of the system. While the student is not at the center of this system, they may be impacted by things that occur within the microsystem (Bronfenbrenner, 1986). Considering the case of May again, an example of an exosystem that affects her occupational engagement is the school's policy on journaling. All students are expected to journal during literacy blocks. This policy contributed to the group encouraging May to write in her journal, and offering her a way to participate, despite her emotional state; thereby supporting her occupational engagement.

The *macrosystem* represents culture and societal structures. In the case of May, an example of a macrosystem impacting her participation in handwriting is the teacher's cultural views on their own role in supporting handwriting skills. If May's teacher values handwriting highly, May will be provided with opportunities to engage in this occupation.

The *chronosystem* addresses the concept of time. It includes aging and maturation of the student, and the time in which they live and develop (Bronfenbrenner, 1986). The COVID pandemic is an example of a chronosystem that has impacted countless children's opportunities to engage in handwriting activities, as much of the educational process took place using a computer. Around the world, students who received their education in a school building, immediately post pandemic, received their education remotely, preventing most children from engaging in rich handwriting instruction and practice (Figure 12.2). This is an example of how a chronosystem can have a profound impact on a student's ability to develop handwriting skills (Garfinkel, 2024).

Motor Acquisition

Motor skill acquisition, which may also be referred to as motor learning, is the process by which individuals acquire and refine voluntary motor skills. It occurs as a result of intentional engagement in the learning process, practice of the motor skill being learned, and feedback. It occurs in stages as follows:

a. In the early stage, the child focuses on understanding what to do and actively problem solves, exploring strategies that match the task and the context or environment. They may gather information about the skill, by observing someone perform the skill, or by receiving verbal instructions. For example, a kindergarten student learning to write the letter "a" may observe their teacher demonstrating how to form the letter, listen to a song describing the steps, and see picture cues in a workbook for how to write the letter "a" (Figure 12.3).

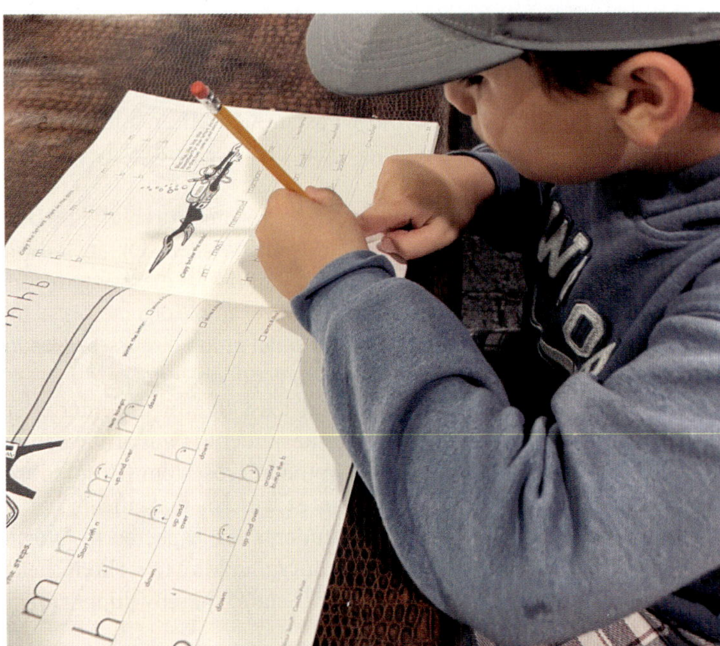

FIGURE 12.3 Child is copying letters in a workbook.

b. Next, the child plans a movement, executes it, and evaluates the effectiveness, based on feedback received. It is during this stage that the child learns to refine their movements by practicing and adjusting their technique. A child in this stage, learning to sign their name in cursive will practice, relying on the tactile, kinesthetic, and visual feedback received to guide them towards mastery.
c. The motor skill is acquired when self-evaluation reveals that motor performance meets the needs of the task within the given context or environment. Further, in this stage, students are able to form letters without intentional thought (automaticity) and efficiency is achieved as evidenced by a student's ability to write letters and words without conscious effort, allowing them to focus on concepts.

When assessing motor acquisition, the occupational therapist considers the child, elements of the task, and the environment/context. It is a dynamic process that does not necessarily follow a specific sequence. The evaluator observes child performance and analyzes the task within the context of the environment in which it needs to be performed.

Schema Theory of Discrete Motor Learning as Related to Handwriting

As children learn how to perform novel motor tasks, they adopt general rules of how to execute that movement. These ideas or rules that evolve from practice are referred to as *schema*. The schema can be expanded by increasing the amount of practice and by varying the contexts and conditions under which the practice takes place (Schmidt, 1975; Schmidt & Lee, 2014). Internalization of these rules allow the child to achieve motor accuracy in different contexts.

Feedback on the accuracy and effectiveness of the motor activity is received during each practice "session," thereby affording the child the opportunity to assess the results of their actions. The concept of knowledge of results refers to the child's assessment of their performance by comparing the expected feedback for the motor activity they are practicing, to the actual feedback received. An example would be a child learning to form a lower case "a." The expected outcome is viewed in the child's handwriting workbook. Each time they practice forming a lower case "a" in the workbook, they gain knowledge of results, as they see how their actual motor act compares to the model in the workbook (expected outcome). With this knowledge of results, they can adjust their movement patterns as they attempt to improve accuracy. "Every time the skill is practiced, and the results of the act are assessed for accuracy, ones schema gets better and more comprehensive and can be used more automatically" (Roston, 2020, p. 432).

An example of how a schema develops during handwriting occurs when a student learns to write their name. When they first learn to write, there are many sub-skills to master; how to form letters, how to leave a space between their first and last names, how to make their letters sit on the line. Each time they write their name, they judge if they have achieved their goal of writing it appropriately. If they have not achieved their goal, they might adjust how they hold their pencil, the type of paper they use, or how they stabilize the paper with their nondominant hand. Over time, students evaluate the results of each attempt and notice which one was the most accurate, thereby enlarging their schema. People who are particularly adept at a specific motor skill, such as a professional athlete or a calligrapher, continue to practice that motor act throughout their lives, thereby expanding their schema even further.

Schmidt (1975) defines the initial conditions in learning a motor skill as

- *Response specifications:* this may include motor variables such as direction, speed, force, height.
- *Sensory consequences of skill performance:* this includes feedback from the senses about the actual performance of the motor activity.
- *Response outcome:* this refers to knowledge of results.

To summarize, schema are sets of internalized rules that receive information during the practice sessions from the response specifications, the sensory information gathered during practice and after, and the knowledge of the results. This information is stored as schemas that can be expanded when more accurate outcomes are produced, or through practice in different contexts.

Interventions that are guided by the motor skill acquisition frame of reference often incorporate functional tasks that are part of the occupation of the child/student. The occupational therapy practitioner facilitates appropriate movement patterns by structuring learning in such a way that it encourages the child to perform the task. There are a number of formalized handwriting interventions used by occupational therapists; and literature shows that adequate handwriting practice must occur in order for learning to happen (Hoy et al., 2011). See Chapter 11, Motor Skill Acquisition Frame of Reference for a more in-depth review of the theory base and intervention from this perspective.

Visual Perception

The sense of vision is critical in learning processes and the development of motor skills. It is part of a system that is dynamic and includes interactions between multiple sensory systems and the environment (Schneck, 2020). Vision is the primary sense through which children learn how to form letters and write. It is also essential to children receiving feedback on their own handwriting skills.

Visual perception is a process by which received visual information is processed and interpreted by the brain (Gibson, 2014; Lieberman, 1984). It includes the following skills:

1. Visual discrimination: the ability to distinguish one shape from another. This helps the writer to proofread. Reversals of letters and numbers occurring after 7 years of age often indicate poor visual discrimination skills.
2. Visual memory: the ability to remember a specific visual stimulus when it is out of the individual's visual field. This aids with automaticity of handwriting.
3. Visual–spatial relationships/Position in space: the ability to recognize that visual stimuli may be the same even if they are in a different spatial orientation. This skill supports appropriate letter formation.
4. Form constancy: the ability to identify shapes/forms as being similar, even though they may be different in size, color, or spatial orientation. This skill allows the child to recognize that a typed "a" is the same as a handwritten "a" whether it is in a word or standing alone.
5. Visual sequential memory: the ability to recall several items in sequence without a visual cue. This helps with letter formation and the automaticity of handwriting. Tseng and Chow (2000) found that proficiency in visual sequential memory is one of the most reliable predictors of handwriting speed.
6. Figure/ground: the ability to identify a target figure amid competing backgrounds. This skill supports a child's ability to use appropriate line orientation and spacing.
7. Visual closure: the ability to recognize familiar shapes/forms that are partially drawn. This skill supports letter formation (Figure 12.4).

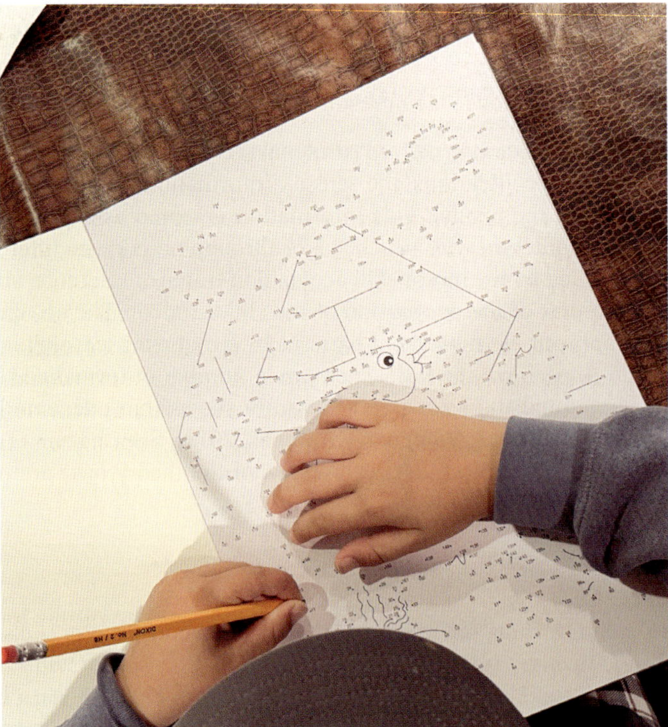

FIGURE 12.4 Doing a connect the dots task.

In addition to *visual perceptual skills*, there are several *visual–cognitive skills* that are essential for handwriting success (Schneck, 2020). They are:

- Visual attention, which includes alertness; selective attention; divided attention; and vigilance, support attention to detail and availability for the writing task.
- Visual memory involves the integration of past lived experiences with visual information. Poor visual memory may lead to children who have difficulty in the areas of spelling, grammar, punctuation, and capitalization. The internal ability to visualize letters and words without visual cues is an essential component to spontaneous production of written language. Visual memory also appears to be essential for *automaticity in handwriting* as children need to automatically recall letter formation patterns to allow for concentrate on *what* to write, not *how* to write. Visual imagery or visualization is the visual cognitive component that allows children to picture things in their mind's eye, such as what a lower case "q" looks like. A study by Slotnick et al. (2012) found that the cognitive processes for visual memory and visual imagery are similar, but not identical.

An intact visual perceptual system contributes to a child's ability to engage in meaningful occupation. This is essential for a child to be able to write with appropriate letter formation, line orientation, and spacing of letters and numbers on paper. Visual perceptual skills are critical to school readiness and to academic performance (Carlson et al., 2013; Pienaar et al., 2013; Schneck, 2020).

Sensory Integration

A. Jean Ayres defined sensory integration as "the neurological process that organizes sensations from one's body and from the environment and makes it possible to use the body effectively in the environment" (Ayres, 1989, p. 22). The sensory processing system includes auditory processing, vestibular processing, proprioceptive processing, tactile processing, and visual processing (Ayres, 2005). The act of handwriting requires organization of all these systems. Good proprioception skills, or the ability to sense where one's body is in space, supports the child's engagement in the fine motor activities inherent in handwriting. Tactile skills are needed to be able to sense and tolerate a writing implement in a child's hand or paper against their skin. Vestibular skills contribute the child's ability to cross midline when writing a sentence across a page; and appropriate vestibular skills allow the child to integrate eye movements, posture, balance, and muscle tone for visual–motor integration and coordinated distal function (Figure 12.5).

An important concept in Ayres Sensory Integration model is *adaptation*. Adaptive responses are actions that an individual uses that are appropriate for the task and a specific environmental demand (Ayres, 2005). An example of an adaptive handwriting response would be the child shifting in their seat to sit more upright to engage in a handwriting task at their desk. Please see Chapter 6, Ayres Sensory Integration Frame of Reference for more information on this theory and its application.

ASSUMPTIONS

There are three underlying assumptions made within the theoretical base of this frame of reference. These assumptions are:

1. The integration of a child's motor, cognitive, sensory, visual, and visual perceptual skill development is essential to engage in handwriting activities.

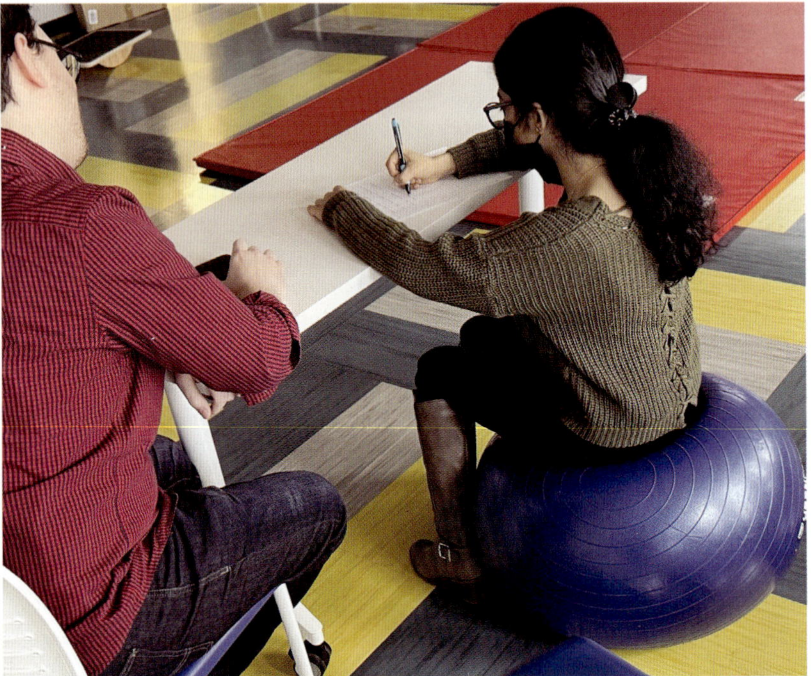

FIGURE 12.5 Sensory-based positioning while seated for writing.

2. The child possesses adequate postural control, or utilizes alternative means to stabilize their head, neck, and proximal musculature to support distal upper extremity function during handwriting tasks.
3. Handwriting skills are developed through instruction, modeling, and consistent practice.

FUNCTION/DYSFUNCTION CONTINUA

This frame of reference has five function/dysfunction continua.

Attention (Visual and Cognitive)

For handwriting, good visual and overall attention is needed so that the child can focus on the various elements implicit in the complex handwriting process and sustain that focus. The child needs to not only attend to the use of visual symbols, but simultaneously attend to ideas and concepts, or content, that they are writing down on paper. Further, their attention needs to be sustained throughout the activity lest the child will neither produce a legible product, nor capture the ideas that they intended to put down on paper. At the functional end of the continuum, the child can sustain attention to all of the elements of handwriting simultaneously and produce a written product that accurately represents what they would like to express. At the dysfunctional end of the continuum, the child is unable to attend to or sustain attention to the mechanics of handwriting, such as letter formation, line orientation, or spacing; and/or they are unable to attend to or sustain attention to the content that they would like to express in a written form (Table 12.1).

Table 12.1 Attention

• The child sustains attention to all the elements of handwriting simultaneously and produces a written product that accurately represents what they would like to express	• The child is unable to attend to, or sustain attention to the mechanics of handwriting, such as letter formation, line orientation, or spacing • Child is unable to attend to or sustain attention to the content that they would like to express in a written form

Visual–Motor Integration (Eye–Hand Coordination)

Visual–motor integration, frequently referred to as eye–hand coordination is a complex skill involving coordination between the visual and motor systems (Law et al., 2016; Schneck, 2020). The literature suggests that children with poor visual–motor integration also have poor handwriting skills (Cornhill & Case-Smith, 1996). While it is possible for an individual with significant visual impairment and/or visual perceptual impairment to produce a handwriting sample, without the use of technology or the assistance of another, they would not be able to evaluate the accuracy and quality of their written work visually. As mentioned earlier, a key component of motor learning is the reception of feedback and refinement of the motor task through the process of practice and feedback. The visually impaired writer would not have knowledge of results without the use of technology or another individual providing the needed visual feedback. Consequently, if a specific motor action is based on information received visually, and that information is inaccurate, we can expect that written output will be inaccurate. At the functional end of the continuum, children with good visual–motor integration skills will integrate visual information about the environment and the writing task with the motor system to produce letters and numerals that are formed correctly, with appropriate size, line orientation, and spacing on the page. At the dysfunctional end of the continuum, children will not be able to integrate both systems adaptively to form legible work with good spacing (Table 12.2).

Cognitive Development—Use of Symbols in Writing

The ability to identify and use visual symbols is a prerequisite for writing letters and numbers. At approximately 2 to 7 years of age, children enter the preoperational stage of cognitive development (Piaget, 1954). It is during this stage that typically developing children experience marked growth in the areas of language development and symbolic play. Recognition that letters and numbers represent concepts and have a different meaning from lines randomly drawn on paper is crucial to a child being able to use those symbols meaningfully in reading and writing tasks.

Table 12.2 Visual–Motor Integration

Function	Dysfunction
• The child can integrate visual information from the environment and the writing task with their motor system to successfully produce letters and numerals that are formed correctly, with appropriate size, line orientation, and spacing on the page	• The child is unable to integrate the visual and motor systems with information received from the environment to adaptively form legible work with good spacing • Letter formation, line orientation, and spacing will not be appropriate for the demands of the writing task

Table 12.3 Cognitive Development—Use of Symbols in Writing

Function	Dysfunction
• The child understands the use of symbols for language and uses letters and numbers to represent words and concepts. • The child can recognize letters and numbers accurately. • The child can use letters and numbers to express the content of their intended message.	• The child acts in a very concrete manner, not recognizing that letters and numerals represent language-based concepts. • A child at this end of the continuum is not able to read or recognize their own name when written.

At 2 to 7 years of age, preoperational stage coincides with a period of rapid physical development of several systems in the young child's body, including the fine motor and visual motor systems, preparing the child to engage in handwriting activities. At the functional end of the continuum, the child cognitively begins to understand the use of symbols and uses letters and numbers to represent language-based concepts. At the dysfunctional end of the continuum, the child acts in a very concrete manner, not recognizing that lexicons and numerals represent other language-based concepts. A child at this end of the continuum would not be able to read or recognize their own name when written (Table 12.3).

Motor Development for Efficient Grasp of a Writing Tool

The term grasp refers to "the manner in which a child holds and utilizes a writing tool" (Schneider et al., 2023, p. 434). As handwriting typically requires the child to grasp a writing tool, such as a pencil, pen, crayon, or marker, the quality of how a child grasps such a tool with their dominant hand is important to the occupation of handwriting. A firm grasp is required for the child's fine motor movements to be effective and efficient. An inefficient grasp is one that interferes with the writer's function, participation and/or performance (Schneider et al., 2023). Factors related to grasp that may negatively impact a child's handwriting include a grasp that is either too loose or too tight, static wrist and fingers, limitations in wrist and/or finger extension or flexion, fatigue, and pain (Schneider et al., 2023). Literature has shown that an inefficient grasp can lead to decreased endurance during writing tasks and illegibility (Feder & Manjrekar, 2007; Schneider et al., 2023; Tseng & Cermak, 1993; Volman et al., 2006). A functional grasp for handwriting is stable, yet dynamic. It allows for a firm grip on the writing utensil, with flexibility at the fingers, wrist, and forearm to allow for coordinated fine motor movements. The child with a functional grasp holds the writing tool with appropriate pressure on the tool, as well as on the paper, thereby allowing the child to write without fatigue or pain; and they can manipulate a writing tool effectively with their dominant hand while crossing the midline of their body. A child is using a dysfunctional grasp when they are unable to write with legibility or speed, and/or they experience fatigue and pain when using a writing tool such as a pencil, pen, marker, or crayon (Figure 12.6A,B; Table 12.4).

Integration for Handwriting Legibility

At its core, handwriting legibility is essential to the reader's understanding of what the writer has put down on paper. When a writing sample is illegible, it poses a barrier between what the writer

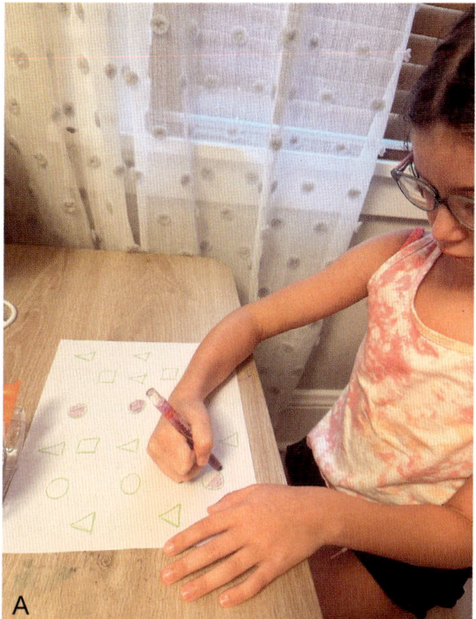
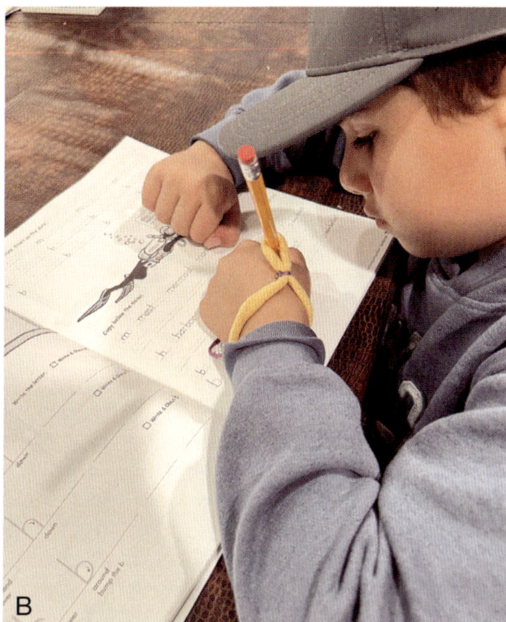

FIGURE 12.6 **A.** Thumb wrap grasp. **B.** Corrected grasp.

intended to say and what the reader interprets the markings on the paper to mean. Reading illegible writing requires increased attention and effort on the part of the reader, something they may or may not be prepared to use. The reader struggles to decode the letters or numbers and will likely misinterpret the intended message. Students receive grades based on their handwritten answers on worksheets, examinations, essays, and projects (Figure 12.7). Consequently, a child's handwritten work may receive a lower grade than their same-aged peers, based on the reader's interpretation of the markings on the page.

Equally as important, children's handwriting is a visual representation of themselves, and as such contributes to the child's sense of self. In schools, handwritten projects are frequently displayed in the classroom and in elementary school hallways, allowing the child, their peers,

Table 12.4 Motor Development for Efficient Grasp of a Writing Tool

Function	Dysfunction
• The child holds the writing tool with appropriate pressure on the tool, as well as on the paper, thereby allowing the child to write without fatigue or pain. • The child can manipulate a writing tool effectively with their dominant hand while crossing the midline of their body.	• The child is unable to write with legibility or speed, and/or they experience fatigue and pain when using a writing tool such as a pencil, pen, marker, or crayon. • The child may drop or lose control of the writing tool because their grasp is too loose; or they may experience discomfort/pain because their grasp is too tight. • The child may have difficulty forming letters and/or numbers because they are not able to adapt their grip on the writing tool.

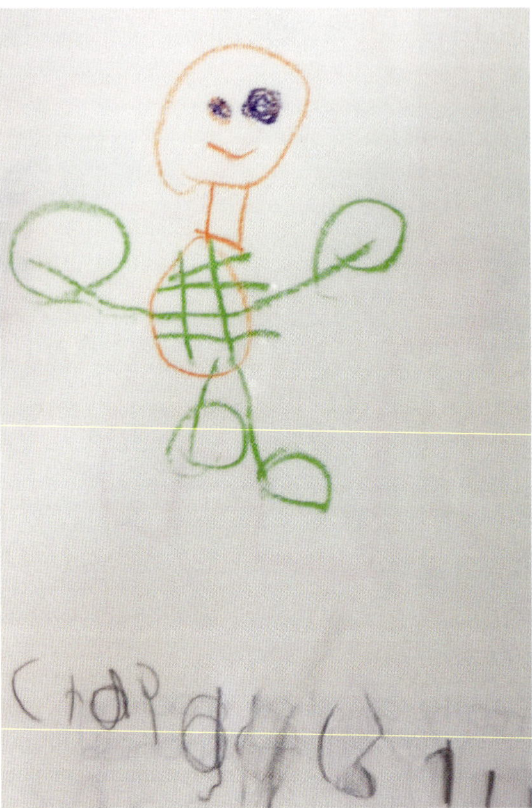

FIGURE 12.7 An example of illegible writing.

teachers, parents, and other stakeholders to judge the quality of the handwriting. A child will measure their own written work against their classmates' and in some cases, judge their work and the work of others as "good" or "bad," based on handwriting legibility and not content. These judgments may lead to a child being labeled "sloppy" or "careless," when they may have put more effort into their handwriting than their same-aged peers.

At the functional end of the continuum, the child uses their handwriting skills to accurately depict their intended message in written form in a way that he or she and their readers can read with ease, using appropriate motor schema. A child with functional legibility will more than likely be pleased with the quality of their handwriting sample. At the dysfunctional end of the continuum, the child displays difficulty producing a handwriting sample with appropriate letter formation, letter size, line orientation, and/or spacing between letters/numbers and words. Consequently, the reader has difficulty understanding the child's intended message, leading to frustration and a decreased sense of self in the child (Table 12.5).

GUIDE FOR EVALUATION

It is important to note that the process of evaluation is dynamic and ongoing. Occupational therapy evaluation must consider the personal skills of the child, the environment/context in which the child will be performing specific occupations, and qualities and attributes of the occupation

Table 12.5 Integration for Handwriting Legibility

Function	Dysfunction
The child uses their handwriting skills to accurately depict their intended message in written form in a way that he or she and their readers can read with ease, using appropriate motor schema.	• Writing poses a barrier between what the writer intended to say and what the reader interprets the markings on the paper to mean. • The child displays difficulty producing a handwriting sample with appropriate letter formation, letter size, line orientation, and/or spacing between letters/numbers and words.

itself (AOTA, 2020). In this frame of reference, evaluation consists of a screening, administration of standardized assessment(s), and analysis of the data collected to either evidence the lack of need for an intervention or to develop an intervention plan with the appropriate stakeholders (Feder et al., 2000; Hammerschmidt & Sudsawad, 2004; Schneider et al., 2023).

Screening

The first step in the evaluation process is to screen the child to determine if there is a need for a complete evaluation. The screening consists of interviews with parents, teachers, and other stakeholders to gather information about the child's handwriting function within their natural environments, and to establish an occupational profile. Crucial to the screening process would be to observe the child's process of handwriting through direct observation in natural environments, thereby providing the screener with information about the context(s) within which the child is required to write, as well as the child's behavior and performance skills. It is also very important to gather handwritten work samples (Case-Smith et al., 2014) to allow the therapist to see the process and product of the child's handwriting.

Supplemental screenings may be used to gather additional information regarding posture, grasp, ergonomics, and other observation-driven skill areas. The *handwriting checklist* (Roston et al., 2008) is one such screen that focuses on a child's posture, components of writing performance, tool use, and grasp patterns. If the screening reveals that the child's handwriting performance is interfering with their function within the context of their day, an evaluation may be warranted.

Standardized Assessments

Governing agencies, school systems, and or other health organizations frequently require standardized, norm-referenced assessments be part of the evaluation process to substantiate the need for skilled services. As handwriting is a dynamic and complex task, there are a wide range of assessment tools that can be used to assess the occupation of handwriting, as well as skill components. In this section, several of these standardized assessments that align with the theoretical underpinnings of the handwriting frame of reference will be discussed. Occupational therapists must be knowledgeable of the most appropriate assessment tools to use for each child given the context within which the intervention may be provided, and the task will be carried out.

Motor and Cognition

During the assessment process, the occupational therapy evaluator assesses the child's motor and cognitive process skills that would likely influence their handwriting skill acquisition (Kaplan,

2020). This may include upper extremity range of motion, strength, and coordination. Standardized assessments might include *The Peabody Developmental Motor Scales, 3rd Edition* (PDMS-3) (Folio & Fewell, 2023) or *The Bruininks-Oseretsky Test of Motor Proficiency, 3rd Edition* (Bruininks & Bruininks, 2024) to assess motor and cognitive skills. The PDMS-3 assesses motor development of children ages 0 to 5 years, 11 months. Therapists are able to use the fine motor portion of the assessment to assess hand manipulation and eye–hand coordination. The BOT-3, is a standardized, norm-referenced measure for children 4 to 21.11 years of age. The assessment has a fine motor portion, which includes assessment of Fine Motor Precision, Fine Motor Integration, Manual Dexterity, and Upper-Limb Coordination. Although these assessments do not provide a standardized score for cognition, the child's ability to understand and follow directions to complete tasks, as well as a child's developmental level will impact their ability to successfully engage in the testing items. An occupational therapy evaluator can use this information to provide insight to a child's cognitive level. Additionally, as an occupational therapist observes the child in these tasks, they can also gain further understanding of the child's cognitive level and ability to participate in activities providing the therapist a better understanding of the fit between the child and their environment as proposed in Bronfenbrenner theory (Figure 12.8).

Visual Perceptual Assessment

A visual perceptual assessment should always begin with gathering information about a child's general vision. In a school environment, this may be accomplished by asking the parent/caregivers

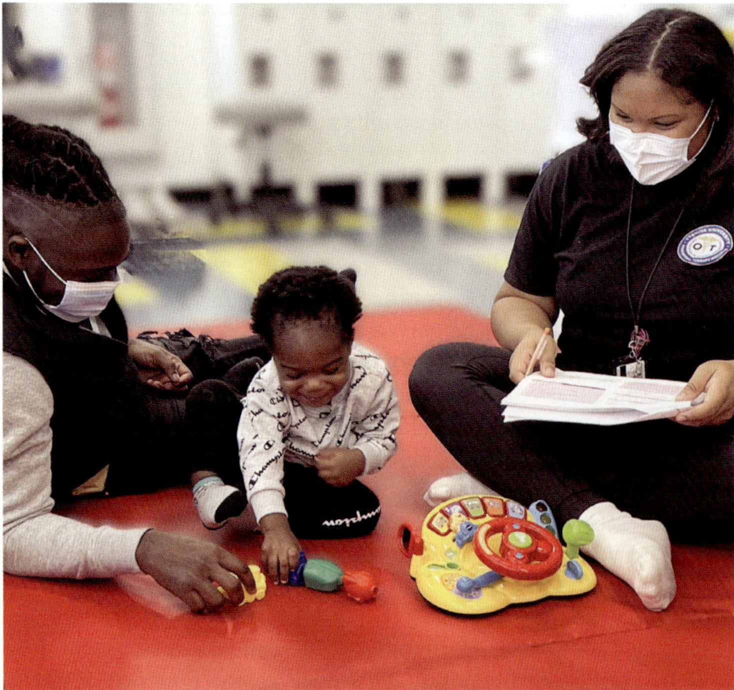

FIGURE 12.8 Family play.

or school nurse about the child's overall vision and eye examination history. The next step may be to observe the child at play, observing how they interact with materials such as Legos, building blocks, coloring books, pegboards, and puzzles. A careful observation of how the child interacts with their environment and objects in their environment will provide rich information about their visual perceptual functioning.

Some commonly used standardized visual perceptual assessment tools include *The Developmental Test of Visual Perception, 3rd Edition* ([DTVP-3]; Hammill et al., 2014), *The Motor Free Visual Perception Test, 3rd Edition* ([MVPT-3]; Colarusso & Hammill, 2003), and *The Test of Visual Perceptual Skills, 4th Edition* ([TVPS]; Martin, 2017).

Visual–Motor Integration Assessment

A widely used assessment of visual–motor integration is the *Beery-Buktenica Developmental Test of Visual-Motor Integration, 6th Edition* ([VMI-6]; Beery et al., 2010). It is a pencil and paper task that can be given individually to a child, or in a small group. It is norm-referenced and requires the child to copy a series of figures. *The Wide Range Assessment of Visual-Motor Abilities* ([WRAVMA]; Adams & Sheslow, 1995) also requires the child to copy a series of figures. It is administered individually.

Sensory-Based Assessments

Although sensory assessments may not provide specific information related to the activity of handwriting, therapists should assess a child's sensory functioning and determine if there are sensory components contributing to handwriting difficulties. Please see Chapter 6, Ayres Sensory Integration Frame of Reference, and Chapter 7, A Frame of Reference for Sensory Integration and Processing Differences: Sensory Therapies and Research (STAR), for more information on standardized assessment for sensory processing and modulation.

Occupation-Based Handwriting Assessments

- *The Minnesota Handwriting Assessment* ([MHA]; Reisman, 1999) is a norm-referenced assessment tool that can be administered quickly to students aged 6 to 8 years, and in the first and second grades. It assesses their handwriting speed and legibility while copying from near point. The test can be administered in less than 5 minutes with approximately 5 to 10 minutes needed for scoring.
- *The Evaluation Tool of Children's Handwriting* ([ETCH]; Amundson, 1995) is a criterion-referenced assessment tool that evaluates a child's handwriting legibility, speed, and pencil grasp/management. The ETCH-C may be used to evaluate cursive handwriting in 3rd to 5th grade students (Amundson, 1995).
- *The Print Tool Evaluation and Remediation Program* (Learning Without Tears, n.d.) assesses a child's ability to correctly form upper- and lower-case letters, and numbers. It targets visual memory, letter and line orientation, placement on the page/line, size of letter/number, starting points for different letters, sequence of motor movements when forming letters, and word spacing.
- *The Test of Handwriting Skills, Revised* ([THS-R]; Milone, 2007) is designed to be administered to children aged 6 years to 18.11 months. It is norm referenced and assesses both manuscript

and cursive handwriting skills. The skills that it assesses are legibility, letter formation, line alignment, and size of the writing sample.

- *The Pediatric Evaluation of Disability Inventory* ([PEDI]; Haley et al., 1992) is an interview-based, criterion-referenced assessment tool that explores a child's functional abilities, their independence levels in a variety of occupations, and the amount of modification needed for them to perform their daily occupations. It was designed for use with children aged 6 months to 7 years. It explores the areas of social function, mobility, and self-care.
- *The School Function Assessment* ([SFA]; Coster et al., 1998) is an occupation-based assessment tool frequently completed by the educational team working with a pediatric student. It assesses how a child is performing their daily occupations within an educational setting relative to their same-aged peers. It requires collaboration of teachers, service providers, and other school-based stakeholders to complete the evaluation. The sections that focus on handwriting skills focus on such skills as the student's ability to: work in an organized fashion from left to right; to identify appropriate starting points for letters and words on the paper; use appropriate line orientation; use adequate spacing on a page with appropriate size; to produce written work at a comparable speed to their peers.
- *The School Assessment of Motor and Processing Skills* ([School AMPS]; Fisher et al., 2007) is an occupation-based assessment wherein the evaluator must be trained and certified in its administration. It is designed to measure the effectiveness of a student's ability to perform school tasks in natural school-based environments.

INTERPRETATION AND DEVELOPMENT OF AN INTERVENTION PLAN

Once a complete evaluation has been performed on a child, a thorough analysis of and interpretation of the findings must be completed to determine the child's strengths, challenges, interests, and motivators. Next, goals that are specific, measurable, attainable, and relevant are developed with the family, teachers, and school team.

Occupational therapy practitioners using this frame of reference to address handwriting can use a variety of approaches to intervention, including developmental, sensorimotor, and motor acquisition/motor learning (Case-Smith et al., 2014; Denton et al., 2006; Schneider, 2023). Research has shown that occupational therapy practitioners indicate they use multiple treatment approaches in their interventions when addressing handwriting deficits (Denton et al., 2006; Feder et al., 2000; Peterson & Nelson, 2003). There is some debate as to whether a top-down approach or a bottom-up approach is more effective when working on handwriting skills with children. In a top-down approach, the occupation in its entirety is completed in the natural setting where the task would be expected to be performed. This is consistent with motor learning theory. An example of a top-down intervention for handwriting would be having the occupational therapist come into the classroom at the end of the day to help the student who has difficulty copying their homework assignments down into their planner, to copy their homework assignments in their planner. When following a bottom-up approach, the focus of the intervention is to address specific child performance skills that may be impacting function (O'Brien & Kuhaneck, 2016). An example of a bottom-up intervention for handwriting would be having the occupational therapist work with the child outside of the classroom to address underlying visual perceptual skills that may be interfering with the child's ability to set their words on a line. The intervention may include drawing paths through a maze. Although literature suggests that using a top-down

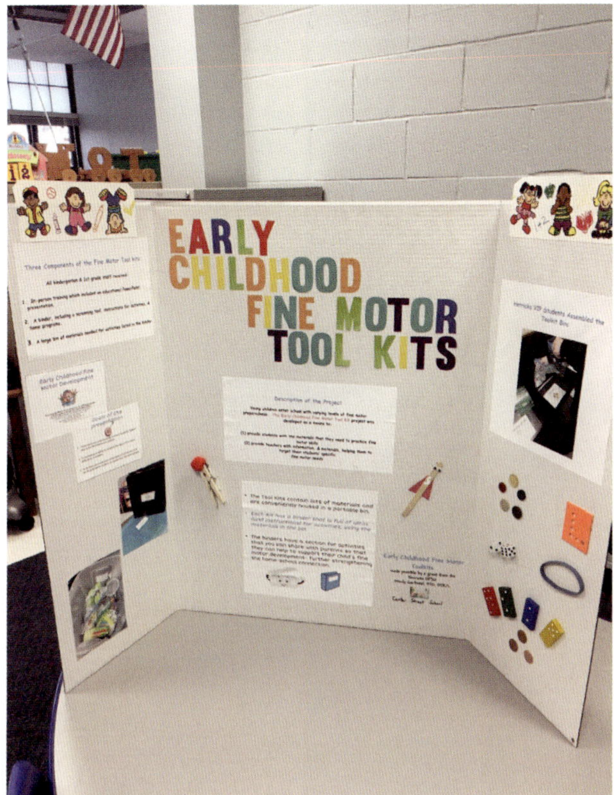

FIGURE 12.9 A bottom-up approach—focusing on the development of fine motor skills.

approach in a natural setting, is the most effective way to increase motor performance (O'Brien & Kuhaneck, 2016), many therapists prefer to use a combined approach, using both a top-down and a bottom-up approach (O'Brien & Kuhaneck, 2016; Schneider, 2023; Weinstock-Zlotick & Hinojosa, 2004) (Figures 12.9 and 12.10). Additionally, O'Brien and Kuhaneck (2016) found that students benefit from teachers and therapists embedding the use of adaptive handwriting tools and strategies in classroom settings. With this type of model, there are more opportunities for rich practice experiences, leading to increased handwriting performance and participation.

Occupational therapy practitioners working with children on handwriting are strongly urged to rely on evidence-based practice to guide decision making for evaluations and interventions (O'Brien & Kuhaneck, 2016).

POSTULATES REGARDING CHANGE

General Postulate Regarding Change

A child will become more proficient in writing letters with appropriate form and size, spacing letters, and words on a page, and using appropriate line orientation, when they are provided with multiple and varied opportunities for handwriting practice while receiving sensory feedback and knowledge of results; thereby expanding their schema for handwriting.

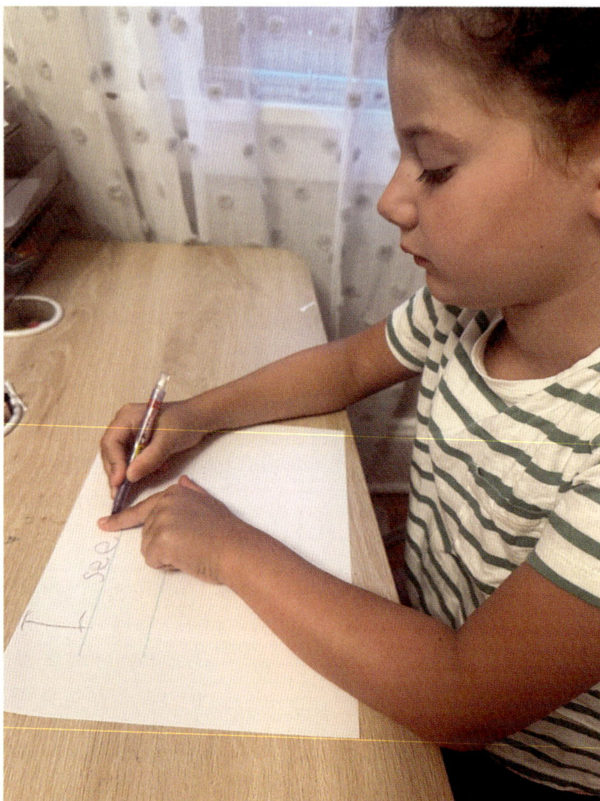

FIGURE 12.10 A top-down approach—actively engaging in writing tasks.

Directional Postulate Regarding Change

1. When visual information about the environment and the writing task is well integrated with the motor system, visual–motor integration skills are optimized and consequently, letters and numbers are formed correctly, with appropriate size, line orientation, and spacing on the page.
2. Pain and fatigue when writing can be avoided when the child grasps a writing tool appropriately and with proper pressure on the tool and the paper.
3. When a child uses the appropriate motor schema for handwriting, their written product accurately depicts their intended message, and readers can read their message accurately and with ease.
4. When a child perceives their handwriting to be poor, their identity as a capable student is lessened.

Specific Postulates Regarding Change

- If a practitioner helps to structure the environment and/or the task to allow for increased attention on the part of the child, the child will be able to focus on the various elements of handwriting and produce a written product that accurately represents what they would like to express.
- If the practitioner supports a child's symbolic play skills prior to and during writing tasks, then they will promote symbol development and facilitate the ability to learn the lexicons of the alphabet.

- If the practitioner addresses visual perception and visual perceptual motor development, then the child will be able to organize and interpret visual information, such as the shape, size, and position of letters to allow for accurate letter spacing, sizing, and orientation.
- If a practitioner provides opportunities to develop postural stability within the trunk, shoulder, forearm, and wrist and addresses fine motor development for dexterity and manipulation, the child will develop efficient grasp patterns to be able to write legibly with greater ease.
- If a practitioner provides consistent opportunities for a child to practice handwriting, with varied practice and feedback, and the results are assessed for accuracy with every trial, then the child's schema or motor understanding, expands and becomes more comprehensive, allowing for more automaticity during writing tasks.

APPLICATION TO PRACTICE

The child's ability to engage in symbolic play is an important component of initial occupational therapy interventions designed to address handwriting dysfunction, as lexicons and numerals are the symbols used when engaged in handwriting occupations (Roston, 2020). Occupational therapy practitioners support children in the occupation of handwriting by creating, providing, and promoting opportunities for children to engage in symbolic play individually, in a dyad, or in a small group. Therefore, identifying the developmental stage of pretend play that the child is in and helping move them through the stage where symbolic play is explored is a foundational element of initial handwriting interventions. Drawing and writing are crucial activities used to help children learn about symbols. Practitioners following this frame of reference will provide the child with varied opportunities to engage in drawing and writing as they are precursor skills to using symbols in writing.

One of the theoretical underpinnings of this frame of reference is motor acquisition, and practice is essential to motor learning. Therefore, practice is essential in the intervention of this frame of reference. Initial practice may involve demonstration and modeling of how to correctly form specific letters. Incorporating a child's interests and motivators into the intervention, will also promote attention—supporting the child in their availability for handwriting instruction. The occupational therapy practitioner must convey to the child and other stakeholders that initially, accuracy is more important than speed. Immediate, specific feedback reinforces motor learning, and it should help the child to identify their best attempt. For example, "The lines on this one are straighter than the others," or "This one is touching the blue line, and the other one does not. Which one do you think is best?" Following a discussion about the best writing sample, the practitioner should reinforce which sample is the best, for example, by putting a sticker or a star next to it.

Occupational therapy intervention focusing on handwriting is most effective when the child has many opportunities to practice the skill in a variety of environments and contexts. Practice need not only occur with the occupational therapist present. In most settings, the occupational therapist is only with the child for a limited amount of time each week, while parents, caregivers, and teachers are with the child for significantly longer periods of time. It is therefore very important that the therapist collaborate with the teachers, parents, caregivers, and other stakeholders so that all members of the team are aware of handwriting strategies that the child uses during practice. The time set aside for collaboration can also be used to discuss potential adaptations that may need to be made to the environment(s) or task(s), such as assuring that desk and chair

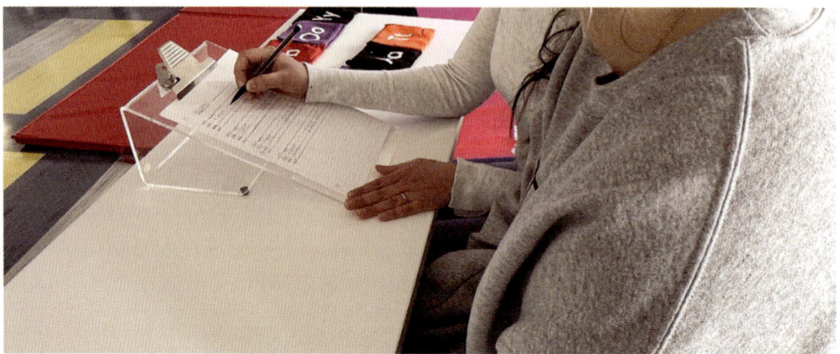

FIGURE 12.11 Using a slant board with modeling for writing.

heights are appropriate for the size of the child, or that children who need pencil grips receive them. The team can also problem solve to support the child's use of appropriate positioning and posture during writing tasks in different contexts (Figure 12.11).

To optimize the likelihood of a child making progress on their handwriting goals, the child must be a willing and active participant in their own learning. Establishing a therapeutic rapport with the child is essential to the success of interventions. The therapist and child develop goals together that are meaningful for the child. At times parents and/or caregivers may collaborate with the child and therapist to develop the goals. Ideally, the child's goals and the therapist's goals align. If they do not, the therapist asks questions of the child, supporting their reflection on their skills and the skills that are needed to enhance participation in daily handwriting-related occupations. Examples of questions asked may be, "Why do you need to write things down? Why do you need to form your letters differently? A therapeutic relationship built on trust and acceptance is crucial to the child being able to reflect on their abilities, share them with the therapist, and willingly participate in the work needed to achieve the agreed-upon goals.

In addition to establishing a therapeutic relationship with the pediatric client, the therapist must incorporate fun and pleasurable intervention activities that will motivate the child to engage actively in the intervention process. One way to do this is to ask children what they enjoy spending their time doing, and whenever possible, add elements of their preferred occupations to their intervention. In addition to making the writing activity more fun for the child, it also helps the child to feel validated because you listened to them, and empowered, because they see that they can have a say in what they do in occupational therapy. An example of this would be asking a young New York Rangers Hockey fan who is working on handwriting skills, to draw a hockey jersey with his name on the back of the jersey. Projects that incorporate holidays or seasons can be motivating for children as well. On the surface, arts and crafts projects do not require handwriting, but the therapist can infuse the activity with opportunities for the child to engage in handwriting. An example would be drawing a turkey from a handprint and then writing something that the child is grateful for on each of the (finger) feathers. Creating greeting cards is another way to motivate a child to engage in handwriting tasks without labeling them as such. Mother's Day, Father's Day, birthdays, thank you cards are all wonderful vehicles for writing. Writing during pretend play can also be a powerful intervention. An example would be to pretend that you are a spy and the only way to get messages to your superior is through written notes. Another way to make writing fun is to use enticing writing tools. Different types of paper with

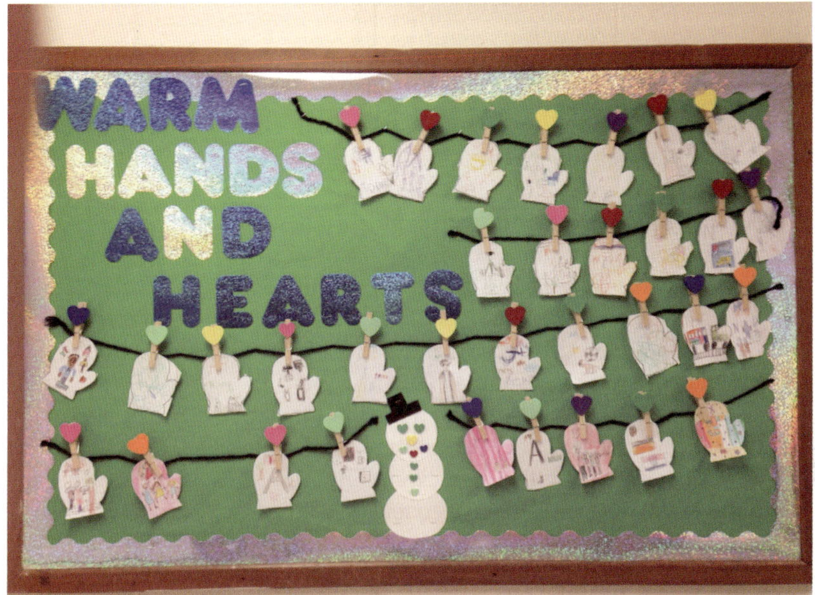

FIGURE 12.12 Bulletin board writing.

and without borders, pencils with brightly colored toys or erasers on the end, scented markers, textured pencil grips, and even finger paint can motivate a child to try writing. Redefining writing can also be helpful in getting a reluctant writer to write. Therapists can use a variety of mediums to introduce the symbols of language, such as molding letters out of clay or playdoh, writing letters in shaving cream, and forming letters out of Legos (Figure 12.12).

There are several individual and multi-player games that can promote handwriting in a fun and engaging way. Players can write the answers to questions posed in a game instead of saying them aloud. An example is 20 questions. Questions and/or answers can be expressed in a written format. This can be graded down by only responding to yes/no questions with pencil and paper. One child can be designated the "score keeper," necessitating them to write down the numbers corresponding to the score. Puzzle books that encourage the child to engage in key elements of handwriting, such as visual–motor integration can be useful and fun vehicles for learning. Identifying letters and words in a word search puzzle, completing an "Eye Spy" or "Where's Waldo" worksheet can help the child to hone their visual perceptual skills and visual attention. Whenever possible, the therapist should set the child up for a successful, fun, experience.

The goal for a child completing a task requiring handwriting is for the handwriting to be an efficient vehicle through which the author conveys a message with accuracy. For this to occur, there needs to be a level of automaticity and legibility so that the writer can put their effort into formulating content. To support the child's attainment of this goal, the therapist must provide the child with feedback on the quality of their performance. This will help them to enlarge their schema with greater accuracy. "The ultimate goal is for the child to be able to transcribe letters in words automatically to support his or her language, composing, and reading proficiencies" (Roston, 2020, p. 448).

CASE EXAMPLES

Christopher

Christopher is a second-grade student who attends an integrated class of 20 students within a public elementary school. Like Christopher, some of his classmates receive special education services; and others do not. Christopher was diagnosed with autism spectrum disorder and receives occupational therapy services focusing on handwriting and sensory regulation. Christopher frequently says that he hates writing because it is hard, and he is bad at it.

Christopher lives with his family in a private home in a middle-class neighborhood. His mother reported that Christopher has one typically developing older sister, and a younger brother with autism spectrum disorder, just like Christopher. His mother, a single parent, stated that she does not receive much help at home.

After reading his Individualized Education Plan (IEP), Christopher was observed on the playground, during his speech session, during physical education class, and in his classroom. He was able to effectively express himself verbally, and frequently participated in classroom activities; however, he frequently bumped into objects and people in his environment and engaged in a lot of in-seat movement. The areas that Christopher displayed challenges in are handwriting, drawing, and sensory integration, as he frequently seeks sensory input and has a decreased sense of where his body is in space (proprioception).

While working with Christopher, I learned that he loved superheroes. He was motivated to draw pictures of his favorite superheroes; however, he was not able to color within the lines when given a large outline for one. He also had difficulty reciting the letters of the alphabet and could only write eight letters in sequence. During our time together, Christopher and I "made a deal." I taught him how to draw superheroes that he had not yet mastered, and he practiced writing the names of the various superheroes that we had drawn together on lined paper. We made a contract that we both signed. I created a chart and Christopher decided that he would get a sticker on the chart each time he completed his handwriting practice.

As I worked with most of the students in Christopher's class, his teacher and I collaborated frequently. We worked together to modify worksheets, and to trial various pencil grips to improve Christopher's grasp on his pencil. We met regularly to provide each other with feedback on each student's response to intervention. We developed routines for the classroom with scheduled times for handwriting practice and set aside space in the classroom designated as "the author's corner" where students could go to engage in writing activities. In the author's corner were a variety of handwriting tools, such as slant boards, pencil grips, different types of pencils, pens, and a variety of writing paper. The routines and handwriting practice included modeling letter formation, line orientation, and spacing on the page. The teaching assistants helped by providing detailed feedback about handwriting samples to each of the students in the class.

As our sessions progressed, Christopher could regularly be found in the author's corner, using author's equipment, a slanted clipboard to secure his writing paper, and a weighted pencil to provide him with increased proprioceptive input throughout the writing process. Christopher worked on drawing larger versions of the superheroes. As the size of the figures got bigger through schema development, Christopher was required to use his visual perceptual skills and motor plan where to fit them on the page in relation to each other. He later needed to adjust the size of his writing to fit on the page along with the drawings.

Christopher and I also worked on other superhero-themed fun activities. Every day, Christopher used a book that I created for him to draw a comic strip involving his superheroes. He practiced writing his name on the comic strip page and then practiced writing the superheroes' names; this practice helped him to enlarge his motor schema. I provided knowledge of the results of his handwriting practice. Once the letters were legible, it was time to further expand Christopher's motor schema. He was asked to dictate what the superheroes were saying in the comic strip. He readily complied and could not wait to copy the words himself, from the dictated model. Christopher drew speech bubbles on his comic strip and practiced fitting the dictated words within the confines of the speech bubbles. As time went on, additional words were added to the comic strip, allowing Christopher to tell a story. Creating a comic strip was a meaningful occupation for Christopher, and it allowed him the opportunity for consistent handwriting practice. He was able to work on letter formation, line orientation, spacing, and size of letters. With continual practice, Christopher's letter recognition improved, and his handwriting schema enlarged. These tasks proved to be very motivating for Christopher who loved writing stories about superheroes.

Over the summer, during the extended school year program, Christopher's new teacher reported that she had difficulty reading his handwriting and she graded his written work harshly. I shared research demonstrating that children with poor handwriting skills frequently receive lower grades than their peers. I suggested that Christopher receive direct handwriting instruction from his teachers so that his content would not be lost due to illegible handwriting. One of the special education teachers was able to work with Christopher using a standardized handwriting program, however, he frequently refused to participate in handwriting practice. I suggested that he practice within the confines of his comic strip book and the special education teacher agreed. She reported back that she was pleasantly surprised by the quality of Christopher's handwriting when he was motivated to write.

During the IEP meeting at the end of the school year, Christopher's mother said that she noticed a big difference in the way Christopher feels about school. He tells her that he is a good artist and writer and that his friends want to read his comics during recess. He is motivated to continue creating comics and writing.

Shawna

At 5 years of age, Shawna began attending kindergarten in a New York City public school. She was diagnosed with cerebral palsy shortly after birth and exhibited increased muscle tone throughout her left upper and lower extremities. In addition, she had impaired visual attention skills.

Shawna was evaluated using the school version of the Assessment of Motor and Processing Skills (AMPS) to see her function in the classroom. Shawna's scores indicated that her schoolwork task performance was moderately inefficient, and she required frequent assistance to complete teacher-assigned classroom tasks. Shawna was unable to manipulate pencils and markers effectively and she had difficulty modulating the amount of force she applied when using classroom materials/tools. Her fine motor percentile rank on the PDMS-2 of 1% was indicative of motor performance that falls below age expectations.

Shawna, a child who loved to come to school, always tried to do everything herself without asking for help. She had a positive attitude, and she made friends easily. She told me that she wanted to be able to write her name all by herself. This aligned with curriculum standards for kindergarten students in her school district as students exiting kindergarten were expected to be able to write their names using upper- and lower- case letters appropriately. Although Shawna was excited about learning to write her name, she exhibited difficulty sustaining visual attention for more than seconds at a time. After working with Shawna for a few weeks, I realized that she did not understand the symbolic characteristics of the letters. In addition, her play was concrete in nature; she did not engage in symbolic play. To help Shawna understand that words were symbols, I began each session with a drawing activity. Shawna gradually began recognizing the symbolism present in her drawing. A bright yellow circle drawn at the top of the page was a symbol for the sun. Slowly, over the course of the school year, Shawna began acknowledging that letters and numbers stood for something other than lines on a page.

As Shawna's symbolic play expanded, I began working with her on practicing writing some of the letters in her name, concentrating on the "S," "A," and "W." These letters were particularly challenging for Shawna to master, given her visual perceptual challenges and the inherent difficulty in producing letters containing diagonal lines and lines that change direction midway. I demonstrated how to form each letter, provided a model, and ample opportunity for practice. Before writing on paper, we made the letters in the air using large arm movements. We then recited a rhyme which reinforced the movement patterns. By incorporating multiple senses, learning is more effective (Syahputri, 2019).

I provided some of Shawna's occupational therapy intervention within the classroom setting during "writing blocks," times when the whole class was engaging in writing tasks. During the writing block, Shawna's teacher chose one student to be "student of the day." The student of the day was asked to write their first name on the board and then to teach the class how to write their name. On their day, the student sat in a special chair and was interviewed by their classmates. The students in the classroom used paper which had a large box at the top and three widely spaced lines underneath. Each student was expected to print their own name at the top of the paper, draw a picture of the student of the day, and write two things about them that they learned during the interview. Given Shawna's challenges, this was an arduous task for her to complete, even with cueing and continual feedback. By providing contextually based occupational therapy services, or interventions within the classroom setting where Shawna was expected to engage in handwriting occupations, I was able to see that Shawna required continual verbal cues from me in order to sustain her visual attention to writing tasks. Further, she did not appear to have the motor schema for most of the letters in her name. Shawna also shared with me that she had never been chosen to be student of the day and that she wanted to be.

As an entering kindergarten student, Shawna had never received formal handwriting instruction, and her classroom teacher provided that instruction, using a formal writing program. The teacher demonstrated how to use writing tools/implements, how to stabilize the paper with one hand and write with the other, and how to form each upper- and lower-case letter of the alphabet. I provided adaptations for Shawna to use as needed, such as a slanted clipboard to stabilize her paper, as she could not use her left upper extremity to do so effectively. Outside of the classroom in our individual occupational therapy sessions, I introduced a variety of alternative lined papers to give Shawna additional sensory input, including raised lines and brightly colored paper. The tactile and visual feedback received from these papers provided additional sensory-based information that could be incorporated into Shawna's developing motor schema and provided her with the knowledge of results.

Once per week, the students were asked to sit on the floor to complete written work. Providing services within the classroom setting allowed me to collaborate with the classroom staff to problem solve ways to give Shawna access to this experience. The teacher had a few bean bag chairs in the classroom and Shawna was able to use one to position herself comfortably on the floor. I showed the classroom staff how to prop up the bean bag chair by stabilizing it against a hard surface, like the wall, to support a more upright posture for Shawna. I provided her with a tray table to stabilize her paper when writing. As we practiced the letters in Shawna's name in and out of the classroom, as she is required to write in both contexts, her motor schema became more accurate.

During the time when I worked with Shawna individually and outside of the classroom, we played games involving symbols and handwriting. This reinforced her recognition of letters and use of them as symbols. An example was playing Tic-Tac-Toe, substituting two letters from her name for the "X" and "O." This was one of her favorite games and she began playing it with classmates during recess, as well. She particularly liked drawing the horizontal and vertical lines of the grid. We provided each other with feedback on letter formation and how the letter fits in its assigned place in the grid. This provided Shawna with knowledge of the results, and it contributed to enlarging the motor schema.

By the end of the school year, Shawna was able to print her name legibly; however, she continued to require a model, verbal, and tactile cues, as well as the visual feedback provided by colored paper. She could not consistently articulate the graphic differences between some of the letters (i.e., "c" and "a") and she did not demonstrate the ability to understand the symbols that make up the alphabet. At the completion of her kindergarten year, Shawna did not own the concept of how letters can be combined to form words. She was able to achieve her goal of printing her own name and as "student of the day," she taught the students in her class how to form the letters in her name. Shawna continued to need support during playtime to engage in symbolic play and increased opportunities to practice the motor aspects of forming letters with feedback and knowledge of the results.

SUPPORTING EVIDENCE

There is an abundance of research on topics related to handwriting assessment, intervention, and processes across the lifespan (Francher et al., 2018; Gillespie & Graham, 2014; Schneider et al., 2023). For the purposes of this frame of reference, only research focusing on children and adolescents will be discussed. In this section, studies providing evidence on the impact of handwriting difficulties on children, adolescents, and their caregivers; the reliability and validity of assessment tools used to evaluate handwriting skills; and the effectiveness of handwriting programs and training, will be summarized as they relate to this frame of reference.

Studies (Francher et al., 2018; Gillespie & Graham, 2014; Schneider et al., 2023) have explored the impact of handwriting difficulties on children, adolescents, and their caregivers. The authors of a meta-analysis of over 40 studies on handwriting concluded that when students needed to focus on forming letters, the content of their writing was not as rich as students who wrote with more automaticity (Gillespie & Graham, 2014). Further, students who take proficient notes during class demonstrate an increased ability to retain academic information, complete work in a timely manner, and perform at grade level (Graham et al., 2000). The research shows that when children find handwriting to be laborious, they have difficulty expressing themselves through handwritten means, and the substance and length of their narratives may be compromised (Francher et al., 2018; Gillespie & Graham, 2014; Schneider et al., 2023).

Effectiveness of Handwriting Programs and Training

There are several commercially available handwriting programs being used in pediatric practice. Some of the more widely used programs include *Handwriting Without Tears* (Learning Without Tears, n.d.), *Size Matters* (Moskowitz et al., 2017), and *Write Start* (Case-Smith et al., 2011; Engel et al., 2018). Each of these programs include materials, such as special papers used for writing, visuals, and protocols for training (Engel et al., 2018). The literature has shown a positive correlation between handwriting legibility and adherence to formal handwriting instruction (Case-Smith et al., 2011; Case-Smith et al., 2014a; Donica & Holt, 2019; Engel et al., 2018; Francher et al., 2018; Graham et al., 2008; Hoy et al., 2011; Learning Without Tears, n.d.; Lust & Donica, 2011; Moskowitz et al., 2017; Pfeiffer et al., 2015; Roberts et al., 2014). Although these formalized occupation-based programs are used broadly, most therapists report using multiple treatment approaches in their interventions, ranging from occupation based, using a top-down approach, to foundational skill development based, using a bottom-up approach (Denton et al., 2006; Feder et al., 2000; Peterson & Nelson, 2003). Research supports the effectiveness of several strategies used to teach handwriting skills. They are: (1) demonstration of letter formation using directional arrows as other visual reminders; (2) the use of visual letter models; (3) continual and consistent practice in various natural settings, such as the home and school; (4) providing students with immediate, accurate, and specific feedback on the results of a student's written product; (5) providing opportunities for students to evaluate their own work; and individualization of instruction based on the student's needs (Case-Smith et al., 2011; Cramm & Egan, 2015; Francher et al., 2018; Hoy et al., 2011; Santangelo & Graham, 2016; Wallen et al., 2013).

These strategies, embedded into the proposed intervention application, are supported by the theoretical base of this frame of reference.

Summary

In summary, the acquisition of handwriting skills is grounded in several factors. The first being the child's ability to learn the concept that letters, words, and numbers are symbols, representing something more than lines on a page. From a developmental perspective, a child must also possess physical, cognitive, sensory, visual perceptual, and socioemotional readiness to carry out the task of handwriting. The next factor is that a child must receive adequate handwriting instruction. They require foundational knowledge on how to form letters of appropriate size with good line orientation and spacing on the page. Children also require significant opportunities to practice writing in varied environments and contexts with feedback on their performance, to develop motor schemas for how letters and words should be written. Once the schema are developed, automaticity must occur to allow the child to concentrate on the content of what they are writing, rather than the mechanics of their handwriting.

This frame of reference provides a framework with which occupational therapy practitioners can take actionable steps to evaluate and provide intervention to children experiencing difficulties in handwriting.

REFERENCES

Adams, W., & Sheslow, D. (1995). *The wide range assessment of visual motor ability (WRAVMA)*. Retrieved https://www.wpspublish.com/wravma-wide-range-assessment-of-visual-motor-ability. Retrieved April 1, 2024.

American Occupational Therapy Association (AOTA). (2020). Occupational therapy practice framework: Domain and process (4th ed.). *American Journal of Occupational Therapy*, *74*(2), 7412410010. https://doi.org/10.5014/ajot.2020.74S2001

American Psychiatric Association. (2013). *Diagnostic and statistical manual of mental disorders* (5th ed.). https://doi.org/10.1176/appi.books.9780890425596

Amundson, S. J. (1995). *The evaluation tool of children's handwriting (ETCH)*. Retrieved https://www.therapro.com/Evaluation-Tool-of-Childrens-Handwriting-ETCH.html. Retrieved April 1, 2024.

Ayres, A. J. (1989). *The sensory integration and praxis tests*. Western Psychological Services.

Ayres, A. J., & Robbins, J. (2005). Sensory integration and the child: Understanding hidden sensory challenges. *Western Psychological Services*. ISBN 0874244374, 9780874244373

Beery, K. E., Buktenica, N. A., & Beery, N. A. (2010). *Beery-Buktenica developmental test of visual-motor integration* (6th ed.). Retrieved https://www.pearsonassessments.com/store/usassessments/en/Store/Professional-Assessments/MotorSensory/Beery-Buktenica-Developmental-Test-of-Visual-Motor-Integration-%7C-Sixth-Edition/p/100000663.html. Retrieved April 1, 2024.

Benbow, M. (2006). Principles and practices of teaching handwriting. In A. Henderson & C. Pehoski (Eds.), *Hand function in the child: Foundations for remediation* (2nd ed., pp. 319–342). Mosby. https://doi.org/10.1016/B978-032303186-8.50018-6

Bonneton-Botte, N., Miramand, L., Bailly, R., & Pons, C. (2023). Teaching and rehabilitation of handwriting for children in the digital age: Issues and challenges. *Children (Basel)*. *10*(7), 1096. https://doi.org/10.3390/children10071096

Bronfenbrenner, U. (1986). Ecology of the family as a context for human development: Research perspectives. *Developmental Psychology*, *22*(6), 723–742. https://doi.org/10.1037/0012-1649.22.6.723

Bruininks, R., & Bruininks, B. (2024). *Bruininks-Oseretsky Test of Motor Proficiency (BOT-3)* (3rd ed.).

Carlson, A. G., Rowe, E., & Curby, T. W. (2013). Disentangling fine motor skills' relations to academic achievement: The relative contributions of visual-spatial integration and visual-motor coordination. *The Journal of Genetic Psychology*, *174*(5), 514–533. https://doi.org/10.1080/00221325.2012.717122

Case-Smith, J., Holland, T., & Bishop, B. (2011). Effectiveness of an integrated handwriting program for first-grade students: A pilot study. *American Journal of Occupational Therapy*, *65*(6), 670–678. https://doi.org/10.5014/ajot.2011.000984

Case-Smith, J., Holland, T., & White, S. (2014a). Effectiveness of a co-taught handwriting program for first grade students. *Physical and Occupational Therapy in Pediatrics*, *34*(1):30–43. https://doi.org/10.3109/01942638.2013.783898.

Case-Smith, J., Weaver, L., & Holland, T. (2014b). Effects of a classroom-embedded occupational therapist-teacher handwriting program for first-grade students. *American Journal of Occupational Therapy*, *68*(6), 690–698. https://doi.org/10.5014/ajot.2014.011585

Cermak, S. A., & Bissell, J. (2014). Content and construct validity of Here's How I Write (HHIW): A child's self-assessment and goal setting tool. *The American Journal of Occupational Therapy*, *68*(3), 296–306. https://doi.org/10.5014/ajot.2014.010637

Cleveland Clinic. (n.d.). *Developmental milestones*. Retrieved https://my.clevelandclinic.org/health/articles/25235-fine-motor-skills. Retrieved April 1, 2024.

Colarusso, R. P., & Hammill, D. D. (2003). *Motor-free visual perceptual test* (3rd ed.). Academic Therapy Publications. https://doi.org/10.1177/0734282906286339

Cornhill, H., & Case-Smith, J. (1996). Factors that relate to good and poor handwriting. *American Journal of Occupational Therapy*, *50*(9), 732–739. https://doi.org/10.5014/ajot.50.9.732

Coster, W., Deeney, T., Haltiwanger, J., & Haley, S. (1998). School Function Assessment. San Antonio, TX: Psychological Corporation.

Cramm, H., & Egan, M. (2015). Practice patterns of school-based occupational therapists targeting handwriting: A knowledge-to-practice gap. *Journal of Occupational Therapy, School and Early Intervention*, *8*(2), 170–179. https://doi.org/10.1080/19411243.2015.1040942

Denton, P., Cope, S., & Moser, C. (2006). The effects of sensorimotor-based intervention versus therapeutic practice on improving handwriting performance in 6- to 11-year-old children. *The American Journal of Occupational Therapy*, *60*(1), 16–27. https://doi.org/10.5014/ajot.60.1.16

Döhla, D., & Heim, S. (2016). Developmental dyslexia and dysgraphia: What can we learn from the one about the other? *Frontiers in Psychology, 6*, 2045. https://doi.org/10.3389/fpsyg.2015.02045

Donica D. K., Goins, A., & Wagner, L. (2013). Effectiveness of handwriting readiness programs on postural control, hand control, and letter and number formation in Head Start classrooms. *Journal of Occupational Therapy Schools & Early Intervention, 6*(2), 81–93. https://doi.org/10.1080/19411243.2013.810938

Donica, D. K., & Holt, S. (2019). Examining validity of the Print Tool compared with Test of Handwriting Skills-Revised. *Occupational Therapy Journal of Research, 39*(3):167–175. https://doi.org/10.1177/1539449218804529

Engel, C., Lillie, K., Zurawski, S., & Travers, B. G. (2018). Curriculum-based handwriting programs: A systematic review with effect sizes. *American Journal of Occupational Therapy, 72*(3), 7203205010p1–7203205010p8. https://doi.org/10.5014/ajot.2018.027110

Feder, K., Majnemer, A., & Synnes, A. (2000). Handwriting: current trends in occupational therapy practice. *Canadian Journal of Occupational Therapy, 67*(3):197–204. https://doi.org/10.1177/000841740006700313

Feder, K. P., & Majnemer, A. (2007). Handwriting development, competency, and intervention. *Developmental Medical Child Neurology, 49*(4):312–7. https://doi.org/10.1111/j.1469-8749.2007.00312.x

Fisher, A. G., Bryze, K., Hume, V., & Griswold, L. A. (2007). *School AMPS: School version of the assessment of motor and process skills* (2nd ed.). Fort Collins, CO: Three Star Press.

Folio, M.R., & Fewell, R.R. (2023). *Peabody developmental motor scales* (3rd ed.). PRO-ED.

Francher, L. A., Priestley-Hopkins, D. A., & Jeffries, L. M. (2018). Handwriting acquisition and intervention: A systematic review. *Journal of Occupational Therapy, Schools, & Early Intervention, 11*(4), 454–473. https://doi.org/10.1080/19411243.2018.153463

Garfinkel, M. (2024). The use of the PC-SCP in school settings. In Waldman-Levi, A. and Bundy A. *Parent/caregiver support of children's playfulness (PC–SCP)*. AOTA Press, 43–50.

Gibson, J. J., (2014). *The ecological approach to visual perception*. Imprint Psychology Press. https://doi.org/10.4324/9781315740218

Gillespie, A., & Graham, S. (2014). A meta-analysis of writing interventions for students with learning disabilities. *Exceptional Children, 80*(4), 454–473. https://doi.org/10.1177/0014402914527238

Graham, S., Harris, K. R., & Fink, B. (2000). Is handwriting causally related to learning to write? Treatment of handwriting problems in beginning writers. *Journal of Educational Psychology, 92*(4), 620–633. https://doi.org/10.1037//0022-0663.92.4.620

Graham, S., Harris, K. R., Mason, L., Fink-Chorzempa, B., Moran, S., & Saddler, B. (2008). How do primary grade teachers teach handwriting? A national survey. *Reading and Writing, 21*(1–2), 49–69. https://doi.org/10.1007/s11145-007-9064-z

Graham, S., Struck, M., Santoro, J., & Berninger, V. W. (2006). Dimensions of good and poor handwriting legibility in first and second graders: Motor program, visual-spatial arrangement, and letter formation parameters. *Developmental Neuropsychology, 29*(1), 43–60. https://doi.org/10.1207/s15326942dn2901_4

Haley, S. M., Coster, W. J., Ludlow, L. H., Haltiwanger, J. T., & Andrellos, P. J. (1992). *Pediatric evaluation of disability inventory (PEDI)*. Retrieved https://www.pearsonassessments.com/store/usassessments/en/Store/Professional-Assessments/Developmental-Early-Childhood/Pediatric-Evaluation-of-Disability-Inventory/p/100000505.html. Retrieved April 1, 2024.

Hammerschmidt, S. L., & Sudsawad, P. (2004). Teachers' survey on problems with handwriting: Referral, evaluation, and outcomes. *American Journal of Occupational Therapy, 58*, 185–192.

Hammill, D. D., Pearson, N. A., & Voress, J. K. (2014). *Developmental test of visual perception* (3rd ed.). PRO-ED. Retrieved https://www.sralab.org/rehabilitation-measures/developmental-test-visual-perception-third-edition. Retrieved April 1, 2024.

Howe, T. H., Roston, K. L., Sheu, C. F., & Hinojosa, J. (2013). Assessing handwriting intervention effectiveness in elementary school students: a two-group controlled study. *American Journal of Occupational Therapy, 67*(1), 19–26. https://doi.org/10.5014/ajot.2013.005470

Hoy, M. M., Egan, M. Y., & Feder, K. P. (2011). A systematic review of interventions to improve handwriting. *Canadian Journal of Occupational Therapy, 78*(1), 13–25. https://doi.org/10.2182/cjot.2011.78.1.3

Jiménez, J. E. (2017). Writing disabilities in Spanish-speaking children: Introduction to the special series. *Journal of Learning Disabilities, 50*(5), 483–490. https://doi.org/10.1177/0022219416633126

Kaplan, M. (2020). Frame of reference for motor acquisition. In P. Kramer, J. Hinojosa, & T. H. Howe (Eds.), *Frames of reference for pediatric occupational therapy* (4th ed., pp. 391–424). Wolters Kluwer.

Karlsdottir, R., & Stefansson, T. (2002). Problems in developing functional handwriting. *Perceptual Motor Skills, 94*, 623–662.

Laszlo, J., & Broderick, P. (1991). Drawing and handwriting difficulties: Reasons for and remediation of dysfunction. In J. Wann, A. Wing, & N. Sovik (Eds.), *Development of graphic skills* (pp. 259–280). Academic Press.

Law, M. C., Baum, C. M., & Dunn, W. (Eds.). (2016). Measuring occupational performance: Supporting best practice in occupational therapy. (3rd Ed.). SLACK Incorporated.

Learning Without Tears. (n.d.). *The print tool.* Retrieved https://shopping.lwtears.com/product/the-print-tool-evaluation-remediation-package/01t4V000007a2pxQAA

Lieberman, L. M. (1984). Visual perception versus visual function. *Journal of Learning Disabilities*, *17*, 182–185. https://doi.org/10.1177/002221948401700311

Lust, C. A., & Donica, D. K. (2011). Effectiveness of a handwriting readiness program in head start: A two-group controlled trial. *American Journal of Occupational Therapy*, *65*(5), 560–568. https://doi.org/10.5014/ajot.2011.000612

Martin, N. A. (2017). *Test of visual perceptual skills (TVPS)* (4th ed.). Retrieved https://www.wpspublish.com/tvps-4-test-of-visual-perception-skills-4th-edition. Retrieved April 1, 2024.

McHale, K., & Cermack, S. A. (1992). Fine motor activities in elementary school: Preliminary findings and provisional implications for children with fine motor problems. *American Journal of Occupational Therapy*, *46*(10), 898–903. https://doi.org/10.5014/ajot.46.10.898

Milone, M. (2007). *The test of handwriting skills, revised*. Retrieved https://www.wpspublish.com/ths-r-test-of-handwriting-skills-revised. Retrieved April 1, 2024.

Moskowitz, B., Carswell, B., Kitzmiller, J., Bushell, M., Neikrug, L., Gottesman, C., Pfeiffer, B., Rai, G., & Murray, T. (2017). The effectiveness of the Size Matters Handwriting Program. *The American Journal of Occupational Therapy*, *71*(4 Supplement 1), 7111520304p1. https://doi.org/10.5014/ajot.2017.71S1-PO5147

O'Brien, J. C., & Kuhaneck, H. (2016). *Case-Smith's occupational therapy for children and adolescents* (8th ed). Mosby.

Pade, M., Liberman, L., Sopher, R. S., & Ratzon, N. Z. (2018). *Pressure distributions on the chair seat and backrest correlate with handwriting outcomes of school children*. IOS Press. Retrieved https://content.iospress.com/articles/work/wor182831. Retrieved April 1, 2024.

Peterson, C. Q., & Nelson, D. L. (2003). Effect of an occupational intervention on printing in children with economic disadvantages. *American Journal of Occupational Therapy*, *57*(2), 152–160. https://doi.org/10.5014/ajot.57.2.152

Pfeiffer, B., Rai, G., Murray, T., & Brusilovskiy, E. (2015). Effectiveness of the size matters handwriting program. *Occupational Therapy Journal of Research: Occupation, Participation and Health*, *35*(2), 110–119. https://doi.org/10.1177/1539449215573004

Piaget, J. (1954). *The construction of reality in the child (M. Cook, Trans.)*. Basic Books. https://doi.org/10.1037/11168-000

Pienaar, A. E., Barhosrst, R., & Twisk, J. W. R. (2013). Relationships between academic performance, SES school type and perceptual-motor skills in first grade South African learners: NW-CHILD study. *Child Care Health Development*, *40*(3), 370–378. https://doi.org/10.1111/cch.12059

Reisman, J. (1999). *Minnesota Handwriting Assessment*, San Antonio, TX: Harcourt Assessment.

Ritty, J. M., Solan, H. A., & Cool, S. J. (1993). Visual and sensory-motor functioning in the classroom: A preliminary report of ergonomic demands. *Journal of the American Optometric Association*, *64*(4), 238–244.

Roberts, G. I., Derkach-Ferguson, A. F., Siever, J. E., & Rose, M. S. (2014). An examination of the effectiveness of handwriting without tears® instruction. *Canadian Journal of Occupational Therapy*, *81*(2), 102–113. https://doi.org/10.1177/0008417414527065

Roston, K. (2020). A frame of reference for developing handwriting skills. In P. Kramer, J. Hinojosa, & T. H. Howe (Eds.), *Frames of Reference for Pediatric Occupational Therapy* (4th ed., pp. 427–460). Wolters Kluwer.

Roston, K. L., Hinojosa, J., & Kaplan, H. (2008). Using the Minnesota Handwriting Assessment and Handwriting Checklist in screening first and second graders' handwriting legibility. *Journal of Occupational Therapy Schools & Early Intervention*, *1*(1), 100–115. https://doi.org/10.1080/19411240802312947

Santangelo, T., & Graham, S. (2016). A comprehensive meta-analysis of handwriting instruction. *Education Psychology Review*, *28*, 225–265. https://doi.org/10.1007/s10648015-9335-1

Schmidt, R. A. (1975). A schema theory of discrete motor skill learning. *Psychological Review*, *82*, 225–260. https://doi.org/10.1037/h0076770

Schmidt, R. A., & Lee, T. D. (2014). *Motor learning and performance: From principles to application* (5th ed.). Human Kinetics.

Schneck, C. M. (2020). A frame of reference for visual perception. In P. Kramer, J. Hinojosa, & T. H. Howe (Eds.), *Frames of reference for pediatric occupational therapy* (4th ed, pp. 319–356). Wolters Kluwer.

Schneider, M. K., Myers, C. T., Morgan-Daniel, J., & Shechtman, O. (2023). A scoping review of grasp and handwriting performance in school-age children. *Physical & Occupational Therapy in Pediatrics*, *43*(4), 430–445. https://doi.org/10.1080/01942638.2022.2151392

Schwellnus, H., Carnahan, H., Kushki, A., Polatajko, H., Missiuna, C., & Chau, T. (2013). Writing forces associated with four pencil grasp patterns in grade 4 children. *The American Journal of Occupational Therapy*, *67*(2), 218–227. https://doi.org/10.5014/ajot.2013.005538

Slotnick, S. D., Thompson, W. L., & Kosslyn, S. M. (2012). Visual memory and visual mental imagery recruit common control and sensory regions of the brain. *Cognitive Neuroscience*, *3*(1), 14–20. https://doi.org/10.1080/17588928.2011.57821

Sudsawad, P., Trombly, C. A., Henderson, A., & Tickle-Degnen, L. (2002). Testing the effect of kinesthetic training on handwriting performance in first-grade students. *American Journal of Occupational Therapy*, *56*(1), 26–33. https://doi.org/10.5014/ajot.56.1.26

Syahputri, D. (2019). The effect of multisensory teaching method on the students' reading achievement. *Budapest International Research and Critics in Linguistics and Education (BirLE) Journal*, *2*(1), 124–131. https://doi.org/10.33258/birle.v2i1.192

Tse, L. F. L., Siu, A. M. H., & Li-Tsang, C. W. P. (2019). Developmental skills between kindergarten children with handwriting difficulties in Chinese and/or English. *Australian Occupational Therapy Journal*, *66*(3), 292–303. https://doi.org/10.1111/1440-1630.12550.

Tseng, M. H., & Cermak, S. A. (1993). The influence of ergonomic factors and perceptual-motor abilities on handwriting performance. *American Journal of Occupational Therapy*, *47*(10), 919–926. https://doi.org/10.5014/ajot.47.10.919.

Tseng, M. H., & Chow, S. M. (2000). Perceptual-motor function of school-age children with slow handwriting speed. *American Journal of Occupational Therapy*, *54*(1), 83–88. https://doi.org/10.5014/ajot.54.1.83

Vico, R., Martin, J., & Gonzalez, M. (2023). Functional assessment of handwriting among children: A systematic review of the psychometric properties. *American Journal of Occupational Therapy*, *77*, 1–9

Volman, M. J., van Schendel, B. M., & Jongmans, M. J. (2006). Handwriting difficulties in primary school children: a search for underlying mechanisms. *American Journal of Occupational Therapy*, *60*(4):451–460. https://doi.org/10.5014/ajot.60.4.451

Wallen, M., Duff, S., Goyen, T. A., & Froude, E. (2013). Respecting the evidence: Responsible assessment and effective intervention for children with handwriting difficulties. *Australian Occupational Therapy Journal*, *60*(5), 366–369. https://doi.org/10.1111/1440-1630.12045

Weinstock-Zlotick, G., & Hinojosa, J., (2004). Bottom-up or top-down evaluation: is one better than the other? *American Journal of Occupational Therapy*, *58*(5), 594–599. https://doi.org/10.5014/ajot.58.5.594

Weintraub, N., & Graham, S. (1998). Writing legibly and quickly: A study of children's ability to adjust their handwriting to meet common classroom demands. *Learning Disabilities Research & Practice*, *13*(3), 146–152.

A Biomechanical Frame of Reference to Position Children for Function

13

Christine Rocchio Mueller ■ Cheryl Colangelo

The biomechanical frame of reference to position children for function is applied when they cannot maintain postural control through appropriate automatic muscle activity due to neuromuscular or musculoskeletal dysfunction. Consequently, external supports are provided, temporarily or permanently, to substitute for the lack of postural control and to provide positions of the body for participation in meaningful activity.

For controlled movement, the human body must provide a stable base from which the head and limbs can move. Every movement creates a shift in the center of gravity that requires a compensatory postural reaction (Figure 13.1) to prevent falling in the direction of the movement. Every time a person moves in relation to another person or object, the person must first move in relation to a greater force (i.e., gravity). This movement is done subtly. Each time a person eats a sandwich, embraces a child, or reaches for a book, they must first shift their bodies position against the earth's gravitational pull.

Gravity affects the human body on physical, mechanical, and physiologic levels. Physically, gravity pulls the body toward the earth. It makes a person tend to fall down. Gravity also makes the movement of limbs away from the earth's surface more difficult to execute. Mechanically, each time a person moves a limb away from the center of the body (e.g., when reaching), a lever arm is created that tends to topple the body by pulling the trunk in the direction of the limb. Fortunately, there are mechanical and physiologic mechanisms that help the body to adapt to the forces of gravity. Responding to the changes of muscle length, body positions, movement speed, or direction, the human body activates an equilibrium reaction to allow the body to remain upright or balanced in a predictable and functional way. The term "biomechanical" is the interaction of external and internal physical forces on the living body.

The biomechanical frame of reference applies the principles of physics to human movement and posture with respect to the force of gravity. There are two general goals of the biomechanical frame of reference to position children for function, they are (1) to enhance the development of postural reactions by reducing the demands of gravity and by aligning the body, and (2) to provide external support for proximal stability to liberate movement of distal body parts and improve skilled activity. By providing proximal external support, we can then directly address functional performance and reduce the need for, or the demands on, postural reactions or less efficient compensatory movements.

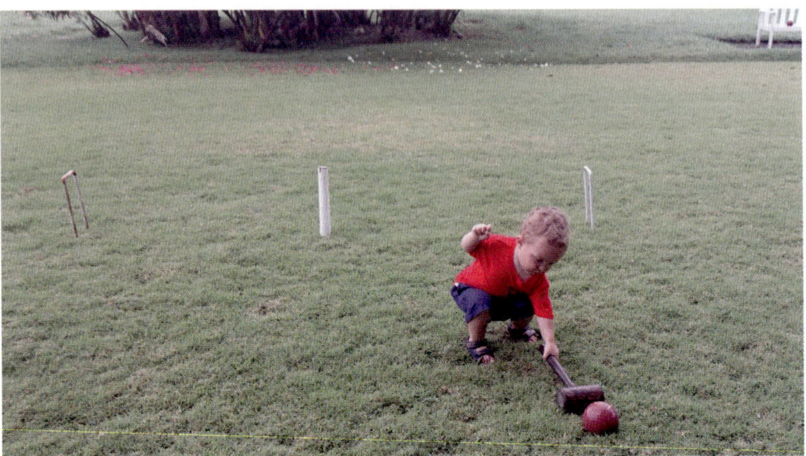

FIGURE 13.1 When the child reaches out with the mallet, his center of gravity shifts. As a compensatory postural reaction, his right shoulder retracts.

The biomechanical frame of reference to position children for function is frequently and successfully used with children who have physical disabilities and to maximize children's potential for movement and function. The biomechanical frame of reference is often tailored to address several areas at the same time, depending on the child's treatment plan and goals. For example, it can be applied to facilitate postural control and minimize children's risk of deformities at the body structure and function level, as well as activity and participation (Costigan, 2011; World Health Organization, 2001). Activity limitations can be addressed using the biomechanical frame of reference to improve stability in sitting, safety, and comfort to enhance fine motor performance such as self-feeding skills or handwriting (Ryan, 2012; World Health Organization, 2001).

Several models in occupational therapy reflect the framework of the World Health Organization, positing that performance is linked to both the child's internal and external environment and the task they are engaged in. They provide an essential foundation for occupational therapists applying biopsychosocial concepts in conjunction with the biomechanical frame of reference for function. The Person-Environment-Occupation (PEO) model considers the person, their environment, and the occupations in which they engage. While these needs may change across the lifespan, the more congruent the relationship among these factors, the higher the quality of occupational performance (Law et al., 1996). Relevant factors for positioning that can facilitate or hinder a child's participation in activities, beyond physical status, include:

- **Person:** motivation, understanding of device use, acceptance, sensory regulation
- **Environment:** physical space, caretaker acceptance and management skills, ambient sensory environment
- **Activity/task:** temporal aspects of length and frequency of participation, contextual factors

The Human Activity Assistive Technology (HAAT), a model developed by an occupational therapist and a rehabilitation engineer, focuses on how technology or positioning aids can be integrated into an activity to enhance an individual's participation and performance with consideration to their physical needs using the principles of the biomechanical frame of reference

(Polgar et al., 2020). A specialized seating system (assistive technology) designed for a child with low tone (human) can provide posture and support requirements to promote better positioning during classroom tasks (activity). Improvement in participation have been shown if at least one factor from each domain has been addressed.

Utilizing these other frames of reference in conjunction with the biomechanical frame of reference to position a child helps to consider the complexity of childhood including their customary environments such as home, school, the community, their family supports, and developmental progression and personal interests.

THEORETICAL BASE

Assumptions

As previously discussed, the biomechanical frame of reference to position children for function maintains the following six major assumptions:

1. This frame of reference contributes to independent participation by providing external supports to substitute for inadequate or abnormal postural reactions, and therefore:
   a. it facilitates the development of some postural control by reducing the effects of gravity, or
   b. it provides a permanent support when the potential to improve seems negligible.
2. Sensory feedback supports children's learning to move effectively, especially through the proprioceptive, vestibular, tactile, and visual systems. Children repeat successful movements based on the sensory cues that the movements provide. In addition, the role of self-regulation, as it relates to sensory processing, influences postural maintenance and control.
3. Normal motor development is predictable and sequential. The development of motor abilities depends on a stable base of support and on the righting and equilibrium reactions that allow a person to respond automatically to the forces of gravity.
   a. Posture depends on the body's response to gravity.
   b. Postural reactions develop sequentially. Each new skill is based on a previously developed skill.
4. Dysfunction or abnormalities of the musculoskeletal, or central nervous system (CNS) may impair the development of normal postural reactions.
   a. Tone affects posture; tone is influenced by many internal and external factors, all of which can be modified.
   b. If normal postural control has not developed, the body compensates by using substitute movements, more effort, and more conscious attention. All of which may interfere with function.
5. The manifestation of postural reactions is influenced not only by neurodevelopment but also by factors related to children, their environments, and tasks. These include, but are not limited to, other body functions; coping styles; motivation; social, cultural, and physical environments; and the characteristics of the task in which children are involved.
6. Occupational therapists must determine the level of postural dysfunction and the external factors that may affect performance. Treatment needs to provide substitutes for absent skills yet still makes demands on the children's existing capacity to function.

The biomechanical frame of reference to position children for function draws from theories in physics and physiology, as well as those addressing motor development. It addresses the implications of physical and physiologic principles on motor development. The biomechanical frame of reference accepts two assumptions for positioning children for functioning in terms of postural control: (1) motor patterns develop from responses to sensory stimulation and (2) automatic motor responses, which maintain posture, develop predictably. This frame of reference also contains the assumption that the practitioner knows and understands normal development and that impairment of musculoskeletal or neuromuscular functions can interfere with effective postural reactions and that motor control emerges not only from neuromuscular functions but also from their interaction with factors such as motivation, personal attitudes, and coping styles, as well as the social, physical, and cultural environments.

Interventions based on the assumptions regarding modifying physical structures of the body for optimal function often require extensive and precise measurements of both the child's body and the supportive device to achieve the optimal match. This process represents the symbiotic relationship between biologic and mechanical elements. Biologic contributors are far more individualized, especially when the CNS is compromised. The biomechanical frame of reference is often utilized to address orthopedic problems that manifest fairly consistently. However, postural needs as a result of CNS dysfunction and/or developmental anomalies tend to be more complex and inconsistent, depending on internal and external factors influencing the individual. While many childhood diagnoses that involve the CNS are not progressive, when left untreated they can affect the musculoskeletal system, leading to orthopedic issues. Thus, assessment and intervention must incorporate a much broader approach.

A comprehensive understanding of typical and atypical motor development is a necessary precursor to the application of this frame of reference. Such a discussion is beyond the scope of this chapter but can be found in numerous textbooks (Bly, 2011; O'Brien & Kuhaneck, 2020).

The following theoretical sections will abbreviate relevant concepts as they apply to biomechanics and positioning for function.

Motor Patterns and Sensory Input

In the developmental continuum encompassing early reflexive movements to mature postural responses, one can consider early reflexes, which are primarily, but not exclusively, elicited by tactile, proprioceptive, and vestibular input, as an opportunity for the infant to experience sensory input via the manifestations of these reflexes. With exploration and maturation comes the integration of stereotypical movement patterns and more selective movements that are motivated by a child's environmental interests. This integration ultimately leads to more choices and control (variability) in the child's movement repertoire.

Mature postural reactions include finding a stable base of support through righting and equilibrium reactions effectively maintaining posture while liberating distal parts (eyes, mouth, arms). For example, placing both feet on the floor and stabilizing at the trunk before reaching with the arms for goal-directed interaction with people and objects.

A postural analysis of a child using the biomechanical frame of reference focuses on range of motion, strength, and endurance, and their influence on the volitional movement. This may be accomplished by modifying sensory input that elicits certain movements or by supporting body parts to provide proximal stability. For example, stabilizing the head at midline or changing classroom placement for midline attention can prevent an asymmetrical tonic neck reflex (ATNR) response through decreased proprioceptive input for improved midline hand use. In addition, mature postural responses may be recruited via positioning in space increasing vestibular and proprioceptive input to enhance righting reactions and increase neck strength.

Postural Control in the Developmental Sequence

The biomechanical frame of reference to position children for function focuses on function within a relatively static position rather than on transitional movements. It is essential, therefore, to be familiar with the developmental sequence of motor characteristics of various positions. Children with neuromuscular dysfunction often have immature motor patterns and need to experience more variability of movement. This allows them to select the most effective movement patterns for goal-directed use. Application of these concepts from evaluation to clinical decision making is an essential component of the biomechanical frame of reference. While use of external supports implies a certain amount of immobility (to provide stability), knowledge of salient features of motor development is essential in determining which positions may be used therapeutically for an individual, and how to modify those positions for proximal stability and distal mobility.

Generally, the ***supine position*** is not a productive position for function, but many movement components can be used effectively in a semireclined sitting position. The way that the child responds to the forces of gravity will influence the decision to use this position or more likely a modification of this position. In the ***prone position,*** the reduced demands on trunk and pelvic control provide early options for head control and the development of shoulder stability and midline use of hands. The ***sidelying position*** provides head stability, supports the shoulders for direct reaching on a horizontal plane, and provides visual access to both hands.

The biomechanical frame of reference considers ***sitting*** as a stable position from which the child can engage in meaningful activities (Figure 13.2A). Moving in and out of positions is better addressed through other frames of reference unless external support or modifications can contribute to this process. For competent sitting, righting and equilibrium reactions must be mature in order to liberate distal body parts (such the head, eyes, mouth, and arms) for functional activity.

When an occupational therapist applies the biomechanical frame of reference to ***the standing position*** (Figure 13.2B), it is to address functional goals rather than the potential for ambulation. The position provides an opportunity for children to experience an upright erect position encouraging a stable trunk as a base for distal control and engagement with people and objects. In addition, depending on the angle of the body's vertical position in space, sensory input can be modified to elicit more effective righting reactions in the head and trunk, enhancing head and shoulder control.

Interference With Postural Reactions That Result From Damage or Dysfunction

Dysfunction of the neuromuscular or musculoskeletal system has serious implications for postural control. Inadequate muscle strength and atypical muscle tone, fixed bony deformities, and soft tissue contractures interfere with freedom of movement. A compensatory movement or posture may result in the body's attempt to make up for inadequate neuromuscular or musculoskeletal actions while responding to disturbance of the base of support, leading to the use of less effective, and inefficient movements that are more accessible. Compensations often decrease

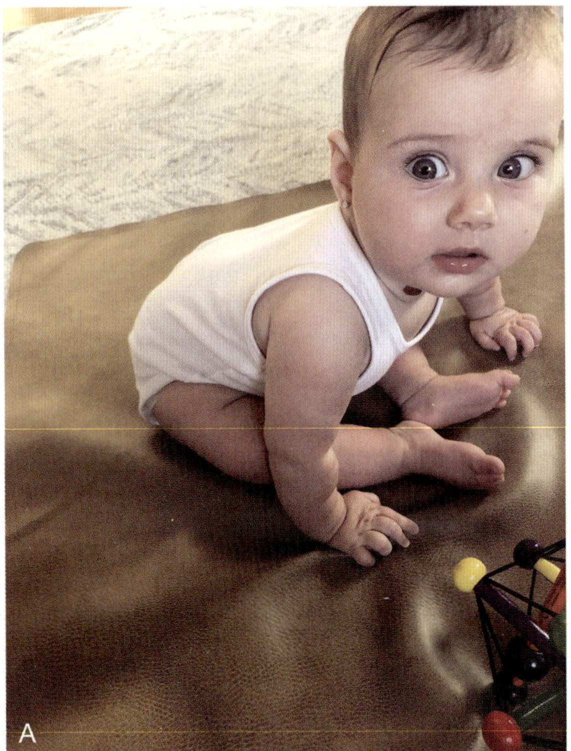

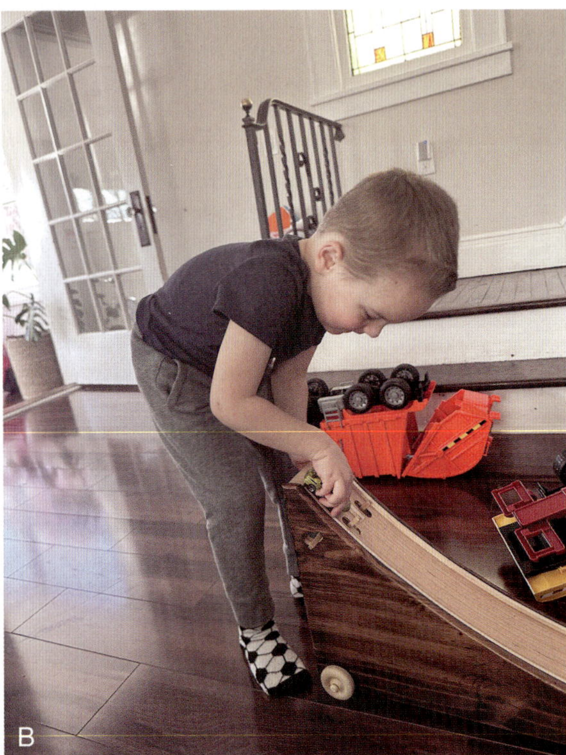

FIGURE 13.2 **A.** The infant must use their arms to prop in an early unsupported sitting. While toys can be motivating for play the arms are not free for active exploration, and the pelvis is forward for stability. **B.** This child has an established base of support and is able to reach toward items for exploration.

mobility in joints that are not affected directly by the initial deforming process because the compensatory positions must be sustained to provide a stable posture. They may result in bony deformities or soft tissue contractions in any situation in which normal movement patterns are consistently compromised.

Motor problems that result from CNS disorders (e.g., cerebral palsy or static encephalopathy) are extremely diverse and complex. This is because such neuromuscular dysfunction is global and is rarely isolated to one specific site in the body. Similarly, motor problems are complex because the manifestations of these dysfunctions can fluctuate depending on a variety of factors, including changes in the child's position in space, effort in activities, affect, and stimulation in the environment.

Muscle tone depends on the ability of motor neurons to activate muscle fibers, and the ability of the CNS to respond to sensory cues by coordinating the activity of agonist and antagonist muscles. Typical muscle tone allows a muscle at rest to react immediately, with enough tension for weight shifting and support yet still have enough "give" to allow for quick changes in movement (Scherzer & Tscharnuter, 1990). Hypotonia, characterized by atypically low tone, produces delayed, and often inadequate, postural responses, giving the child a "floppy" appearance. Hypotonicity should not be confused with weakness. Maintaining upright positions is impaired and, while many joints may be hypermobile, there may be shortening and decreased flexibility in muscle groups that are enlisted as compensations.

Table 13.1 Biomechanical Risk Factors

Tone Abnormality	Biomechanical Risk Factors	Effect on Postural Control
Low tone (hypotonia)	Decreased joint stability	Joint laxity, leading to reduced postural stability and increased risk of joint hypermobility
	Overstretched or lengthened muscles	Difficulty maintaining upright posture and controlling movements due to weak muscles
	Difficulty initiating or sustaining muscle contractions	Poor proprioception and muscle coordination, affecting balance and coordination
High tone (hypertonus)	Increased muscle stiffness and resistance to movement	Decreased joint mobility and flexibility, leading to restricted range of motion and joint contractures
	Muscle tightness and contractures	Difficulty achieving and maintaining neutral posture, contributing to postural misalignments
	Difficulty relaxing or releasing muscle contractions	Abnormal muscle cocontractions, affecting postural control and movement efficiency

Hypertonia, characterized by spasticity or rigidity, manifests in overreaction to stretch. Affected muscles appear "tight," with exaggerated responses to quick stretch and resistance to passive stretch. Hypertonicity primarily affects antigravity muscle groups (flexion in upper extremities and extension in lower extremities), though it may not affect all muscles in these groups. The interaction of hypertonic and normal muscles results in atypical postural patterns. Additionally, normal muscles working in synergy with hypertonic muscles tend to become shortened because spastic muscles limit the range of movement, preventing full lengthening of the muscles they are attached to.

Many medical conditions (such as cerebral palsy, Down syndrome, myasthenia gravis) can affect a child's tone. Specific diagnostic information should be incorporated into intervention planning for positioning. Table 13.1 provides a brief overview of biomechanical risk factors based on differences in tone and their effect on postural control.

An anatomical component of movement that contributes to postural challenges is the action of muscles that serve two joints (diarthrodial), such as hamstrings and biceps. When these muscles are shortened by the action of atypical tone and compensatory movement, it is difficult for children to execute full movement over both joints simultaneously. In the case of hamstrings, in sitting, knee extension may mechanically interfere with hip flexion, preventing a neutral pelvic position with compensatory trunk flexion to remain upright. Similar effects can be observed with other diarthrodial muscles.

Movements and postures are affected by a multitude of internal and external factors. Postural stability relies on the integration of information from the musculoskeletal and nervous systems which includes sensory inputs from the visual, somatosensory, and vestibular systems (Woollacott et al., 2005). The influences of these factors are exaggerated in children who have CNS disorders. These include, but are not limited to:

Position in space of head or body: As a result of vestibular and proprioceptive input, changes of position in space in vertical and horizontal positions (upright, supine, prone, semireclined, sidelying), as well as head position, may elicit early reflexive responses (such as the tonic labyrinthine or the ATNR), affecting movements and posture, particularly in children with CNS impairments. Whereas postural tone related to position may change imperceptibly in typical populations, these changes may be observable and dramatic in children with hypertonicity. Not only can tonal changes interfere with posture and control, but when unanticipated by the child they may be startling, adding further unwelcome changes in postural tone as well as to the child's sense of safety.

Tactile stimulation: As with changes in position, early reflexes may be elicited by light touch, affecting head or body position. For example, head position changes when the rooting reflex is elicited by light touch and that may be further complicated if the ATNR is elicited by that change in head position, potentially impacting both arm and trunk. The Gallant response results in a lateral curve of the trunk. Because a simple touch or change in position can interfere with postural control, it is important to assess the impact on each child so as to avoid inadvertently eliciting them in the course of providing positioning equipment.

Pain: There is evidence that over 60% of children with cerebral palsy experience chronic pain due to factors such as immobility, gastrointestinal symptoms, orthopedic impairments, and spasticity (McKearnan et al., 2004). Pain is directly associated with poor sleep and functional complications associated with this, such as executive function deficits, emotional issues, and impaired capacity for learning (Buckhalt, 2011). There are so many ways to inadvertently cause more pain by immobilizing a child in an unfamiliar position when providing postural supports. Because of this such possibilities should be constantly assessed by the practitioner.

Stress and effort: As these factors increase, movement and posture can be impacted. An isolated movement may be accompanied by involvement of the entire body, such as the effort of righting one's head may result in an extension pattern throughout the body. Or, the effort of controlling one body part may produce an unwanted associated movement in a nonrelated body part, such as the fisting of the nondominant hand when the child is attempting to write. Environmental factors contributing to sensory overload (noise, visual field) can affect tone, as can the child's emotional reaction to internal or external events.

Ambient temperature: Neutral warmth (which approximates body temperature) promotes muscle relaxation, whereas colder temperatures tend to increase muscle tone. This can be used therapeutically by attending to the child's layers of clothing and room temperature.

Examples of poor responses to various internal and external changes are listed in Table 13.2.

Finally, the effects of neuromuscular dysfunction on postural reactions and function can also be illustrated using Rood's concept of phasic and tonic muscles and their functional purposes (Stockmeyer, 1967). Tonic muscle groups are best suited to postural maintenance via sustained contractions and are located proximally. When these muscles are unable to perform their tasks adequately, the phasic muscles act as substitutes. Because the primary functions of phasic muscle groups are mobility and skill, they are far less effective in maintaining postures. For example, children with CNS dysfunction may retract their shoulders and extend their humeri to "hold themselves up" because of inefficient tonic muscle groups for trunk extension. This results in fatigue as the phasic muscles are not well equipped for sustained use impairing the development of volitional skills as the extremities used to maintain posture are not free to engage in skilled activity.

The fundamental goal of the biomechanical frame of reference to position children for function is to provide artificial postural stability. With such external support, children may interact more freely with their environment as effort is decreased and distal muscles do not need to be used to maintain and upright position. For one child, this may mean providing enough head

Table 13.2 Postural Responses to Internal and External Changes

Internal and External Factors	Changes in Postural Responses
Elements of movement	Active movement and rapid passive movement of a joint in a hypertonic child may increase tone. Rapid changes in speed can increase tone, particularly when unexpected. Slow, gentle rocking often decreases tone.
Reflexive reactions	Tonic labyrinth can cause total extension pattern in the supine position, with the child unable to tuck their chin, or close their jaw, or bring their hands together or up to their mouth. Head extension in hypertonic children can create a strong, total extension pattern with shoulder retraction, arched back, and extended hips. Passive neck extension often leads to rotation of the entire body with complete relation or full body flexion. The rooting reflex response takes the head out of the midline and may also elicit an asymmetrical tonic neck reflex, causing the entire body to be asymmetrical. The Gallant reflex causes the trunk to laterally flex toward the source of touch on the lateral trunk, creating a temporary asymmetry of the spine.
Tactile stimulation	Light touch often elicits phasic movements, which is undesirable in maintaining a static posture.
Stress of effort	Children can right their heads easily when they are tipped forward 5 degrees, but have more difficulty when they are tipped forward 20 degrees. Exaggerated mirror movements may occur in the nondominated arm while writing with the dominant arm.
Temperature	Cool temperatures increase muscle tone. Neutral warmth (which approximates body temperature) is provided by warm clothing or ambient temperature, promotes muscle relaxation.
Surface support	Hard surfaces tend to be alerting and, therefore, may increase postural tone.
Intensity of environmental stimulation	Frequent changes and high intensity of environmental stimulation often increase tone. Monotony and low levels of intensity have lulling effects and generally are associated with a decrease in muscle tone.
Affect	Strong affectual responses increase tone, regardless of their positive or negative associations.

support to allow the child to make and maintain eye contact with a care provider or providing enough tone reduction to enable the child to breathe deeply and easily while listening to a story. For another, it may mean providing sufficient support to enable the physical capacity to manipulate toys. This biomechanical approach assumes consistent and effective postural control is essential for optimal participation in occupation for all children. When assisted via modifications of position, the potential for participation is enhanced.

The contemporary focus on health outcomes emphasizes an intervention shift from principles that suggest there is a "right way" of performing activities to principles that allow people to perform in their own way as long as it is effective (Imms et al., 2017). Thus, the practitioner working from the biomechanical frame of reference is tasked with determining, with children and their families, when to address improving capacities and when to support alternative strategies through substitutions.

Postural Responses to Facilitate Participation in Occupation

While the goal of this frame of reference is to enhance function through the use of artificial supports, success is dependent upon attention to other factors that influence the development of postural control. These include, but are not restricted to, other body functions, environmental factors, and activities. As mentioned previously the biomechanical approach cannot be applied in a vacuum; simply providing a good fit between the supportive device and the child will not adequately address functional goals. Here are some examples of situations where other factors must be addressed simultaneously when applying artificial support:

- Introduction of positioning equipment is disruptive to the child's familiar routines, regardless of whether these routines facilitated, or were barriers to, participation.
- An adapted toilet corrects posture, provides children with a sense of safety, and reduces hypertonicity. However, children with impaired digestive functions may have little success with bowel control because a diet with adequate fiber is sometimes difficult for children to manage orally.
- Students have better control during graphomotor tasks when positioned in a standing device but feel isolated from the rest of the class who work and talk together at their desks.
- Babies have better oral control when supported in an adapted chair, but their mothers prefer to hold the baby in her arms during feeding.

FUNCTION/DYSFUNCTION CONTINUA

There can be many causes of delays or dysfunction in children's ability to interact with their environment. Only those issues related to compromised postural reactions that interfere with skill development are appropriate targets for the biomechanical frame of reference. For example, the inability to use both hands at midline may be related to delayed sitting skills, which may result in retracted shoulders or the need to always prop on one arm for support. Conversely, that same inability may be the result of poor bilateral integration or tactile defensiveness, which is unrelated to postural competence. If children have delayed postural reactions due to weak, exaggerated, or poor performance of improper muscle groups, a therapist should consider the biomechanical frame of reference to position children for function.

The goal of a positioning aide for children with neuromuscular dysfunction is to facilitate engagement in meaningful tasks or to maximize their ability to participate by providing them with a secure postural base. Providing artificial support allows children to engage in task-oriented activities which may promote neuroplasticity (Kliem & Jones, 2008; Novak, 2014; Wittenberg, 2009).

Range of Motion

Range of motion is the ability to move a child's head and extremities through their full span of movement. Problems in this area are evident when a child has limitations in range of motion or contractures (Table 13.3).

Head Control

In this continuum, function is represented by children who can maintain their head in a righted position, when moving, and who can direct head movements as desired. This provides stability

Table 13.3 Indicators of Function: Range of Motion

Function	Dysfunction
Able to passively move head and extremities through their full movement potential of their joints	Contractures, deformities
Indicators of Function	**Indicators of Dysfunction**
Full, passive range of motion	Fixed contractures, deformities
Full, active range of motion	Functional limits of range of motion

for ocular tasks such as eye control and visual fixation and for oral motor control and mobility for turning the head toward a source of stimulation. Limited neck mobility or stability represents dysfunction. This may occur primarily through inadequate muscular control or secondary to compensatory movements, such as stabilizing the head through the use of shoulder elevation, which limits active range in the neck and shoulders (Table 13.4).

Trunk Control

Function is represented by children who demonstrate equilibrium reactions in the trunk as they reach and interact with the environment in an upright position. These children should also have full thoracic range for inspirations and expirations. Note that respiration function is only analyzed related to tone and position of the trunk within biomechanical approach. With less trunk control, dysfunction appears as (1) an inability to remain upright once distal limb movements are initiated or (2) an inability to maintain any upright position at all. Abnormal muscle tone in the trunk can compromise respiratory capacity. Trunk deformities may occur from the force of gravity curving the spine, asymmetrical muscle tone or muscle innervation, or constant use of compensatory movements. Lateral, forward, and/or rotational curvatures of the spine (e.g., scoliosis and lordosis) reduce the thoracic space and may impair respiration with detriment to health, energy, and phonation (Table 13.5), as well as limit freedom of arm/hand use.

Table 13.4 Indicators of Function: Head Control

Function	Dysfunction
Age-appropriate head control and mobility	Poor head control and mobility
Indicators of Function	**Indicators of Dysfunction**
Maintains head in a righted position in all planes	Maintains head in an upright position but loses head control when initiating a movement
Turns head as desired	Unable to right head or control any head movements

Table 13.5 Indicators of Function: Trunk Control

Function	Dysfunction
Demonstrates trunk control	Lack of trunk control
Indicators of Function	**Indicators of Dysfunction**
Trunk is righted and stable in an upright position	Trunk is righted but unstable when limb movements are initiated
Trunk is symmetrical when seated	Trunk is not righted but unable to remain symmetrical posture when seated
Trunk is symmetrical when standing	Trunk is not righted but unable to remain symmetrical posture when standing
Trunk provides normal respiratory capacity	Respiratory capacity is compromised by decreased size of thoracic cavity and because of trunk and shoulder position
Trunk control muscle tone supports respiratory capacity	Respiratory capacity is decreased because of abnormal muscle tone on respiratory muscles, such as tightness of intercostal muscles

Control of Arm Movements

At the functional end of the continuum, children can reach in all planes, regardless of body position. These children also demonstrate the ability to maintain their hands as they desire. Dysfunction is an inability to direct arm movements due to the following possible three reasons. First, the shoulders and arms are involved in supporting the trunk (as a result of tone in the trunk interfering or being inadequate). Second, arm movements against gravity are difficult to execute. Third, children have difficulty maintaining the position of their hands in relation to an object. Providing trunk support or changing the children's position in space can enhance function (Table 13.6).

Table 13.6 Indicators of Function: Control of Arm Movements

Function	Dysfunction
Ability to reach in all planes	Inability to reach in all planes
Indicators of Function	**Indicators of Dysfunction**
Reaches in all directions, regardless of position	Unable to use arms for reaching; they are used for other compensatory support (propping, aid in upper trunk stability)
Places, maintains, and controls hands as desired when in an upright position	Cannot place or maintain hands in place as desired due to having difficulty moving arms against gravity

Table 13.7 Indicators of Function: Mobility

Function	Dysfunction
Smooth mobility through space	Slow, effortful mobility, or immobility
Indicators of Function	**Indicators of Dysfunction**
Child is mobile through space in all planes (walking; climbing in, out of, and over obstacles)	Child cannot move their body through space
Child can navigate in a horizontal position (crawling or creeping) on a flat surface	Child can only navigate in space by rolling

Mobility

While mobility is the ability to reach or adjust your position, the ability to move through space to attain a goal, explore an environment, or experience movement in many planes is at the functional end of this continuum. Mobility that is stressful or slow is dysfunctional because children often may feel that the effort is not worth the goal or the children may be too fatigued to interact with the person or object once they attain their goal. Lack of mobility deprives children of essential sensory experiences, particularly vestibular and proprioceptive, which are provided by movement through space (Table 13.7). Last, a child whose mobility patterns do not meet their developmental needs across all environments may require additional supports. For example, an 8-year-old who can crawl independently in the home is unsafe to do this in public settings.

Participation in Life Activities

The goal of the biomechanical frame of reference to position children for function means providing a secure postural base through positioning or with the assistance of external support. The previous section addresses specific components of motor development that provide a foundation for controlled movement. The following are examples of function and dysfunction continua that are specific to participation in life activities, including eating, toileting, and accessing switches for technologic aids.

Eating

The functional end of this continuum includes adequate oral-motor control to ingest food safely in an average amount of time without choking and aspirating. Although feeding difficulties may exist despite the development of postural control, the absence of good head and trunk control exacerbates oral motor dysfunction. Dysfunctional eating patterns (e.g., lack of jaw stability; poor tongue, cheek, and lip control; and disorganized swallowing) are affected by poor head control, compensatory movements in the shoulder girdle, irregular respiration, and abnormal tone associated with certain postures (Table 13.8).

Table 13.8 Indicators of Function: Eating

Function	Dysfunction
Safe, efficient eating	Difficulty with chewing and swallowing
Indicators of Function	**Indicators of Dysfunction**
Child can chew and swallow food successfully without choking and aspirating	Child is unable to grade jaw movements or control lips and tongue when eating
	Child frequently chokes on or aspirates food

Toileting

Function in toileting includes the ability to sit independently on a toilet or commode and the ability to void. Dysfunction, with its concomitant lack of comfort and dignity, is represented by a lack of awareness or control of the voiding process or the inability to relax enough to void when sitting unsupported on a toilet. Awareness and control may be affected by abnormal tone, and postural control has a direct effect on the ability to relax when sitting independently (Table 13.9).

Accessing a Switch for Technologic Aids

Children who can make and maintain contact with a device (e.g., switch, button, or joystick), move it in a controlled fashion, and release it at will are at the functional end of this continuum. The selection of switches to control augmentative communication devices and power wheelchairs, environment control, and other technologic devices is extensive. The highest level of function consists of controlling the switch rapidly and efficiently without fatigue. Ideally, children would accomplish this with high-level controlled arm and hand movements. However, movement in virtually any part of the body can be harnessed to drive a device. Switches may be controlled,

Table 13.9 Indicators of Function: Toileting

Function	Dysfunction
Independence on toileting	Inability to void in toilet
Indicators of Function	**Indicators of Dysfunction**
Child can empty bowel and bladder when seated on toilet	Child can only void intentionally when lying down
Child can maintain sitting balance on a toilet	Child cannot maintain sitting balance on a toilet
Child can maintain sitting balance on a toilet and direct the flow of urine into the bowl	Child can maintain sitting balance on a toilet but cannot direct the flow of urine into the bowl
Child can indicate the need to go to the potty	Child has no conscious bowel and bladder control

Table 13.10 Indicators of Function: Accessing Switch for Technologic Aids

Function	Dysfunction
Ability to independently use technologic aids	Inability to independently use technologic aids
Indicators of Function	**Indicators of Dysfunction**
Child can approach, contact, and release switch with adequate speed and control using hand	Child cannot approach, switch, or maintain contact and control release using hand
Child can sustain approach or release sequence for duration of activity	Child cannot sustain approach or release sequence for duration of activity
Child can approach, contact, and release switch using body part other than hand without affecting other skill related to movement of that body part	Child can approach, contact, and release switch with a body part, but the action impedes another function

for example, by inspiration/expiration or movements of the head, neck, eyelids, shoulders, or feet. Function is decreased if, by harnessing one of these movements, another skill related to that movement is impaired. For example, does a breath-driven device interfere with speech or create excessive drooling? Or, does the child use a shoulder movement with significant postural asymmetry or with compensatory movements that eventually impair posture or mobility (Table 13.10).

Each of these functions depends on the interaction of numerous factors. Cognition, perception, and behavior, as well as fine motor and organization abilities, contribute to these skills. Evaluation of the postural components necessary for function will determine whether and, specifically, which biomechanical assists are appropriate.

GUIDE FOR EVALUATION

The purpose of the evaluation is to assess the postural components of a given dysfunction to plan an intervention. Within the biomechanical frame of reference, the child's potential for change in postural reactions is a major focus because it helps the therapist determine what type of postural aids to provide and how they will be most effective. Ideally, assessment is often completed over months to fully understand all factors (internal and external) impacting a child's movement. This may include trial and error based on positioning needs and implementation success in a child's natural environment and may evolve due to cognitive and physical development.

At times, the assessment of a child's needs within this frame of reference may be done by an assessing therapist who has expertise in this area or through a clinic, as opposed to the therapist who is providing ongoing treatment. This is most likely to be considered when a seating system is being provided as part of durable medical equipment such as a wheelchair. A team approach in these situations provides the assessing therapist with additional insight into the environment in which they will be using a seating system. The practitioner(s) who provides ongoing treatment to the child should be actively involved in equipment decisions because of their long-term interaction with the child and understanding of the child's potential for change, both during the day and over an extended period. This involvement is particularly important for the child who needs a positioning device for the classroom. In these cases, the child's parents or at-home caregivers do not have the opportunity to observe their child's performance, needs, and responses in the context of the school, so the school-based practitioner's observations and assessments, as well as input from teachers, may be a critical resource during an off-site evaluation.

The assessment of the child begins by considering all contributing factors to the child's potential for change including age, therapeutic history, physical status, prognosis, and environment. Age is an important consideration because of the plasticity of the CNS. Therapeutic history is relevant because it indicates the types and focus of the child's previous contact with therapy and the child's responsiveness to intervention. Physical status indicates the child's general health, medication regimen, and surgical history. Prognosis indicates the progression expected in relation to the child's diagnosis. The environment influences the child's potential for growth and motivation.

The therapist needs to carefully observe any sequence of specific elements of postural control when evaluating a child's positioning options. The outline in this section is intended to assist with this process.

- Can the child move all body parts through full range against gravity?
- Can the child right their head and is it mobile in all planes?
- Can the child visually focus and scan their environment?
- Can the child right their trunk and maintain stability in all positions?
- Can the child place, maintain, and control the position of their hands?
- Is the child mobile through space in all planes?
- Can the child chew and swallow food successfully without aspirating?
- Can the child void when seated on a toilet or commode?
- Can the child access a switch to activate a technologic device?

It is important during this scrutiny to remember, however, that all elements of movement are interrelated, and that the therapist must step back and view the child's body as a whole. Furthermore, it is imperative to apply the evaluation and intervention process to the child's life—the end goal is not that the child is seated with complete postural symmetry with hip and knees at 90 degrees, but so the child can perform meaningful activities.

While assessments include range of motion and strength testing, the child should also be observed participating in an activity. This provides the therapist with an opportunity to analyze movement as it relates to posture and gravity as well as to the activity. It is essential to look at the child's ability to make rapid, unconscious postural changes within the context of an activity. References and charts are available to assist in this evaluation of the sequential development of motor skills (Bly, 1994; Fiorentino, 1981; Green, Mulcahy, & Pountney, 1995). Concentration is on those central postural skills needed to support movement of the head and limbs to interact with the environment. In addition, wheelchair seating assessment forms are found in textbooks (Barnes, 1991; Batavia, 2010; Bergen & Colangelo, 1985; Polgar et al., 2020; Rothstein, 2005). The Segmental Assessment of Trunk Control (SATCA) assesses trunk control by progressively adjusting trunk support levels from fully supported to independent sitting, evaluating control from the head to the lumbar spine to identify specific postural issues (Butler et al., 2010). The Posture and Postural Ability Scale (PPAS) assesses an individual's quality and ability to stabilize body segments in various positions: supine, prone, sitting, and standing (Rodby-Bousquet et al., 2016).

The following questions provide some guidelines for evaluating motor development in terms of functional posture, as derived from the function and dysfunction continua. In all cases, a therapist must determine if dysfunctional movement is delayed (slow to develop) or pathologic (influenced by abnormal tone or reflexes). Each of the following questions is directed toward the functional end of the continuum.

Can the Child Move All Body Parts Through Full Range Against Gravity?

Passive Range of Motion and Contractures

Assessment of passive range of motion typically begins in the supine position, this involves the assessment of the child's passive range of motion and the presence of fixed or dynamic contractures. Practitioners should be aware of not just how much range a child has in the particular joint but if other parts of the body are compensating. For example, a posterior pelvic tilt marks the end of available hip flexion range of motion. The effects of movement and changes in position on functional range of motion are just as important as passive range of motion.

- Is muscle tone high, low, or fluctuating? What kinds of stimuli increase pathologic tone and, possibly, interfere with active range of motion?
- Does the effect of gravity prevent certain ranges of movement mechanically or physiologically?
- Does gravity change postural asymmetries in the trunk and pelvis?
- Can movement be enhanced by changing position to decrease the effects of gravity or by using gravity to assist movement?
- What movements or positions elicit reflexes that compromise full range?

If the functional range is influenced by position, then the therapist needs to know how much of each day the child spends in different positions. A positioning log can be completed with the help of parents, care providers, and educators, this can be completed using a written log or photographs that meet privacy regulations.

- How is the child fed, transported, toileted, and positioned for rest, recreation, and school?
- Which positions have been selected with function in mind?
- Which can be modified to enhance movement, and which are selected to reduce stress on the family or care providers? In addition to the time spent in school chairs, highchairs, and wheelchairs, the child's time being carried in backpacks; placed in baby swings, car seats, beanbag chairs, on the floor, and in bed should also be assessed.
- From the positioning log, the therapist can make modifications or suggestions to promote independent movement for the child and to minimize the caregiving responsibilities for his or her family and school staff.

Can the Child Right Their Head and Is the Head Mobile in All Planes?

Supine

- In the supine position, can the child maintain their head in the midline, turn it to either side, and tuck their chin to observe people?
- Can the child maintain their head to look at one's own body parts, for example, look at their own hands? Is the child presenting with development delayed yet following a typical sequence, or is pathology present?
- Is difficulty with movement caused by low tone, struggle against gravity, or is immobility caused by high tone?

- Is there increased extension in this position because of the influence of the tonic labyrinthine reflex?
- This may include neck hyperextension, an open jaw, retracted lips, or upward gaze. Does the rooting reflex cause the child to press one side of their face against the floor?
- Does the inability to maintain the head in midline elicit an asymmetric tonic neck reflex?
- When attempting to lift their head from the supine position, does the child use peripheral, phasic musculature (e.g., the sternocleidomastoids) to substitute for deep tonic musculature work?

Prone Position

- In the prone position, can the child lift their head to 90 degrees and maintain it in the upright position, or can he or she turn the head freely to either side without flipping over caused by primitive reflex?
- Can the child raise and lower their head with graded movements?
- Functionally, can the child turn their head to examine the world visually, and can the child control his or her mouth for age-appropriate speaking and swallowing in this position?
- If delay or pathology is present, is neck hyperextension necessary to keep the head upright?
- If so, is it accompanied by increased extensor tone throughout the body? Can the child close their mouth when the head is righted, or is the jaw pulled open as part of extension patterning?
- When the child attempts to lower their head, does the child simply collapse to the floor?

Sidelying

- In sidelying, where the effects of gravity on the head are minimized, can the child look up and to the side without flipping into a prone or supine position?
- Can the child use lateral neck flexion against gravity to right their head or initiate movements of his or her body?

Upright Position

- In an upright position (either sitting or supported standing), is the child's head aligned in space? Is it aligned with the child's body? It should be noted that the head may be righted, but the neck may be flexed laterally or hyperextended to compensate for poor trunk position (e.g., in children with scoliosis or kyphosis).
- If head control is poor, is shoulder elevation used to "nestle" the head for stability, thereby limiting neck mobility? Or is the head generally thrown back or flopping forward? What is the controlled range of head movements? For example, can the child flex their neck forward 5 degrees and right it again but loses control if they flex 10 degrees or more?
- Does the position of the trunk affect head control? For example, if head control is inadequate, does tipping the trunk slightly forward or backward activate righting reactions or change muscle tone so that head stability is enhanced?
- If head control is minimal, how far back must the therapist tip the child's seat or stander until the child's head rests on a supporting back piece without flopping forward?
- If the practitioner supports the head by tipping the seat back in space, is this a functional position for viewing the world and a safe position for swallowing?

Can the Child Right Their Trunk and Maintain Stability in All Positions?

In this context, the trunk is seen not in terms of mobility but as a stable base of support for the head and arms. This is not meant to minimize the importance of the whole body in learning but to establish priorities for someone who is limited in functional movement. That is, providing optimal trunk support allows the primary parts of the body, the head and arms, to seek stimuli and manipulate the world. The therapist, therefore, examines the trunk's capacity to stay upright in response to displacement (Hadders-Algra et al., 1996) and its ability to support the head and arms as they change position in relation to the trunk. The roles of the pelvis, legs, and feet are observed in conjunction with the trunk as part of the support basis for the body rather than in their roles of providing mobility through space.

Upright Position

- In an upright position (i.e., seated or standing at rest), is the trunk righted, stable, and symmetrical?
- Are adequate space and mobility evident in the chest for effective respiration?
- Can the child sit in various positions, or is the child limited to a particular position because of their lack of stability (e.g., ring sitting or "W" sitting)?
- Are equilibrium reactions fully effective in all planes and ranges or only within a limited range of displacement?
- Are the arms liberated; can the child reach in any plane without losing balance, or does the child need to use the compensatory movement of the shoulder girdle or arms to maintain an upright trunk? For example, retracted shoulders and arms may assist upper back extension, or there may be a need to prop on one or both arms.
- Can the trunk support the head and itself but not the weight of the arms? This can be determined if the child can sit erect only when resting, not when leaning, with their arms placed lightly on a tabletop.

Positions of the Pelvis and Legs

- How does the position of the pelvis and legs affect the trunk?
- Is weight distributed equally on both sides of the pelvis?
- Is the pelvis in a relatively neutral position or tilted in the anterior or posterior direction?
- Is the pelvis too far forward, requiring compensatory lumbar hyperextension or shoulder retraction to remain upright?
- Is the pelvis posteriorly tilted creating a rounded back, possibly combining with protracted shoulders and a hyperextended neck?

Sitting

- In the sitting position, does tightness or contractures of hip extension cause the child's back to press against the back of the chair, sliding the child toward or off the front edge of the chair?
- Are the hips adducted in such a way that the child has no lateral stability, or abducted in such a way that they have little anterior stability?
- Can hips, knees, and ankles be maintained in a position that allows feet to be planted firmly on the floor?
- Does the child seem to be more functional in a standing or sitting position?

Can the Child Place, Maintain, and Control Position of Their Hands?

In this area, the practitioner's concern is not fine motor skill but the ability to get the hands where they need to be, keep them there as long as necessary, and change their position through controlled movements of the shoulders and arms from a stable base. Improving function in this area may have secondary effects on fine motor skills in two ways; first, alteration of muscle tone in the trunk and shoulders often improves tone in the extremities and, second, control of hand placement provides more opportunities for manipulation and the sensory experiences that contribute to fine motor control.

As with previous areas, the therapist must assess the quality of muscle tone. How can gravity impede or improve movement mechanically and physiologically? Mechanically, the concern is how gravity weighs limbs down in various positions. Physiologically, the concern is how it elicits righting or reflex activity in various positions. Also, what compensatory movements or associated reactions interfere with function?

Supine Position

- In the supine position, can the child reach in all planes against gravity and maintain their hands away from their body without the need to stabilize by grasping an object? For example, can the child reach up and touch a mobile or does the child need to hold onto it to keep their hand in that position in space?
- Can the child bring their hands to the midline or does gravity or the response of the ATNR or tonic labyrinthine reflex prevent this?
- Can the child get their scapulae off the floor by protracting them for an upward reach?
- Can the child look at and reach their tummy, knees, or toes, or must the child look up and initiate a symmetrical tonic neck reflex to reach down?

Prone Position

- In the prone position, can the child lift their chest off the floor by using the interaction of their flexors and protractors to bring arms forward as supports or with extensors to bring the child's head and back up so that their elbows are beneath the shoulders?
- In the absence of flexor activity, is the chest raised by back extensors with little or no weight bearing on the forearms?
- Can the child shift weight onto one arm to reach out with the other?
- Does the child collapse onto their chest when attempting to reach out, or compensate with neck and back hyperextension to keep from collapsing?
- Is shoulder stability adequate for sustained play in this position?

Sidelying Position

- In the sidelying position, is the upper arm fully mobile in the sagittal plane?
- Can the child reach up from the floor against gravity?
- Are shoulder movements isolated, or does the child need to initiate them with changes in the position of their head?
- Is the child's shoulder trapped in an internally rotated position by the effects of gravity in this position?

Upright Position

- In an upright position, are the shoulders and arms free to move in all planes?
- Are there compensatory movements such as elevation, retraction, and external rotation or protraction and internal rotation to assist an ineffective control of head or trunk?
- Is the shoulder girdle mobile enough for full range of arm movements but stable enough to maintain arms in a certain position against gravity?
- Can the child use their arms only when supported by a tabletop?
- How does the position of the shoulder girdle affect mobility of the humeri and forearms? For example, protraction often is accompanied by internal rotation and adduction of the shoulder with elbow extension, and forearm pronation in children who have tone problems.
- How do the positions of the trunk and pelvis affect the position of the shoulders?

Is the Child Mobile Through Space in All Planes?

In this area, the concern of the practitioner who uses the biomechanical frame of reference to position children for function is not ambulation but mobility through space for two purposes: participation, and body structures and function development. (1) Can the child move to attain a goal such as a toy, a person, or food? (2) Can the child move to gather proprioceptive and vestibular input to enhance the development of body schema and spatial awareness? The practitioner assesses how the child moves independently through space and if mechanical assistance would be beneficial.

Can the Child Get to a Desired Goal by Walking, Creeping, Crawling, or Rolling?

Walking, Creeping, Crawling, or Rolling

- If so, does the child use pathologic movements to achieve the goal?
- Is the amount of time needed for the movement too extreme, or is the effort too exhausting?
- What alternatives for goal-oriented movement are realistic?
- Does the child have the potential to propel a wheelchair (either mechanical or powered), tricycle, or scooter board based on their functional range, postural reactions, and ability to maintain and control their hands?
- If the child has independent, but not optimal locomotion, is the potential improvement gained through a piece of equipment worth the extra training required for the child, family, and care providers? Furthermore, the therapist should explore with the child, family, and care providers their feelings about the use of this piece of equipment and their ability to follow through with its use. Finally, the therapist should consider the expense of the equipment in relation to its need and the potential for reimbursement.
- If the child has no independent movement through space, which one of several methods is most appropriate for his or her physical and emotional growth and his or her lifestyle?
- In addition to goal-directed movement through space, what kinds of passive movement through space can be provided?
- How can the child's position be modified so that they feel comfortable and secure?

Can the Child Chew and Swallow Food Successfully Without Aspirating?

Feeding skills are assessed by the impact of posture on oral-motor function. The assessment of hand placement and control, as previously discussed, should yield similar information in relation to self-feeding skills. Although assessment of posture is critical to effective feeding intervention, it is only one part of a sophisticated evaluation of sensory, fine motor, cognitive, and behavioral skills that goes beyond the scope of this chapter.

Posture and Tone

Without describing an in-depth feeding evaluation, the following explanation gives examples of how posture and tone are incorporated into oral-motor assessment.

- Are the trunk and neck stable to provide a base for movements and stability of the jaw?
- Can the head be maintained in a neutral or slightly flexed position?
- Is the neck extended so that the airway is open, but the child is more likely to aspirate the food, or is the neck flexed in such a way that swallowing is difficult?
- Is the trunk in an optimal position for respiration so that it does not interfere with the coordination of swallowing and breathing?

Hypertonicity

- Does the presence of hypertonicity contribute to oral reflexes such as rooting or the bite reflex?
- Does it prevent isolated movements, such as separation of the tongue from the jaw? Does the child have difficulty bringing the tongue forward or lips together because of their increased extensor tone?

Gradation of Oral Movements

- Is gradation of oral movements affected? Does the jaw just open and snap shut when food is presented?
- Can oral-motor control be optimized by modifying high muscle tone with support of the head and trunk or changes in body position in space?
- How does gravity affect oral-motor control in the presence of hypotonicity?

Eating

- Does the child bite on the spoon because of ungraded jaw movements or because they are trying to keep their head from wobbling?
- Do the tongue and lips fall backward in a passively retracted position when the head is tipped back?
- Can the child create enough lip pressure to keep food from falling out of their mouth?
- Is there enough activity in the cheeks to keep food from spilling over the teeth and pocketing in the cheeks?
- Does the child manage better in supported standing or reclined sitting positions?
- Does a change in position increase postural tone, or is extra support needed to accommodate for lack of tone?

Can the Child Void When Seated on a Toilet or Potty?

As with feeding, an evaluation using the biomechanical frame of reference is part of a complex evaluation, including independent toileting. Information about the child's levels of cognition and sensory awareness is essential. Furthermore, it would be helpful for the therapist to know about the child's diet and behavior patterns.

The postural component addresses comfort, trunk stability, and the ability to relax hip extensors and abductors that otherwise may interfere mechanically with controlled elimination. The assessment is the same, then, as an evaluation of the child's capacity to sit in a stable, comfortable position with hips flexed and slightly abducted. In addition, the child should be assessed for the ability to direct the flow of urine into the toilet rather than onto the floor. This can be an issue with boys and girls alike and often is related to pelvic position. An additional, extremely important component of the assessment is consideration of the family's or care provider's acceptance of any toileting aid or device in terms of size, management, and cosmesis.

Can the Child Access a Switch to Activate a Technologic Device?

Again, the components of this task from a biomechanical frame of reference refer to the capacity to control the head, trunk, and arms. Regardless of their complexity, most devices can be driven by either intermittent or sustained contact with a switch. However, the fewer demands on motor output when accessing a switch, the greater the cognitive or perceptual demands. When a child uses a complex device (such as augmentative communication or powered wheelchairs), the therapist needs to identify what one action the child can perform with accuracy and control in a specific sequence. For example, does the child demonstrate the sequencing and memory needed to access a control menu? The process of selecting the best match for the child and switch is dependent upon skilled team assessment of a multitude of performance components.

Physical Components

- Does the child need additional postural supports (such as supports for shoulders and humerus) while mastering the fine control necessary for this skill?
- Where in space can the switch be placed to maximize control? This is referred to as the "sweet spot." If using the hand, is position at the midline or to the side the most successful placement for learning to activate the switch? If using movement of a body part other than the hand, in what position can the body activate the switch with the least energy and minimum of compensatory movements?
- Can the necessary movements for activation of the switch be performed against gravity, or does the switch need to be placed where movements are performed in a gravity-eliminated position?
- Can the child produce adequate force to activate the switch that is selected?
- Can the child release the switch in a timely manner?
- Does the child have a variety of movements available to activate the device (e.g., keyboard, joystick) or must the child rely on one movement to activate a switch in a coded fashion?
- Is the child able to sustain the movement of a momentary switch (e.g., holding the joystick in a forward position to "drive" forward) or does the child require a latching switch? A latching switch is a switch that maintains its state after being activated until the switch is actuated again.

Once the child's postural components have been assessed, the primary intervention plan addresses the need for and type of postural support. However, designing the positioning device using only the biomechanical framework to facilitate change cannot be effectively provided in a vacuum. As mentioned earlier in this chapter, the incorporation of PEO and/or HAAT models allow for further assessment of internal and external factors to ensure the device meets all the needs of the child, not just physical. The following questions can guide this process:

What Personal Factors Might Restrain or Support the Use of Equipment?

Personal style will influence how a child adapts to the use of postural supports. As liberating as it may ultimately be, the use of adapted positioning devices creates changes in routines, physical sensations, habits, and patterns of movement. The child's coping style and level of motivation will influence their ability to adapt to these changes. Age and prior experience with positioning devices are other personal factors that need to be considered when choosing equipment. A young child may be less likely to tolerate the limitations of movement through space imposed by equipment than a student whose daily routines include longer periods of sitting in the classroom. It is important to note that any child may balk at new interventions if they have had similar but negative experiences in the past.

What Activities Will the Child Engage in When Positioned in the Device?

The appropriately selected activity will enhance the effectiveness of biomechanical intervention when it is selected in collaboration with the child and is set up in a way that makes reasonable demands on the motor skills that are being addressed. The positioning of the objects involved in the task is part of the therapeutic design. For example, if the goal of a prone positioner is to promote the development of weight shifting in the shoulders, an activity that requires the child to reach forward and upward with one arm (such as block constructions) is more demanding than one that can be accomplished with both forearms resting on the floor (such as coloring). The child's participation in choosing the activity will affect the extent to which they engage in it.

Will the Device Support Participation in Life and Social Engagement?

While addressing postural goals, is the equipment functioning as a support or barrier to the child's routine or interactions? When the child is in a stander or seating unit, can they transition (or be assisted with transitions) between activity stations in the classroom in a timely fashion with peers in the school? Should they be in a manual wheelchair during recess? Can they receive spontaneous hugs of comfort or glee, or does the lap tray, head support, and protraction wings make the child physically inaccessible?

Will Physical, Cultural, and Social Environmental Factors Be Supports or Barriers to the Use of the Device and Vice Versa?

- How does the device fit into the space available in home, school, or other customary environments?
- Is it cumbersome to move when the locus of activity changes?
- How does it look—does it have visual appeal or does industrial construction hide the presence of the child within it?

- Do the parents feel that the device helps their child engage with their environment or does its presence exacerbate their sense of their child's differences and special needs?
- Does the classroom teacher resent the time and space that the device requires, or appreciate the equipment optimizing his or her student's participation in the classroom?

In addition, a practitioner also needs to be aware that the culture and goals of school programs vary widely in relation to the appropriateness and acceptance of supportive devices in the classroom. Some programs for physically challenged students prioritize sensory and motor skills in their curricula. On the other end of the continuum, schools that practice full inclusion are more likely to emphasize social and academic participation, relegating the more intensive physical intervention to the home. The attitudes and priorities of families and systems play a significant role in how, if, and when the device is used.

POSTULATES REGARDING CHANGE

The biomechanical frame of reference to position children for function uses external devices to promote the child's performance. Based on the results of the evaluation, the occupational therapist establishes functional goals for the child that may be developmental or task specific. For example, a developmental goal may be to provide the child with a device to facilitate weight bearing on the forearms during floor play in preparation for controlled mobility. A task-specific goal may be for the child to control a switch to activate their communication device. In the biomechanical frame of reference, specific guidelines for the design, fabrication, and fitting of special devices are found in the Application to Practice section.

General Postulate Regarding Change

Adapted equipment provides essential support allowing the child to practice skills. An increase in practice results in an increase in skill. Intervention focuses on environmental opportunities, specifically how often the child uses equipment and at what point its use restricts the child's participation in life.

Directional Postulate Regarding Change

Intervention begins with the focus on optimal position for functioning followed by specific postural support. The best way to help the child engage in functional activities and maintain as much normal postural activity as possible is by providing as much support as the child needs, but no more.

Specific Postulate Regarding Change

1. If the therapist combines knowledge of the developmental progress of postural skills along with an awareness of the effects of gravity and sensory stimulation on normal and compensatory movement, then the therapist can determine appropriate positions to enhance a child's function.
2. If the therapist handles the child in a variety of ways, the therapist can determine how best to enhance normal postural responses in any one position.

3. If the therapist first provides control proximal to the body, then the distal parts of the body may be freed from the compensatory patterning or the influence of associated reactions.
4. If the therapist uses the effects of gravity to the child's benefit, then the therapist may reduce the need for more intrusive pieces of equipment.
5. If the therapist can identify an effective position through handling, the therapist can attempt to simulate that handling by using an adapted device.
6. If the therapist modifies the child's sensory environment, the therapist may enhance the postural control supported by adapted equipment.
7. If a child's practice time for a skill is increased, then the skill is developed more rapidly.
8. If the therapist considers the needs of the child's care providers, the therapist may provide equipment that is more likely to be used consistently.
9. If the occupational therapist engages in team decision making to prescribe a piece of equipment, then this equipment is more likely to fulfill the child's needs from different perspectives.

APPLICATION TO PRACTICE

During therapy sessions, the practitioner often provides physical contact to assist a child to perform a task directly. A significant increase in therapeutic handling time generally is as impractical for the staff as it is intrusive for the child. It may also unintentionally increase the child's dependence on the adult. Adapted equipment provides essential support allowing the child to practice skills, an increase in practice results in an increase in skill. The practitioner must use clinical judgment to determine how often the child uses equipment and at what point its use restricts the child's participation in life. Without moderation and consistent reassessment of a child's skills, a good tool can become counterproductive. It is also important to acknowledge Wittenberg's (2009) work that skill acquisition can continue into teenage years and that at this time, there are no specific guidelines to determine the most effective protocol.

Once the practitioner determines an optimal position for function, they often find that the child cannot maintain the position independently without using compensatory movements. Because compensatory movements result in significant secondary complications (including permanent deformity which may ultimately decrease function), it is usually counterproductive to use these compensatory movement patterns to enhance function. However, sometimes these compensatory movement patterns may be the only option with what the child has available to themself. The practitioner must identify the best way to help the child engage in functional activities and maintain as much typical postural activity as possible. This should be done by providing as much support as the child needs, but no more.

The process of determining an effective way to enhance a child's ability to tolerate an upright sitting position includes a combination of handling and manipulation of the child, an understanding of theoretical information, and trial and error. The understanding of theoretical information helps the practitioner gain initial insights into what may be happening as a child moves or is moved. Objective observation is essential so that the practitioner sees and responds to what is happening, not what is expected to happen. This is the point at which trial and error becomes essential: the practitioner adjusts the child's position based on theoretical handling principles (e.g., proximal over distal handling) and then evaluates the child's response. If a child cannot prop in the prone position, it may be because their body weight is shifted onto their chest. Before supporting them under the chest, the practitioner should help the child shift weight back over the hips by decreasing hip flexion by pressing down on their buttocks. With weight shifting back over the hips, the child may now be able to bear weight on the forearms and prop themself up. If the response is not a desired one, the practitioner continues to experiment and evaluate until the desired response is attained.

Translating Handling to Positioning

The practitioner translates a position from handling to a durable piece of equipment by recording exactly what supports are provided by practitioner's hands or body (e.g., minimal or moderate support), and at exactly which body location the supports contact the child's body. This record will provide a blueprint for constructing or ordering equipment. General principles that apply to all positioning devices:

- The surface of support units should be solid and stable so that it does not "give" or change with the child's movements. Flexible surfaces, such as large bean bag chairs or sling seats on wheelchairs, accommodate to the child's weight shifting, can result in instability, and as a result, can exacerbate asymmetries or compensatory postures.
- Surfaces that provide more contact or contour to a child's body will provide more support. Depending on the child's tone this may facilitate posture or lead to decreased muscle activation.
- Ancillary supports, such as lateral trunk supports, leg abductors, or protraction blocks, should be assessed in a proximal to distal method, and the least amount of support necessary to facilitate postural control should be used.
- Ancillary supports should be both small and thin enough so that they "fit" the child. However, at the same time, they should be large enough to distribute pressure over the contacting surface of the body part. In this way, the controlling support does not dig in and cause discomfort or, in some cases, active resistance. Whenever possible, blocks rather than straps should be used to support posture or control movements.

Equipment Selection Considerations

There are advantages and disadvantages to every piece of equipment. The challenge is finding the best piece of equipment to meet each child's specific needs. The positioning devices should be fitted to the child; the child should not be fitted to the device. Measurements must be accurate when trailing equipment, however the configuration may vary based on the child's needs and the physical components of the accessories. Once in the equipment, ill-fitting parts may be difficult to observe. In addition to proper fit and positioning, the material qualities of the equipment play a role in the potential for pressure sores, especially for individuals who have increased tone or decreased ability to weight shift. Therapists must consider the interaction of forces between the child's body and the material.

Environmental and Sensory Factors

The practitioner makes changes in the environment to complement the postural device and the child's responses to sensory factors (e.g., ambient noise and light, temperature, and the texture or firmness of a supporting surface). For example, a child who responds with a negative startling reaction and increased extensor tone to being placed on a cold hard plastic chair may exhibit more postural control with a lightly padded surface. A child who becomes lethargic in the presence of soft, slow music may maintain an upright position more easily with an increase in the volume and tempo of the music.

Family and Caregiver Attitudes Toward the Use of Equipment

The practitioner should be aware of the many factors that may influence the attitudes of families and caregivers toward a piece of equipment. Caregivers are integral to this process. Discussing the benefits of early application of a seating system to produce long-term benefits can assist in the consistent use of equipment (Pérez-de la Cruz, 2017). Often, parents can make immediate improvements in their child's posture in the home by carrying over handling or small modifications. However, for some parents it may take time for parents to understand the benefits of incorporating supports. Practitioners are recommended to provide clear and comprehensive information about the equipment, its purpose, and potential benefits that specifically focus on their child's potential or goals (Byrne et al., 2019). Caregivers who understand the reason or future benefit of equipment are more likely to have positive attitudes toward recommended equipment. Conversations when recommending equipment may occur over numerous sessions. Some questions the practitioner should ask and discuss with caregivers regarding the logistics of equipment include:

- Is the equipment pleasing to the eye? How much space does the equipment take up?
- Will this piece of equipment stay in one place or travel with the child?
- How difficult it will be to position the child and to transfer the child in and out of the equipment? (McDonald et al., 2003)
- How much assistance does the child need to use the device?
- How does the device enhance or interfere with social interaction?
- Finally, the practitioner also needs to be aware of what the cost–performance ratio of the devices is. For example, does the adapted commode fit in the bathroom at home? Or does the chrome and plastic standing device look too industrial? If the equipment is offensive to those persons expected to use it, it is less likely to be used.

Team Collaboration

Working with family members, physical therapists, speech pathologists, teachers, teaching assistants, physicians, and equipment vendors as a team provides more information about the child and makes the problems easier to solve. Each member of the team has a unique area of expertise and concern for the child. Accordingly, each team member provides distinctive input. All team members, including the family, should participate whenever appropriate in goal setting and problem solving. This is an effective way to address complex factors such as cultural, social, and physical environment.

In-depth Discussion of Biomechanical Interventions

The following are two sections that discuss in-depth: (1) common positions in which central stability can be provided artificially and (2) postural components or pieces of equipment as they relate to functional skills. Specific biomechanical interventions discussed in this section are based on the best available evidence. Much of the current evidence is based on small samples and with subjects who vary regarding the severity of cerebral palsy (Stavness, 2006). Keeping in mind that "every child with cerebral palsy is different and every intervention plan and each child's outcome will be unique" (Novak, 2014, p. 1146). Application of these principles should be applied with a good dose of clinical judgment and problem solving.

Central Stability

Intervention related to central stability covers the function and dysfunction continua of range of motion, head control, and trunk control. In these interventions, the practitioner takes a primary role in determining the appropriate position and equipment. Any one position may be appropriate for a variety of goals, depending on where supports are provided and how the equipment and, subsequently, the child's body is oriented in space. Is the equipment perpendicular or parallel to the floor or tilted, and how does this affect the child? The following section provides an outline of what general goals may be approached in various positions, and how to fit equipment to the child. Each section contains a brief review of expected skill development in each position, along with the therapeutic advantages of the position.

Supine Position

- Flexor activity develops head control: midline control and chin tuck
- Shoulder protraction and flexion against gravity
- Hands to the midline
- Reduced demands on trunk; more effort can be given to head, oral, ocular, and shoulder control

Although supine is not a functional position beyond infancy, practicing some movements in a restful supine position may be beneficial for a child who has severe physical impairments. Keeping in mind how gravity affects the child who has low tone and how reflex activity may increase hypertonicity in the supine position, the practitioner may alleviate these effects by providing passive flexion. A pillow may be placed beneath the head and shoulders of a child so that it enhances neck flexion, supports the head laterally, and protracts the shoulders passively. A roll beneath the thighs can place the hips in a flexed position and yet allow the soles of the feet to be in contact with the floor. Positioning materials for the child to engage with is challenging in this position. Often it may simply provide an opportunity for the child to bring their hands to the midline to explore the body. If the child is able to reach up against gravity, the activity must be suspended or supported above the child's body using an easel or rod. Oral-motor control is taxed in this position, as it is more difficult to bring the tongue forward and lips together and to stabilize the jaw.

Prone Position

- Head righting in a horizontal plane
- Interaction of dorsal extensors and ventral flexors for propping on forearms
- Shoulder stability during weight bearing (propping), and mobility on stability during weight shift

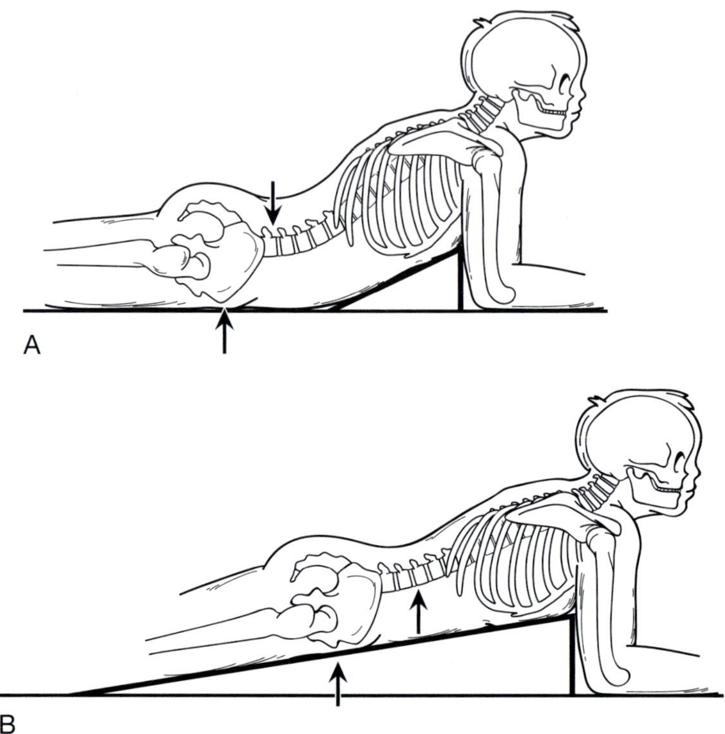

FIGURE 13.3 **A.** Lumbar spine can be extended passively in prone by having the lower portion of the wedge end at the child's waist. **B.** A wedge that extends well beyond the hips can prevent an exaggerated lumbar curve.

- Increased necessary range of shoulder flexion when reaching from horizontal position
- Decreased effects of gravity on lateral asymmetries that occur with upright positioning
- Hands more likely to be in the visual field by nature of shoulder position when propping

A wedge provides the basic support unit to enhance prone positioning for a child who cannot prop independently. The wedge should be wide enough so that it does not tip if the child starts to roll over. The length of the wedge is determined by the point of support at the chest and hips (Figure 13.3). The demand on the shoulder for weight bearing is influenced by the amount of contact of the wedge on the chest. Consequently, the lower the contact of the wedge on the chest, the greater the demands on the shoulder girdle for weight bearing. However, for some individuals, if the front edge is too far back, the child may flex their trunk and curl over it. The front edge of the wedge, where it contacts the child's chest, may also affect respiration. This should be monitored carefully to ensure that weight bearing on the chest is not compromising respiration.

If a child tends to be kyphotic in the upright position but has a mobile, flexible spine, then the lumbar spine can be extended passively in prone. This can be accomplished by having the lower portion of the wedge end at the child's waist. Conversely, a lordotic child who lies in the prone position with an anteriorly tipped pelvis should be provided with a wedge that extends well beyond the hips so that the lumbar curve is not exaggerated. In addition, the pelvis can be stabilized further by strapping an "X" across the buttocks, each strap beginning at the iliac crest and crossing down to the opposite hip. This pelvic position, assisted by the straps, keeps the center of gravity at the hips. The straps also can prevent the child from pulling themself forward over the front edge of the wedge. It should be noted that the use of a single strap often results in the strap sliding up to the lumbar area, causing an increase in lumbar extension and pelvic tilt (see Figure 13.3).

The distance of the front edge of the wedge from the floor determines the demands placed on the shoulder girdle (Figure 13.4). A very low wedge provides support to the chest as the child fatigues but places high demands for weight bearing on the arms and allows more upper trunk mobility for weight shifting. A higher wedge that fully supports the chest but is low enough so that the forearms contact the floor reduces stress on the shoulders, provides proprioceptive feedback, and allows the child with less shoulder girdle control to reach out without collapsing. A very high wedge may be used to eliminate demands on upper extremity weight bearing. In this position, a child's arms may dangle downward, in the same direction as the force of gravity. As the influence of gravity is minimized on the arms by the position, when the child makes a slight shoulder movement, it results in a larger movement of their hands in their visual field. It is important to remember that the activity provided and the height of the activity relative to the child determine how the child uses their arms. For example, the child may play with small figures when weight bearing on both elbows but must weight shift to place rings on a stack pole.

When used in conjunction with hip straps, lateral supports to the trunk can help provide midline guidance and, if necessary, align the spine in the prone position. With some children, head raising in a prone position is accompanied by associated extensor patterns in the lower extremities, including hip adduction and ankle plantar flexion. This pattern can be modified by placing an abductor wedge between the knees to abduct and externally rotate the hips, distributing pressure along the inner legs. It is important to remember that too much abduction creates an anterior pelvic tilt. A small roll beneath the ankle supports the instep so that the ankles are not stretched passively into plantar flexion.

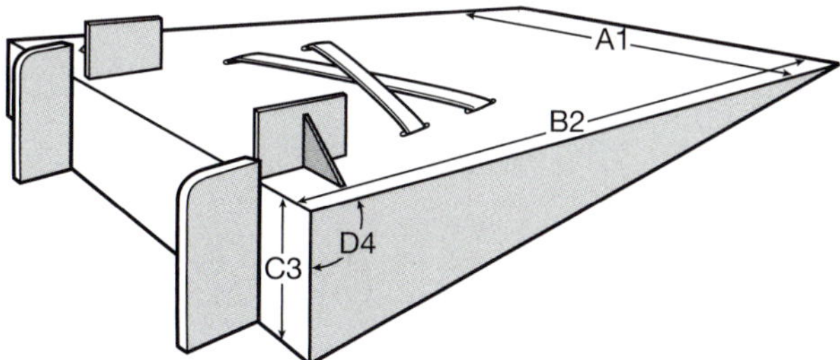

FIGURE 13.4 A, The prone-lyer provides hip control, lateral controls, and wings to prevent shoulder abduction and extension, keeping the arms forward of the shoulders. B, Measurements to consider for a prone wedge. 1, Width: unit should be wide enough so that it will not tip over if the child rolls over when strapped to it. 2, Length: contact of the front edge with the chest will determine how much shoulder stability is needed; the lower on the chest, the more the child is taxed. Lumbar curve and pelvic tilt are determined where the back edge ends in relation to the child's trunk or legs. C, 3, Height of wedge will determine if weight is borne on forearms or extended arms. D, 4, Depending on which side of the wedge is chosen as the top surface, shoulders will be placed in either 90-degree flexion or a lesser degree of flexion.

Maintaining the head upright when in a horizontal position can be stressful. The practitioner must carefully monitor the amount of time a child is in this position. In addition, the child's options for social interaction in this position are limited. Other people need to be sitting or, preferably, lying, on the floor to engage with the child. While prone lying opposite the child maximizes interaction, this is a difficult position for many parents and teachers to maintain. The plan to provide a prone-lyer needs to include appropriate activities and realistic expectations for parent/peer interaction when the child is in this position (Figure 13.4).

Sidelying Position

- Lateral head righting (a component of neck stability in the upright position)
- Differentiation of two sides of the body (bottom side weight bearing, top side mobile)
- Hands easily placed in the visual field
- Hypertonicity reduced; tonic labyrinthine reflexes inhibited
- Effects of gravity on shoulder flexion/extension reduced

The child who cannot maintain the sidelying position independently will benefit from front or back supports to prevent inadvertent rolling. The back support can be a wall or a board perpendicular to the floor. The front support can be a block (towel roll, stuffed animal) that contacts the trunk but allows movement of the shoulders and hips. A block is preferred to straps because it distributes pressure more evenly (Figure 13.5).

The child's head should be supported by a pillow or padded block that keeps the head and neck aligned laterally with the spine to prevent asymmetry and to facilitate lateral head righting. This also helps relieve pressure on the lower, weight-bearing shoulder. It is important to make sure that the pillow is wide enough so that the child's head does not fall when the child flexes their neck. If the child tends to extend their neck, slight padding can be attached to the back support behind the head to encourage a more neutral anterior/posterior neck position.

If the child tends to retract their shoulders, the practitioner can use gravity to facilitate protraction by rolling them slightly forward. This can be done by angling the back support slightly forward. As the child's upper arm falls toward the floor, the shoulder tends to adduct horizontally and rotate internally. If this is not a desirable position, the top of the trunk support block can be lengthened to serve as an armrest. This does, however, eliminate functional hand use in this position.

The lower, weight-bearing leg is extended, and the upside leg is flexed. If necessary, the weight-bearing leg can be extended by blocking the knee, distributing pressure along the thigh. The child who has lower tone generally does not need this blocking at the lower knee because the leg will stay where you position it. In addition, the upside leg can be flexed easily, adducted, and rotated internally. This is important because the child who has low tone tends to position their hips in abduction and external rotation. When placing the child who shows extensor hypertonicity in sidelying, their hips generally are positioned more appropriately in neutral abduction/adduction and neutral rotation. This is accomplished by supporting the higher knee, calf, ankle, and foot with a long block to position the hip properly and, simultaneously, to prevent the tibial torsion and ankle inversion/plantar flexion caused by the lack of support to the foot.

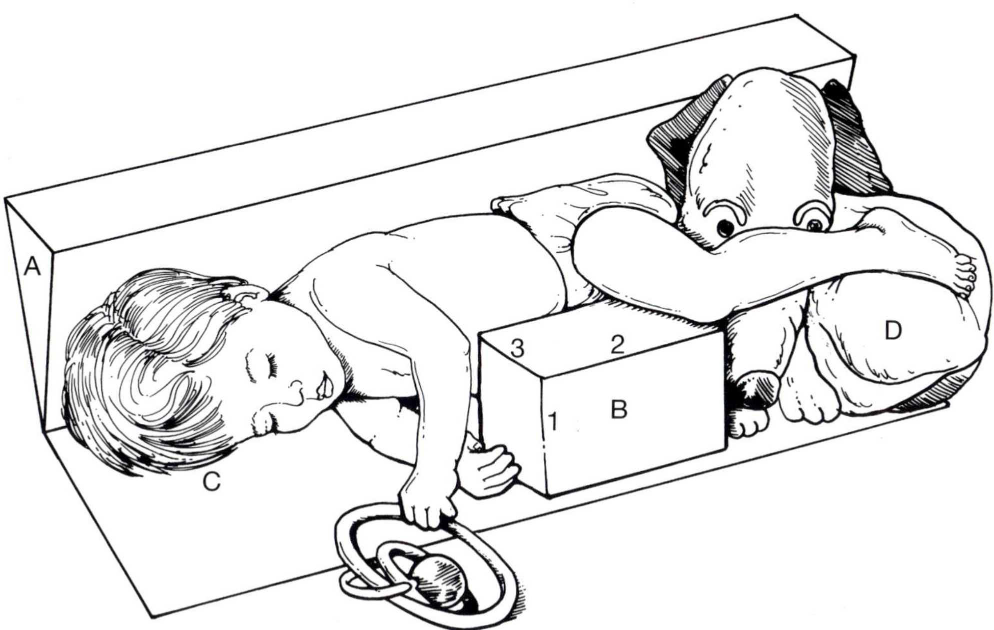

FIGURE 13.5 Possible components of a side-lyer: A, Wedged back tips child forward and assists in passive protraction. B, Chest block/leg support. 1, Height determines the position of the upper hip (adduction/abduction; internal/external rotation). 2, Length determines if chest alone is supported or if the hip, leg, and foot of upper leg are supported while lower leg is held in extension. 3, Depth is an issue only if the block also is used to maintain the position of the lower arm in shoulder flexion and elbow extension. C, Surface is padded beneath this child's head, but no pillow is used because his head is proportionately large in relation to his body. A pillow would flex his neck laterally. D, Stuffed animal acts as a leg block to extend the lower leg while supporting the upper leg in flexion. A longer chest block/leg support could have been used.

It is important that the child be positioned in sidelying on both sides equally in most cases. A side-lyer is a positioning aide that can be provided with detachable parts so that head and leg supports switch, allowing the child to be placed on either side (Figure 13.6). One exception is the child who has functional scoliosis; generally, the scoliosis is reduced when the "C" curve faces down and is exaggerated when the "C" faces up. The goal for sidelying with a child with functional scoliosis (the posture is only assumed for stabilization upright against gravity) is to elongate the "shortened" side by lying on that side to facilitate elongation. Another consideration for determining on which side to place a child is to encourage specific arm and hand use: the upside arm is more liberated and most likely to be used.

The sidelying position places the child in a very dependent position and limits the child's visual field due to restrictions in head movements. It offers excellent opportunities for the severely involved child to practice components of movement in a comfortable position with decreased influence of abnormal tone. Those benefits must be weighed against restrictions to engagement with others and the environment when determining when and where the side-lyer would be best used. For the less involved child who might benefit from the sidelying position, temporary and softer supports such as foam blocks and pillows might be used so that the child might volitionally and independently roll out of the position.

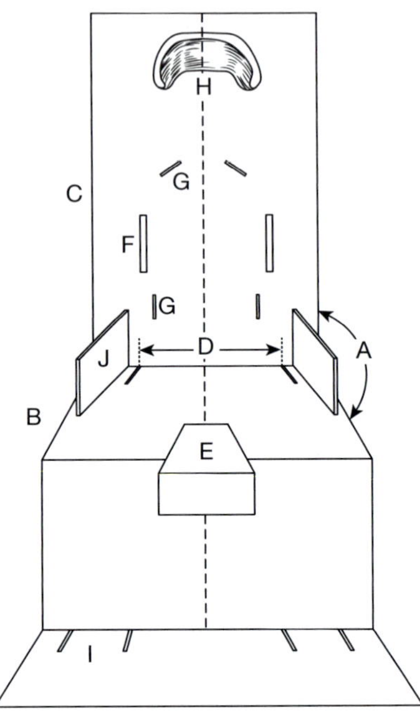

FIGURE 13.6 Possible components of an adapted chair: A, Hip angle is commonly 90 degrees, open more if hamstrings are very tight and close angle slightly if it helps to reduce extensor hypertonus. B, Seat depth should support thighs fully without digging into calf behind knee. C, Seat height is determined by need for trunk/head support. D, Hip straps generally come from seat bottom to hold bottom of pelvis back. Slots or attachments should be placed directly alongside the body to prevent lateral shifting of pelvis. E, Abductor wedge serves to keep legs centered; amount of abduction is determined once the pelvis is secured in seating unit. Abductor wedge starts at midthigh, distributing pressure out to the front of the knees, beyond the front edge of the seat. F, Lateral trunk supports are placed only as high as necessary to assist with trunk control. Lateral trunk supports should not interfere with humeral mobility because of height or thickness. G, Slots or attachments for harness come in contact with shoulders without digging into the child's neck, and lower placement should be below the rib cage to allow for thoracic expansion during inhalation. H, Placement and angle of head support should be determined after hip and trunk controls are provided with decisions regarding tilt in space. I, Foot straps may be needed if knee extension keeps feet from providing a base of support. J, Hip guides may be necessary to keep the pelvis centered and may help keep pelvic weight bearing symmetrical.

Sitting Position

- Anterior/posterior and lateral stability of the neck and trunk
- Weight shift on hips; hips in a slight anterior tilt
- Arms liberated; shoulder position independent of trunk
- Shoulders girdle: provide stable base for arm movements

The biomechanical frame of reference to position a child for function posits that independent functions can be increased if overall alignment and postural stability are provided via external supports. This claim is supported by numerous studies. Researchers reported that increased alignment via adaptive seating devices increased head control (Hulme et al., 1987), improved femoral head position (Soo et al., 2006), and decreased scoliosis deformity (Heller, Forst, & Hengtler, 1997). In addition, this increased postural alignment and support can led to increased communication (Clarke & Redden, 1992), mental performance (Miedaner & Finuf, 1993), feeding, breathing, bowel movement (Sahinoğlu et al., 2016), and the ability to play (Vekerdy, 2007).

Supported sitting for function is not a passive position, it requires active postural control of the trunk and pelvis to provide the foundation for visual attention, cognitive focus, and the dynamic movements of the head, arms, and at times, legs. A child who is unable to sit independently needs stability in the pelvis and lower body to actively use the upper trunk, arms, and head (Blair et al., 1995; Colbert et al., 1986; Myhr et al., 1995). Trunk supports and pelvic positioning should be selected individually to best support static and dynamic control and upper extremity function (Sahinoğlu et al., 2016; Seyhan & Kerem-Günel, 2019). Children who have limited ability to reposition themselves are at risk of developing pressure ulcers when seated for prolonged periods, which can significantly impact their quality of life. Practitioners should consider the materials used when selecting seating aids, positioning protocols, or the variety of seating aids used to improve their quality of life.

Compensatory movements often occur in response to an inadequate central base of support, and controlled upper extremity movements are restricted (Boehme, 1998). practitioners must first correct any inadequacies in the base by providing support, especially at the pelvis (Reid & Rigby, 1996). This may decrease tone, compensatory movements, or associated reactions elicited by stress, giving practitioners a better idea of what, if any, corrections need to be made in the more mobile, upper parts of the body. It is important to provide the least amount of artificial support necessary, providing flexibility for the development of dynamic movement (Brogren et al., 1996; Myhr et al., 1995)

Various studies have hypothesized and supported various seat positions for optimal posture in a child with cerebral palsy. The optimal posture is one that allows a child to function as independently and efficiently as possible without significant compensatory movements. There is a positive relationship between trunk control and reaching quality (Carlberg & Hadders-Algra, 2005), researchers have proposed that different seating positioning affects upper extremity functions. Within the literature, various postures have been promoted including a slightly reclined posture (Hadders-Algra et al., 1999) which can decrease the forces of gravity and a straddle posture occasionally combined with a forward leaning of the trunk (Reid, 1996) which is often observed using a bolster and wedge in therapy sessions. Following a review of the literature, Stavness (2006) utilization of various supportive elements such as a pelvic belt, hip abductors, footrests, and upper extremity support (tray) with cutouts for improved fit can support most individuals. However, more individualized modifications include a posterior tilt of the seating system ranging between 0 degrees and 15 degrees (Stavness, 2006), and a neutral to anteriorly included seat (McNamara & Casey, 2007; Stavness, 2006).

However, as noted earlier in this chapter, the results of seating and positioning may vary for different children depending on each individual's specific postural control and ability to use their extremities for function. It is also important to note that if compensatory postures are used for function, a home exercise program to elongate the "tightened" musculature is essential to minimize a child's risk of increased deformity and secondary complications.

Another way to modify tone to enhance the child's function is to consider the padding on the support unit (Figure 13.7). Sitting on firmer support tends to increase arousal level. Adding medium-density foam to create softer support, which conforms to and supports the curves of the child's body, tends to reduce postural stress and hypertonicity.

The child's pelvis should be supported on a solid surface, padded if necessary, that extends to just behind the knees to support the thighs. Careful measurements must be taken when designing

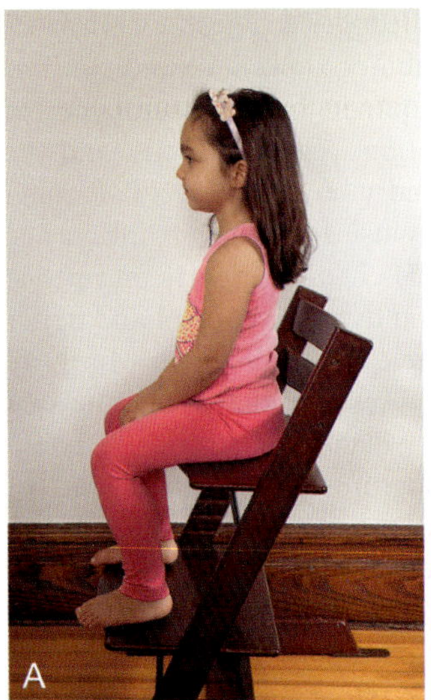

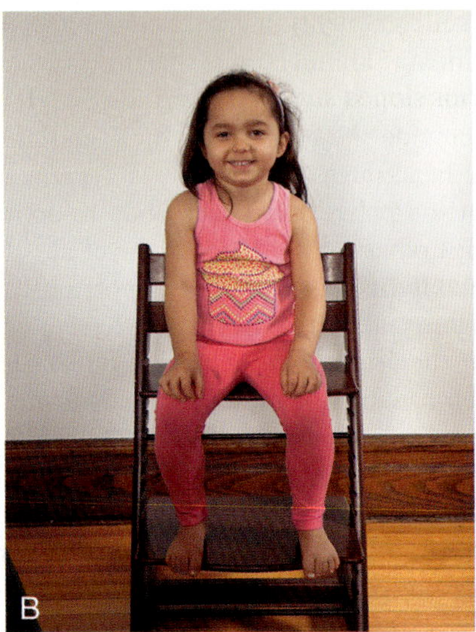

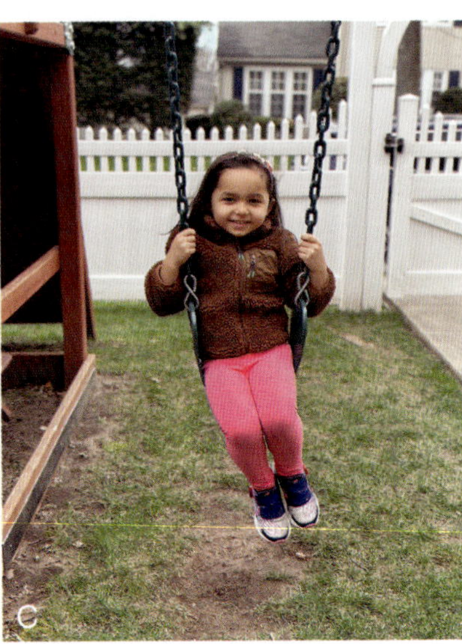

FIGURE 13.7 A solid seat (**A**) encourages upright posture from the pelvis through the head (**B**) and facilitates the hips to assume a relatively neutral position. The sling seat (**C**) places the hips into adduction and internal rotation and shifts weight laterally.

and ordering seating equipment. A seat that is too deep causes the edge to dig in behind the child's knees, pushing the legs and the bottom of the pelvis forward. A seat that is too shallow does not support the child's thighs, and the weight of their legs pulls their thighs downward and the bottom of the pelvis forward.

The back support should be no higher than necessary to discourage postural dependency. A child, for example, might do with back support that stops at the level of the pelvic crests or with no back support at all. If the goal is to increase anterior shoulder movement, care should be taken to leave the scapula area clear for upward and downward scapular rotation with humeral movement. If a practitioner considers a high back that also supports the head, attention should be given to the shape of the child's head. A young child and a child with hydrocephalus often have large occipital regions. The high back support may push a large head forward, causing a compensatory curve in the neck. In such cases, back support to shoulder height and separate head support may be more appropriate to accommodate the child's head and allow for neutral cervical alignment.

The position of the child's pelvis also is controlled by the seat-to-back angle (the angle of hip flexion) and the angle of the seating unit in space (the amount that it tilts in relation to the floor). These two factors should be explored simultaneously. Conventionally, the hip angle generally is maintained at 95 degrees to 100 degrees in a seating system. For individuals with increased extensor tone, increasing hip flexion or decreasing the seat-to-back angle to 80 degrees or 90 degrees may control or decrease severe extension hypertonicity. A child's tolerance for this position should be carefully evaluated. This may be a good position to attempt to increase strength in the trunk musculature via therapeutic activities. When a child's high tone is reduced with support, they may still have minimal postural tone in the trunk. In another situation, when a child has very tight hamstrings, opening the hip angle slightly (5 degrees to 10 degrees) to extend the hips may reduce the posterior pelvic tilt caused by the pull of their hamstrings. Opening the seat angle also can be effective with a low tone child. This can be accomplished by having the back perpendicular to the floor and using an anterior sloped seat. This position may facilitate increased proprioceptive input to the feet and consequently, postural alertness.

Pelvic Belt

A pelvic positioning belt is often used to ensure the proper position of the child's pelvis. Coming up from the point at which the seat meets the back of the chair, the belt is generally at a 60-degree to 90-degree angle to the hips and holds the pelvis in place. The belt itself should be appropriately sized and wide enough so that it does not dig into the child's flesh but narrow enough so that it places control only where desired and does not further limit a child's movement and functional potential. Rather than coming from the outside edge of the seat, it should be attached alongside the hips to keep the child's pelvis centered. The angle and type of pelvic belt are dependent upon the child's trunk and pelvic control, ability to weight shift, muscle tone, and positioning support needs. The various angles and types of belts can support the continuum of pelvic mobility to full pelvic stabilization.

A pelvic belt on a child with good trunk and pelvis control should be positioned below the anterior superior iliac spine and comes from the seat at a 90-degree angle, perpendicular to the floor. A belt at this position will adequately support the child's pelvis and will allow anterior tilt of the pelvis for a forward reach. If a child's pelvis can achieve a neutral alignment position, but they cannot keep that position because of weakness, a pelvic belt that is positioned below the anterior superior iliac spine at a 60-degree angle to the seat is the general rule of thumb.

If a child has an anterior pelvic tilt tendency, the belt should be positioned directly over the anterior superior iliac spine and anchored on the back support parallel to the floor. This will hold back the top of the child's pelvis. This is helpful when an exaggerated anterior pelvic tilt exists; however, in most cases, it is contraindicated because it does not allow for the trunk to shift forward over the hips. For a child without an anterior pelvic tilt tendency, positioning the belt directly over the anterior superior iliac spine encourages a posterior pelvic tilt and a subsequent compensatory forward curve of the trunk (kyphosis) and therefore should be avoided.

If a child has a pelvic rotation or pelvic obliquity tendency due to muscle tone or muscle strength asymmetry, a more aggressive four-point, padded pelvic belt can be utilized to control the pelvis. The belt itself should be positioned directly over the anterior superior iliac spine, and the secondary attachment straps can be anchored at 45-degree and 90-degree angles for optimal support.

Regarding pelvic positioning belts, size does matter. As noted in many pediatric seating systems, a too-wide strap placed at a 45-degree angle significantly limits pelvic mobility and can cause a posterior pelvic tilt by pulling the top of the child's pelvis backward.

If the child's pelvis tends to move laterally on the seat despite the seat belt, pelvic blocks also known as hip guides can be used for midline guidance and centering. These blocks can come from the seat cushion or the back support to nestle the child's pelvis in place. This is particularly important for a child who uses lateral trunk supports because if the pelvis moves laterally while the trunk is positioned between the lateral trunk supports, a scoliotic position is created. In accordance with proximal to distal support principle, pelvic blocks should always be considered before lateral trunk supports are considered.

For a child with significant spasticity where an aggressive pelvic belt and hip guides are insufficient other options are available. A leg harness provides increased surface area for control by individually wrapping around each leg, extending from the rear to the front of the chair. It supports the legs from the lateral thigh to the medial thigh. This provides increased surface area for control. A rigid pelvic stabilizer has been found helpful for anterior pelvic stabilization (Ryan et al., 2005). The rigid pelvic stabilizer is reported to increase a child's independence with bimanual tasks (Rigby et al., 2002) and is preferred by the user and caregivers (Reid et al., 1999). This is a very aggressive way to manage the pelvis and should be considered only after all other options have been exhausted.

Tilting the Seat

Depending on the degree to which it is done, tilting the seat unit slightly backward may increase or decrease postural demands. The stress and extensor tone that accompanies an upright position can be decreased with a backward tilt. This provides the child with back support on which they can lean intermittently. The same position may encourage activity in the neck or trunk flexors when the child comes forward into an upright position from a partial recline. When a reclining position is used to reduce the effects of gravity on the trunk and the child is incapable of flexing their neck or trunk forward into a righted position, it is important to support their head so that it is upright to facilitate a forward visual gaze. It is important to note that tilting back or reclining the seat back is a good position for increased stability. It is a good resting position for more sedentary activities such as watching television or being mobilized in a car/van. The tilted slightly back position should not be used exclusively as it does not facilitate engagement in activity. For individuals who can tolerate more upright sitting, tilting the seating system to a more upright position or not reclining the back is important for activity engagement and participation in dynamic activities such as feeding or writing. Carlberg and Hadders-Algra (2005) suggest tilt of the seating may depend on specific postural or diagnostic criteria, with a forward-tilted position benefiting children with spastic hemiplegia, and a horizontal sitting position is optimal for children with bilateral spastic cerebral palsy.

Abductor

The child's thighs contribute to their base of support. Too much abduction reduces anterior/posterior stability. Too much adduction reduces lateral stability and contributes to a pattern of extensor hypertonicity. Adductors are supports that run laterally along the child's thighs to reduce abduction. In general, the child's pelvis should be horizontal, and the hips should be in neutral abduction/adduction, with the limbs parallel to each other (Aroojis et al., 2021). For a child with high extensor tone in the hips, moderate hip abduction may be used to reduce tone and provide a wide base of support to help reduce extensor tone in the hips for orthopedic stabilization reasons (Howard et al., 2006; Manolikakis, 1992; Scrutton, 1991) or to facilitate an anterior pelvic tilt (Reid, 1996).

Pommel

Medial thigh support, also known as a pommel, is a rhombus-shaped wedge that can be used to maintain the child's hips in abduction. When used, it should start at the middle of the child's thighs and extend to their knees, beyond the edge of the seat, to distribute pressure. A rhombus-shaped wedge also may be needed to keep the child's thighs symmetrical if one hip tends to abduct or to rotate externally while the other adducts or rotates internally. This support is often misused, and it should not be used to keep a child's hips back in the wheelchair.

Height of the Chair

Care must be taken to ensure that the seat is not too high from the floor so that the child's feet can be placed firmly on the floor or on the foot support. Generally speaking, positioning the knees and ankles at 90-degree angles is a good guideline for weight bearing for postural stability. If the seating unit is in a wheelchair, the seat height should be just high enough for 2 to 3 inches of footplate clearance from the ground. This will enable the child to better access the same tables and desks as their peers. This will also allow the child to come to the front edge of the seat and have their feet stabilized on the ground for an alternative, possible assisted, seating position. Foot orthotics should be considered to correct ankles that are unstable or pathologically positioned so that the child's feet can contribute to stability.

Lateral Trunk Supports

Once the child has been positioned so that their pelvis is aligned in a relatively neutral position, the practitioner is better able to determine the positioning needs of the trunk, shoulders, and head. Lateral trunk supports provide lateral stability and increased postural alignment (Reid, 2002). They should be as thin as possible so that they do not interfere with upper extremity movement and function. They should be as shallow as possible and as low as possible if the child has decent postural control and the potential to continue to gain postural control. Lateral supports should not be placed slightly away from the body to encourage the child to do more postural "work" because they will make contact with the sensitive area on the inside of the humerus and will cause the humerus to work in an abducted position, which will compromise the movement pattern. A child may not be able to control their trunk and arms simultaneously. The higher the lateral supports, the more control they provide. Care should be taken to ensure that the lateral supports are 1 to 2 inches below the axilla so that they are not suspending the child by the armpits. The two supports should be opposite to each other, unless muscle control or tone in the trunk is asymmetrical. In that case, one support should be at the apex of the curve, and the contralateral side should be higher to either "correct" or accommodate scoliosis. Care should be taken to ensure that the supports are not so high that they press into the axilla where they may put pressure on the brachial plexus, nor so far apart that they hold the humeri in an abducted position. It is important to remember that improperly placed lateral supports interfere with shoulder mobility and hand use.

Custom-Molded Seating System

At times, a custom-molded seating system or a thoracic lumbar sacral orthosis is used to provide maximum trunk support to "correct" or support a child with a scoliosis or rotational scoliosis. Vekerdy (2007) found that wearing the nonrigid custom-molded trunk support several hours a day resulted in a significant change in posture of the trunk, extremities, head, chin, and mouth. This improvement of alignment and trunk support also resulted in a change in performance skills including improvement in eye–hand coordination, feeding, and ability to play. Shoham et al. (2004) noted a decrease in scoliosis on the contralateral side of the pelvic obliquity with orthosis use and Holms et al. (2003) and Heller et al. (1997) found an improvement in posture for the duration of use of the support.

Lap Tray

Lap trays or table surfaces can be designed to contribute to the child's more neutral shoulder and trunk positioning. It is important that they are provided only after optimal positioning has been attained through the design of the seating or standing unit. With an improperly fitted basic unit, a lap tray may be used by a child to "hang" by their arms or to rest their head and upper trunk, rather than enhance arm position and function.

A lap tray should provide enough surface area to support the full length of the child's arms during all movements. Hands or fingers should not hang off the edge of the tray. If the tray trunk cutout is deep enough, the tray almost "wraps around" the child's trunk. The cutout should be large enough so that it does not dig into the child's chest or interfere with their breathing or slight weight shifts. It should be snug enough so that the arms do not slip and become wedged between the trunk and the tray. In general, it is preferable to provide a transparent tray for two reasons: (1) a child can see the rest of their body and (2) in a wheelchair, a child or care provider can see the floor through the tray to maneuver more easily through space.

The child's use of a lap tray can enhance arm and hand function by diminishing pathology in the shoulders. Although it cannot directly affect humeral rotation when supporting the humeri in slight forward flexion, this position modifies the pattern of external rotation, extension, and retraction. In addition, the humeri can be adducted horizontally, bringing the arms toward the midline, by using humeral "wings" also known as protractor blocks. These are rectangular surfaces attached perpendicular to the lap tray. They push the humeri forward, preventing humeral extension and horizontal abduction. They also help to correct the position of humeri that are extended as part of a retraction/external rotation pattern. The humeral wings provide contact along the length of the humeri and should be high enough so that the child cannot lift their arms over them and get trapped behind them. The desired position for humeral wings can be determined by holding the child's humeri in slight flexion and running a pencil mark along the back of the elbows on the tray.

The child's use of a lap tray can contribute to trunk control by supporting the arms, thereby relieving the trunk of the weight of the arms. In this situation, the tray supports the arms, not the trunk. The position of a lap tray should be at or slightly above elbow height and be on height-adjustable armrests for optimal glenohumeral support. For a child who habitually experiences excessive trunk flexion, passive shoulder flexion that places the humeri in an almost horizontal position helps to elongate the thoracic spine as long as the child is not hanging by their arms on the tray.

It may be difficult for a child who demonstrates inadequate shoulder flexion or tightness in shoulder extension to keep their elbows and forearms on the tray surface because the arms are inclined to slide back from the tray edge and get trapped between the seat back and the back edge of the tray. Two possible solutions include the use of a "wraparound" tray and the use of humeral wings. A more proximal approach to the problem of excessive shoulder retraction/extension would include the use of scapula wings also known as "protraction wedges." These are small wedges placed on the seat back to bring the scapulae forward slightly. If the child retracts and pushes against the wedges, using a harness helps to maintain the trunk against the seat back, allowing the wedges to provide the scapulae with a gentle nudge forward.

Two issues prompt concern when using a lap tray on a seating or standing unit that tips back. First, if the lap tray is perpendicular to the back of the unit, it will be angled toward the child in an easel-like fashion when the unit is tilted back. The tilt of the lap tray can be controlled with adjustable hardware to keep it horizontal when the unit is tipped back. Second, by tipping the child slightly backward, gravity tends to push the humeri backward. It may be necessary to consider humeral wings that may not be otherwise needed when the child sits in a full, upright position.

The practitioner may choose to tilt the lap tray like an easel if it helps correct trunk or head position. By resting the forearms on an easel surface, the child may use greater degrees of shoulder flexion. This may elongate the upper trunk, enhancing the upright position. Also, tilting the lap tray places visual stimuli closer to eye level. This may encourage the child to keep their head in a more upright position, rather than looking downward and initiating a flexion pattern in the neck and trunk when reading or drawing (Figure 13.8).

A lap tray should not be used exclusively. Its primary function is to support a child's arms and provide them with a surface to reach and access items when a standard table or desk is not available (e.g., in the park) and, when necessary, to support functional positioning of the arms for specific activities. As often as possible, it is important to remove the tray to allow the child to get close to others to interact more normally and close to tables and objects for manipulation and learning (e.g., books on bookshelves). Hopefully, the child's wheelchair seat height will be low enough to provide them access to the same tables and desks as their peers. The issue of wheelchair height for small children presents a bit of a dilemma. If the lower height allows them to approach classroom tables and be at peer height when seated in the classroom, it will be too low for tables in the home and for matching height with peers when they are standing to work or play. In one environment or the other, the child would need to be transferred to another chair to be at the more appropriate level. The seat elevation function on a power wheelchair provides an option of adjustable seat height. It allows a child or caregiver to meet different environmental demands and to maximize a child's ability to participate.

Harness

If a child's control of the trunk is so limited that they continually falls forward and cannot right themselves, a harness may be provided. This is an anterior trunk support that is traditionally made of a chest plate with four straps. Often, when a harness is used, the child's sitting unit is tipped slightly backward so that the child rests against the back and does not hang into the harness. The top two straps attach to the back support directly over the shoulders. Slots may be cut into the back for proper strap placement. This ensures a snug fit and, simultaneously, discourages shoulder elevation. It also discourages lateral upper trunk flexion by keeping the shoulders at the same level. The lower straps should attach to the back or through slots on either side of the trunk, below the level of the rib cage, so they are less likely to interfere with thoracic expansion during respiration. The chest plate should be at a midchest level so that there is no danger of it digging into a child's neck. It is critical to note that a harness must always be used in conjunction with a pelvic belt. This is essential to prevent the child from sliding forward and down into the harness, possibly risking strangulation.

For a child with more complex positioning issues due to muscle strength or tone asymmetries, a harness can assist the other seating supports, such as the hip guides and lateral supports, by facilitating a "correction" of the flexible deformities. This includes "correction" of trunk lordosis, kyphosis, scoliosis, and rotational scoliosis. There are various styles of

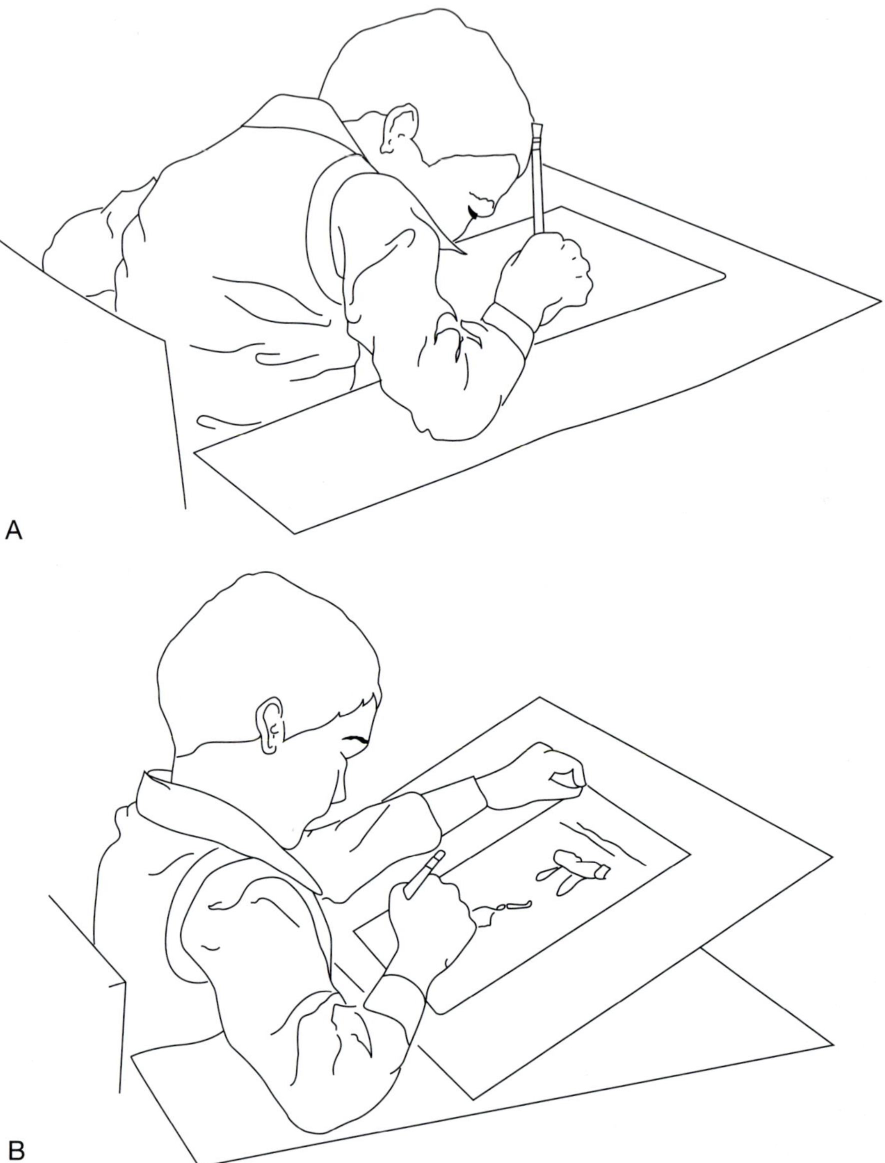

FIGURE 13.8 **A.** Flexion pattern, including overflow into hands, is created when this child looks down at his work. **B.** Angling the work surface changes the position of the head and modifies the associated tone.

harnesses along with strap length and direction modifications that can facilitate optimal alignment. If the harness causes the shoulders to retract, protraction wedges can be used. Care should be taken that the sizes or positions of the wedges do not create rounding of the upper trunk. If retraction is mild and the scapulae are mobile, then the protraction wedge may be used without a harness.

Because of the complexity of the head, shoulder, and arm interaction, the practitioner must be flexible and try several approaches to meet the child's needs. Supported alignment in the child's shoulders for more neutral positioning may provide more freedom of head movement or, conversely, may create a need for external head support. For example, by "correcting" a pattern of shoulder retraction and external rotation and straightening of the upper back, the child may no longer need compensatory neck extension to align their head with their body. Another child, with the same "corrections," however, may require head support.

Head Control

The first approach to improve inadequate head control or poor head alignment caused by tone problems is to correct total body position. Given enough external body support and reduction of physical stress, the child may be able to exercise control over their head on their own (Hulme et al., 1987). Properly aligning the child's body with subsequent "normalization" of tone can reduce associated reactions and the need for compensatory movements in the neck. Conversely, it is important to remember that head movement elicits many pathologic reflexes. In such cases, correction of head position can enhance body position. For example, slight flexion of a hyperextended neck may reduce extensor tone throughout the body, and support midline head positioning may eliminate body asymmetry caused by the influence of an ATNR. These are small gentle positioning techniques. Aggressive head positioning should not be a primary goal of any child who exhibits issues with head control.

A child needs to change head position continually throughout the day to gather visual or auditory information and receive and respond to environmental stimulation for function. Many children hyperextend their necks when seated in a chair to look at and speak with an adult who stands before or next to them. The position of the child in relation to their environmental surroundings must be considered when attempting to correct head position.

If a child has head control and a prominent ATNR that is used for function, such as to reach a water bottle on the table, then as long as the child can independently utilize this to access the water bottle and bring it to the mouth for drinking, then restricting their head movement with aggressive head support is not recommended. Conversely, if the child cannot control the ATNR, and their limb movements are compromising environmental access with the risk of injury upon entrance into a standard door, then a more aggressive head support is recommended for safety. Also, if these uncontrolled limb movements result in injury to others and intimidate others from socially interacting with the child, then a more aggressive head support is recommended for these times.

Aggressive head positioning is a goal only for a child who has no head control when upright against gravity. Head supports have various posterior and lateral components to assist with head alignment. In addition, cervical collars are often utilized in conjunction with aggressive headrests for optimal support.

A child with no head control may not be able to turn the head even when supported by a headrest. The caregivers must attend to the child's position in the environment to assure that they have visual access to the important events.

The simplest support for the head may be a small posterior headrest. This provides a resting place but no lateral or anterior controls. In conjunction with a slight tip back of the unit, gravity assists in preventing passive, floppy forward flexion yet still encourages active neck flexion against slight resistance. The latter example may enhance active control of the head. Another child may use an undesirable pattern of total flexion to right their head when tipped back. Care should be taken with head support because the headrest may provide a tactile cue that stimulates neck extension against the surface, which may be contraindicated.

Another simple control consists of adding lateral support pads to the headrest. With all head supports, care should be taken that these supports do not interfere with the visual field or cover the ears. In addition, if the lateral contours of head support touch the cheeks, a rooting reflex may be elicited.

The suboccipital support is an attempt to simulate the shape of the therapist's hand where the practitioner places their thumb and forefinger around the back of the child's neck with the occiput resting on the web space and the base of the temporal bones on thumb and fingertips. A suboccipital pad and neck collars contribute to head control with little interference to sensory inputs received from head and face. A suboccipital pad attaches via headrest hardware to the seat back and cradles the base of the cranium. A child should be seated as upright as possible, and the suboccipital pad should be placed at a height to support the base of the skull. A neck collar made of medium-density foam, cut in width to fit between the shoulders and the base of the skull snugly, supports and elongates the neck and can be used independently of the seating unit. The front of the neck collar should be connected in a yoke-like or V fashion to allow for slight neck flexion or jaw movements.

If a child requires the support of a multicomponent headrest, the major headrest manufacturers offer a wide array of pad shapes, sizes, and contours to customize a head support for more aggressive contact. This aggressive support of the head and neck is essential for a child who has no head control and is unable to prevent their head from falling forward, sideways, or backward when in an upright position. A slight backward tilt of the seating unit assists in keeping the head in contact with the support. When a child is tipped back more than 5 degrees or 10 degrees for the sake of trunk control, however, it is necessary to right the head as much as possible by angling the head support or pushing it forward to flex the neck and align the head in space. The therapist must experiment with the child and caregivers to find the optimal balance among the head, trunk, and angle in space.

In extreme cases, a child may have a complete lack of head control. This child will also most likely have poor or absent trunk and lower extremity control. For this child, it is essential first to ensure that the trunk and pelvis are aggressively supported. Once that is accomplished, head support needs can be the primary focus. Along with the multicomponent headrest and cervical collar, a head strap or head cap (similar to a baseball cap appearance) can be utilized to stabilize a child's head adequately. Just as it is important only to utilize aggressive head supports after the trunk and pelvis are adequately stabilized, it is important only to use a head strap or head cap if the other components are insufficient to stabilize a child's head in the anterior direction.

Three notes of caution with more aggressive head and neck supports: (1) the head support lateral components should not compromise circulation in the neck; (2) a full neck collar immobilizes the head and may interfere with jaw movements or swallowing; and (3) a severe recline of the seating unit (up to 40 degrees tipped back) to provide head support limits the child's visual access to the environment and ability to interact with people in the environment and can compromise swallowing.

In general, demands on active head control in the severely involved child should be minimized when the child is seated. The child will then able to direct their efforts toward intake of information, interaction with the environment, and fine motor or oral-motor skills. The practitioner should keep in mind that developing active components for head control may be addressed by using various positions and equipment such as standers, scooter boards, and prone wedges.

Supported Standing Position

- Erect spine, liberated arms
- Neutral or slightly posterior pelvic tilt
- Hips extended with neutral rotation
- Knees stable but not locked in hyperextension
- Ankles in 90-degree flexion, neutral eversion/inversion
- Improved circulation and bone growth from upright weight bearing
- Increased alertness from an upright position and extensor activity
- Decreased effects of flexor hypertonicity in the neck and trunk when weight bearing on extended hips and knees

The supported standing position should not be used for potential ambulators exclusively. This position provides increased opportunities for function for a child who is least likely to walk by enhancing circulation, growth, and alertness. It also provides opportunities for a child who has moderate to severe disabilities to perform some degrees of head and arm control and serves as an alternative to long-term sitting (Manley & Gurtowski, 1985; Motloch & Brearley, 1983; Noronha et al., 1989). Standing programs are one way to reduce sedentary behavior in a child with cerebral palsy (Verschuren et al., 2014); they have a positive effect on bone mineral density (Caulton et al., 2004; Stuberg, 1992), hip stability (Macias, 2005; Pountney et al., 2009), and range of motion of hips, knees, and ankle, and spasticity (Martinsson & Himmelmann, 2011; Salem et al., 2010). In addition, regarding constipation that plagues many children with cerebral palsy, standing programs have been shown to reduce the need for induced evacuation (Rivi et al., 2014). The therapist first must decide which surface of the child's body is to be supported in standing.

The height of the stander determines how much support is provided to the trunk (and head in a supine position) and how much postural work must be done by the child. The practitioner's goal is to challenge the postural system without causing fatigue or undesirable associated reactions that result from physical stress.

As with sitting, the pelvis should be positioned first. If lateral shifting of the pelvis occurs, which would create a compensatory curve in the trunk, lateral pelvic blocks also known as "lateral hip guides" should be placed on either side of the pelvis. With hips in neutral, the knees should be directly below the hips. Occasionally, some hip abduction is desired. In either case, depending on the degree of abduction desired, a rectangular- or trapezoid-shaped block should be placed between the knees. This spacer or abductor should extend above and below the knees to distribute pressure. Its primary purpose is to keep the legs aligned and symmetrical. If the child abducts and rotates their hips externally, then the front of their knees is no longer blocked by the surface of the stander because the knees will be facing laterally. In this case, lateral supports at the level of the knees can be used to bring the hips into a more neutral abduction/adduction position and prevent collapse at the knees or allowing for slight hip and knee flexion.

Padding in front of the knees on a stander is necessary to relieve pressure and prevent knee flexion. This should be done judiciously because too much padding can cause the knees to hyperextend. If the knees hyperextend regardless of padding, the joint can be flexed by slightly realigning the feet so that the ankle is slightly behind the knee. If a child wears foot orthoses, then the upper straps of the foot orthoses must be loosened to allow necessary ankle dorsiflexion in this position.

Blocks placed laterally or medially to the child's feet or shoe holders can maintain the foot position if necessary. A nonskid surface could be just as effective. The integrity of the ankle and foot must be evaluated in standing. Although full discussion of this is beyond this chapter, ankle/foot orthoses must be provided for standing if pathology exists.

The need for and placement of lateral trunk supports can be determined once the lower-body position is corrected and stable. The chest support or upper edge of the prone stander may end anywhere between the bottom of the sternum to just below the clavicle, depending on the need. If the chest support is cut high, it should be narrow and contoured (something like the end of an ironing board) to free the shoulder girdle for movement.

As in the sitting position, height and angle of the lap tray contribute to facilitating postural control and alignment. A low lap tray may encourage weight bearing on extended arms. A child who has inadequate extension, however, may flex over the top of the chest support in an attempt to rest on the lap tray. In such cases, a lap tray at nipple level helps elongate the upper trunk and provides support for the arms as the child masters head control. The need for humeral wings on the lap tray should be assessed if retraction and extension are the dominant shoulder movements.

Standers offer versatile support options, catering to individuals' needs whether in a prone or supine position. Additionally, sit-to-stand standers present an alternative for those unable to sustain hip and knee extension, either due to prolonged discomfort or muscle contraction, but would benefit from weight bearing in a modified standing position.

Prone Stander

Providing support to the ventral surface of a child's body by using a "prone" stander at an 80-degree to 85-degree angle to the floor provides a close-to-normal standing position and requires slightly more extensor activity (Figure 13.9). If upright at 90 degrees, the prone stander tends to throw the child's body backward in space, and they may flex over the top edge of the stander to compensate.

Through a series of trials and observations, the practitioner can determine the optimal angle of a standing board to the floor. Postural demands and responses change as the stander is tipped farther forward or backward. In a prone stander, demands on head righting are less in this upright position than in a horizontal position. In the prone stander, crossed straps should stabilize the pelvis in the same way as in the prone position. The child who cannot maintain a righted head in a full prone-lying position may be successful in a prone stander at 75 degrees upright. In this case, with head control and tolerance in the prone position as the primary goal, the prone stander actually may be lowered as the child develops head control in increasingly higher horizontal positions.

Supine Stander

A supine stander provides full dorsal support with the body tilted back slightly for a child who has very high or very low tone. In the supine stander, a child may use slight neck flexion to right their head and lean back against the head support when fatigued. In the supine stander, a pelvic strap is unnecessary because the chest and knee straps tend to encourage extension against the back support. Care should be taken to ensure that the chest strap does not dig into the axillary area. Hip blocks may be desirable to prevent lateral movement and any resultant asymmetries. As with the prone stander, abductor/spacer blocks or lateral adductors should be considered to align hips and legs. Padding should be placed behind the knees if there is any indication of hyperextension at that joint. Ankle straps that come from behind the heel over the instep at a 45-degree angle or medial or lateral foot blocks may be needed to maintain foot placement.

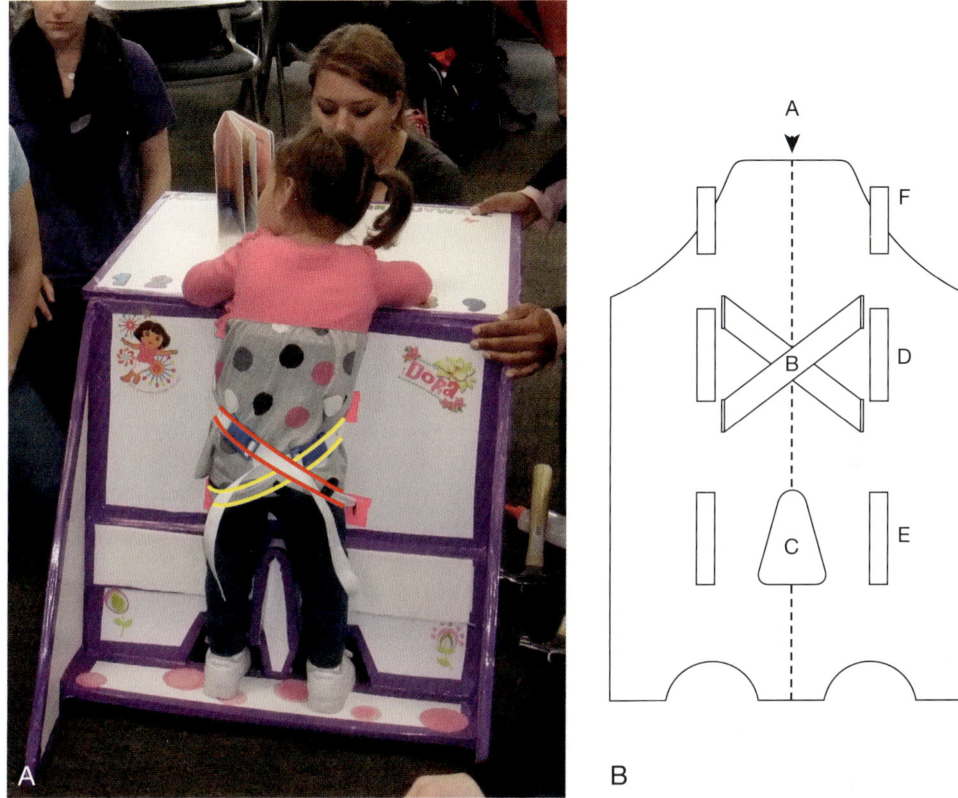

FIGURE 13.9 **A.** Example of a prone stander with hip straps. **B.** Possible components of a prone stander. A, Height is determined by the child's need for ventral support, anywhere between the waist and sternoclavicular joint. When the support is cut high (as in this example), sides must be cut out to allow for shoulder mobility. B, Hip straps come through slots right alongside the hips. They cross from the posterior crest of one side to the hip joint of the other side, placing pressure over the sacrum. C, Abductor wedge keeps the legs aligned symmetrically and determines the amount of hip abduction. It runs above and below the knees but does not come in contact with the perineum. D, Hip guides may be added for additional lateral stability, especially in the presence of a functional scoliosis. E, Lateral leg guides prevent the external rotation/knee flexion pattern that often causes children with low tone to collapse in standing. F, Lateral trunk supports may be necessary and should be placed as low as possible.

A supine stander that has a lap tray supports the arms, provides a working surface, and encourages the child to use some active neck and upper trunk flexion to right the head and come forward to the working surface. Because the supine stander is tilted backward to some extent, protraction wedges on the stander or humeral wings on the lap tray may be necessary to assist the child in keeping their shoulders and arms forward against gravity. If head supports are needed, this is determined in the same way as for the partially reclined sitting position.

Sit-to-Stand Stander

Sit-to-stand standers offer many of the same features as prone standers but are particularly beneficial for children who struggle to tolerate extension at the hips and knees due to muscle contraction, joint deformities, or general fatigue associated with standing positions. The stander can be adjusted progressively from a seated position to a fully extended standing position, aiding children in building strength and endurance in various positions. Sit-to-stand standers can be controlled by the user to provide independence to adjust their position via a manual hydraulic pump or a battery-operated lift.

Often two people are needed to safely transfer and position a child into an upright stander. Facilitating transfers into a sit-to-stand stander reduces the demands for both the caregiver and child while still encouraging a weight-bearing position for individuals.

Functional Skills

The previous section discussed several common positions in which central stability is provided artificially to decrease pathologic movement, encourage components of postural responses, and liberate the head and arms. Intervention in this section addresses the function–dysfunction continua that relate to hand control, mobility, feeding, and toileting, all of which involve more than postural responses. These functions also require cognition, perception, attention, motor planning, and fine motor skills. Postural control is a foundation for the development of these functions. The absence of postural control impedes the development of skills in these areas. The following sections describe postural components or equipment related to these functions.

Ability to Place, Maintain, and Control Hand Position

Although it is desirable to have shoulder and arm mobility in all planes, this is not always a realistic goal. If expectations must be graded or limited, then the most functional ranges of shoulder and arm movement are those that contribute to midline activity so that the child can bring objects toward their eyes, ears, and mouth for learning and survival. In this case, desirable ranges of volitional movement include neutral toward slight protraction; 30 degrees of external rotation toward full internal rotation; 0-degree to 90-degree shoulder flexion, abduction, adduction, and horizontal adduction; and midranges of elbow flexion/extension and forearm rotation. The development of control in these ranges can be addressed in two ways: (1) by establishing skill in shoulder and elbow mobility and stability in developmental positions (enhancing the development of components of movement) and (2) by providing as much support as necessary to the body and proximal upper extremities to enable the child to perform a few distal isolated movements (providing proximal stability via external support reduces the need for postural reactions).

With a child who has moderate to severe disabilities, the practitioner may choose to devise a specific pattern of movement related to one function. Examples of specific patterns of movement may be a hand-to-mouth pattern for feeding or a simple elbow movement to activate a switch. The first step is to provide an optimum base of support to modify tone, reduce demands on the rest of the body, and enhance attention to task. Sidelying, sitting, and supported standing are positions that should be considered. The second step is to determine how many arm movements the child can control, and which ones need to be supported artificially by a table, lap tray, or other equipment components. For example, humeral wings on a tray minimize the child's ability to protract actively or to adduct horizontally when bringing their hand to the mouth. If the practitioner raises the lap tray to axilla level, the child's movements are then limited to the horizontal plane, and demands for shoulder and elbow movements against gravity are eliminated.

In extreme cases, if a child has no control over arm movements (i.e., such as a child who has severe athetoid movements), one arm can be positioned so that movement is channeled in one direction. For example, blocks may be placed laterally and medially along the child's arm, creating a channel on the lap tray. With such an arrangement, the hand can move only in the vertical plane, regardless of extraneous shoulder, elbow, or forearm movements. In this way, the child may successfully depress a switch plate. Following a training period, supports should be withdrawn to assess the potential for performance without aggressive supports.

Ability to Move Through Space

Postural stability is the foundation for movement. Mobility contributes to the development of the brain and has been shown to improve cognitive and perceptual skills, reduce learned helplessness, increase confidence, and increase participation with peers in everyday activities (Rosen et al., 2009; Rousseau-Harrison & Rochette, 2012). Mobility promotes environmental exploration through play and social interactions, eventually enabling children to access settings beyond their homes, such as school and public spaces.

Mobility devices for children with postural difficulties may be appropriate for a child who has less severe involvement but whose ability to perform a task efficiently or whose ability to participate in activities with their peers is impaired. When choosing a mobility device for a child, it is important to consider both the duration of use and the level of postural support required. Various devices facilitate mobility, ranging from basic tools (scooters) that facilitate active exploration during a specific activity to more complex devices (wheelchairs) that become integral to everyday life. For instance, while a folding stroller might facilitate transportation from home to the clinic, it may lack adequate postural support for prolonged periods. Conversely, in settings like classrooms where supports are needed for extended times, a wheelchair base with customizable seating would be a better fit.

If present, pathologic tone may be increased through passive movement because of the intensity of the stimulation but effectual responses are positive, it is up to the therapist to provide a position in which unwanted overflow of tone can be controlled. For example, a child who hyperextends when swinging may be nestled in a flexed position within an inflatable tube placed on a platform swing.

Scooter Boards

Scooter boards may be effective in enhancing self-initiated movement, providing opportunities for weight bearing and weight shifting. For a child with milder limitations, it can provide the sensory experience of rapid movement through space. Directed, forward movement is not the goal in this case. The goal is to experience movement and interact with the environment for sensorimotor (weight bearing, movement over stability, visual perceptual) and cognitive development. The child begins to initiate movement through space whenever their hands begin to bear weight through the arms. For a child who cannot roll or crawl, this may be their only opportunity to experience active movement through space.

The scooter board consists of an appropriately fitted prone wedge placed on highly responsive ball-bearing casters. Several modifications to the prone wedge can enhance its effectiveness. These include a chest wedge to provide the correct shoulder-to-floor distance and a narrower front wedge cutaway to support only the chest and liberate the shoulder girdle (which is "ironing board" shaped). The length of the back end of the wedge determines the amount of support provided, with a back edge ending at the hips providing less support than one ending before the ankles. This design allows the child's feet to hang freely over the end of the board. A child who has more severe disabilities may need an extension of the front edge of the wedge for intermittent head support.

Tricycle

A child who is nonambulatory or who walks slowly with crutches may be less taxed when using a tricycle. A tricycle also allows them to engage socially with peers in gross motor activity and increases opportunities for physical activity. Tricycles can be purchased with back supports, hip straps, abductors along the handlebar uprights, and footplates with straps (Fernandes, 2006). The therapist's role is to determine the tricycle measurements and provide appropriate support for a particular child's sitting and mobility skills. Positioning of the arms and hands, as well as lower extremity, should be assessed. The handlebars can be raised to encourage an upright trunk. Adapted vertical hand grips that place the forearm in a neutral rotation also encourage an erect trunk, provided there is forearm mobility. Appropriate seat height and abductor wedge can facilitate a more neutral lower extremity alignment. For children who are unable to utilize a foot petal bike, there are adaptive tricycles that can be propelled using the hands that have seating modifications as well.

Wheelchair

Functional mobility is the primary purpose of a wheelchair. Selecting and building a wheelchair involves more than just addressing mobility concerns, considerations regarding biomechanical factors and optimal positioning are crucial. If a manual wheelchair does not provide efficient mobility, it may impede a child's independence. A properly fitting wheelchair has been shown to have a significant and positive impact on quality of life. For individuals who do not have the mobility control to maneuver a manual wheelchair functionally and efficiently, a powered wheelchair can be an alternative. This is an important consideration for the nonambulatory client who finds a manual wheelchair painstakingly slow to propel and requires excessive effort to move. It is important to emphasize to the full team, parents, children, teachers, and other clinicians, that propelling a manual wheelchair is not exercise.

As long as a child demonstrates some spatial awareness and judgment about their safety and the safety of others, they have the potential to be trained using a power wheelchair. There is a wide range of electronic modifications, "joystick" and switch access devices to provide mobility to a child with more severe disabilities. Just as an 18-month-old child can direct their body through space with reasonable safety, a child of the same developmental age can learn to negotiate a power chair using a switch.

An occupational therapy practitioner's role is to understand a child's positioning needs for optimal function which includes evaluation of a child's seating and mobility needs based on the activity and the environment (Short et al., 2023). For mobility outdoors and playing with their peers, a child may need more aggressive postural support and posterior support. However, for mobility on level surfaces, eating, or writing at a desk, a child may need less aggressive supports and more anterior positioning. Even for a child with more severe involvement, a seating system must allow for easy modification to accommodate more active and more passive activities that make up an average child's day. Device abandonment or dissatisfaction often occurs when individuals' contextual factors are not considered. The Wheelchair Outcomes Assessment Tool for Children (WATCh) was developed to help therapists work with children to identify the main outcomes of importance to young wheelchair users (Tuersley et al., 2018).

Ability to Feed

Positioning in a feeding program is designed to reduce the influence of muscle tone (low or high) on oral-motor activity, minimize situations that may trigger primitive reflexes, and provide central stability to enhance controlled distal mobility, such as sucking, biting, chewing, and swallowing (Larnet & Ekberg, 1995). Before initiating a total seating position for feeding, practitioners should use concepts regarding central postural supports in sitting or standing.

During feeding some children may benefit from the physical warmth, touch, and social interaction when positioned properly in an adult's lap. While using the practitioner or caregiver's body as a support surface can be applied in other situations, for feeding it may support the child with regulation during an experience that requires a variety of demands on the child.

For more involved individuals, head support may be needed to provide a stable base for jaw movements. A neutral or slightly flexed position of the neck reduces extensor hypertonicity, contributes to controlled swallowing, and prevents a child who has a disability from throwing their head back and "bird feeding," which is uncontrolled swallowing that uses gravity rather than musculature to get the food down. The appropriate position of the head can be accomplished by reclining the trunk partially and bringing the head forward to an almost-righted position.

The head support should not contact the face to avoid a rooting reflex, which might turn the child's head toward the source of food and initiate asymmetries because the turning of the head can produce ATNR activity. Special attention should be paid to shoulder position during feeding (Figure 13.10). High tone in elevation, retraction, protraction, or humeral rotation can compromise swallowing and the coordination of swallowing with respiration.

Ability to Void When Seated on a Toilet or Potty

The primary goal of equipment in this area is to provide support and modify tone so that the child can relax. Postural challenges should not be the issue here; instead, comfort is essential. Special attention should be paid to providing adequate hip flexion and abduction in supported sitting (Figure 13.10).

Potty training for a young child who has severe disabilities frequently requires a long period. Diversional activities are sometimes helpful to motivate and engage the child. If a younger child's potty training program includes diversional activities, then a lap tray or light table can serve the dual purpose of arm support and a play surface.

Ability to Activate the Switch for a Technology Aid

The goal of positioning here is to facilitate effortless and reliable switch control. Once an optimal sitting position has been established, a therapist may find that a child benefits from additional supports (e.g., head support, harness) while learning the refinements of this task. If the hand has the potential for switch activation, it may help to temporarily provide additional supports to limit degrees of freedom of arm movements (e.g., using protractor blocks to limit shoulder retraction

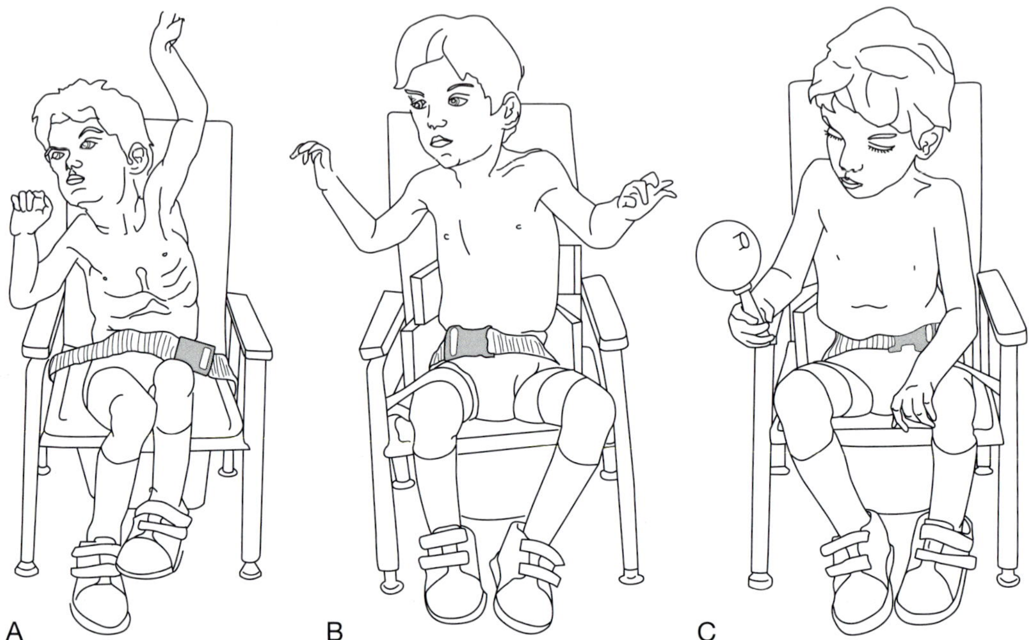

FIGURE 13.10 **A.** Child in commercially available adapted potty with seat belt. **B.** Child sitting with additional control facilitated by lateral trunk supports, hip guides, and abductor straps. **C.** Relaxation is enhanced by the use of an activity.

and extension to enable the child to develop control of a wrist or finger movement). Another way to reduce motor demands for a severely involved child when beginning switch activation training is to approach the task from a sidelying position.

The therapist and child must find the best position in space for the switch, where access to it is most efficient. If the child is using their hand, a graphic way to identify this "sweet spot" may be to cover the lap tray with paper and attach a marker to the child's hand. The most heavily colored portion of the paper usually represents the most accessible place for the switch. With a child who is less involved, clinical observation can determine this spot. The "sweet spot" may be at the midline for one child and to the side for others. Once access skills emerge, it is good to gradually move the switch off to the side, leaving midline space for the placement of other activities and table and desk access. If the child does not have the potential to use their hand, the therapist and child must explore together the options for a reliable movement in other body parts (e.g., the head).

A variety of switches that can be activated via contact and noncontact methods are available commercially (Leung et al., 2013). If a child can control more than a single movement, they have the potential to access more standard switches such as joysticks and keyboards. These tend to be more efficient switch methods. If a child cannot efficiently operate a standard or modified joystick or keyboard, the therapist must find a match between the child's motor ability and the type of switch, in terms of force and speed needed, the distance traversed to activate/deactivate, and the cognitive/perceptual components to plan coded sequences of single movements (such as the attention and discrimination necessary to select one word from a vocabulary of hundreds on a communication device).

When using any switch, a critical goal is to limit accidental switch activation by the user (Leung et al., 2013). If the child has an adequate agonist musculature to activate a switch but inadequate antagonist to release it (or a similar scenario), the switch can be placed in a gravity-eliminated position to facilitate the weaker movement. If a similar modification does not provide consistent success in activation, noncontact technology such as gaze-based, webcam-based systems, or facial thermography has been used for children with physical limitations as well as hygiene concerns and switch placement limitations (Borgestig et al., 2017; Leung et al., 2013).

Making Custom Positioning Devices More Accessible

The purchase of durable medical equipment is costly, and financial resources are often limited, especially when the child needs a variety of custom-designed positioning devices. In addition, the process of getting funding can involve quite a bit of time, and often equipment that is funded cannot be replaced until a certain period has elapsed. Devices made from alternative materials can offer a solution for a child who needs frequent changes in adaptations due to growth or changes in capacity. They can also benefit children who require a variety of positioning devices and adaptations to school or home furniture. Additionally, they can be useful for children living in locales where access to durable medical equipment is limited. Alternative materials can include readily available items, such as foam or batting for small adjustments to current furniture or creating devices via cardboard or three-dimensional (3D) printing.

In addition to cost-effectiveness and limited wait time, using alternative materials to make positioning modifications has the following benefits:

1. Modifying existing durable devices to improve fit in responses to growth or changes in physical status
2. Assessing function and fit of desired positioning device before ordering durable equipment
3. Providing progressive positioning for a child whose physical status is changing, before finalizing the design of the device
4. Providing equipment for an infant or small child whose size and positioning needs change rapidly.

Often practitioners are limited to items available within the environment they work in or affordable options from distributors. For some children, an additional piece of equipment is too cumbersome for their home, or they are able to use the same equipment as their classmates but need slight modifications for postural support (Figure 13.11). Practitioners can often create effective adaptations using readily accessible materials. Common items such as foam, batting, bean bags, or towel rolls can be repurposed to make subtle yet impactful adjustments such as lateral guides or a foot base, ensuring that children receive the tailored support they need without overburdening their environment or compromising their inclusion in social settings. These skills require the application of the above principles paired with creativity and adaptability. Often families have come up with creative adaptations in the home, communication around this empowers the family and assists the therapist in problem solving.

Triple-wall cardboard, which has one more layer than cardboard commonly used in boxes, or common cardboard layers glued together can be used to make equipment. It provides a custom fit at a low cost and in a timely fashion. Positioning devices constructed of cardboard have been provided in the United States since the 1970s. There are various not-for-profit or for profit companies with the goal of providing custom low-cost items to families both in the United States and

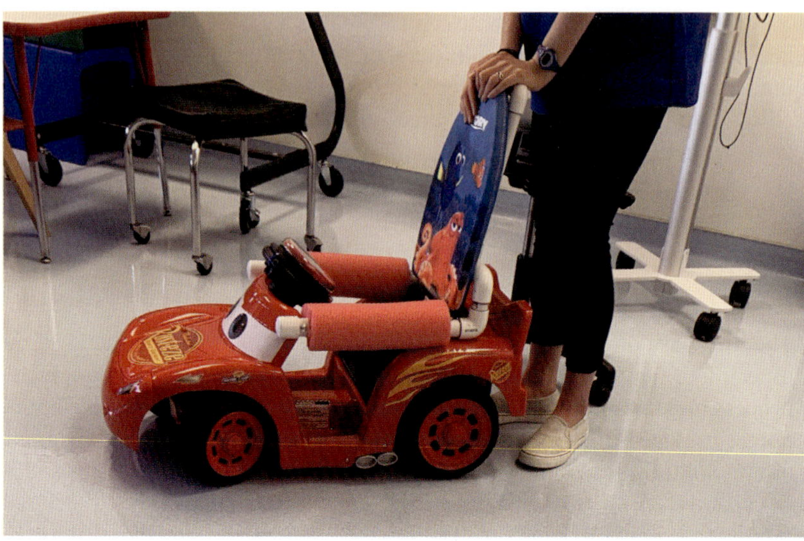

FIGURE 13.11 This adapted electric car utilizes PVC pipe and pool accessories for back and lateral trunk support.

in developing countries. While a practitioner must determine the best option for fit using a cardboard device, the construction can be a shared enterprise. Often families, or local volunteer agencies, can help with the actual construction of these devices, as only simple hand tools are required.

With the increasing affordability and accessibility of 3D printing for health care professions (Hunzeker & Ozelie, 2021), 3D printing has become more affordable and accessible for health care professions, offering individualized and reproducible products at relatively low costs. However, despite the potential benefits, 3D printing still presents barriers including limited awareness, experience, and training, as well as the time required to master computer-aided design (CAD) software and 3D printers (Patterson et al., 2020). The Emerging Tech Lab (ETL) at Rancho Los Amigos National Rehabilitation Center (RLANRC), is one resource for assistive tech related to 3D printing for individuals with abilities.

The last part of this chapter has addressed the more technical aspects of the biomechanical frame of reference to position a child for function (i.e., the practical problems of translating a therapeutic intention into a piece of equipment). This process requires some mechanical skills and an ability to manipulate 3D space mentally. Although it is only one component of treatment implementation, the actual prescription or design of equipment often makes greater demands on the novice practitioner. Frequent hazards involved in this process include that concentration becomes too focused on the product (i.e., adaptive device) and the multitude of other factors that enhance posture and function are overlooked.

While assistive technology recommendations are often made within a collaborative team, occupational therapy practitioners should feel confident in their role within the team which includes application of the biomechanical frame of references to position for function and how these changes may impact habits, roles, and routines of the child (Sarsak et al., 2023). The role of the occupational therapy practitioner is to apply this knowledge and articulate those specifications to a vendor. This is highlighted by practitioner identification that a lack of time and staffing often affects addressing the needs of the individual (Sarsak et al., 2023) and awareness of funding source logistics (Long et al., 2007). The vendor can then assist with their knowledge of the pros and cons of various products and product selection.

CASE EXAMPLE

Adelina

Adelina, a social, 7-year-old child diagnosed with mixed athetosis and hypotonic cerebral palsy, attends a public school in the inclusion classroom. Her mother walks with her to school in an adaptive stroller and she transfers into an adapted chair with trunk supports at school. Adelina smiles and laughs often, but her speech is slow and laborious. She has a basic communication board for when she is overexcited and cannot get her needs across quickly. She is at grade level for academics and has begun to integrate a laptop and tablet to complete her work with less assistance from her full-time aide.

Adelina presents with decreased central tone (hypotonic neck and trunk) and increased fluctuating peripheral extensor tone. Adelina shows minimal equilibrium reactions and no functional protective reactions—she can maintain an unsupported upright posture for short bursts of time safely on the floor. This peripheral tone is usually precipitated by the initiation of voluntary movement or by changes of affect, such as when Adelina is excited, frustrated, or startled. In unsupported sitting, she frequently falls backward due to increased neck and back extension which occurs in response to fatigue or environmental stressors. Adelina sits with hip extension, adduction, and internal rotation with a posterior pelvic tilt and prefers knee extension. Adelina can accomplish graded arm movements at end-range movements but does not have a functional grasp and often has difficulty with targeted reach.

The fluctuating tone in her legs makes it difficult to maintain weight bearing through her feet on the floor to contribute to a stable postural base. Adelina turns her head to the side especially when she is communicating her needs but can focus on people and objects without head movement on when she is engaged.

She attends school in an inclusive classroom with some pullouts for special services. These occur during lunch as she does not have functional independent mobility through space in the same plane as her peers. Her developmental delays influence posture and mobility, speech/language, and play skills. Her preferred activities include movement through space (primarily through independent creeping; also using unsteady ambulation using furniture and walls for support) and music. Adelina is motivated by her peers but often is not able to join in during recess and physical education due to access and pull-out services.

The biomechanical frame of reference to position children for function was used to increase Adelina's occupational performance in the areas of communication and mobility. A supportive seating system, including a solid seat and back, seat belt, lateral trunk supports, hip guides, a chest harness, an anterior knee block to maintain hips and thighs in a stable, symmetrical position, and sandal footplates with Velcro straps were provided. This, with the addition of a lap tray for upper extremity support, enabled Adelina to exercise sufficient postural and head control to drive a power wheelchair by using a modified joystick. After training with an occupational therapist, Adelina was able to maneuver her chair through busy school hallways.

However, Adelina expressed feeling constricted by the tray, limiting her interaction with peers during playground activities. Additionally, she experienced discomfort from the straps on her footplates. Removing the tray posed challenges in maintaining upright trunk control, and her driving arm frequently slipped off the armrest laterally, raising safety concerns. Adjustments were made to the Velcro straps, positioning them diagonally across Adelina's feet to permit a slight heel lift when she became excited. Adelina reported relief from discomfort, and no changes to her posture were noted. To enhance Adelina's safety and independence, a system was devised to address several key needs: providing trunk support, maintaining her arm on the armrest, and ensuring enough freedom for interaction with her peers. While Adelina was successful in propping her arms on the tray for trunk support, it was determined that this would primarily be used for academic work, mealtime, and self-care routines. Instead, an anterior chest support was installed to assist Adelina in maintaining an upright position. This offers a tactile cue to encourage trunk extension or provides support when fatigue sets in. Additionally, a padded lateral block was installed to prevent Adelina's elbow from slipping laterally while driving, aiding in keeping her arm on the armrest. These adaptations have enabled Adelina to safely maneuver her wheelchair and engage with her peers.

SUPPORTING EVIDENCE

There has been limited research done in this area as every child with cerebral palsy and movement disorders is quite unique, as are their intervention plans and the outcomes of interventions (Novak, 2014). Much of the current evidence is based on small samples and with subjects who vary regarding the severity of cerebral palsy (Stavness, 2006). The primary goal of this frame of reference is to facilitate postural control and minimize the risks of deformities to promote meaningful activity and participation in life (Costigan, 2011; World Health Organization, 2001). When considering this population, it is critical for the practitioner to keep in mind that the optimal posture is one that allows a child to function as independently and efficiently as possible without significant compensatory movements. Data has shown that providing artificial supports allows children to engage in task-oriented activities which may promote neuroplasticity (Kliem, 2008; Novak, 2014; Wittenberg, 2009). Further, a positive relationship has been found between trunk control and reaching quality (Carlberg & Hadders-Algra, 2005), thereby increasing the child's function performance and independence. Additionally, Wittenberg's (2009) work identified that skill acquisition can continue into teenage years. Considering this data, it is still recommended that practitioners should consider providing the least amount of artificial support necessary for allowing the development of dynamic movement (Brogren et al., 1996; Myhr et al., 1995)

Increased alignment via adaptive seating devices was found to increase head control (Hulme et al., 1987), improved femoral head position (Howard et al., 2006), and decreased scoliosis deformity (Heller et al., 1997). Additionally, increased postural alignment and support was also found to increased communication (Clarke & Redden, 1992), mental performance (Miedaner & Finuf, 1993), feeding, breathing, bowel movement (Sahinoğlu et al., 2016), and the ability to play (Vekerdy, 2007).

The following is evidence found related to specific areas of positioning. Stavness (2006) reviewed the literature and found that the utilization of various supportive elements such as a pelvic belt, hip abductors, footrests, and upper extremity support (tray) with cutouts for improved fit can support most individuals. However, more individualized modifications include a posterior tilt of the seating system ranging between 0 degrees and 15 degrees (Stavness, 2006), and a neutral to anteriorly sloped seat (McNamara & Casey, 2007; Stavness, 2006). It has also been found that with some children a slightly reclined posture decreases the forces of gravity, which promotes more independent movement (Haddars-Algra et al., 1999). Vekerdy (2007) found that the use of the nonrigid custom-molded trunk support several hours a day resulted in a significant change in posture of the trunk, extremities, head, chin, and mouth. Further, the resultant improvement of alignment and trunk support promoted improvement in eye–hand coordination, feeding, and ability to play. Shoham et al. (2004) noted that this orthosis resulted in a decrease in scoliosis on the contralateral side of the pelvic obliquity, and Holms et al. (2003) and Heller et al. (1997) found an improvement in posture for the duration of use of the support.

Finally, it is important for practitioners to include caregivers and parents in the use of any positioning equipment. Pérez-de la Cruz (2017) found that discussing the benefits of use of a seating system produced long-term benefits in the consistent use of equipment, while Byrne et al. (2019) recommended that practitioners provide clear and comprehensive information about the equipment, its purpose, and potential benefits that specifically focus on their child's potential or goals, to promote effective usage.

Summary

In summary, the biomechanical frame of reference is utilized to position children for function when they are unable to maintain posture due to neuromuscular or musculoskeletal dysfunction, employing external supports or equipment to compensate for the lack of postural control. This approach is often employed primarily with children exhibiting severe physical disabilities and in combination with other frames of reference. The first goal of this frame of reference is to enhance the development of postural reactions by reducing gravity's demands and properly aligning the body. The second goal is to enhance functional performance by utilizing external supports, thereby reducing the need for postural reactions and compensatory movements. Understanding this frame of reference requires a thorough grasp of the typical sequence of development.

While this approach is the primary one, it should not be used in isolation or at the expense of function. Function–dysfunction continua encompass measures of central stability, including range of motion, head control, and trunk control, as well as functional skills such as head and arm movement control, mobility, feeding, and toileting. It should be noted that while concepts are consistent application varies on a variety of factors including diagnosis and individualized movement patterns. The Application to Practice section involves translating therapeutic intentions into equipment that enhances posture and function. Through the use of external supports, posture and central stability can be improved, enabling children to engage in functional activities and participate more actively in their home, school, and community environments. This intervention aims to facilitate development, functional gains, and participation in meaningful occupations.

REFERENCES

Aroojis, A., Mantri, N., & Johari, A. N. (2021). Hip displacement in cerebral palsy: The role of surveillance. *Journal of Indian Orthopedics, 55*, 5–19. https://doi.org/10.1007/s43465-020-00162-y

Barnes, K. J. (1991). Modification of the physical environment. In C. Christiansen & C. M. Baum (Eds.), *Occupational therapy: Overcoming human performance deficits* (pp. 701–745). Slack.

Batavia, M. (2010). *The wheelchair evaluation: Clinician's guide* (2nd ed.). Jones & Bartlett Learning.

Bergen, A., & Colangelo, C. (1985). *Positioning the client with central nervous system deficits*. Valhalla Rehabilitation Publications.

Blair, E., Ballantyne, J., Horseman, S., & Chauvel, P. (1995). A study of a dynamic proximal stability splint in the management of children with cerebral palsy. *Developmental Medicine and Child Neurology, 37*(6), 544–554. https://doi.org/10.1111/j.1469-8749.1995.tb12041.x

Bly, L. (1994). *Motor skill acquisition in the first year*. Psychological Corp.

Bly, L. (2011). *Components of typical and atypical motor development*. Neuro-Developmental Treatment Association, Inc.

Boehme, R. (1998). *Improving upper body control*. Therapy Skill Builders.

Borgestig, M., Sandqvist, J., Ahlsten, G., Falkmer, T., & Hemmingsson, H. (2017). Gaze-based assistive technology in daily activities in children with severe physical impairments: An intervention study. *Developmental Neurorehabilitation, 20*(3), 129–141. https://doi.org/10.3109/17518423.2015.1132281

Brogren, E., Hadders-Algra, M., & Forssberg, H. (1996). Postural control in children with spastic diplegia: Muscle activity during perturbations in sitting. *Developmental Medicine and Child Neurology, 38*(5), 379–388. https://doi.org/10.1111/j.1469-8749.1996.tb15095.x

Buckhalt, J. A. (2011). Children's sleep, sleepiness, and performance on cognitive tasks. *WMF Press Bulletins, 2011*(2), 1–12. https://pmc.ncbi.nlm.nih.gov/articles/PMC4180085/

Butler P., Saavedra, M. S., Sofranac, M. M., Jarvis, M. S., & Woollacott, M. (2010). Refinement, reliability and validity of the segmental assessment of trunk control (SATCo). *Pediatric Physical Therapy, 22*(3), 246. https://doi.org/10.1097/PEP.0b013e3181e69490

Byrne, R., Duncan, A., Pickar, T., Burkhardt, S., Boyd, R., Neel, M. L. & Maitre, N. (2019). Comparing parent and provider priorities in discussions of early detection and intervention for infants with and at risk of cerebral palsy. *Child: Care, Health and Development, 45*(6), 799–807. https://doi.org/10.1111/cch.12707

Carlberg, E. B., & Hadders-Algra, M. (2005). Postural dysfunction in children with cerebral palsy: Some implications for therapeutic guidance. *Neural Plasticity, 12*(2–3), 221–228. https://doi.org/10.1155/NP.2005.221

Carlberg, E. B., & Hadder-Algra, M. (2015). Postural dysfunction in children with cerebral palsy: Some implications therapeutic guidance. *Neural Plasticity, 12*(2–3), 221–228.

Caulton, J., Ward, K., Alsop, C., Dunn, G., Adams, J., & Mughal, M. (2004). A randomized controlled trial of standing programme on bone mineral density in non-ambulant children with cerebral palsy. *Archives of Disabled Children, 89*(2), 131. https://doi.org/10.1136/adc.2002.009316

Clarke, A. M., & Redden, J. F. (1992). Management of hip posture in cerebral palsy. *Journal of the Royal Society of Medicine, 85*(3), 150–151.

Colbert, A. P., Doyle, K. M., & Webb, W. E. (1986). DESEMO seats for young children with cerebral palsy. *Archives of Physical Medicine Rehabilitation, 67*(7), 484–486.

Costigan, F. A. & Light, J. (2011). Functional seating for school-age children with cerebral palsy: An evidence-based tutorial. *Language Speech Hearing Services in School, 42*, 223–236. https://doi.org/10.1044/0161-1461(2010/10-0001)

Fiorentino, M. (1981). *A basis for sensorimotor development—normal and abnormal*. Charles C. Thomas.

Fernandes, T. (2006). Independent mobility for children with disabilities. *International Journal of Therapy and Rehabilitation, 13*(7), 329–333. https://doi.org/10.12968/ijtr.2006.13.7.21410

Green, E. M., Mulcahy, C. M., & Pountney, T. E. (1995). An investigation into the development of early postural control. *Developmental Medicine and Child Neurology, 37*(5), 437–448. https://doi.org/10.1111/j.1469-8749,tb12027.x

Hadders-Algra, M. (2005). Development of postural control during the first 18 months of life. *Neural Plasticity, 12*(2–3), 99–272. https://doi.org/10.1155/NP.2005.99

Hadders-Algra, M., Brogren, E., & Forssberg, H. (1996). Training affects the development of postural adjustments in sitting infants. *Journal of Physiology, 493*(Pt. 1), 289–298. https://doi.org/10.1113/jphysiol.1996.sp021383

Hadders-Algra, M., van der Fits, I. B., Stremmelaar, E. F., & Touwen, B. C. (1999). Development of postural adjustments during reaching in infants with CP. *Developmental Medicine & Child Neurology, 41*(11), 766–776. https://doi.org/10.1111/j.1469-8749.1999.tb00537.x

Heller, K. D., Forst, R., & Hengtler, K. (1997). Scoliosis in Duchenne muscular dystrophy. *Prosthetic Orthotic International, 21*(3), 202–209. https://doi.org/10.3109/03093649709164558.

Holms, K. J., Michael, S. M., & Solomonidis, S. E. (2003). Management of scoliosis with special seating for the non-ambulant spastic cerebral palsy population – a biomechanical study. *Clinical Biomechanics, 18*(6), 480–487. https://doi.org/10.1016/S0268-0033(03)00075-5

Hulme, J. B., Gallacher, K., Walsh, J., Niesen, S., & Waldron, D. (1987). Behavioral and postural changes observed with use of adaptive seating by clients with multiple handicaps. *Physical Therapy, 67*(7), 1060–1067. https://doi.org/10.1093/ptj/67.7.1060

Hunzeker, M., & Ozelie, R. (2021). A cost-effective analysis of 3D printing applications in occupational therapy practice. *The Open Journal of Occupational Therapy, 9*(1), 1–12. https://doi.org/10.15453/2168-6408.1751

Imms, C., Granlund, M., Wilson, P., Steenbergen, B., Rosenbaum, P., & Gordon, A. (2017). Participation, both a means and an end: A conceptual analysis of processes and outcomes in childhood disability. *Developmental Medicine and Child Neurology, 59*(1), 16–25. https://doi.org/10.1111/dmcn.13237

Kliem, J. A., & Jones, T. A. (2008). Principles of experience-dependent neural plasticity: Implications for rehabilitation after brain damage. *Journal Speech, Language, and Hearing Research, 51*, S225–S239. https://doi.org/10.1044/1092-4388(2008/018)

Larnet, G., & Ekberg, O. (1995). Positioning improves the oral and pharyngeal swallowing function in children with cerebral palsy. *Acta Paediatrica, 84*(6), 689–692. https://doi.org/10.1111/j.1651-2227.1995.tb13730.x

Law, M., Cooper, B. A., Strong, S., Stewart, D., Rigby, P., & Letts, L. (1996). The person-environment-occupation model: A transactive approach to occupational performance. *Canadian Journal of Occupational Therapy, 63*, 9–23. https://doi.org/10.1177/000841749606300l

Leung, B., Jessica, A. B., & Chau, T. (2013). Learning and mastery behaviors as risk factors to abandonment in a pediatric user of advanced single-switch access technology. *Disability and rehabilitation. Assistive Technology, 8*(5), 426–433. https://doi.org/10.3109/17483107.2012.754955

Long, T. M., Woolverton, M., Perry, D. F., & Thomas, M. J. (2007). Training needs of pediatric occupational therapists in assistive technology. *American Journal of Occupational Therapy, 61*, 345–354. https://doi.org/10.5014/ajot.61.3.345

Macias, L. (2005). The effect of the standing programs with abduction on children with spastic diplegia. *Pediatric Physical Therapy, 17*(1), 96. https://doi.org/10.1097/01.PEP.0000155630.54603.B6

Manley, M. T., & Gurtowski, J. (1985). The vertical wheeler: A device for ambulation in cerebral palsy. *Archives of Physical Medicine and Rehabilitation, 66*(10), 717–720.

Manolikakis, G. (1992). Individual care of adduction contractures and threatening paralytic hip dislocations in cerebral palsy using sitting and lying expanding casts. *Orthopedic Technique, 43*, 810–815.

Martinsson, C., & Himmelmann, K. (2011). Effect of weight-bearing in abduction and extension on hip stability in children with cerebral palsy. *Pediatric Physical Therapy, 23*(2), 150–157. https://doi.org/10.1097/PEP.0b013e318218efc3

McDonald, R., Surtees, R., & Wirz, S. (2003). A comparison between parents' and therapists' views of their child's individual seating systems. *International Journal of Rehabilitation Research, 26*(3), 235–243. https://doi.org/10.1097/01.mrr.0000088449.78481.7c

McKearnan, K. A., Kiekhefer, G. M., Engel, J. M., Jensen, M. P. & Labyak, S. (2004). Pain in children with cerebral palsy: A review. *Journal of Neuroscience Nursing, 36*(5), 252–259. https://doi.org/10.1097/01376517-200410000-00004

Mcnamara, L., & Casey, J. (2007). Seat inclinations affect the function of children with cerebral palsy: A review of the effect of different seat inclines. *Disability and Rehabilitation: Assistive Technology, 2*(6), 309–318. https://doi.org/10.1080/17483100701661314

Miedaner, J., & Finuf, I. (1993). Effects of adaptive positioning on psychological test scores for pre-school children with cerebral palsy. *Pediatric Physical Therapy, 5*(4), 177–182.

Motloch, W. M., & Brearley, M. N. (1983). Technical note—a patient propelled variable-inclination prone stander. *Prosthetic Orthotics International, 7*(3), 176–177.

Myhr, U., Von-Wendt, L., Norrlin, S., & Randell, U. (1995). Five year follow-up of functional sitting position in children with cerebral palsy. *Developmental Medicine and Child Neurology, 37*(7), 587–596. https://doi.org/10.1111/j.1469-8749.1995.tb12047.x

Noronha, J., Bundy, A., & Groll, J. (1989). The effect of positioning on the hand function of boys with cerebral palsy. *American Journal of Occupational Therapy, 43*, 504–512. https://doi.org/10.5014/ajot.43.8.507

Novak, I. (2014). Evidence-based diagnosis, health care, and rehabilitation for children with cerebral palsy. *Journal of Child Neurology, 29*(8), 1141–1156. https://doi.org/10.1177/0883073814535503

O'Brien, J. C. & Kuhaneck, H. (2019). *Case-Smith's occupational therapy for children and adolescents* (8th ed.). Elsevier.

Patterson, R. M., Salatin, B., Janson, R., Salinas, S. P., & Mullins, M. J. (2020). A current snapshot of the state of 3D printing in hand rehabilitation. *Journal of Hand Therapy, 33*(2), 156–163. https://doi.org/10.1016/j.jht.2019.12.018

Pérez-de La Cruiz, S. (2017). Cerebral palsy and the use of positioning systems to control body posture: current practices. *Neurología, 32*(9), 610–615. https://doi.org/10.1016/j.nrleng.2015.05.015

Polgar, J. M., Cook, A. M., & Encarnação, P. (2020). *Assistive technologies* (5th ed.). Mosby.

Pountney, T. E., Mandy, A., Green, E., & Gard, P. R. (2009). Hip subluxation and dislocation in cerebral palsy – prospective study on the effectiveness of postural management programmes. *Physiotherapy Research International, 14*(2), 116–127. https://doi.org/10.1002/pri.434

Reid, D. T. (1996). The effects of the saddle seat on seated postural control and upper extremity movement in children with cerebral palsy. *Developmental Medicine and Child Neurology, 38*(9), 805–815. https://doi.org/10.1111/j.1469-8749.1996.tb15115.x

Reid, D. T. (2002). Critical review of the research literature of seating interventions focusing on adults with mobility impairments. *Disability and Rehabilitation. Assistive Technology, 14*(2), 118–129. https://doi.org/10.1080/10400435.2002.10132061

Reid, D., & Rigby, P. (1996). Towards improving anterior pelvic stabilization devices for pediatric wheelchair users with cerebral palsy. *Canadian Journal of Rehabilitation, 9*, 147–158.

Reid, D., Rigby, P., & Ryan, S. (1999). Functional impact of a rigid pelvic stabilizer on children with cerebral palsy who use wheelchairs: Users' and caregivers' perceptions. *Pediatric Rehabilitation, 3*(3), 101–118. https://doi.org/10.1080/136384999289513

Rigby, P., Reid, D., Schoger, S., & Ryan, S. (2002). Effects of a wheelchair-mounted rigid pelvic stabilizer on caregiver assistance for children with cerebral palsy. *Disability and Rehabilitation. Assistive Technology, 13*(1), 2–11. https://doi.org/10.1080/10400435.2001.10132029

Rivi, E., Filippi, M., Fornasari, E., Mascia, M. T., Ferrari, A., & Costi, S. (2014). Effectiveness of standing frame on constipation in children with cerebral palsy: A single subject study. *Occupational Therapy International, 21*, 115–123. https://doi.org/10.1002/oti.1370

Rodby-Bousquet, E., Persson-Bunke, M., & Czuba, T. (2016). Psychometric evaluation of the Posture and Postural Ability Scale for children with cerebral palsy. *Clinical Rehabilitation, 30*(7), 697–704. https://doi.org/0.1177/0269215515593612

Rosen, L., Arva, J., Furumasu, M., Harris, M., Lange, M. L., McCarthy, E., Kermoian, R., Pinkerton, H., Plummer, T., Roos, J., Sabet, A., Schaaf, P. V., & Wonsettler, T. (2009). RESNA Position of the application of power wheelchairs for pediatric users. *Assistive Technology, 21*, 218–226. https://doi.org/10.1080/10400430903246076

Rothstein, J. M. (2005). The *rehabilitation specialist's handbook*. F.A. Davis.7.

Rousseau-Harrison, K., & Rochette, A. (2012). Impacts of wheelchair acquisition on children from a person-occupation-environment interactional perspective. *Disability and Rehabilitation: Assistive Technology, 8*(1), 1–10. https://doi.org/10.3109/17483107.2012.670867.

Ryan, S. E. (2012). An overview of systematic reviews of adaptive seating interventions for children with cerebral palsy: where do we go from here? *Disability and Rehabilitation: Assistive Technology, 7*(2), 104–111. https://doi.org/10.3109/17483107.2011.595044

Ryan, S., Snider-Riczker, P., & Rigby, P. (2005). Community-based performance of a pelvic stabilization device for children with cerebral palsy. *Assistive Technology, 17*(1), 37–46. https://doi.org/10.1080/10400435.2005.10132094

Sahinoğlu, D., Coskun, C., & Bek, N. (2016). Effects of different seating equipment on postural control and upper extremity function in children with cerebral palsy. *Prosthetics and Orthotics International, 1*:85–94. https://doi.org/10.1177/0309364616637490

Salem, Y., Lovelace-Chandler, V., Zabel, R. J., & McMillan, A. G. (2010). Effects of prolonged standing on gait in children with spastic cerebral palsy. *Physical & Occupational Therapy in Pediatrics, 30*(1), 54–65. https://doi.org/10.3109/01942630903297177

Sarsak, H. I., von Zweck, C., & Ledgerd, R. (2023). Wheeled and seated mobility devices provision: Quantitative findings and SWOT thematic analysis of a global occupational therapist survey. *Healthcare (Basel, Switzerland), 11*(8), 1075. https://doi.org/10.3390/healthcare11081075

Scherzer, A., & Tscharnuter, I. (1990). *Early diagnosis and therapy in cerebral palsy* (2nd ed.). Marcel Dekker.

Scrutton, D. (1991). The causes of developmental deformity and their implication for seating. *Prosthetic and Orthotic International, 15*(3), 199–202. https://doi.org/10.3109/03093649109164289

Seyhan, K., & Kerem-Günel, M. (2019). Does stable sitting influence upper limb function in children with cerebral palsy? *The Turkish Journal of Pediatrics, 61*(1), 79–84. https://doi.org/10.24953/turkjped.2019.01.012

Shoham, Y., Meyer, S., Katz-Leuer, M., & Weiss, P. L. (2004). The influence of seat adjustment and a thoracic lumbar sacral orthosis on the distribution of body seat pressure in children with scoliosis and pelvic obliquity. *Disability & Rehabilitation, 26*(1), 21–26. https://doi.org/10.1080/09638280410001645940

Short, N., Peters, H. S., Eckert, J., Grady, N., Kline, E., & Weber, H. (2023). Impact of seating and mobility services for individuals with disabilities in El Salvador. *American Journal of Occupational Therapy, 77*, 7704205140. https://doi.org/10.5014/ajot.2023.050150

Soo, B., Howard, J. J., Boyd, R. N., Reidt, S. M., Lanigan, A., Wolfe, R., Reddihough, D., & Graham, H. K. (2006). Hip displacement in cerebral palsy. *Journal of Bone & Joint Surgery, 88*(1), 121–129. https://doi.org/10.2106/JBJS.E.00071

Stavness, C. (2006). The effect of positioning for children with cerebral palsy on upper-extremity function: A review of the evidence. *Physical & Occupational Therapy in Pediatrics, 26*(3), 39–53. https://doi.org/10.1080/J006v26n03_04

Stockmeyer, S. A. (1967). An interpretation of the approach of Rood to the treatment of neuromuscular dysfunction. *American Journal of Physical Medicine, 46*(1), 900–956.

Stuberg, W. A. (1992). Considerations related to weight-bearing programs in children with developmental disabilities. *Physical Therapy, 72*(1), 35–40. https://doi.org/10.1093/ptj/72.1.35

Tuersley, L., Bray, N., & Edwards, R. T. (2018). Development of the Wheelchair outcomes Assessment Tool for Children (WATCh): A patient-centered outcome measure for young wheelchair users. *PLoS One, 13*(12), e0209380. https://doi.org/10.1371/journal.pone.0209380

Vekerdy, Z. (2007). Management of seating posture of children with cerebral palsy by using thoracic-lumbar-sacral orthosis with non-rigid SIDO frame. *Disability & Rehabilitation, 29*(18), 1434–1441. https://doi.org/10.1080/09638280601055691

Verschuren, O., Peterson, M. D., Leferink, S., & Darrah, J. (2014). Muscle activation and energy-requirements for varying postures in children and adolescents with cerebral palsy. *Journal of Pediatrics, 165*(5), 1011–1016. https://doi.org/10.1016/j.jpeds.2014.07.027

Wittenberg, G. F. (2009). Neural plasticity and treatment across the lifespan for motor deficits in cerebral palsy. *Development Medicine & Child Neurology, 51*(s4), 130–133. https://doi.org/10.1111/j.1469-8749.2009.03425.x

Woollacott, M., Shumway-Cook, A., Hutchinson, S., Ciol, M., Price, R., & Kartin, D. (2005). Effect of balance training on muscle activity used in recovery of stability in children with cerebral palsy: a pilot study. *Developmental Medicine and Child Neurology, 47*(7), 455–461. https://doi.org/10.1017/s0012162205000885

World Health Organization (WHO). (2001). *ICF: International classification of functioning, disability and health.* Author.

A Frame of Reference for Social Participation

Shawna Gigliotti ■ Margaret Folkes

This chapter outlines the elements and factors that impact a child's ability to engage in healthy social participation. Factors such as human development, attachment and self-regulation, trauma, disability, and temperament are considered as well as the elements that influence these factors. Additionally, the chapter serves to provide occupational therapy practitioners with a framework for assessment and intervention of the multifaceted human factors that may impact a child's ability to engage in social participation. This chapter is designed to support clinicians in providing effective interventions and education for children and caregivers for successful social participation and engagement in occupations the child/caregiver may want and need to do throughout daily life. For the purpose of this chapter, a child is defined as a person from birth through 17 years of age. Therefore, the application of this perspective is focused on individuals within the stated age range.

THEORETICAL BASE

The theoretical base serving as the foundation for assessment and intervention as related to social participation is made up of theories of human development, social participation, attachment and regulation theories, temperament, and caregiver and child relations.

Human Development

There are a variety of human and behavioral development theories that focus on individualized and group human behavior. Many of the theories conceptualize development as a series of hierarchical stages. For example, Erik Erikson has been influenced by Freud's work and describes socialization over the course of a lifespan. His theories encompasses the impact of socialization and relationship's impact on growth over time (Orenstein & Lewis, 2022). Other theorists such as Piaget and Vygotsky discuss how children learn through hands-on experiences and actively learn within their environments (Matusov & Hayes, 2000). These basic theories of growth and development have influenced the way occupational therapy practitioners use developmental theories in practice. For the purpose of this frame of reference (FOR), human development is defined as the process of growth and change that takes place in the individual between birth and maturity (www.britannica.com).

This FOR is intended to further support the bridge of human development, socialization, relationships, learned behavior, etc., and how all these very human factors and experiences influence function. Further, these theories will be applied to assist practitioners with assessment and intervention strategies to support functional outcomes for the children seeking occupational therapy (OT) services to facilitate independence in social participation.

Developmental theory helps to understand how social development and human development should be considered. Synthesizing stage-specific, ecologic, and acquisitional development are essential to OT practitioners (OTPs) as they evaluate a child's social participation. Considering physiologic, biologic, environmental, and social factors interconnectedness will impact a child's ability to develop healthy social attachments, therefore, occupational therapists must be prepared to evaluate all factors with a child who may be exhibiting limitations in social functioning (Olson, 2020).

Biologic development is a foundation of a child's ability. However, the social environment can support or hinder appropriate social–emotional learning and connectedness. The most significant piece of social development is the impact of the child's environment including how the child is nurtured from parents, caregivers, family, and the community (Figure 14.1). Social environmental factors such as housing circumstances, interpersonal interactions among children, caregivers, and peers, daycare/school system supports, safety in community, and sociopolitical settings also impact healthy social development (Olson, 2020). See Chapter 2, Developmental Perspective: Fundamentals of Developmental Theory.

Attachment, Self-Regulation, and Resiliency

Coined the "First Core Strength" by Perry, *attachment* is identified as the capacity to form and maintain healthy relationships throughout the lifespan. Infants are not born attached to their caregivers (Perry, 2020). However, throughout infancy (birth to 2 years old), infants experience

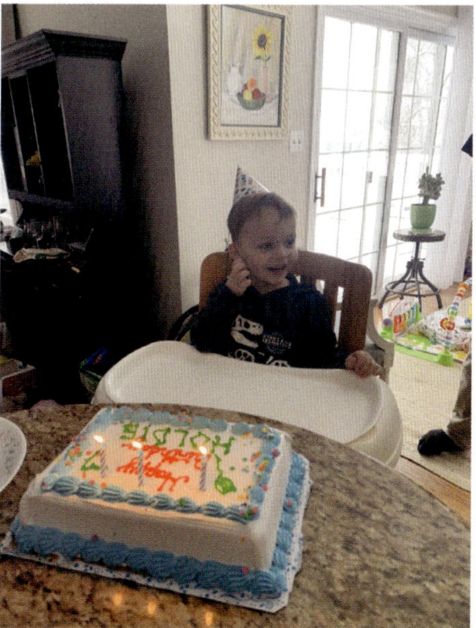

FIGURE 14.1 A child enjoying his birthday in a nurturing home environment.

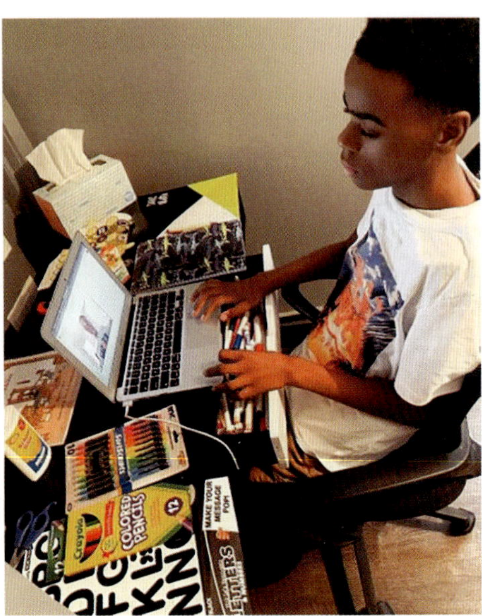

FIGURE 14.2 A child demonstrating good self-regulation when engaged in a task.

an intense period of neurologic development through repetitive patterned experiences that form attachment to one's caregiver (Perry, 2020). Through the attachment cycle, a caregiver lays the foundation for the child's developing social and emotional capacities. For example, a caregiver feeding or changing the diaper of crying infant in a consistent and nurturing pattern allows the child to begin to understand safety (Lynch et al., 2021). Attachment and self-regulation are vital to understanding the development of social participation as it is the first understanding of relating to another. It assists with learning the first rules and nature of social interaction and understanding how to maintain relationships/friendships (Dorman & Williamson, 2002). Self-regulation is when a child has the ability to understand and manage one's own behavior and reactions (American Psychology Association [APA], 2018) (Figure 14.2). Additionally, the child is beginning to create a foundation for coregulatory abilities through their caregiver meeting biologic needs paired with feelings of comfort. Coregulation is the interaction between two individuals to help each other regulate their emotions. It is also used to mean when adults help teach children how to manage their emotions on their own (Hagen, n.d.).

Therefore, the infant attachment cycle provides the foundation for an individual's ability to form and maintain healthy emotional bonds with another individual (Lynch et al., 2021). Furthermore, laying the foundation for future relational development with classmates, peers, teachers, and community members. Resiliency is being able to adapt to difficult or challenging life experiences, especially through mental, emotional, and behavioral flexibility and adjustment to external and internal demands (APA, 2018).

Trauma

Adverse childhood events (ACEs) or trauma is viewed as a subset under human development as it does not apply to all children, yet trauma has been shown to have a significant impact on social–emotional development. It is important to note that while trauma may be experienced as a child, it can have a significant impact on a child's ability to function well into adulthood. Trauma is defined as the experience of violence and victimization including sexual abuse, physical abuse, severe neglect, loss, domestic violence, and/or witnessing violence, terrorism, or disasters (Ukeru, 2020). The severity of trauma is person specific therefore making it difficult to generalize the impact of a particular traumatizing event. Trauma has been noted to change cognitive functioning, effect brain development, increase health comorbidities, and ultimately result in an earlier death. Further, trauma can affect the ability to make attachment with others, resiliency, and successful interactions with others. Trauma may affect many aspects of social participation. As occupational therapy practitioners, the clinician should assess how the trauma symptoms are impacting the child's ability to engage in healthy, age-appropriate social participation if the practitioner believes there may have been ACEs to which the child was exposed (Wilcox, 2012).

Sensory Modulation as It Relates to Trauma

Trauma has also been noted to change the way in which a child can engage in effective sensory modulation. Sensory modulation is a balance of both inhibitory and excitatory inputs to the sensory system (Joseph et al., 2021; Yochman & Pat-Horencyzk, 2019). This process reflects as behaviors and functionality. It has been noted that children with repeated traumas or neglect have demonstrated neuroanatomical changes to the sensory cortex impacting sensory modulation. When sensory modulation is functional for a child, the child can adaptively respond to the environment as well as engage in healthy ways socially (Joseph et al., 2021). Conversely, a child can demonstrate impulsivity, distractibility, increased activity level, disorganization, anxiety, and decreased ability to self-regulate when experiencing sensory modulation dysfunction (Yochman & Pat-Horencyzk, 2019). Refer to Chapter 6, Ayres Sensory Integration Frame of Reference and Chapter 7, A Frame of Reference for Sensory Integration and Processing Differences: Sensory Therapies and Research (STAR) of this book for a more in-depth discussion of sensory integration and sensory modulation.

Temperament

The psychological literature is filled with varying discussions and definitions of temperament (Goldsmith et al., 1987; McCrae et al., 2000; Shiner et al., 2012; Strelau, 1987; Yilmaz, n.d.). Temperament is described as the basic dispositions of the person that underlie behavior as it relates to activity, reactivity, emotionality, and sociability. It is thought to be present early in life and influenced by both biologic and environmental factors. Over time, temperament is influenced by environmental context and experience (Goldsmith et al., 1987).

As it relates to social participation, differences in temperament have been associated with social competence (e.g., socially appropriate behaviors and social success, or peer likeability), parent–child relations, and self-regulatory abilities (Sanson et al., 2004). Children who exhibit characteristics like adaptability, positive affect, ability to be soothed or comforted, and demonstrate personal effortful control, including self-regulation have increased opportunities for social interaction. This is believed to be because their temperament supports regulated interactions with others (Shiner et al., 2012). Conversely, those children who exhibit behaviors such as fear, frustration, sadness, and a low ability for self-control may reduce their opportunities for social interaction and a positive response (Salley et al., 2013). Additionally, temperament may impact one's willingness to cope with unfamiliar situations and manage associated stress response. This all impacts one's willingness to pursue a variety of social scenarios and peer interaction (Salley et al., 2013).

Caregiver and Child Relationship

Both attachment and temperament styles impact the caregiver–infant interactions and relationship. In secure attachment patterns, the child seeks out closeness with their caregiver. For example, a securely attached child will feel safe exploring their environment while turning to check in with their caregiver as they move throughout the environment. In this way, the child learns to access items in their environment to self-soothe when the caregiver is not present (e.g., teddy bear, blanket, eating a snack) (Perry, 2001). This is learned through what a caregiver personally provides and the items they provide access to when the child experiences discomfort. This supportive parent–child relationship creates the development for responding to each other in ways that reflect the emotion and need of one another (Dorman &Williamson, 2002). This is the infant's first opportunity for learning reciprocal communication for relating to others (Dorman &Williamson, 2002) further supporting early self-regulatory skills required for successful peer-to-peer interactions and engagement with others throughout childhood and adolescence. This is the beginning of the development of resilience.

In a supportive caregiver–child relationship and stable environment, children are more likely to develop healthy habits and routines for functional social participation (Taylor, 2011). The Occupational Therapy Practice Framework 4 (OTPF 4) defines routines as sequence of activities that provide structure for daily life (American Occupational Therapy Association [AOTA] (OTPF-4), 2020). This includes family and child-specific activities such as homework, sports, self-care, bedtime, and mealtimes. Regular routines allow for family organization and cohesion for childhood well-being (Spagnola & Fiese, 2007) (Figure 14.3). Further, research has shown that routine helps to manage familial stress and transition (Spagnola & Fiese, 2007). Additionally, it has been shown that consistency in daily structure and activities contributes to the development of positive social behaviors. It has also been theorized that taking on responsibilities as a child teaches one how to respond to the needs of others (Taylor, 2011). Consistency and predictability created by the caregiver through

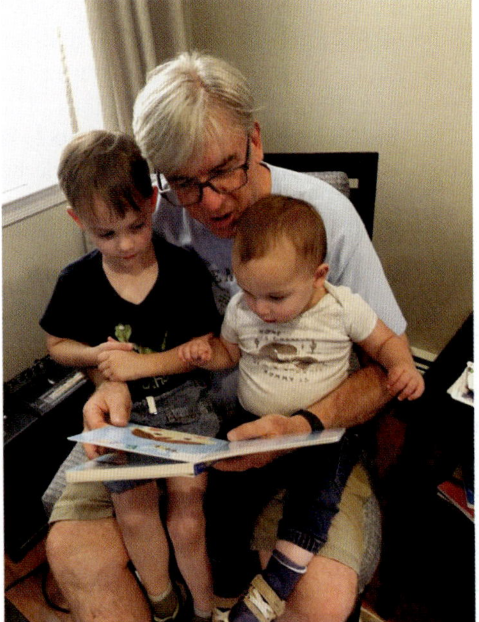

FIGURE 14.3 Children enjoying a bed-time story with a caregiver.

routines and structure, allows for a child to practice responding to variety of situations that build self-confidence and resiliency, or the capacity to tolerate stressors and challenges, with a functional outcome (Perry & Winfry, 2021). Therefore, resiliency is developed through experiences and interactions where the stressor is mild, predictable, and has some consistency (Perry & Winfry, 2021).

The routines and rituals established within the context of parent–child relationship allow for scaffolding to build resiliency. This is also done through interactions between family members who can structure the child's environment and activities with the "just right challenge" for the successful completion of the task (Martini, 2002). Self-regulation and resiliency are critical components for engaging in effective social participation.

Children begin to practice developmental and social skills in a safe predictable environment. It is important for caregivers to create opportunities for children to engage in social activities with others from a young age (Martini, 2002). Often, family routines are disrupted when one or more children in the family unit require more care and additional resources for daily activities (Spagnola & Fiese, 2007). When this occurs, a child may not have the chance to engage in social activities with others, interfering with their skill development in the area of social participation.

The Environment

As the child grows the experiences in the environment affect temperament and performance. The external environment refers to the physical, social, and attitudinal surroundings in which people live and conduct their lives. For children, this includes the natural environment and human-made changes, including the home, community, school, and other areas to which the child may be exposed (AOTA, 2020).

The environment outside of the home is often critical in the lives of children and refers to environmental factors including:

- Products and technology—natural or human-made products of systems
- Support and relationships—people or animals that support, nurture, protect, assist, and provide connection in home, workplace, school, or at play or other aspects of daily occupations
- Attitudes—observable evidence of customs, practices, ideologies, values, norms, factual beliefs, and religious beliefs held by people around the child
- Services, systems, and policies—benefits, structured programs, and regulations for operations provided by institutions in various sectors of society designed to meet the needs of persons, groups, and populations (AOTA, 2020).

Social Participation

It is critical to understand that for children and adolescents, social participation primarily begins within the context of everyday activities with adult caregivers (e.g., family and service providers) and social settings with peers (i.e., school, sports, daycare, etc.). Social participation influences social–emotional development and physical and psychological health, and supports experiences in gaining competence while growing up (Bärwalde et al., 2023). Research has shown that forming positive relationships with peers, family members, and teachers improves one's sense of safety and belonging in school and social environments (Leigers et al., 2016) (Figure 14.4). As children grow older their sense of belonging also changes, which is greatly impacted by feelings of "belonging" in social scenarios. This helps to internalize feelings of self-confidence, self-efficacy, and socioemotional development (Bärwalde et al., 2023).

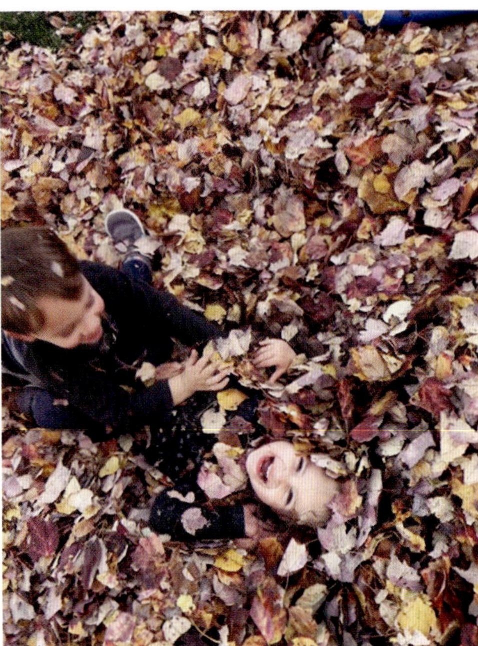

FIGURE 14.4 Children enjoying playing together.

The Infinity Perspective

When considering the theoretical basis of this FOR, the authors have developed a perspective to aid in visualizing how the various foundational components affect the child's social–emotional capacity for social participation. It is clear that these concepts are interrelated. When the child is in a well-supported, nurturing environment, without noted areas of dysfunction, the infinity symbol is balanced (Figure 14.5).

If there is any area lacking balance, the infinity sign will be skewed. Figure 14.6 demonstrates possible deficits in the area of human development, and how the infinity perspective would be skewed, with diminished self-regulation and resiliency and less functional behavior in social

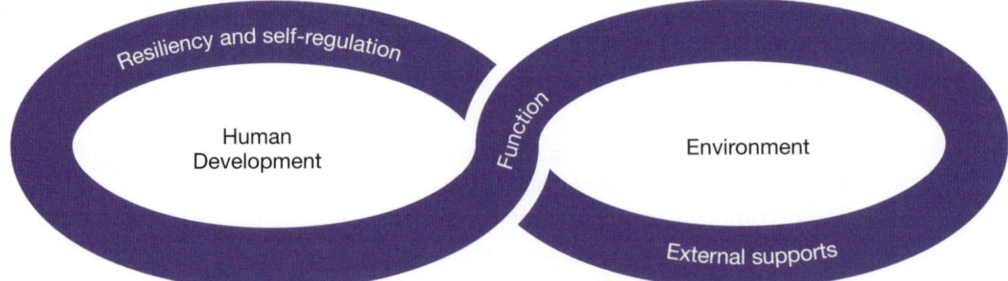

FIGURE 14.5 The balanced infinity symbol demonstrates a situation without areas of dysfunction, with typical development, resiliency and self-regulation, and a well-supported, nurturing environment, resulting in strong abilities in social participation.

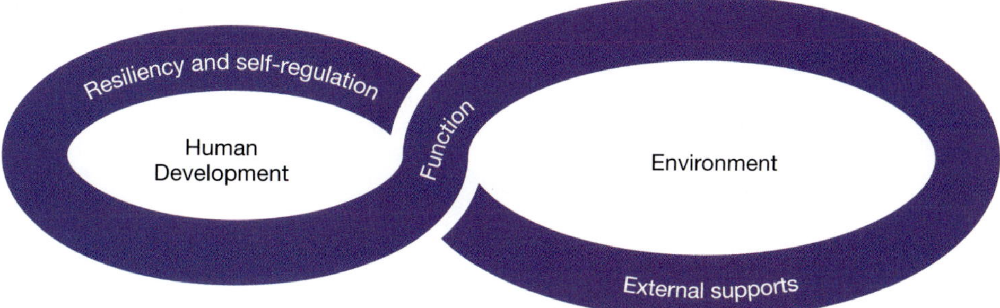

FIGURE 14.6 This infinity symbol shows deficits in the area of human development, and this perspective would be skewed, with diminished self-regulation and resiliency and less functional behavior in social participation.

participation. When there is a lack of support in the home/school/daycare environment, the infinity perspective will be skewed as shown in Figure 14.7. When the child is experiencing deficits in multiple areas that have been previously described, the infinity perspective demonstrates overall distortions in functioning (Figure 14.8). When there are deficits in the balance of the infinity symbol, this may result in difficulty with their overall functioning and in skill development in the area of social participation.

Dynamic Theory

In order to develop adequate social participation and peer-to-peer interaction, intervention in this perspective relies on Yalom's perspective (1995) on the critical therapeutic power of groups, and Bandura's social cognitive theory (1977, 2006).

Most of the interventions in this FOR rely on group process and their usefulness as part of the change process. Groups provide an opportunity for modeling, imitation, various types of learning, and social interaction. The focus is on positive change (Yalom, 1995). This approach can be used with children, adolescents, and with parents in this FOR.

Social cognitive theory (Bandura, 1997, 2006) focuses on personal motivation for improvement and successful performance. This includes observing the positive behaviors of others,

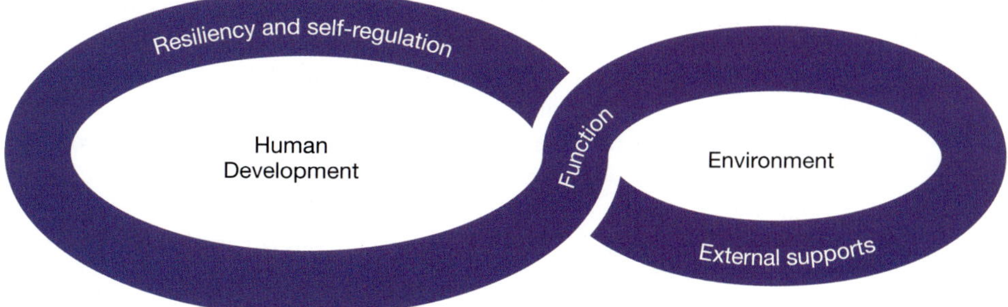

FIGURE 14.7 This demonstrates how the infinity perspective would be skewed with deficits in the environment, affecting social participation performance.

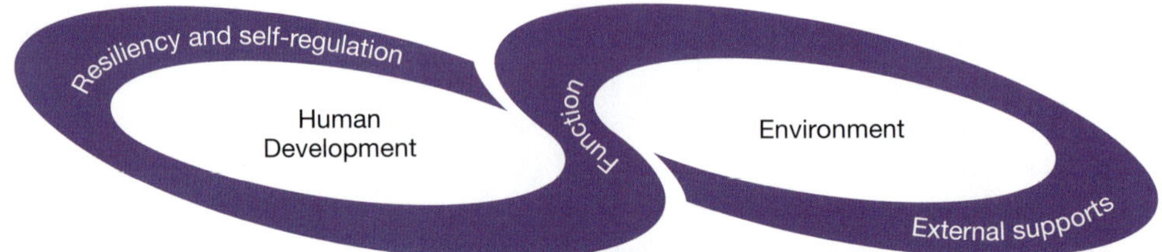

FIGURE 14.8 This demonstrates how the infinity perspective would be skewed with deficits in several areas, affecting social participation performance.

modeling positive behaviors so that children can learn. Children are supported in the belief that they can grow and change to improve their interactions with others, including and especially peers. This can also be effective when working with parents.

GUIDE TO EVALUATION

Since social participation is highly individualized, it is important for an occupational therapist to consider the ideal method for capturing a child's social engagement and participation in occupations. This will allow for the therapist to identify what factors (environment, economic, skill) are either hindering or facilitating engagement. Therefore, using a wide variety of assessment methods is recommended including both formal and informal assessment methods for gathering information will support better understanding of how to promote engagement in desired activities. Utilizing observation as well as a standardized assessment tool is best in assessment and monitoring patient outcomes (Stigen et al., 2023). Further, informal methods of data collection can often provide more qualitative information for intervention and goal development.

Informal Assessment

There are several informal methods of evaluation that can be used to learn more about a child's social participation. These include an occupational profile, clinical observation in several different social settings, and interviewing.

An occupational therapist should begin the assessment process by completing an occupational profile with the child and parent/caregiver. The occupational profile is a summary of a client's (person's, group's, or population's) occupational history and experiences, patterns of daily living, interests, values, needs, and relevant contexts (AOTA, 2014).

Clinical observation of a child's behavior in a variety of social situations and environments is a very important component of the assessment. Observing a child in various settings with different people and varying task requirements exposes differences in performance as they relate to skill performance and environmental context. This can give the therapist insight into the child's ability to engage in social participation in a large group setting versus a smaller more intimate social scenario. For example, a child may appear to enjoy working with preferred peers when in their favorite class with a teacher that they have an established relationship. This same child's behavior may appear very different and inappropriate with peers during large group activity during gym class or the recess yard. Therefore, it would be important to observe the child in a variety of settings during their daily routine.

Interviewing methods provide many benefits to the assessment process. Interviews allow the clinician to form a collaborative relationship with the caregiver and child. It also lets the clinician learn more about the child–parent interaction and attachment style. Interview questions can be highly targeted or open-ended which can provide more insight into familial perspectives of social roles, self-regulatory, and communication skills for social engagement (Dorman & Williamson, 2002). It is recommended that both types of questioning be used. Interviewing can also supplement data gained from the occupational profile.

Interviews also provide time to learn more about both child and parent goals for intervention, education, and change. Through observations during interview, the clinician can gather more information related to the caregiver's values, beliefs, habits, family routines, and rituals. Additionally, during an interview, the practitioner can observe reciprocal child–caregiver interactions, verbal and nonverbal expressions of emotions (adequacy, enjoyment, frustration, etc.), expression of mutual needs, and the caregiver's ability to both structure and problem solve with their child during activities. An occupational therapist should identify what social demands and expectations caregivers' place on a child and their vision for the child's social occupational performance (Olson, 2020). For example, the therapist might ask what activities the parent/caregiver would like their child to participate in and how does that fit with their overall goals for the child.

Standardized Methods

During the interview, the occupational therapist can also begin to create individualized family goals, using a more formal assessment tool. The *Family Goal Setting Tool* (Jones, 2013) is a standardized assessment tool that supports collaborative goal setting between parents and therapists about a young child's occupational participation including social participation. Additionally, the *Canadian Occupational Performance Measure* (Law et al., 2014) will be useful to assist the caregiver and child in identifying and prioritizing occupational performance issues that are of importance to parent/caregiver and the child.

Table 14.1 provides a list of applicable evaluation tools to assess social participation functioning and factors impacting engagement and provides information on a variety of rating scales and questionnaires. Some of the listed assessments do not exclusively assess social participation, rather functioning in cognitive, motor, and sensory processing skills to understand how these client factors impact social participation. Additionally, some of the recommended assessments focus on performance in specific settings or skill area (i.e., School Function Assessment, Sensory Processing Measure). These types of measures can provide insight into the child's overall occupational performance, as well as their social participation, as provided by additional personnel who come in contact with the child, such as teachers, social workers, and other clinicians.

FUNCTION/DYSFUNCTION CONTINUA

This FOR has four function/dysfunction continua. The first is self-regulation and resiliency. Self-regulation focuses on the child's ability to understand and manage their own behavior, while resiliency relates to adapting to challenging experiences and adjusting to internal and external demands (Table 14.2). The second continuum relates to the daily environments which encompasses the various environments in which the child participates on a regular basis such as home, school, and daycare, and also includes those individuals within these environments that have an impact on the child (Table 14.3). The third continuum relates to the environments for socialization that

Table 14.1 Evaluation Tools for Social Participation

Evaluation Tool	Purpose	Highlights
Social Profile (Donohue, 2013)	*Social Profile* is a psychosocial instrument designed to assess behavioral interactions. *Social Profile* assesses whether groups or individuals participate appropriately at a level suitable for the activity or development stage. This assessment includes a Children's version and an Adult/Adolescent version.	Assesses participation and social cooperation across five levels (i.e., being with others, interacting with others, collaborating with others, and helping others).
The *Children's Assessment of Participation and Enjoyment (CAPE) and Preferences for Activities of Children (PAC)* (King et al., 2007)	The CAPE/PAC is a 55-item questionnaire designed to examine how children and youth participate in everyday activities outside of their school classes.	Assesses five dimensions of participation, including diversity (number of activities done), intensity (frequency of participation measured as a function of the number of possible activities within a category), and enjoyment of activities. Additionally, the CAPE/PAC provided qualitative information related to social participation (i.e., where they participate and who they participate with).
Sensory Processing Measure-2 (SPM-2) (Parham et al., 2021)	The Sensory Processing Measure (SPM-2) is multienvironment assessment to evaluate praxis, social participation, and five sensory systems (visual, auditory, tactile, proprioceptive, and vestibular functioning).	SPM-2 assesses children in a variety of settings (home, school, and community). Utilized for children ages 5 to 12 y of age.
Sensory Profile 2 (SP2) (Dunn, 2014)	The SP2 contains parent and teacher questionnaires designed to assess the sensory processing patterns of children from birth through 14 y, 11 mo across settings.	SP2 Identifies how sensory processing may contribute to or interfering with a child's participation at home, school, and the community. Specifically, contributes information of both child's strength and weakness based on the environment. Additionally, offers congruent assessment, Adolescent/Adult Sensory Profile, to assess sensory processing patterns and effects on functional performance from 11 y and older.
The Short Child Occupational Profile (SCOPE) (Bowyer, 2007)	The SCOPE is an occupation-focused assessment that determines how a child's volition, habituation, skills, and the environment facilitate or restrict participation. Based on the Model of Human Occupation including the personal actors of volition, habituation, communication and interaction process, and motor skills as how the environment impacts occupational participation and performance. The SCOPE can be used with children birth–21 y of age with a range of abilities and diagnosis.	Practitioners can gather information to rate the SCOPE in a variety of ways (observation, interviews, chart review, and other assessments). SCOPE ratings are based on each child's "individual developmental" trajectory, or the capacities a child has the potential to acquire in the future given the child's age, impairment, prior life experiences, and environmental context.

Table 14.1 Evaluation Tools for Social Participation (Continued)

Evaluation Tool	Purpose	Highlights
School Function Assessment (SFA) (Coster et al., 1998)	SFA is a questionnaire-based assessment that is completed by one or more school professional known to have observed their typical performance. The assessment evaluates students on three scales: Participation, Task Supports, and Activity Performance. It is utilized for children from kindergarten through 6th grade.	SFA evaluates activity performance of functional communication, following social conventions, compliance with adult directives and school rules, positive interaction, and behavior regulation. It can be utilized to establish eligibility for special services.
Pediatric Interest Profiles (PIP) (Henry, 2000)	The PIP is a self-report questionnaire completed by the client to evaluate their interest and participation in a variety of play and leisure activities. It includes three activity scales: the kid play profile, the preteen play profile, and the adolescent leisure Interest profile based on the child's age. Utilized for individuals aged 6 through 21 y old.	The self-report feature assists a therapist in assessing a child's leisure participation from their point of view relative to preferences, actual participation, and their perceptions about that participation.
Family Goal Setting Tool (FGST) (Jones, 2013)	The FGST is designed to support family-centered, holistic child-focused treatment goals an OT can utilize throughout evaluation for children birth to early school years.	The FGST facilitates goal setting in collaboration with the family or caregivers around nine categories influencing active participation in the community. Those areas are as follows: communication, social participation, emotional regulation, play and learning, self-care, motor skills, community access and participation, information, and support.
Canadian Occupational Performance Measure (COPM) (Polatajko et al., 2014)	The COPM is a semistructured interview used to help individuals and their families identify goals. The COPM can be used for individuals throughout their lifespan. For children under the age of 8, a caregiver will assist with completion.	The COPM evaluates everyday activities such as self-care, attending school or work, and participating in leisure or play. Additionally, the COPM can be utilized as an outcome measure following intervention to self-rate performance and satisfaction with intervention.
Social Skills Improvement System (Gresham & Elliot, 1990)	The Social Skills Improvement System (SSIS) is used to measure social behaviors, problem behaviors, and academic competence at the preschool, elementary, and secondary developmental. It captures positive social behaviors of cooperation, empathy, assertion, self-control, and responsibility. Additionally, the problem Behaviors Scale measures behaviors that can interfere with the development of positive social skills. The assessment can be used for children from 3 to 18 y old.	The SSIS allows for multiple practitioners to provide clinical perspective of child's social skills. This includes a Parent Form, a Student Form, or a Teacher Form.

Table 14.2 Indicators of Function: Self-Regulation and Resilience

Function	Dysfunction
Self-Regulation: The child understands and manages their own behavior and reactions	The child does not understand or manage their own behavior
Resiliency: Adapts to difficult or challenging life experiences, being flexible and responding appropriately to external and internal demands	Has difficulty adapting to difficulty and challenging life experiences, is not flexible, and does not respond appropriately to internal and external demands
Identifies feelings and emotions in the self and others based on both verbal and nonverbal communication	Difficulty recognizing emotional responses in the self and others and self, and recognizing emotional responses in others and self
Awareness of physical, behavioral, cognitive, and emotional responses to emotions	Difficulty with awareness of self and own emotional responses
Exercises emotional and behavioral control in response to intense emotions	Cannot control emotional and behavioral responses to intense emotions

are outside of the home or school settings (Table 14.4). The final continuum is the development of positive peer-to-peer interactions (Table 14.5). The effect of trauma on behavior is covered with various continua, however, behaviors seen in children with sensory modulation issues is covered in Chapter 6, Ayres Sensory Integration Frame of Reference and Chapter 7, A Frame of Reference for Sensory Integration and Processing Differences: Sensory Therapies and Research (STAR).

Table 14.3 Indicators of Function: Environment—Home/School/Daycare

Function	Dysfunction
Environment is stable, predictable, safe, and secure to support development of the child	Environment is unsafe, unpredictable, unstable, and unsecure therefore not supporting development of the child
Environment has sufficient materials to engage child in developmentally appropriate activities facilitating appropriate socialization based on the context	Environment lacks materials and structure to facilitate developmentally appropriate tasks and activities
Environment contains a nurturing caregiver who communicates effectively validating child's emotions, meeting their needs, and supporting peer interaction	Caregiver does not demonstrate nurturing behaviors or positive communication styles, does not validate child's emotions or allow for positive peer interactions
School/daycare contains supportive teachers and staff members who support appropriate and positive interactions with child peer to peer	School/daycare staff and teachers do not support positive peer interaction for child
Caregiver in the home models positive, appropriate behaviors for secure and safe social bonds with family, friends, and community. Teachers and staff work with the child to facilitate positive learning and support rapport to allow positive learning and social interactions	Caregiver in the home does not model positive, appropriate behaviors for secure and safe social bonds with family, friends, and community. Teachers and staff are not able to work with the child to facilitate a supportive learning environment and promote the development of trusting safe social interactions
Child can adapt to various personalities within home, school, and daycare environments to benefit from teaching and parenting styles	Child demonstrates difficulty with adaptations to various personalities, teaching and parenting styles, which hindering learning

Table 14.4 Indicators of Function: Environments Outside of the Home, School, or Daycare

Function	Dysfunction
Access to environments where the child can positively interact with peers	Limited or no access to environments that support positive social interactions with peers
Opportunities for participation in choice of activities, and informal and formal community activities	Limited or no opportunities for participation in choice of activities, and informal, and formal community activities
Child has safe spaces and dedicated time to develop friendships with peers	Limited or no access to safe spaces and no dedicated time to develop friendships with peers
Has supportive relationships with caregivers to guide child in conflict resolution and negotiation with peers	Does not have supportive relationships with caregivers to guide child in conflict resolution and negotiation with peers

POSTULATES REGARDING CHANGE

General Postulate for Change

Based on the evaluation, the therapist needs to determine which area (or areas) as described in the theoretical base may be contributing to difficulties in social participation. Then the intervention can be directed towards those specific area(s) to improve performance.

Specific Postulates Regarding Change

Resiliency and Self-Regulation

1. If a practitioner can support the child in identifying their emotions, as well as how the child specifically responds to various emotions, the child will increase their awareness of self.

Table 14.5 Indicators of Function: Development of Peer to Peer Interaction

Function	Dysfunction
Seeks out and is accepted into developmentally appropriate peer groups	Does not seek out and is not accepted into developmentally appropriate peer groups
Can initiate age-appropriate activities with peers	Cannot or does not initiate age-appropriate activities with peers
Child's nonverbal and verbal communication is appropriate for setting, activity, and social context with peers	Child's nonverbal and verbal communication is not appropriate for setting, activity, and social context with peers
Demonstrates and sustains eye contact, body posture, reciprocal communication, tone and volume of voice	Does not demonstrate or sustain eye contact, body posture, reciprocal communication, tone and volume of voice
Can adapt nonverbal and verbal responses based on context and environmental changes	Cannot adapt nonverbal and verbal responses based on context and environmental changes
Is able to share and take turns with peers	Is not able to share and take turns with peers
Can adhere to rules of established activities determined by both the peers participating and social norms	Cannot adhere to rules of established activities determined by both the peers participating and social norms

2. If a practitioner can support a child in identifying and recognizing verbal and nonverbal signals indicating emotions in others, the child can assess emotional response of others in everyday functioning over time.
3. If a practitioner can support the child in developing skills and strategies to manage intense emotions during social participation, the child will more readily be able to effectively manage emotional responses over time increasing positive social participation.
4. If a practitioner can support a caregiver in providing the "just right challenge" for the child throughout daily routines, a child will begin to foster self-confidence and mastery, foundational skills of resilience.

Developing Supportive Daily Environments

1. If a caregiver and occupational therapy practitioner can provide support and comfort when a child is feeling overwhelmed, a sense of security and stability will support healthy development.
2. If a practitioner and caregiver can effectively communicate with the child regarding behaviors inhibiting positive social interaction and demonstrate a more positive way of approaching the situation, mutual problem solving can occur to support decreasing the impact of the problem hindering positive social interaction.
3. If a practitioner can support caregivers in increasing self-awareness, a caregiver can better understand the situation and self-regulate and see how their behavior impacts relationship building as well as the child's ability to self-regulate.
4. If a practitioner can support caregivers in developing positive routines with the child, balancing activities that have to occur with activities the child find enjoyment in, then enhancement of the caregiver–child relationship will be achieved.
5. If a practitioner can model a positive, supportive play environment for the caregiver, the caregiver can utilize modeled strategies to create this within the home and throughout routines with the child.

Developing Supportive External Environments

1. If the practitioner can enlist the support of teachers and significant others in the child's environment outside of the home, the child is more likely to engage successfully in social activities.
2. The child's performance in social participation might be improved if the practitioner can advocate for resources and support in the external environment from governing bodies/school-based resources/insurance companies, etc.

Peer-to-Peer Interaction

1. A child is more likely to engage in positive peer-to-peer interaction within an environment that is safe, stable, and supportive to the child.
2. If the practitioner can support a child in managing social demands of various environments, the child is more likely to generalize positive engagement with others in a variety of spaces.
3. If a practitioner can support a child in learning how to share, help others, and follow directions/expectations set for specific activities, the child is more likely to form reciprocal bonds and friendships.

APPLICATION TO PRACTICE

Following completion of assessments, an occupational therapy practitioner should begin the intervention process by creating goals with the child and caregiver. These goals would be based on the evaluation data, which can determine where to start with skill building and/or contextual interventions for the child and/or caregiver.

Utilizing the infinity perspective can assist with identifying which factors are impacting successful social participation.

Occupation-Based Groups

Group intervention is the preferred method for intervention with this FOR as group dynamics naturally foster peer interactions and the use of self-regulatory skills through social participation (Brown & Tilley, 2019). Yalom (1995) notes the critical therapeutic power that groups have for positive change. Occupational therapy practitioners lead groups to develop and support a child's social participation in various settings including schools, after-school programs, community centers, mental health facilities, children's hospitals, or private practices. Group interventions allow for reciprocal social interactions to promote self-regulatory skills, social skills and communication skills, and developmental skill building. Additionally, groups allow a child to coregulate with peers or therapist to practice social skills in real time. Repeated positive social interactions in groups assist in fostering relational skill building.

Occupational therapy practitioners (OTP) can use a group intervention to assist with developmental skill acquisition and deficits. During the assessment process, it would be determined if a physical, cognitive, or communicative delay/disruption is impacting the child's ability to engage in preferred social occupations. Additionally, informal observations from the evaluation would assist with indicating deficits in self-regulation, impulse control, and attention which need to be addressed. Group goals can be developed to provide cohesion among all participants and also address challenges seen among all the group members. Activities selected for group intervention should be therapeutically graded to facilitate engagement from all of children involved.

Further, practitioners can design groups based on mutual needs or challenges to support development by the scaffolding of various skills across a window of time. Examples of these interventions include groups based on life skills, shared interests, and needs. Groups can also be formed based on a topic of shared interest or activity. For example, the practitioner can create a group in which the children work cooperatively to participate in an identified project to be completed over a series of weeks, or months (e.g., large-scale art projects, exercise programming, or celebration preparations).

Cole's Seven Step Protocol for running groups (2017) provides occupational therapy practitioners with an outline for facilitating group therapy sessions. The seven steps outline predictable group process and stages showing individual and group development over time. These steps include introduction, activity, sharing, processing, generalizing, application and summary. The seven steps serve to guide practitioners through the evolution of the group process.

When working with vulnerable populations, relationship building, and structure is essential to support group cohesion. Psychologists Purvis et al. (2013) developed a trauma informed intervention method for children who have experienced early adversity. The components to their model, *Trust Based Relational Intervention* (TBRI), emphasize the need for regulation and self-safety in relationships to successfully engage in chosen occupations (Purvis et al., 2013). Elements of their model support successful group intervention as a both a highly nurtured and highly structured environment. This is achieved through levels of intervention they recommend (Purvis et al., 2013):

1. **Empowering:** Creating both a safe ecologic (e.g., transitions and rituals) and physiologic environment (hydration, healthy touch, rhythmic and sensory-focused activities).
2. **Connecting:** Strategies that facilitate building trust and replicate secure attachment through mindfulness and engagement (creative problem solving, proactive response, playful interaction).
3. **Correcting:** Utilizing proactive strategies to build new skills and social competence (behavioral scripts, consistent terminology, systematic level of responding to behavior).

Sensory Modulation Interventions

When a child demonstrates sensory modulation issues, there are several areas that can be useful with these behaviors. Sensory rooms are used to describe therapeutic spaces that may have multiple types of sensory inputs in a specific space. These therapeutic spaces are strategically designed to promote self-organization and positive functional change in behaviors through experience that are comforting to the child. These spaces allow for crisis de-escalation, and prevention of negative behaviors that may harm the child or others around them. The use of these spaces has been shown to decrease the occurrence of restraint and seclusion episodes in inpatient behavioral health settings (Champagne, 2011).

In addition to sensory rooms, other sensory modulation interventions such as sensory kits or bins that are individual specific, utilizing specific items tailored to an individual's needs to support grounding and coping with intense emotions. These bins can focus on safety, reduction of self-injurious behavior, and relaxation (Champagne, 2011). Additionally, structured sensory strategies are believed to support self-organization and function. Safety must be considered with the use of any sensory interventions. For additional information on sensory modulation, see Chapter 6, Ayres Sensory Integration Frame of Reference and Chapter 7, A Frame of Reference for Sensory Integration and Processing Differences: Sensory Therapies and Research (STAR).

Caregiver Involvement in Intervention

It is just as essential to form a therapeutic relationship with the child's caregiver, as well as building a therapeutic rapport with the child. This can create a situation of "felt safety," which refers to a situation when an adult creates a supportive environment fostering a feeling of safety and security within the home for the child (Purvis Institute, 2023). When felt safety is achieved, both the caregiver and child can establish mutual support as part of the intervention methods and education. A safe learning environment is created when there is trust among all parties. Family goals should be collaborative and achievable.

When working with children with social–emotional challenges, it is important to include caregivers. In this way, they will have a better understanding of the child's behaviors. Coaching can be an effective tool to use with caregivers. A scoping review done by Seruya et al. (2022) highlighted the various methods used by occupational therapy practitioners to provide caregiver coaching within early intervention settings. The review highlighted that caregiver coaching falls within the OT Practice Framework 4 to create interventions in appropriate physical and social contexts so that children can participate to the best of their abilities in meaningful occupations (AOTA, 2020). Additionally, the research served to further highlight the use of co-occupations as a natural coaching method to involve caregivers and children within a family's existing routines and environments (Seruya et al., 2022). Occupational therapy practitioners can learn about the family's role, habits, routines, and rituals to more successfully coach caregivers. Additionally, the review found that play was utilized to support engagement in chosen co-occupations (Seruya et al., 2022). While play is a primary occupation for children, it also aids in creating a safe and positive atmosphere for learning (Gaskill & Perry, 2014). It allows parents to continue building a healthy relationship with their child (Schultz-Krohn & Cara, 2000).

The OTP can begin intervention by helping caregivers to understand their child and their own attachment and interaction styles. Understanding attachment style can teach the caregiver about their own responses to their child and develop mindfulness during teachable moments (KPID, 2023). Specifically, when working with families of children with social participation challenges, caregiver education should focus on building positive relationships within the family unit and teaching caregivers to be active participants in their child's chosen occupation (Dempsey et al., 2009).

The practitioner may also serve as a role model by demonstrating effective ways of working with dysregulation through educating caregivers to focus on coregulation (with caregiver and/or family) first, then self-regulation (self) to build connection and social–emotional learning (KPID, 2023). Emphasizing coregulation, the caregivers and child can attune to each other's needs. Additionally, occupational therapy practitioners can provide relational activities that will match the child's developmental and emotional functioning. When a child feels successful in an activity, it is more likely to promote positive engagement and in return a positive response from the caregiver. Therefore, the child and caregiver can express joy in their co-occupations (Olson, 2020).

In addition to direct caregiver coaching, Kramer et al. (2018) developed an approach defining how occupational therapy practitioners can support parents' ability to identify environmental barriers to their child's participation in occupations inside and outside the home. This included problem solving beyond the home environment, including community and policy levels. This approach focuses on caregiver skill building in areas of leadership and advocacy to support their children from a larger systematic lens. This example broadens the understanding of caregiver coaching as more than just a 1:1 direct intervention method (Seruya et al., 2022).

CASE EXAMPLE

Maddie

Maddie is a 12-year-old female with no known physical or cognitive delays. Her home environment has been unstable for the past 6 years. Her mother struggles with addiction and has been institutionalized in rehabilitation centers on and off over the past 6 years. During those periods of time, she has been with various relatives and grandparents, so parenting has been inconsistent. While Maddie feels she has a relationship with her mother, she doesn't feel a strong connection with her other relatives or grandparents. Her school is concerned about her as both her grades and her behavior are erratic. While she has consistently attended the same school, she does not seem to have friends in her class or get involved in any school activities. When her mother is available, Maddie's school performance is better.

The Child Study Team in her school referred her for a complete evaluation including an OT evaluation. The occupational therapist started out with an occupational profile and found that Maddie liked school but was often uncomfortable with her peers because of her home situation. She was hesitant to talk with others about it and when they asked her questions, she started avoiding them and picking fights. She stated she liked crafts, drawing and puzzles, and preferred activities she could do alone. Mostly, she wanted her mother to be around more and be more reliable. Utilizing standardized assessment, it was found that she had no sensory deficits as per the Sensory Profile 2 (Dunn, 2014). However, the Social Profile (Donahue, 2012) indicated she had difficulty with social engagement, participation, and cooperation with others. Using the infinity perspective, Maddie's results look most like Figure 14.7, with deficit noted in her environment, resulting in personal problems with resiliency and social participation. The occupational therapist's recommendation was to have Maddie participate in a group that focused on peer interaction and social participation. She also recommended a weekly individual session to address the development of a greater sense of self-awareness to build resilience and emotional regulation.

In her individual session with the OTP, Maddie indicated she wanted to learn how to better control her emotions and not get so upset when people asked her questions about her home life. Individual sessions focused on cognitive behavioral strategies to identify emotions and problem solve solutions and strategies to manage emotions, addressing the function/dysfunction continuum of self-regulation and resiliency. Maddie felt breathing exercises and positive self-talk were strategies that helped her when she felt emotionally dysregulated.

Maddie participated in a group with five other girls of her age, addressing the last function/dysfunction continuum of peer-to-peer interactions. Each of the girls set goals individually with the practitioner. The girls determined the goals of the group together, which were to develop positive interactions and engage in cooperative activities with each other. The group planned art projects together and then carried them out weekly. This was followed by discussions of their project outcome and their interactions. Through the interactions in the group and with facilitation by the OTP in their individual sessions, Maddie was able to develop skills that allowed her to demonstrate increased resiliency such as increasing her emotional self-awareness, and improved peer-to-peer interactions. Maddie's increased resilience also provided a more stable base on which she was able to trust the other girls and form attachments to support her peer interactions. The OTP was also able to build on skills of self-regulation worked in individual sessions, through various interactions during the group. For example, when topics were upsetting, the OT was able to direct the conversation to allow for the sharing of thoughts and feelings in a safe environment while also problem solving with the girls on how to manage emotions when they seemed overwhelming.

The OTP also wanted Maddie to utilize the skills she developed within the context of the safe individual session and group environment, into the larger classroom environments. Therefore, she consulted with Maddie's teacher to provide additional support and share the strategies Maddie was working on within OT sessions to facilitate the carryover of those skills to other school environments successfully. Via consistent collaboration, the OTP and the teacher identified particularly challenging times and classroom activities that Maddie found difficult to develop support strategies such as creating small groups or building in breaks when appropriate to allow Maddie to practice the self-regulation strategies she had worked on in her sessions. The OT also provided suggestions for verbal cues the teacher could use to help Maddie initiate self-regulating strategies. The teacher reported success with implementing strategies in the classroom and she was able to observe Maddie making more mindful decisions and demonstrating better self-regulation throughout the day and even when there were more challenging activities.

SUPPORTING EVIDENCE

There have been various studies synthesizing the current literature regarding occupational therapy interventions for the improvement of mental health and social–emotional development for children and youth (Arbesman et al., 2013; Cahill et al., 2020; Case-Smith, 2013). These studies have attempted to demonstrate the efficacy of both individualized as well as group interventions across various settings (including schools and home-based contexts), ages, and diagnoses to address the development and use of social–emotional skills. It is inherent that improving mental health and social–emotional development will improve social participation in children.

In a systematic review, Case-Smith (2013) examined the types of interventions targeting the social–emotional development of younger (birth to 5) children utilized by occupational therapists. The findings of this review provided support for the inclusion of parents and caregivers in the intervention process regardless of the interventions utilized. Several types of interventions were most utilized with this age group including the use of touch-based interventions, relationship-based interventions, interventions requiring joint attention, instruction-based interventions, and those interventions occurring within naturalistic settings. The findings support utilizing sensory-based strategies as touch-based interventions (e.g., use of deep pressure and massage) can improve parent bonding and child behavior. Likewise, the provision of intervention within natural settings via the use of play activities was noted to improve social interactions among the child and their peers. Regardless of the type of intervention, the coaching of caregivers was noted to be an essential component when addressing parent–child bonding and relationship development, both of which have been identified in this FOR to be significant factors that can affect social–emotional skills as children mature. The interventions utilized were deemed to support the development of social–emotional skills in at-risk young children.

Evidence also supports the use of activity- and occupation-based group interventions (Arbesman et al., 2013; Cahill et al., 2020) to address social–emotional development in children and youth. In a systematic review, Arbesman and colleagues (2013) reviewed the literature to assess the effectiveness of activity-based interventions in addressing mental health and social–emotional skills in children utilizing a public health framework. Their findings indicate activity-based approaches are efficacious in various settings and tiers of intervention. Interventions at the population level, such as in schools, were deemed to be effective in promoting social–emotional development. Examples include bullying prevention programs and facilitating participation in arts programming. At a more individualized and targeted level, interventions focused on life skills, play, leisure, and recreation led to positive social–emotional outcomes for children. A systematic review by Cahill and colleagues (2020) further supports the use of activity and occupation-based interventions to support the development of appropriate social–emotional skills in children and youth. Findings demonstrated participation in activities such as life skills training, yoga, and sports facilitated improvement in mental health, positive behavior, and social participation. Providing activity- and occupation-based interventions in both individualized and group service delivery models were determined to be efficacious with some activities naturally lending themselves to the use of groups such as sports or whole school programming (Arbesman et al., 2013; Cahill et al., 2020). The use of groups has been a hallmark of the profession since its inception (Meyers, 1922/1977).

These studies have demonstrated practitioners can address social–emotional and mental health challenges for children and youth through targeted interventions inclusive of activity-based groups, sensory-based activities, and by utilizing coaching models in natural settings. These intervention strategies can facilitate the development of emotional self-regulation and appropriate attachment and relationship skills, thereby supporting the participation of children and youth in developmentally appropriate social activities within their natural home and school environments.

REFERENCES

American Occupational Therapy Association (AOTA). (2014). Occupational therapy practice framework: Domain and process (3rd ed.). *American Journal of Occupational Therapy*, *68*(Suppl 1), S1–S48. https://doi.org/10.5014/ajot.2014.682006

American Occupational Therapy Association (AOTA). (2020). Occupational therapy practice framework: Domain and process (4th ed.). *American Journal of Occupational Therapy*, *74*(Suppl 2), 7412410010. https://doi.org/10.5014/ajot.2020.74S2001

American Psychology Association. (2018). In *APA dictionary of psychology*. Retrieved February 3, 2024, from https://dictionary.apa.org

Arbesman, M., Bazyk, S., & Nochajski, S. M. (2013). Systematic review of occupational therapy and mental health promotion, prevention, and intervention for children and youth. *American Journal of Occupational Therapy*, *67*, e120–e130. https://doi.org/10.5014/ajot.2013.008359

Bandura, A. (1977). *Social learning theory.* Prentice Hall.

Bandura, A. (2006). Toward a psychology of human agency. *Perspectives on Psychological Science, 1*(2), 164.

Bärwalde, T., Hoffmann, L., Fink, A., Völlm, C., Martin, O., Bernard, M., Gebhard, B., & Richter, M. (2023). The adolescent concept of social participation—A qualitative study on the concept of social participation from adolescents with and without physical disabilities. *Qualitative Health Research*, *33*(3), 143–153. https://doi.org/10.1177/10497323221146414

Brown, C., & Tilley, S. (2019). Group development theory. In C. Brown, V. C. Stoffel, J. P. Munoz (Eds.), *Occupational therapy in mental health: A vision for participation* (2nd ed., pp. 407–408). F.A. Davis Company.

Cahill, S. M., Egan, B. E., & Seber, J. (2020). Activity- and occupation-based interventions to support mental health, positive behavior, and social participation for children and youth: A systematic review. *American Journal of Occupational Therapy*, *74*, 7402180020. https://doi.org/10.5014/ajot.2020.038687

Case-Smith, J. (2013). Systematic review of interventions to promote social–emotional development in young children with or at risk for disability. *American Journal of Occupational Therapy*, *67*, 395–404. https://doi.org/10.5014/ajot.2013.004713

Champagne, T. (2011). *Sensory modulation & environment: Essential elements of occupation* (3rd ed. Rev.). Pearson Assessment.

Cole, M. B. (2017). *Group Dynamics in occupational therapy: The theoretical basis and practice application of group intervention* (5th ed.). Slack, Inc.

Coster, W. J., Deeney, T. A., Haltiwanger, J. T., & Haley, S. M. (1998). *School function assessment*. Psychological Corporation/Therapy Skill Builders.

Dempsey, I., Keen, D., Pennell, D., O'Reilly, J., & Neilands, J. (2009). Parent stress, parenting competence and family-centered support to young children with an intellectual or developmental disability. *Research in Developmental Disabilities*, *30*(3), 558–566. https://doi.org/10.1016/j.ridd.2008.08.005

Donahue, M. (2012). *Social profile: Assessment of social participation in children, adolescents, and adults*. AOTA Press.

Dorman, W., & Williamson, G. (2002). *Promoting social competency*. Therapy Skill Builders.

Dunn, W. (2014). *Sensory profile 2 manual*. Pearson.

Gresham, F. M., & Elliot, S. N. (1990). *Social skills rating system*. American Guidance Service.

Gaskill, R. L., & Perry, B. D. (2014). The neurobiological power of play: Using the neurosequential model of therapeutics to guide play in the healing process. In C. A. Malchiodi & D. A. Crenshaw (Eds.), *Creative arts and play therapy for attachment problems* (pp. 178–194). The Guilford Press.

Goldsmith, H. H., Buss, A. H., Plomin, R., Rothbart, M. K., Thomas, A., Chess, S., Hinde, R. A., & McCall, R. B. (1987). Roundtable: What is temperament? Four approaches. *Child Development*, *58*(2), 505–529.

Hagen, M. (n.d.). What is co-regulation? Retrieved September 1, 2024, from https://childmind.org/article/what-is-co-regulation/#full_article

Henry, A. D. (2000). *Pediatric interest profiles*. Therapy Skill Builders.

Jones. (2013). *The family goal setting tool: ASD version*. https://autismqld.com.au/product/family-goal-setting-tool-asd-version/

Joseph, R. Y., Casteleijn, D., van der Linde, J., & Franzsen, D. (2021). Sensory modulation dysfunction in child victims of trauma: A scoping review. *Journal of Child & Adolescent Trauma*, *14*(4), 455–470. https://doi.org/10.1007/s40653-020-00333-x

Karen Purvis Institute of Development (KPID). (2023). *TBRI training notebook and reference manual*. Texas Christian University.

King, G. A., Law, M., King, S., Hurley, P., Hanna, S., Kertoy, M., & Rosenbaum, P. (2007). Measuring children's participation in recreation and leisure activities: construct validation of the CAPE and PAC. *Child: Care, Health and Development*, *33*(1), 28–39. https://doi.org/10.1111/j.1365-2214.2006.00613.x

Kramer, J. M., Hwang, I. T., Levin, M., Acevedo-García, D., & Rosenfeld, L. (2018). Identifying environmental barriers to participation: Usability of a health-literacy informed problem identification approach for parents of young children with developmental disabilities. *Child Care, Health and Development*, *44*, 249–259. https://doi.org/10.1111/cch.12542

Law, M., Baptiste, S., Carswell, A., McCall, M. A., Polatajko, H., & Pollack, N. (2014). *Canadian Occupational Performance Measure* (4th ed.). COPM, Inc.

Leigers, K., Myers, C., & Schneck, C. (2016). Social participation in schools: A survey of occupational therapy practitioners. *American Journal of Occupational Therapy*, *70*, 7005280010. https://doi.org/10.5014/ajot.2016.020768

Lynch, A., Ashcraft, R., & Tekell, L. (2021). *Trauma, Occupation and participation: Foundations and population considerations in occupational therapy*. AOTA Press.

Martini, M. (2002). How mothers in four American cultural groups shape infant learning during mealtimes. *Zero to Three*, *22*(4), 14–20.

Matusov, E., & Hayes, R. (2000). Sociocultural critique of Piaget and Vygotsky. *New Ideas in Psychology*, *18*(2–3), 215–239. https://doi.org/10.1016/S0732-118X(00)00009-X

McCrae, R. R., Costa, P. T. Jr., Ostendorf, F., Angleitner, A., Hřebíčková, M., Avia, M. D., Sanz, J., Sánchez-Bernardos, M. L., Kusdil, M. E., Woodfield, R., Saunders, P. R., & Smith, P. B. (2000). Nature over nurture: Temperament, personality, and life span development. *Journal of Personality and Social Psychology*, *78*(1), 173–186. https://doi.org/10.1037//0022-3514.78.1.173

Meyer, A. (1977). The philosophy of occupational therapy. *American Journal of Occupational Therapy, 37*(10), 639–642. (Original work published 1922).

Olson, L. J. (2020). A frame of reference for enhancing social participation. In P. Kramer, J. Hinojosa & T. Howe (Eds.), *Frames of reference for pediatric occupational therapy* (4th ed., pp. 461–495). Wolters Kluwer.

Orenstein, G. A., & Lewis, L. (2022). Eriksons stages of psychosocial development. In *StatPearls [Internet]*. National Library of Medicine. https://www.ncbi.nlm.nih.gov/books/NBK556096/

Parham, L. D., Ecker, C. L., Kuhaneck, H., Henry, D. A., & Glennon, T. J. (2021). *Sensory processing measure, second edition (SPM-2)*. Western Psychological Services.

Perry, B. (2001). Bonding and attachment in maltreated children. *The Child Trauma Center*, *3*, 1–17. The childtrauma academy. www.childtrauma.org

Perry, B. (2020). *Six core strengths for healthy childhood development*. www.childtrauma.org; https://attachmentnetwork.ca/wp-content/uploads/2020/08/Six-Core-Strengths-for-Healthy-Child-Development-B.-D.-Perry.pdf

Perry, B. D., & Winfry, O. (2021). *What happened to you? Conversations on trauma, resilience, and healing*. Flatiron Books.

Polatajko, H., Carswell, A., Baptiste, S., Law, M., McColl, M., & Pollock, N. (2014). *Canadian occupational performance measure (COPM)*. Canadian Association of Occupational Therapists (CAOT).

Purvis, K. B., Cross, D. R., Dansereau, D. F., & Parris, S. R. (2013). Trust-based relational intervention (TBRI): A systemic approach to complex developmental trauma. *Child & Youth Services*, *34*(4), 360–386. https://doi.org/10.1080/0145935X.2013.859906

Salley, B., Miller, A., & Bell, M. A. (2013). Associations between temperament and social responsiveness in young children. *Infant and Child Development*, *22*(3), 270–288. https://doi.org/10.1002/icd.1785

Sanson, A., Hemphill, S. A., & Smart, D. (2004). Connections between temperament and social development: A review. *Social Development, 13*(1), 142–170. https://doi.org/10.1046/j.1467-9507.2004.00261

Schultz-Krohn, W., & Cara, E. (2000). Occupational therapy in early intervention: Applying concepts from infant mental health. *The American Journal of Occupational Therapy*, *54*(5), 550–554. https://doi.org/10.5014/ajot.54.5.550

Seruya, F. M., Feit, E., Tirado, A., Ottomanelli, D., & Celio, M. (2022). Caregiver coaching in early intervention: A scoping review. *American Journal of Occupational Therapy*, *76*(4), 7604205070. https://doi.org/10.5014/ajot.2022.049143

Shiner, R. L., Buss, K. A., McClowry, S. G., Putnam, S. P., Saudino, K. J., & Zentner, M. (2012). What is temperament now? Assessing progress in temperament research on the twenty-fifth anniversary of Goldsmith et al. *Child Development Perspectives*, *6*, 436–444. https://doi.org/10.1111/j.1750-8606.2012.00254.x

Spagnola, M., & Fiese, B. H. (2007). Family routines and rituals: A context for development in the lives of young children. *Infants & Young Children*, *20*(4), 284–299. https://doi.org/10.1097/01.iyc.0000290352.32170.5a

Stigen, L., Bjørk, E., & Lund, A. (2023). The power of observation. Occupational therapists' descriptions of doing observations of people with cognitive impairments in the context of community practice. *Scandinavian Journal of Occupational Therapy*, *30*(1), 21–33. https://doi.org/10.1080/11038128.2020.1839966

Strelau, J. (1987). The concept of temperament in personality research. *European Journal of Personality*, *1*(2), 107–117. https://doi.org/10.1002/per.2410010205

Taylor, C. L. (2011). Scaffolding the development of early self-regulation: The role of structure and routine in children's daily activities. *Dissertations and Theses*. Paper 287. https://doi.org/10.15760/etd.287

Ukeru. (2020). *Ukeru training manual*. Ukeru systems: https://www.ukerusystems.com/how-we-can-help/training/.

Wilcox, P. (2012). *Trauma-informed treatment: The restorative approach*. NEARI Press.

Yalom, I. D. (1995). *The theory and practice of group psychotherapy* (4th ed.). Basic Books.

Yilmaz, E. (n.d.). Temperaments: Definition, examples, & types. Retrieved September 1, 2024, from https://www.berkeleywellbeing.com/temperaments.html

Yochman, A., & Pat-Horenczyk, R. (2019). Sensory modulation in children exposed to continuous traumatic stress. *Journal of Child & Adolescent Trauma*, *13*(1), 93–102. https://doi.org/10.1007/s40653-019-00254-4

A Strength-Based Frame of Reference for Autistic Individuals

Dora D. Onwumere ▪ Joana Nana Serwaa Akrofi ▪ Kavitha Murthi
Lauren Melissa Ellzey ▪ Kristie K. Patten

"Autism is not a processing error; it's a different operating system. Strengths come from our differences, not deficits."

Stuart Duncan (personal communication, 2024)

The fundamental tenets of occupational therapy prioritize holistic, client-centered, evidence-based, and culturally responsive approaches. However, there remains room for growth regarding how we support autistic individuals within the therapeutic contexts. This frame of reference is designed for occupational therapy practitioners (OTPs) dedicated to supporting the participation of autistic individuals and their families in daily activities across their lifespan.

Autistic individuals are frequently perceived through a deficit-oriented lens, which focuses on interventions aimed at mitigating the primary challenges associated with autism. This perspective is criticized as ableist and can hinder the adoption of practices that embrace neurodiversity. Ableism refers to discriminatory attitudes or practices that devalue individuals considered disabled compared to those individuals who are not (Bottema-Beutel et al., 2024). Engaging in neurodiversity-affirming practices (Dallman et al., 2022; Shaw et al., 2022) entails taking a stance against this discrimination and advocating for accommodations and inclusive opportunities that respect the varied identities within the neurodivergent community (Patten, 2022). This approach acknowledges various abilities and unique ways individuals engage with the world, emphasizing that differences should be celebrated rather than viewed as deficits needing correction.

Neurodiversity-affirming practices center on the idea that OTPs have the power and responsibility to advocate for neurodiverse individuals (Patten, 2022). OTPs who see themselves as agents of change view their environments as opportunities to promote social equality and advocate for autistic individuals' rights and well-being. They actively challenge and transform the status quo to better meet diverse needs, recognizing the impact of environmental factors and power dynamics in their practice settings. Instead of being passive, they work to dismantle barriers to inclusion and access, aiming to support individuals to reach their full potential (Table 15.1).

Neurodiversity-affirming practices acknowledge individual differences and address unmet needs without judgment or pressure to conform (Chapman, 2021; Fletcher-Watson, 2022). They respect diverse ways of thinking and avoid labeling autistic individuals as abnormal, focusing

Table 15.1 Occupational Therapist Agency–Enhancing Practice

Effective Practice	Ineffective Practice
Combines focus on using strengths to develop skills and competence further and addressing areas that require support	The sole focus of services is the remediation of weakness
Assumes competence and capabilities of nonspeaking autistic individuals	Does not assume competence or capabilities of nonspeaking autistic individuals
Uses interests to foster the development of competence	Only uses interests to reward or control behavior
Uses language that reframes some of the autistic characteristics as neutral or positive	Does not use language that reframes some of the autistic characteristics as neutral or positive
Does not attempt to "fix" or make the autistic individual more "normal"	Does attempt to "fix" or make the autistic individual more "normal"
Provides services that promote positive mental health and well-being	Does not provide services that promote positive mental health and well-being
Provides environmental modifications, including sensory adaptations where necessary, to ensure that the autistic individual has all they need to the best of their ability	Does not make any environmental modifications to facilitate the autistic individual's ability in the space
Provides interventions that promote positive mental health and well-being	Does not provide interventions that promote positive mental health and well-being

instead on personal characteristics, social perspectives, and autonomy (Bottema-Beutel et al., 2024; Cook, 2024). OTPs using these practices leverage strengths, presume competence, and provide support that affirms and respects neurodivergent identities.

If OTPs only identify differences as deficits and maladaptive functioning in autistic individuals, it narrows the scope of both practice and research to the challenges that autistic individuals experience. This approach gives little to no attention to the positive attributes or unique qualities that autistic individuals possess, many of which directly relate to their autistic neurotype (Table 15.2). Consequently, the services provided may not fully address the broader aspects critical for long-term outcomes such as quality of life, well-being, and the ability to live self-determined lives. To achieve more comprehensive success and outcomes over time, there is a pressing need to shift away from a deficit-focused approach (Patten Koenig & Shore, 2018).

The strength-based frame of reference for autistic individuals represents a shift away from deficit-based thinking toward recognizing their strengths (Table 15.3). Occupational therapist (OT) practitioners can put this frame of reference into practice by focusing on strengths. However, it is crucial to avoid overly prioritizing strengths. Cook (2024) points out that exclusively valuing functionality might hinder growth by overlooking the inherent value of each person, regardless of how they perform. Therefore, a balanced approach is essential. This approach recognizes both strengths and challenges, offering a comprehensive view of how autistic individuals experience the world. By embracing this balanced perspective, OTPs can create environments that support flourishing and overall well-being.

OTPs who adopt a strength-based frame of reference for autistic individuals shift their focus from problems to challenges, from pathology to strengths, and from dwelling on the past to

Table 15.2 Strengths and Characteristics of Autistics

Strengths	Autistic Indicators
What people have learned about themselves (life experiences, successes, and failures)	Using self-stimulatory behaviors to cope with the stressful environment, stay in an interaction, or express joy, happiness, and interest
Personal qualities, traits, and virtues that people possess (sense of humor, loyalty, spirituality, patience, insight, and independence)	Honesty when questioned and loyalty to groups, people, and causes
What people know about the world around them (formal and informal learning, perceptions, self-taught, or "do it yourself" learning)	Nonspeaking individuals who have taught themselves to read by flipping through books, reading television credits, and using echolalia to understand the structure and function of language
The talents that people have	Attention to visual details, perfect pitch, mechanical knowledge of how things work, innovative technologic thinking, and understanding
Cultural, personal stories, and lore (cultural stories, myths, narratives, accounts of origin, trauma, and survival)	Autistic individuals recounting the impact of discrete trial training support interventions on stress and trauma
The pride of people (often buried under labeling, shame, and deficit models)	Autistic self-advocacy groups leading the way in forming new narratives that are voiced by autistic individuals

Adapted from List of common strengths taken from Saleeby, D. (2001). *The strengths perspective in social work practice* (3rd ed.). Allyn and Bacon.

Table 15.3 Contrast Between Deficit-Lens and Strength-Based Perspectives

Low-Functioning Environments

- Deficit-lens perspective
- Fails to accommodate strengths, abilities, and preferences
- Neglects to provide required accommodations and supports
- Ableist or deficit-based language, focusing on challenges rather than strengths
- Contributes to overwhelming sensory experiences
- Lack of understanding about multiple means of communication (e.g., speaking, Augmentative and alternative communication (AAC), Visual communication, and Assistive technology (AT))
- Risks supporting unsafe environments that impede meaningful engagement
- Lacks proactive measures to optimize the environment
- Exhibit disorganized spatial factors, clutter, and lack of visual supports
- Utilizes unsupportive systems perpetuating ableism, disregarding individual needs
- Lack of support and understanding of autistic needs from families, administration, employers, teachers, service providers, and staff

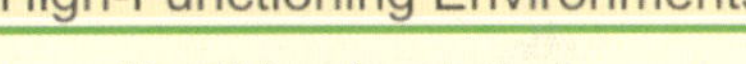

High-Functioning Environments

- Strength-based perspective
- Supports individual strengths, abilities, and preferences
- Provides necessary accommodations and resources
- Respectful and uses anti-ableist language
- Supports sensory regulation
- Understanding of multiple communication methods (e.g., speaking, Augmentative and alternative communication (AAC), Visual communication, and Assistive technology (AT))
- Creates safe and supportive environments
- Optimizes environment for better engagement
- Employs supportive spatial and sensory factors
- Employs supportive systems understanding individual needs
- Supportive and understanding of autistic needs from families, administration, employers, teachers, service providers, and staff

Courtesy of Dora Onwumere.

looking toward the future. These shifts require OTPs to perceive the individual, their environments, and their current situations in a fundamentally different way. This perspective marks a significant departure from traditional problem-focused approaches. By adopting this strength-based frame of reference, OTPs equip themselves with the knowledge, skills, and supportive strategies to integrate strength-based practice into their work with autistic individuals.

Before delving into the theoretical base, it is necessary to discuss the difference between identity-first versus person-first language. Language preference stems from sociolinguistic research principles, which recognize that terminologies and discourses are impinged by subjective judgments and values rather than being purely objective (Bloemmaert, 2005; Bottema-Beutel et al., 2023). Since the 1970s and 1980s, person-first language has been advocated to combat negative attitudes toward individuals with disabilities (Dunn & Andrews, 2015) and to emphasize a person's unique strengths, challenges, and experiences (Vivanti, 2020). Over time, person-first language became widely accepted as the "appropriate" mainstream terminology in professional settings such as schools, hospitals, and clinics. It was endorsed by various organizations, including the American Psychological Association, the American Medical Association, the American Psychiatric Association, and the American Speech-Language-Hearing Association (Gernsbacher, 2017).

In contrast, identity-first language places the disability at the forefront when describing a person. This approach is considered less ableist as it signifies acceptance of the disability as part of an individual's identity, acknowledging it as a natural aspect of who they are (i.e., autistic and Deaf communities). Identity-first language has garnered acceptance among health care professionals and researchers (Bottema-Beutel et al., 2021; Kenny et al., 2016; Murthi et al., 2023). Identity-first language is seen as a way to empower and show respect in the autism community because it focuses on recognizing and validating individuals' identities as autistic. In the words of Sinclair (1993), a known advocate for autism awareness, "Autism isn't something a person *has*, or a 'shell' that a person is trapped inside. There's no normal child hidden behind autism. Autism is a way of being. It is *pervasive*; it colors every experience, every sensation, perception, thought, emotion, encounter, and aspect of existence. It is not possible to separate the autism from the person, and if it were possible, the person you'd have left would not be the same person you started with." Referring to someone as an "autistic person" highlights autism as a part of who they are, rather than portraying it negatively or separately from their essence. Identify-first language values individuals' self-determination and self-identification, acknowledging their unique experiences and viewpoints.

In 2023, Taboas et al. surveyed autism stakeholders in the United States to ascertain whether current preferences mirrored those in the United Kingdom, where different stakeholder groups preferred both person-first and identity-first language, as reported by Kenny et al. (2016), or the more polarized pattern found in Australia by Bury et al. (2023). Their findings indicated that a majority of autistic adults (87%) preferred to self-identify using identity-first language. Given that our language shapes our conscious and unconscious perceptions and beliefs about autistic individuals, it is imperative to ascertain the terminology preferred by members of the community (Taboas et al., 2023).

Currently, there is a move toward dismantling ableism in autism research and the language associated with research in this community. However, critics argue that eliminating terminologies such as "comorbidities," "severe," and "suffer" might inadvertently limit the support available to autistic individuals with significant needs, questioning the rigor of such changes (Bottema-Beutel et al., 2021; Tan, 2023). Self-advocates from the community have underscored that these terminologies are humiliating (Natri et al., 2023). As mentioned, terminologies and language infuse values and societal norms derived from social and temporal ideologies. Botteuma-Botel et al. (2023) assert that many such presumed scientifically rigorous approaches are ableist in nature. In this way, OTPs can break the current stereotype of upholding presumed scientific rigor and accuracy through the use of value-laden terminologies by adopting anti-ableist and neuroaffirming language and approaches in practice.

Therefore, this chapter will use identity-first language, which is aligned with strength-based or ability-based perspectives. Terms like "autistic individuals" will be utilized deliberately to emphasize the strengths and abilities of individuals and to respect the preferences of autistic communities and self-advocates.

THEORETICAL BASE

The strength-based approach offers a practical, supported framework that strives to address these strengths and challenges associated with autism, recognizing them as intertwined components of the individual's identity, and lived experiences. This holistic approach promotes acceptance, understanding, and empowerment, fostering an environment where autistic individuals can thrive while embracing their neurodiversity. Therefore, this frame of reference gives OTPs the knowledge, skills, understanding, and strengths to incorporate into their practice.

A strength-based frame of reference for autistic individuals draws its theoretical foundation from the double empathy theory (DET) (Milton, 2012), the monotropism theory (Murray & Lawson, 2005), and the minority stress model (Meyer, 2003). Together, these theories and related concepts converge to provide a comprehensive understanding of the factors influencing the strengths, challenges, and overall well-being of autistic individuals (Figure 15.1).

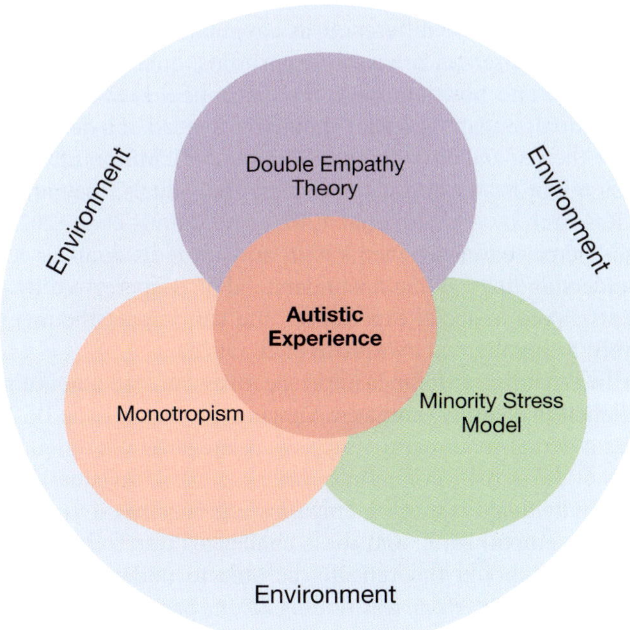

FIGURE 15.1 The interconnected dynamics of double empathy theory, monotropism, and minority stress in autistic individuals.

Assumptions

This frame of reference accepts five key assumptions that influence the way OTPs engage with autistic individuals:

1. OTPs perceive strengths as closely related to autism rather than as solely personal characteristics. Conversely, difficulties are viewed as both personal challenges as well as attributed to autism.
2. In an inclusive and compassionate social context, where everyone is valued and understood, autistic people's lived experiences can be valued as legitimate and significant contributions to society.
3. Both autistic and non-autistic individuals may struggle to interpret each other's perspectives. Social relationships are bidirectional and different based on group preferences. Autistic individuals may prefer socializing based on their interests, whereas non-autistic individuals generally prefer socializing based on social group positioning (Chen et al., 2022).
4. To optimize productivity and effectiveness within the autistic individual's endeavors, it is essential to maintain focus, attention, and engagement, particularly in tasks or activities that align with the individual's specific interests or areas of expertise.
5. Due to societal stigma and discrimination related to their neurodivergent identity, autistic individuals face stressors beyond ordinary daily life.

The Double Empathy Theory

Milton (2012) developed the DET to describe a disconnect in mutual understanding and reciprocal relationships between individuals with different social dispositions. This disconnect becomes evident when there are significant differences in how these individuals perceive the social environment. While non-autistic individuals may perceive this disconnect as a "deviation from the norm," autistic individuals experience these differences as a regular and often challenging aspect of their daily reality. Due to the differences in social dispositions, quality of experiences, worldviews, communication patterns, and positionalities, the disconnect is evident mutually when autistic and non-autistic individuals engage in social situations, instead of a deficit in the autistic individual's understanding of their social environment (Figure 15.2). Milton (2023) underscores that while these experiences might be novel for non-autistic individuals, they are common for many autistic individuals. Research by Alkhaldi et al. (2021) and Camus et al. (2022) has shown that non-autistic individuals perceived engagements with autistic individuals as less desirable, which could result in misunderstandings. Being misunderstood or misperceived by other people could create a barrier to participate in social experiences and can impact the mental health of autistic individuals negatively, as highlighted by Murthi et al. (2023).

Chapman (2019) described that this difference in perspectives can lead non-autistic individuals to perceive autism as a deficit in cognitive empathy. Viewing this through the DET framework, such labeling can be seen as a deficit in empathy itself, as it disregards the unique perspectives, worldviews, and experiences of the autistic community. Milton et al. (2023) question the concept of "deficit" traits in autistic individuals regarding empathy, arguing that if autistic individuals indeed demonstrated deficits in empathizing, and these challenges were related to their understanding, non-autistic individuals should theoretically be able to understand, recognize, and empathize with these deficits. However, empirical findings from Sasson et al. (2017) indicated that non-autistic individuals tended to rate autistic children and adults less positively across

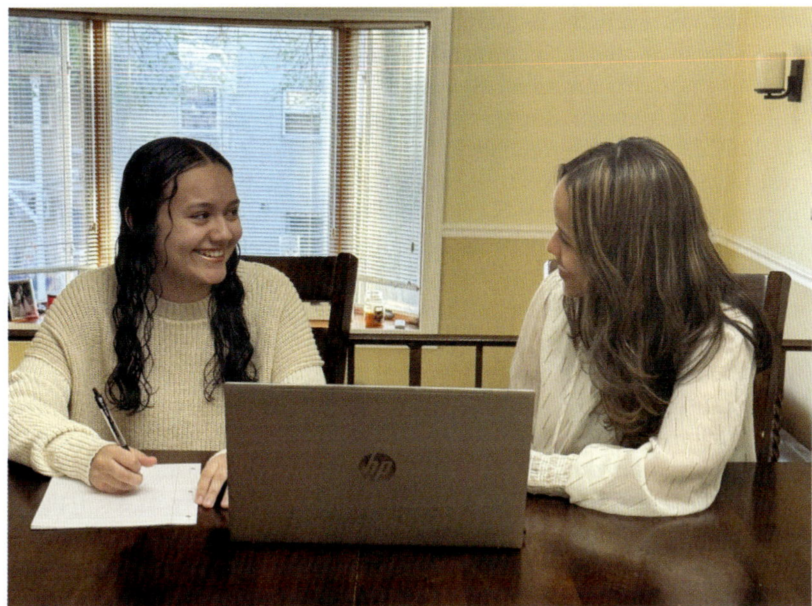

FIGURE 15.2 When an autistic individual interacts with a non-autistic individual, it is important to recognize the presence of the double empathy theory (DET). (Courtesy of Jackeline Ortiz.)

various measures and expressed a decreased willingness to engage in interactions with them. Similar results were replicated by other researchers, such as Alkhaldi et al. (2019) and Scheerer et al. (2022).

Crompton et al. (2020) showed in their study that autistic individuals possess the ability to transfer information among themselves with similar quality and quantity as non-autistic individuals. That is, the misunderstanding may predominantly occur in interactions between autistic and non-autistic individuals. The DET can serve as a foundation for explaining the social disconnect between practitioners and the autistic individuals they work with. OTPs can adopt a strength-based approach to both research and practice, informed by DET, which emphasizes understanding the nature of social reciprocity in relationships. This approach involves supporting non-autistic individuals in gaining a deeper understanding of the autistic perspective.

Monotropism Theory

The monotropism theory proposes that attention, as a cognitive process, is limited in quantity for all individuals. It suggests that attention may be broadly distributed over many interests in non-autistic individuals or concentrated on a few interests in autistic individuals (Murray et al., 2005). Instead of interpreting this difference as an abnormality requiring correction, the theory posits it as a natural neurologic variation between non-autistic and autistic individuals.

The classification of monotropic traits as "restricted, repetitive patterns of behavior, interests, or activities" in the DSM-V can lead to a pathologizing view of autism, framing it solely in terms of deficits or abnormalities. However, embracing a neurodiversity-affirming approach challenges this perspective by recognizing monotropism as a natural variation in human cognition that can offer its own strengths and abilities. Klin et al. (2007) surveyed parents of autistic individuals regarding their children's special or passionate interests, termed as circumscribed interests, finding that these circumscribed interests were more frequent among autistic children. The researchers also observed that attempts to restrict children's circumscribed interests were associated with a higher degree of interference in other activities. Consequently, autistic children showed higher resistance when interrupted, less flexibility regarding their interests, and less interest in involving other people (Turner-Brown et al., 2011). These studies portray these circumscribed interests negatively and do not represent the autistic perspective.

In contrast, a survey of eighty autistic adults highlighted overwhelmingly positive perspectives on how they characterized and used these circumscribed interests (Patten Koenig & Hough Williams, 2017). It was reported that engaging in preferred interests helped these autistic adults to calm themselves and mitigate stress. These refer to what is often condisered circumscribed interests as they are highly focused, intense, and often narrow areas of interest, whereas preferred interests in a general sense, refer to activities or subjects that an individual enjoys and prefers to engage with—less about the intensity and more about personal enjoyment. Additionally, they found that these preferred interests did not interfere with or produce anxiety. As such, these preferred interests can be viewed as a valuable and meaningful aspect of their identity, challenging dismissive labels such as "obsessions" or "fixations." Instead, these interests were recognized for their role in foster learning, development, and autonomy (Patten Koenig & Hough Williams, 2017). Therefore, by reframing monotropism as a strength associated with autism, we can redirect the focus from attempts to "fix" or treat these differences and instead focus on supporting individuals in leveraging their unique attentional profiles to thrive in their own unique way. This approach aligns with the neurodiversity-affirming principles that emphasize the value of diverse neurologic perspectives and experiences.

Minority Stress Model

The minority stress model, as proposed by Meyer (2003), offers a perspective on understanding the challenges experienced by marginalized groups, including autistic individuals. Hatzenbuehler (2009) further developed this model, highlighting how minority stress influences cognitive and interpersonal processes that are linked to mental health problems. Minority stress models aim to explain the increased vulnerability of minoritized groups, including disabled and autistic individuals, to various mental health issues. At its core, the minority stress model explores the health disparities observed between majority and stigmatized minority groups. It identifies the additional stressors experienced by marginalized communities, such as autistic individuals, going beyond typical day-to-day stressors. These stressors include internalized stigma, bullying, discrimination, and ableism, stemming from living in a world that fails to accommodate them and is worsened by inadequate representation (Patten, 2022).

The minority model of disability challenges the traditional medical model perspective by attributing societal inflexibility to social institutions and norms rather than innate traits. The minority stress model explains unfavorable outcomes within autistic individuals, as demonstrated by research by Botha and Frost (2020). In the past, autism has been linked to a lower quality of life, frequently overlooking the influence of harmful social variables such as minority stress. Viewing autism through the lens of minority stress recognizes a change from attributing mental health problems as innate to the condition itself. Research demonstrates that minority stresses significantly contribute to poorer mental health outcomes among autistic individuals (Botha & Frost, 2020).

Overall, by integrating the DET, monotropism, and minority stress models into a strength-based framework, OTPs can play a critical and forward-thinking role in supporting autistic individuals in their daily lives (Figure 15.1). OTPs can promote social interactions by fostering empathy and mutual understanding between themselves and autistic individuals. By applying the monotropism principle, OTPs can assist autistic individuals in identifying and utilizing their unique interests to motivation, self-control, and engagement in activities. Moreover, OTPs can design sessions that are meaningful, aiming to increase engagement, foster a sense of autonomy and well-being, and improve daily activities. Finally, OTPs can promote inclusive environments and advocate for reducing the stigma and discrimination experienced by autistic individuals using the insights from the minority stress model. Collaborating with community groups and legislators, OTPs can advocate for advanced resource accessibility, promote social inclusion, and improve supportive services. Ultimately, OTPs can support the strengths of autistic people, fostering a sense of empowerment that supports meaningful participation in daily tasks and social interactions.

THEORETICAL POSTULATES

A strength-based frame of reference for autistic individuals is grounded in maximizing the autistic individual's holistic experience. This framework considers various aspects of the individual's life, including environment, social, and societal contexts, through a fundamentally different lens than the traditional deficit-based approach. In the frame of reference, there is an interaction between the individual and the environment, coupled with a shift in the OTP's mindset to make changes based on the autistic individual's strengths and challenges.

1. Supporting the attentional styles of autistic people—such as intense focus on a single topic or scattered attention—will encourage various forms of expertise and learning patterns (Murray et al., 2005).
2. Creating opportunities for shared activities and experiences that appeal to the interests and strengths of both autistic and non-autistic individuals can facilitate empathy and mutual understanding, fostering meaningful connections and relationships (Milton, 2012).
3. Empowering autistic individuals to advocate for their rights and needs will help them amplify their voices and experiences in decision-making processes, thus helping combat the effects of minority stress and foster a sense of belonging and empowerment within the community (Meyer, 2003).

Many non-autistic individuals in a given society may not feel compelled to understand the perspectives of autistic individuals unless they share a social bond or a deeper relationship. Recognizing and addressing this issue is vital when working with autistic individuals. OTPs can better understand the challenges faced by autistic individuals and acknowledge that difficulties in social interactions often arise from mutual misunderstandings rather than inherent deficits within autistic individuals. This insight can guide OTPs toward adopting inclusive approaches to service delivery.

OTPs can prioritize promoting mutual understanding and reciprocal communication among neurodiverse individuals when they use the DET. This focus can help autistic individuals and their non-autistic peers develop empathy and mutual understanding. Ultimately, this strategy can foster relationships and social exchanges while giving OTPs a sense of fulfillment for their support. OTPs can help create environments that support autistic individuals by validating their experiences and promoting greater understanding and acceptance. Understanding the subtleties of the DET can enhance OT services by fostering cooperation between autistic individuals and those who serve them in creating support plans that address their unique needs, preferences, and capabilities.

It is misguided to assume that an OTP would create therapy plans for individuals without directly involving them in setting their priorities. However, OTPs who support neurodiversity must question if their goals aim to change behaviors that are essential to the autistic individual's identity and well-being. Being autistic is not an objective in itself but a reason to seek therapy if needed. Therapists should focus on identifying the specific support needs of the individual rather than viewing autism as inherently negative and requiring therapy. Additionally, not all autistic individuals will necessarily need occupational therapy, which should not be seen as a problem or a reason for seeking therapy, and therapeutic objectives should not focus on changing the autistic individual's ways of being. Embracing neurodiversity means accepting and valuing individuals' behavior, expression, and communication styles as essential to their identity. OTPs should prioritize individualized concepts, respect differences in participation, and enhance capabilities for individuals.

FUNCTION/DYSFUNCTION CONTINUA

This chapter acknowledges that autistic individuals face real challenges such as executive functioning issues, self-care difficulties, and sensory sensitivities. From a strength-based perspective, we view the function–dysfunction continuum as encompassing both strengths and areas for improvement. Therefore, we have chosen to relabel "function" as strengths (in parentheses) and "dysfunction" as challenges (in parentheses). The therapist's reflexivity, reflection, and interaction with the individual all influence this dynamic. By adopting a strengths-focused approach, OTPs can better encourage and support autistic individuals, leading to more positive outcomes in their therapeutic journey. Our approach avoids labeling autistic individuals as simply "functional" or "dysfunctional," instead emphasizing the importance of examining the OTP's mindsets and potential biases in order to foster a more nuanced and supportive perspective (Table 15.4). We confront the ramifications of years spent framing supports predominantly around deficits rather than innate strengths.

Additionally, OTPs can cultivate awareness through reflective practices, examining their assessments to evaluate individuals. However, reflection generally critiques past events using critical evaluation methods, adjusts their decision making, and aligns with certain policies while also questioning and contesting others (Cook, 2024). OTPs must also engage in critical reflexiveness. This process involves practitioners adapting and adjusting to unfolding events by embracing openness, willingness to unlearn and learn, and demonstrating humility through their practice.

Within this framework, a dysfunctional approach emerges when OTPs excessively rely on deficit-based paradigms. OTPs often default to a "dysfunctional mindset" in their interactions. However, recognizing indicators of dysfunctional thinking, such as overreliance on deficit-based framing, is a crucial step toward growth and improvement. This realization can serve as a powerful motivator for change. This approach, which consistently frames interactions and supports around limitations rather than strengths, can hinder the progress of autistic individuals. In contrast, a holistic practice involves identifying issues requiring support and viewing them through the lens of autistic individuals' inherent strengths, abilities, and aspirations. By scrutinizing these tools and processes, OTPs can identify areas dominated by deficit-based thinking and strategize ways to shift toward a more balanced and strengths-focused approach. This shift enhances therapeutic effectiveness and fosters a more empowering and inclusive environment for autistic individuals.

Table 15.4 Supportive Practice of the Occupational Therapist

Effective Practice	Ineffective Practice
Provides intervention that supports the development of autistic individuals' goals, preferences, and interests	Does not provide services that support the development of autistic individuals' goals, preferences, and interests
Uses assessments that comprehensively identify autistic individuals' interests and preferences	Does not use assessments that comprehensively identify autistic individuals' interests and preferences
Once interests are identified, develop goals, and use support services that are centered around specific interests, and preferences	Fails to develop goals and uses support services that are centered around specific interests and preferences
Uses multiple means of engagement and observation to develop a communication system that can assist with revealing interests, preferences, and goals with both verbal and nonspeaking autistic individuals	Does not use multiple means of engagement and observation to develop a communication system that can assist with revealing interests, preferences, and goals with both verbal and nonspeaking autistic individuals
Facilitates autonomy by offering choice in activities that incorporate interests, and preferences	Does not facilitate autonomy by offering choice in activities that incorporate interests, and preferences
Provides services in a safe environment that supports the development of an autistic individual's strengths, interests, preferences, and goals	Does not provide services in a safe environment that supports the development of an autistic individual's strengths, interests, preferences, and goals

Environment Support

This continuum is related to the autistic individual's positioning within the environment and the reciprocal influences between the individual and the environment. OTPs should first assess the environment to determine whether it is high functioning or low functioning (Patten, 2022). The environment's functionality depends not on the autistic individual but on the environmental context, which includes physical and social environment. Spatial factors, organization of materials, reduction of clutter, use of visual supports, and foreground–background color match are components that impact the physical environment. Support from families, administration, teachers, related service providers, and employers constitute social environments (see Figure 15.1).

In a high-functioning environment, where the individual's needs are adequately met on an environmental and systemic level, it can be assumed that their well-being is supported. However, in a low-functioning environment that does not accommodate their strengths, abilities, and preferences, the harmony between well-being and motivation is disrupted. At the functional end of the continuum, the OTP focuses on optimizing the supportive environment for the autistic individual. This may involve fine-tuning existing structures and systems to better accommodate the individual's strengths, preferences, and needs. Additionally, the OTP may provide guidance and resources to enhance communication and collaboration among stakeholders, strengthening the individual's sense of safety and ability to engage effectively within their surroundings. Through this proactive approach, the OTP fosters an environment where autistic individuals can thrive and fully leverage their strengths to participate meaningfully in daily activities. A high-functioning environment also enables an autistic individual to thrive, as the language used to describe them will be according to their preferences and adopt anti-ableist terminologies (Table 15.5).

At the dysfunctional end of the continuum, barriers within the environment are described as hindering the autistic individual's well-being and participation. This could mean neglecting

Table 15.5 Indicators of Function: Environmental Support

Function (Strengths)	Dysfunction (Challenges)
Can identify environments that support their sensory needs (e.g., a high-functioning environment)	Cannot identify environments that support their sensory needs (e.g., poorly adapted environments)
Indicators of Function (Strengths)	**Indicators of Dysfunction (Challenges)**
Demonstrates strengths with support within a dysregulated environment	Does not demonstrate strengths even with support within a dysregulated environment
Seeks an environment that is physically and socially accessible, taking into account sensory sensitivities, communication differences, and/or mobility challenges	Does not seek an environment that is physically and socially accessible, neglecting considerations for sensory sensitivities, communication differences, and/or mobility challenges
Seeks accommodations such as sensory-friendly spaces, flexible work arrangements, and/or communication supports	Does not seek accommodations such as sensory-friendly spaces, flexible work arrangements, and communication supports
Supports collaboration and partnership, and recognizes that they are a key part of the decision-making process	Does not support collaboration and partnership, and fails to recognize themselves as a key part of the decision-making process
Offers feedback on how to improve the environment for their own needs	Does not offer feedback on how to improve the environment for their own needs
Advocates for their needs and environmental modifications, creating effective and high-functional environments	Does not advocate for their needs and environmental modifications, which would create effective and high-functional environments

to provide the required accommodations and support for autistic individuals. Examples might be ignoring the impact of an overwhelming sensory environment or failing to understand the importance of multiple means of communication, or supposing they neglect to address these environmental issues that contribute to "dysfunctionality." In that case, these unsafe environments may impede individuals' capacity to interact meaningfully with their surroundings. In a low-functioning environment, the language used to describe autistic individuals will be ableist or deficit based, highlighting their challenges (see Table 15.3).

Social Connection and Mutual Understanding

The social component of the DET is covered in the second continuum. At the dysfunctional end of the continuum, social situations between the OTP and the autistic individual are complicated by a lack of empathy and understanding. OTPs who are not autistic could view interactions with autistic individuals as less desirable, which could result in misinterpretations and misunderstandings. Because of this false perception, autistic individuals are often harshly judged and misunderstood, which can seriously harm their mental health. The disparity is further exacerbated by the non-autistic OTP's propensity to characterize autism as a lack of "theory of mind"—the inability to deduce the thoughts and feelings of others. This definition undervalues the distinct viewpoints and experiences of the autistic population.

Table 15.6 Indicators of Function: Social Connection and Mutual Understanding

Function (Strengths)	Dysfunction (Challenges)
The autistic individual and the therapist demonstrate connection and mutual understanding of each other, valuing each other's autonomy and competence	The autistic individual and the therapist do not demonstrate a connection or mutual understanding nor do they value each other's autonomy and competence
Indicators of Function (Strengths)	**Indicators of Dysfunction (Challenges)**
Feels recognized and valued as an individual	Does not feel recognized or valued as an individual
Does not feel pressured to conform to non-autistic social patterns (e.g., making eye contact when speaking)	Feels pressured to conform to non-autistic social patterns (e.g., making eye contact when speaking)
Feels accepted, safe, supported, and has a sense of belonging during the therapeutic process	Does not feel accepted, safe, supported, or a sense of belonging during the therapeutic process
Feels connected to their school or community environment	Feels disconnected from their school or community environment
Shares interests with others and is provided with opportunities to do so	Does not share interests with others and is not provided with opportunities to do so
Advocates for needs and environmental modifications	Does not know how to advocate for their needs, support, and environmental modifications

Despite empirical evidence demonstrating similarities in the quality and quantity of information exchanged between autistic and non-autistic individuals, non-autistic individuals still rate autistic individuals less favorably and are reluctant to interact with them (Chen et al., 2021; Milton et al., 2022). The OTP at the functional end of the continuum uses a strength-based approach influenced by DET to provide solutions for bridging the gap between social interactions by understanding the nature of social reciprocity in relationships. This approach places a heavy emphasis on recognizing and understanding the unique perspectives and experiences of autistic individuals in order to foster empathy and understanding among people, with a focus on the OTP changing their mindset and being agents of change (Table 15.6).

Stress

The third continuum pertains to societal factors and the additional stress experienced by autistic individuals, which extends beyond typical day-to-day stressors. At the dysfunctional end, the nuanced stressors experienced by autistic individuals within the framework of the minority stress model may not be recognized and addressed. This could result in a lack of understanding or acknowledgment of the impact of societal factors such as discrimination, stigma, bullying, indifference to their challenges, and a lack of representation of the mental health and well-being of autistic individuals. Additionally, individuals who fail to receive appropriate support and accommodations, or undermining or ignoring the stress may further marginalize or exacerbate the adverse effects of minority stress. This issue is compounded if the OTPs fail to provide appropriate sensory support for the individual (Table 15.7).

At the functional end of the continuum, autistic individuals are able to acknowledge and identify the unique pressures that they experience, including societal components like stigma and discrimination. Working alongside OTPs, other professionals, and community resources, autistic individuals will be able to develop strategies to lower stress and foster resilience.

Table 15.7 Indicators of Function: Stress

Function (Strength)	Dysfunction (Challenges)
Acknowledges and identifies strategies that help alleviate autism-related stressors	Unable to identify autism-related stressors and mitigating strategies
Collaborates with therapists to identify stressors and develop coping strategies tailored to their specific needs and preferences	Passively accept services without providing inputs or preferences, leading to resistance or disengagement
Advocates for systemic changes to reduce societal barriers and discrimination, such as advocating for inclusive policies and accessible measures	Remains passive in challenging societal norms and discrimination, perpetuating stressors
Fosters a supportive and validating therapeutic relationship, seeking a safe space for expression and exploration of emotions and experiences	Unable to establish supportive and validating relationship with therapists. Feelings of alienation and isolation
Able to develop self-awareness and self-advocacy skills with support	Unable to develop self-awareness and self-advocacy skills
Engage in mindfulness and relaxation techniques to regulate emotions and manage stress	Fails to engage in mindfulness and relaxation techniques to regulate emotions and manage stress
Addresses sensitivities and environmental stressors effectively	Does not address sensitivities or environmental stressors

Occupational Therapy Agency–Enhancing Practice

OTPs must embrace a reflective self-assessment and strategy to align their behaviors relevant to the evaluation and application to practice facilitating a strength-based approach for autistic individuals (refer back to Tables 15.1 and 15.4). OTPs can use Tables 15.1 and 15.3 to 15.5 as a reference to assess and consider where their actions fall on the continuum. Adopting a strength-based approach means developing habits that help to move away from a deficit mindset, in which the autistic individual is blamed, and toward an approach that weighs strengths and challenges about an individual's personhood as well as their experiences with autism.

GUIDE FOR EVALUATION

In a strength-based frame of reference, deliberate use, and careful selection of standardized and non-standardized evaluations are required. Standardized evaluations can both support and hinder strength-based practice for autistic individuals. On the one hand, they offer an organized and uniform framework for evaluating different facets of skills, which can aid in identifying areas of strength and improvement. Because these assessments frequently include established norms and benchmarks, OTs can use them to compare an individual's performance to that of a wider community and adjust their support plans accordingly. Standardized assessments can also yield important quantitative data that helps communicate with families and other professionals and track progress over time. Therefore, this section aims to guide OTs through reflective self-assessment, a necessary part of professional development, prompting significant adjustments in order to adopt a strength-based perspective (Table 15.8).

Table 15.8 Sample Assessments for a Strength-Based Evaluation

Assessment	Objectives/Contents	Strength-Based Information Provided
AIR Self-Determination Scale (Wolman et al., 1994)	Parent, teacher, and student forms that examine capacity and opportunity to apply knowledge, abilities, and perceptions to becoming self-determined	• Identify and express own needs, interests, and abilities • Set goals • Make choices and plans for goal achievement
Child Occupational Self-Assessment (Kramer et al., 2014)	Self-assessment of occupational competence and value of everyday activities in children	• Identify interests • Self-report on competence • Identify goal areas
Canadian Occupational Performance Measure (Law et al., 2014)	Self-endorsed goals and satisfaction related to occupational performance in youth and adults	• Self-determined goals that indicate autonomy and individual goal priorities
Behavioral and Emotional Rating Scale: A Strength-Based Approach to Assessment Scale, 2nd Edition (Epstein, 2004)	Self-evaluation of strengths for children aged 11–18 y Parent evaluation of strengths for children aged 5–18 y Addresses relatedness and competence	• Interpersonal strengths • Family involvement • Intrapersonal strengths • School functioning • Affective strength • Career Strength
The Survey of Favorite Interests and Activities (Smerbeck, 2017)	Identifies interests, including potential benefits of interests in competence development and relationship building specifically to the autistic population	• Adaptive Coping Subscale that looks at how interests foster happiness, emotional coping, and skill development
Self-Determination Inventory (Shogren & Wehmeyer, 2017)	Student report (SDI:SR) and parent/teacher report (SDI: PTR) measures designed for individuals aged 13–22, encompassing both those with and without disabilities	• Choice making • Goal setting • Decision making
Gallup's Clifton StrengthsFinder 2.0 (Rath, 2007)	Assessment of personal aptitude pinpoints the areas where an individual's highest potential for cultivating strengths lies. It is used to evaluate an individual's traits and natural talents. The 34 strength traits are categorized into four domains: executing, influencing, relationship building, and strategic thinking	• Provides top 10 themes to help integrate talents into a more informed view of self

We acknowledge that OT identities and beliefs are shaped by societal and cultural experiences, as these encounters can create implicit attitudes and assumptions, potentially leading to a fixed mindset and hindering change (Cook, 2024). OTs can question using two approaches: reflection and reflexiveness. A thorough reflection on one's beliefs, goals, and self-perceptions concerning one's practice can broaden one's viewpoints, which is an effective way to bring about learning changes.

However, it is crucial to remember that standardized assessments can miss the distinctive qualities and skills of autistic individuals. They are created using non-autistic norms, which might not fully take into consideration autism as well as the range of abilities, supportive needs, and skills among autistic individuals. This can lead to an incomplete or inaccurate assessment of an individual's capabilities, potentially resulting in services failing to leverage their strengths fully. Nonstandardized assessments, on the other hand, provide a distinct set of benefits for evaluating the needs and strengths of autistic individuals. The methods of informal assessments, interviews, and observations offer increased flexibility and adaptability, and produce detailed qualitative insights into an individual's preferences, interests, and skills in real-world situations. Incorporating information gaining from both standardized and nonstandardized assessments can help OTPs create individualized and successful treatments by fostering a more comprehensive understanding of an individual's strengths and weaknesses. For example, Kenworthy et al. (2022) noted that when they implemented the Behavior Rating Inventory of Executive Function (BRIEF) (2013) with autistic youth and their parents, parents rated their children's executive function (EF) challenges more significantly than what the youth themselves rated. While they both underscored cognitive flexibility as a challenge, youths were more considerate as they rated themselves more holistically by viewing their deficits in the light of their capabilities and adaptability. Hence, asking the youth directly enhances their knowledge and understanding of the EF challenges. In contrast, when open-ended approaches like the Engineering Design Process (https://www.sciencebuddies.org/science-fair-projects/engineering-design-process/engineering-design-process-steps, n.d.) are used, autistic youth feel more comfortable sharing their experiences related to problem-solving and EF challenges due to the flexible and adaptable nature of these approaches (Murthi & Patten, 2023).

Nonstandard evaluations lack generalizability but can be applied across different contexts. Comparing individual outcomes or monitoring progress over time with nonstandardized assessments may be challenging due to concerns about reliability and precision. Furthermore, administering and interpreting nonstandard evaluations may require more time and resources. However, when selected carefully and thoughtfully, both standardized and nonstandardized assessments can enhance strength-based practice. Promoting strengths-based support for autistic individuals may be best achieved through a well-rounded strategy that combines components of both assessment types.

So, how do OTPs characterize strengths and evaluate them systematically? Strengths vary from person to person. Saleebey (2001) identifies that there is an exhaustive list of strengths but outlines that "some capacities, resources, and assets do commonly appear on any roster of strengths" (p. 84). These strengths are summarized in Table 15.2, along with specific examples of autistic characteristics.

OTPs should select specific evaluations (as detailed in Table 15.8), as discussed later in this chapter, that target the identification and understanding of the individual's strengths in addition to assessing their support needs. This approach makes it easier to conduct a thorough assessment that highlights the individual's abilities, either on their own, independently, or in conjunction with standardized test scores. When writing the evaluation, OTPs should consider using strength-based language (Table 15.9) and identifying specific strengths and preferences, not solely based on the individual's deficits. Thus, the assessment, whether explicitly strength-based or informed by strengths, anchors its recommendations to the individual's inherent strengths (Cosden et al., 2006).

Strength-informed assessments that focus on the cognitive strengths of autistic individuals, can significantly impact the estimation of their cognitive potential, especially for those who are nonspeaking (Barbeau et al., 2013; Courchesne et al., 2015; Dawson et al., 2007). For instance, traditional IQ testing may lead to an overidentification of significant cognitive delays. However, by engaging an autistic individual's atypical autistic strengths, especially with older autistic children who speak minimally or not at all, strength-informed assessments can yield a more accurate indication of potential. For example, Courchesne et al., (2015) performed strength-informed assessments on 30 autistic children aged 6 to 12 years, who had little or no spoken language.

Table 15.9 Inclusive Language

Say This	Not This	Explanation
Autistic individual	Individuals with autism Individuals afflicted with autism	Using identity-first language is often favored for students with disabilities like autism. Research shows this choice is more respectful and helps avoid negative associations. Terms like "special needs" can be offensive and patronizing (Cokley, 2020). When unsure, ask the individual which term they prefer.
Students with Individualized Education Programs (IEPs), students with disabilities, or describe the student's educational needs	Special Education Students/ Special Needs Students, or Students with special needs	"Students with disabilities" is a comprehensive term that includes those with IEPs, 504 plans, and recognized disabilities without formal documentation. Person-first language promotes inclusivity and equality.
Student who uses a wheelchair	Wheelchair-bound, confined to a wheelchair	A student who uses a wheelchair relies on it for mobility, but they are not "confined" or limited by it.
Most inclusive environment	Least restrictive environment (LRE)*	This term emphasizes celebrating inclusion rather than battling restrictions.
More specialized settings	More restrictive environment (MRE)	This term highlights the extra help individuals receive to succeed in specialized settings, moving away from the idea of restriction.
d/Deaf or hard-of-hearing	Hearing impaired*	This terminology aligns with feedback from the d/Deaf and hard-of-hearing communities despite being inconsistent with regulatory language.
Students with emotional disabilities (EDs)	ED students/emotionally disturbed students/students with emotional disturbance	Many states have evolved from "emotional disturbance" to "emotional disability." Focus on describing specific supportive needs instead of potentially exclusive terms.
Students without IEPs	General Education Students*/ nondisabled peers*/typically developing peers	"Students without IEPs" is a more neutral, inclusive term acknowledging diverse growth and learning paths. Terms like "typically developing peers" can imply normalcy and exclusion, impacting a sense of belonging.
Discuss whether the student can access grade-level content with minimal academic support or whether the student is participating in standard or alternate assessments	High/low functioning typically developing	These subjective terms vary by perspective and fail to recognize unique strengths and support needs. Instead, focus on the specific support required.
In class or at a separate location as an alternative: For primary instruction or supplementary instruction	Push in/pull out	Using terms like "in class" or "separate location" avoids making students feel separated from peers and emphasizes the integration of OTPs and staff in the classroom.

(*continued*)

Table 15.9 Inclusive Language (Continued)

Say This	Not This	Explanation
More specialized settings	MRE	This term emphasizes the extra help received in specialized settings, moving away from the idea of restriction.
Describe the class needs of the individual	Self-contained class* Special Class*	"Self-contained class" suggests unnecessary separation from peers. Despite regulatory use, this term needs to be adjusted to avoid exclusion.
High-functioning environments, low-functioning environments, and inclusive environments	High-functioning student or low-functioning student	Terms like "high functioning" and "low functioning" fail to capture the diverse experiences within the autistic community. Describing the environment's support for individual needs is more constructive. Try focusing on the specific strengths, needs, and support needs of the individual (Bottema-Beutel et al., 2021)
Describe what the individual is doing	"Nonresponders" or "unresponsive students"	These terms imply that learning difficulties lie solely within the student, overlooking the possibility of ineffective intervention. Instead of labeling the student, focus on the effectiveness of the intervention and improving/adapting it.
Describe the behavior	Challenging behaviors Problem behaviors	Consider describing the specific behavior and the context in which it occurs and what it prevents the individual from doing.

Adapted from "Inclusive and Interdependent Language Initiative Glossary" by New York City Public Schools, 2024.

They compared their performance obtained from strength-informed assessments, which are more visually based, including *Raven's Colored Progressive Matrices* (Raven et al., 1998), the *Children's Embedded Figures Test* (Karp & Konstadt, 1963), and a visual search task with traditional intelligence testing such as the *Wechsler Intelligence Scale for Children,* 4th Edition (Wechsler, 2005). The study found that none of the autistic children were able to complete the *Wechsler Intelligence Scale for Children*, which would indicate a "low functioning" profile and limited cognitive potential, whereas all the typical children could complete the *Wechsler Intelligence Scale for Children,* 4th edition. In contrast, 26 autistic children completed the *Raven's Colored Progressive Matrices* and *Children's Embedded Figures Test*, and their performance was better compared to non-autistic peers (Courchesne et al., 2015). Even autistic students in the study who were not highly verbal outperformed in visual-based assessments compared to their non-autistic counterparts.

Similarly, another study conducted by Jaswal et al. (2024) examined autistic adults and adolescents who spoke little or nothing in terms of phrases. The findings suggest that nonspeaking autistic individuals can indeed acquire basic literacy skills. Through this study, they discovered that autistic individuals who are nonspeaking run the danger of being undervalued, as their lack of speech and other nontraditional behaviors and demeanors might lead to misconceptions about their abilities, including their ability to read and write. It was concluded that nonspeaking autistic individuals should be given access to written communication as an alternative to speech, with the proper training and assistance. This study underscores the importance of presuming competence in autistic individuals. Furthermore, considering the implications of Jaswal et al.'s findings, OTPs must advocate strongly for alternative and comprehensive assessments that integrate deeply into the individual, particularly for nonspeaking autistic individuals. These assessments are crucial for capturing the diverse nuances of autism and ensuring that the capabilities of autistic individuals are accurately recognized and supported.

Inadequate selection of assessments may underestimate autistic individual's abilities. As a member of school-based teams, OTPs should advocate for alternative assessments for their nonspeaking students, especially when psychological testing determines programming and educational pathways. Furthermore, OTPs can contribute to a strength-informed and ultimately strength-based evaluation by utilizing specific assessments and conducting observations that highlight autistic strengths. These strategies could offer insight into the child's strengths and potential avenues for development. OTPs can also use this opportunity to support students' self-advocacy and incorporate the students' perspectives of interests, preferences, and concerns when developing and implementing OTP support plans. Additionally, OTPs may observe the environment, activities, objects, interactions, and events that the autistic individual spends the most time with as an indicator of potential interests, including sensory interests (Figure 15.3). Refer back to Table 15.8 to identify specific assessments that OTPs can utilize in a strength-based evaluation.

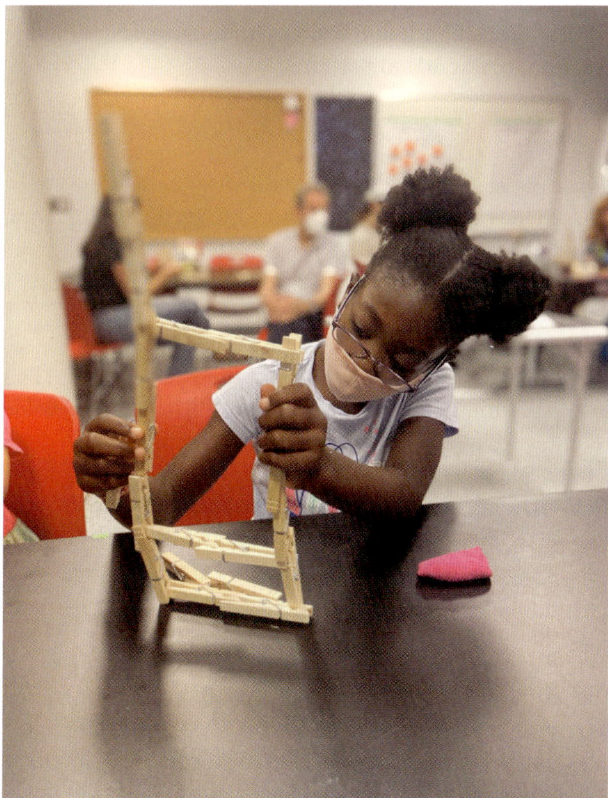

FIGURE 15.3 In occupational therapy, focusing on tasks without considering the individual's monotropic interests may overlook valuable opportunities for engagement and skill development. Therefore, therapy should strive to balance the need for task completion with the individual's interests, promoting both competence and well-being. (Courtesy of Dora Onwumere.)

POSTULATES REGARDING CHANGE

The autistic individual will feel a sense of belonging, safety, and connection if the OTP understands the autistic way of being and provides support that fosters mutual understanding, high-functioning environments, and encourages the individual's strengths.

General Postulates Regarding Change

Autistic individuals will experience a greater sense of safety, connection, identity, trust, and overall mental well-being when they have supportive environments, meaningful social connections, mutual understanding, and effective strategies to manage autism-related stress.

Specific Postulates Regarding Change

Environment Supports

The autistic individual can improve their overall well-being if they are supported in a high-functioning environment or in a socially and physically acceptable environment.

Social Connections and Mutual Understanding

The autistic individual can engage in social connection if there is mutual understanding when interacting with someone and they are supported in expressing themselves authentically without being pressured to conform to non-autistic social patterns.

Stress

The autistic individual can experience a sense of safety and belonging if they are provided with inclusive and affirming therapeutic environments and opportunities to develop coping strategies to manage autism-related stress.

APPLICATION TO PRACTICE

While it is true that autistic people face challenges in some of their activities, OTPs should avoid relying on assumptions about disabilities. Instead, OTPs should listen to the voices of autistic individuals and their families and work together by championing their voices to determine meaningful goals, as they are experts in their lives. The focus should be on supporting goals that are personally meaningful to the individual rather than trying to modify or replace behaviors just because they are labeled as "autistic." Instead, these actions should be considered based on how the individual lives and what they find meaningful to them. OTPs should actively collaborate with autistic individuals to understand the significance of their actions, daily activities, and goals.

OTPs can gain insights into the meanings behind specific behaviors or activities by engaging with the individual about their experiences and, if need be, seeking input from their families. Autistic individuals deserve the autonomy to engage in ways that feel comfortable for them. OTPs who are not autistic should strive to learn about the individuals' norms, values, rules, strengths, challenges, preferences, goals, and communication styles to provide adequate support (see Table 15.4). This aligns with a key tenet of OTP philosophy, which is culturally sensitive practice.

Ableist values, which are practices that subtly discriminate against people with disabilities, including autistic individuals (Patten, 2022), can significantly impact the quality of care provided by non-autistic OTPs. These biases, if not recognized and addressed, can lead to a deficit-based focus, where autism is viewed in terms of what individuals lack rather than their strengths and abilities. Imposing typical norms and expectations without considering the unique needs and preferences of autistic individuals, assuming one-size-fits-all approaches, and neglecting the individual's self-identity and strengths can also result from these values.

To address these ableist values, OTPs should practice cultural humility, approaching each individual with an open mind and valuing their unique experiences. Understanding how ableism affects service delivery is crucial, as it provides individualized care tailored to the autistic individual's specific needs and preferences. Embracing a strength-based perspective, focusing on the individual's strengths, and ensuring empowerment and autonomy in the therapeutic process can help mitigate the impact of ableist values. Specific strategies for recognizing and addressing ableist values in occupational therapy include regular self-reflection on personal biases, seeking feedback from autistic individuals and their families, and continuous learning about the experiences and needs of autistic individuals. These strategies can lead to more respectful and effective care for autistic individuals.

OTPs must reflect on how their understanding of norms aligns with or differs from each individual. Additionally, OTPs must be open and accommodating of different external and augmentative communication devices and strategies to support and enhance the autistic individual's preferred choice of communication rather than emphasizing normative standards of spoken language.

The OT services begin with the OTP reflecting on the values and interests of the autistic individual. OTPs foster a sense of self-determination by nurturing the development of independence rather than self-endorsed actions from an autistic perspective (Onwumere et al., 2021). OTPs should provide support to autistic individuals who develop competence by leveraging the individuals' strengths to build skills while also addressing areas where they require support. OTPs should assume competence with nonspeaking autistic individuals, use their interests to foster the development of competence, and use language that reframes some of the characteristics of autism as neutral or positive, not attempt to "fix" or make the autistic individual more "normal."

Incorporating neurodiversity-affirming practices, OTPs engage in self-reflection to highlight strengths and validate the identity of autistic individuals. Dallman et al. (2022) outlined the principles of neurodiversity-affirming practice, offering guidance for OTPs in their work with autistic individuals. As an illustration, OTPs are encouraged to shift their focus away from "challenging" behaviors such as meltdowns or aggressions. Instead, they can support individuals through coregulation and by identifying environmental triggers. This approach views these behaviors as possible responses to fight/flight mechanisms in low-functioning environments. Implementing sensory strategies can aid individuals return to a state of calm while also facilitating the identification and management of their emotions. Additionally, this approach acknowledges the potential differences in emotional experiences among autistic individuals.

Similarly, instead of aiming to reduce stimming behaviors, OTPs acknowledge the significance of self-stimulation as a valuable neurologic behavior for autistic individuals. Stimming serves multiple purposes, including providing enjoyment, aiding in information processing, and facilitating self-regulation. The OTP's role is to support individuals in engaging in nonharmful stimming activities while also exploring whether these behaviors may be linked to sensory discomfort or feelings of overwhelmingness, and making appropriate adjustments to the environment as needed.

When using the strength-based frame of reference with autistic individuals, OTPs must have a central focus that stems from their understanding of and the ability to address the particular strengths and challenges associated with autism: (1) The OTP recognizes the social difficulties and potential miscommunications that may occur, as well as the gap in mutual understanding and reciprocal interactions between autistic and non-autistic individuals; (2) the OTP applies a strength-based approach, utilizing the principles of the DET to encourage social interactions that respect the viewpoints and experiences of autistic individuals; (3) the OTP is mindful of the attentional patterns specific to autistic individuals, valuing intense focus and specialized interests; (4) to foster a sense of identity and self-control, the OTP enables the autistic individual to explore and engage with their interests independently; (5) the OTP uses strategies to address the additional stressors and challenges faced by autistic individual due to societal stigma and discrimination; and (6) the OTP advocates for inclusive environments that provide access to supportive services.

The OTP, who adopts a strength-based perspective for autistic individuals in their daily work, moves away from "normalization" supports and toward neurodiversity-celebrating services that highlight the person's strengths and abilities and foster autonomy, well-being, and self-acceptance. OTPs are prompted by this change in viewpoint to reflect on themselves and ask themselves questions regularly, such as:

- Does my evaluation and support strike a balance, focusing on strengths and weaknesses?
- Am I incorporating activities and choices that align with the individual's restricted interests?
- Am I assuming that the autistic individuals who cannot speak are competent?
- Am I assessing high-functioning environments?
- Am I advocating for and supporting the individual within the most inclusive environments?
- Am I actively working with other professionals to create universally understood and presumed competent communication systems?
- Am I seeing the interests of autistic individuals as cognitive assets and motivators instead of seeing them as maladaptive behaviors?
- Am I addressing the individual's difficulties while incorporating a strength-based approach?

There are many ways of thinking, doing, and reflecting that will allow the OTP to make this shift. Specific strategies to make this shift may include the following:

1. Focus interactions (parent–child, OTP–child) on enrichment and access to nonsocial interests as a goal of services versus focusing on developing typical social interaction as the goal (Mottron, 2017).
2. Nonacademic periods, such as lunchtime, recess, and after school, can offer structured, supported interaction around interests rather than the unstructured social time that autistic students can find stressful (Koegel et al., 2012).
3. Rather than employing a traditional social skills group focusing on discrete social abilities, an OTP would opt for an interest-based group where students are intrinsically motivated to engage. Participants possess a solid knowledge foundation in this setting, facilitating exploring connections, relationships, and social involvement, which inherently holds a deeper meaning and mutual understanding (Milton, 2012).
4. Utilize the individual's attentional profiles and concentrated interests in their learning environments, routines, and social dynamics (Murray et al., 2005). Adopt a creative mindset while integrating these hobbies, and use them to understand complex ideas and improve abilities.
5. Establish clear schedules that indicate when to explore hobbies and when to work on other assignments, while appreciating the student's requirement for deep concentration. This will help when a specific interest starts to interfere with class activities. These schedules

Table 15.10 Examples of Incorporating Interests Into School, Routines, and Relationships

Airplane interest	A child is interested in airplanes and has difficulty in math; there is plenty of mathematics involved in calculating distances, speeds, amount of time, etc., and when considering flight paths of airplanes. Where an airplane lands can be used to introduce subjects related to social studies. Similarly, comparing the need for careful scheduling of flights or maintenance of airplanes can be compared to the scheduling of the day, week, or another period for the student. Finally, this interest could be used as a topic of conversation in developing social interactions with others. For example, a protocol could be developed where one talks about their interests (in aviation) for a few minutes before handing over control of the subject matter to the other person by talking about their interest.
Train interest to the exclusion of all their interests	A student is fascinated with train schedules to the exclusion of other activities or topics of conversation. This interest can be used as a jumping-off point where, after a short time of discussion schedules, other questions can be introduced as "excursions" from the central topic of train schedules. Some possible "excursions" can include characteristics of various stations, time it takes to get between stations, the history of particular stations, what employment opportunities exist getting the train from one place to another, etc. Some students may become overwhelmed with anxiety when these conversation excursions become too long, so it may be necessary to return to the central topic of interest periodically. However, the time spent on these peripheral topics can slowly increase and may even generate new areas of interest and tap into unknown areas of strength.

Shore, S. (2013). *Keeping it real.* Retrieved from http://www.projectkeepitreal.com/

can be communicated by accommodating different attentional preferences and promoting inclusivity.

6. Echolalia, hyperlexia, and intense interests are related to information seeking and processing and should be encouraged (Mottron, 2017). These behaviors serve as pillars for fostering motivation and self-regulation of behavior. The OTP is urged to perceive special interests as meaningful activities that can enhance occupational performance. Table 15.10 offers illustrative examples of integrating these passionate interests into school routines and relationships.
7. Work with autistic ways of learning, not against them (Murray et al., 2005). Embrace and accommodate autistic learning styles instead of opposing them. For some individuals, maintaining eye contact may be distracting and not essential for comprehension. According to Mottron (2017), autistic individuals often exhibit a strong affinity for and proficiency in nonsocial language and interactions, which should be acknowledged and respected.

CASE EXAMPLES

The implementation of a strength-based frame of reference for individuals is presented in two case examples that represent aspects of autistic being. An OTP may have more difficulty applying this frame of reference because the individual's behaviors would be considered extremely challenging versus applying the frame of reference to a highly verbal elementary school student who has an interest in astronomy, for example. These two cases are presented intentionally to show how an OTP can apply this frame of reference to a wide range of autistic individuals. In addition to the case information, a key postulate regarding the change will be demonstrated within the case; that is, if the OTP shifts from deficit- to strength-based neurodiversity-affirming practice, then areas of engagement, competence, interests, and strengths will be valued and used to address challenging areas.

Remi

Remi, a 16-year-old nonbinary student at a specialized school for autistic individuals, is in a small classroom with a special education teacher and three paraprofessionals who are 1:1 aide for several students, including Remi. The OTP began to see Remi's strengths and abilities when they stopped framing Remi's experience through a deficit lens and instead adopted a strength-based approach to understand and support Remi's unique abilities. To contrast this perspective with a traditional approach, Remi will first be briefly described in terms of a deficit paradigm to illustrate to OTPs how they can, when shifting to a strength-based description, discuss a person's status without sacrificing the necessary information to plan an intervention.

Remi is *nonspeaking* and does not use gestures to communicate. They have a picture exchange system that they do not use consistently but can respond with *"yes," "no,"* and *"I need help, please."* Remi perseverates on electronics, including a Harry Potter book on the iPad that they listen to on the bus ride to school, and gets extremely agitated and aggressive when staff tries to remove the headphones when they arrive in their classroom. Remi frequently engages in repetitive and restricted behavior, especially around the videos that are brought from home of a football game are being announced. This behavior interferes with Remi's daily routines, as they get very agitated if they cannot watch the videos first thing in the morning. Remi is dependent on most activities of daily living, especially dressing and grooming. They do not communicate verbally, but the staff reports that they are aware of their environment and appear to be very observant before acting out in their classroom. Remi would often drop to the floor and not continue walking with their class when they were moving throughout the building. Staff would then be called in to walk with them on either side until they got to their destination.

The above represents a typical introductory paragraph that would be seen in a standard OT evaluation. When adopting a strength-based paradigm, the words and framing matter from the very first interaction with families, children, and adults. To contrast the above description, strength-based language is utilized not only to describe Remi more accurately but also to begin to uncover strengths and abilities that may be autistic specific.

Remi can understand directions, especially those related to their preferred activities, including watching television. Further discussion with Remi's mother and staff identified that they spent most of their days, whether at home or at school, engaged in watching television and listening to the same audiobook over and over again, an audio version of a *Harry Potter* book. The OTP explores Remi's preferences for television viewing with their mother in-depth, and she identifies that Remi always wanted to keep the television on the channel that showed the mass or religious programming. They get upset whenever someone attempts to change the channel, especially when an Irish priest is speaking, which they enjoy. Additionally, Remi would rewind the TV of sports announcers who were calling a Monday night football game and would do this repetitively, becoming upset if they had to switch activities. They were very accurate in rewinding these videos, and they would rewind to the point where the three male announcers were chatting back and forth with unique voices. For communication, Remi uses a simple board with responses, including "yes," "no," and "help," which they use with 100% accuracy. They use this board very quickly and often with a sense of humor, replying "yes" or "no" incorrectly as they smile and laugh.

From this contrast in describing Remi, OTPs begin to see abilities that may not have been evident if they looked solely at Remi's challenges. For example, they are drawn to male voices that have different accents, attending to and listening to Harry Potter books on iPad, which are complex, stopping to watch a man with an Irish brogue speak and sports announcers with distinctive dialects and a common theme. They spend a significant amount of time doing this type of activity. By carefully observing what Remi does with their time, if given a choice, the OTP can begin to understand Remi's preferences and likes. By evaluating who they are holistically and identifying their strengths and challenges, the OTP can begin to identify specific and detailed strengths and challenges in the assessment process.

Remi's preference for specific audio, such as listening to a Harry Potter audiobook on their iPad and rewinding videos of sports announcers on TV, provides insight into their unique attentional profile and interests, which aligns with the principles of monotropism theory. Remi's extreme interest in a specific audio piece indicates their monotropic attentional style, in which they find that particular auditory stimuli significantly increase their engagement and enjoyment. In Remi's case, intense interest in specific audio content reflects their monotropic attentional style, where they derive significant pleasure and engagement from specific auditory stimuli. This preference for certain sounds and voices demonstrates their distinct cognitive processing style, characterized by deep immersion and fascination with certain auditory experiences.

In addition, their ability to precisely rewind and interact with these audio sources demonstrates their proficiency with technology and media content navigation. A neurodiversity-affirming viewpoint acknowledges Remi's special interests as significant and valuable expressions of their individuality and interests instead of seeing them as weaknesses. The OTP can capitalize on Remi's preferences for particular audio content to boost engagement, improve communication, and encourage autonomy by noting and implementing these preferences into their services. This method celebrates Remi's neurodiversity and validates their unique abilities while promoting their independence and general well-being.

The DET draws attention to the possibility of miscommunication and misinterpretations while interaction occurs between autistic and non-autistic individuals. Since Remi is nonspeaking and uses a photo exchange system and a communication board, even with these methods of communication, it can still be difficult for Remi to express their feelings and ideas in a way that a non-autistic individual can understand. This lack of mutual understanding may make Remi feel more alone and frustrated. The OTP, staff, and families can approach their interactions with empathy and understanding, acknowledging the role of the DEP. This will help close the communication gap and create meaningful connections based on mutual respect and acceptance of differences in social dispositions. Using this strategy is in line with neurodiversity-affirming approaches, which emphasize respecting and appreciating the variety of ways people connect with one another and the outside world.

In Remi's case, the minority stress model offers valuable insights into the challenges they may face as an autistic individual navigating a predominantly non-autistic world. Remi's experiences of being nonspeaking and relying on alternative forms of communication, such as a picture exchange system, may subject them to social and environmental stressors stemming from a lack of understanding and accommodation for their communication needs. The frustration and agitation they exhibit when staff attempts to remove their headphones or interfere with their preferred activities suggest potential sources of stress related to sensory sensitivities and special interests. Remi's dependence on others for activities of daily living, such as dressing and grooming, may contribute to feelings of disempowerment and social exclusion, further exacerbating their stress levels. Additionally, their engagement in "repetitive and restricted behaviors," while meaningful to them, may be perceived as socially deviant or abnormal by others, leading to increased stigma and discrimination. By applying the principles of the minority stress model, the OTP can recognize the systemic barriers and social inequalities that impact Remi's well-being and occupational participation. Therapeutic services can mitigate these stressors by promoting acceptance, fostering a supportive environment, and advocating for accommodations that honor Remi's independence and unique needs, including updating communication methods. For example, support for Remi may include sensory modulation strategies to manage sensory overload, engagement in coping strategies to promote self-advocacy skills in order to communicate preferences and boundaries, and facilitating social inclusion through peer education and awareness-building activities.

In the assessment and subsequent services to foster independence, the OT must evaluate whether they have predominantly focused on remedying Remi's challenges or embraced and capitalized on their strengths. Many assessments tend to emphasize deficits without adequately acknowledging areas of competence, limiting the effectiveness of service provision. The OTP must adopt neurodiversity-affirming practices to transcend this limited perspective, particularly for individuals like Remi. If the OTP adopts a strength-based perspective, it becomes easier to identify areas of competence within the case that can be utilized to address challenging areas. These include:

- can effectively use nonverbal cues to communicate with others.
- can easily pick up on the emotional state of another person.
- intense focus and absorption in activities.
- can become totally absorbed in an activity.
- enjoys learning about different cultural traditions.
- enjoys listening to audiobooks or to someone telling a story.
- is sensitive to the visual world around them.
- enjoys listening to music.
- is proficient in setting up and operating audiovisual or computer equipment.
- can express their preferences and assert their choices in certain contexts.
- knows how to set up audiovisual or computer equipment.

This list of potential strengths can provide a good starting point for support to build upon these strengths and utilize them to address behaviors. Although it requires more observational skill and interpretation of these observations to reveal strengths and interests in a nonspeaking individual, once found, they are powerful ways to support and begin to develop a sense of autonomy, mutual understanding, and independence.

Annie

Annie is a 5-year-old girl in a general education kindergarten classroom. She was diagnosed with autism at 30 months old and has received early intervention services since she was 2, when her parents became concerned about her limited social engagement with peers, siblings, and adults. Annie is hyperlexic, and very verbal; she has been reading since she was 3 years old. She is interested in maps and directions and often spends time on the computer exploring the locations of different fast-food restaurants using Google Earth. When riding in the car, Annie directs the driver on which roads to take and often becomes agitated and anxious if there is road construction, if her parents take a different route, or if there is an unplanned stop. She repeatedly asks her teachers at school about their addresses and then gives directions from the school to their homes. In response, her classroom teacher has initiated a behavior plan that rewards her with computer time when she refrains from asking questions about maps or directions, a strategy supported by all school team members. Annie also demonstrates hyperresponsiveness to auditory and visual stimuli; she often covers her ears during the school day, and has been known to yell at her classmates, saying "Keep it down. I am reading." She is easily distracted by unpredictable changes in her environment, including new classroom materials and decorations. Based on these behaviors, the school psychologist recommended an OT evaluation to assess her self-regulation, sensory processing, and participation in the general education curriculum.

Standardized testing using the *Sensory Processing Measure-2* (Parham et al., 2013) revealed that Annie received a rating of "definite difference" in vision, touch, hearing, and planning and ideas. This indicates that she needed external support to participate with significant awareness and attention within her learning environment. She also received a rating of "probable difference" in social participation, as well as balance and motion. Structured clinical observations were conducted within the school context to assess Annie's self-regulation, social communication, play skills, and participation in classroom activities. Annie's teacher has reported that her primary concerns in the classroom include keeping Annie engaged in classroom activities and managing her overall negative interactions with peers. During circle time and table activities, Annie often leaves the circle or the activity to trace her finger over long words found in materials hanging up in the classroom. She requires prompting to complete most tasks.

Observations of play and social participation on the playground revealed limited interaction with both playground equipment and her peers. Annie often sits by herself on the playground or tries to engage the adult recess monitor in conversation about where they live and how to get there. From a neurodiversity perspective, which emphasizes affirming strengths, the OTP can further develop areas of independence and address challenging areas. The information gathered in this case highlights several key areas for focus, which include:

- enjoys working independently.
- can pay close attention to details.
- has a good short-term and long-term memory.
- enjoys reading books.
- can read maps well.
- reports being able to visualize images clearly.
- gets information more easily through pictures than words.
- is sensitive to the visual world around her.
- has a good sense of direction.
- is curious about the world around her.
- likes to spend time using a computer, tablet, or smartphone.
- has good reading comprehension.
- has a large vocabulary.
- can become absorbed in an activity.

The DET plays a significant role in Annie's interactions with others, particularly her peers. Annie's hyperlexia and intense interest in maps and directions may lead to communication and socialization challenges with non-autistic individuals who do not share her specific interests or communication style. From the DET's perspective, non-autistic individuals may need help understanding Annie's unique way of processing information and engaging with the world. They may misinterpret her behaviors, such as her intense focus on maps or her hyperresponsiveness to sensory stimuli, as odd or disruptive, leading to negative interactions or misunderstandings. Similarly, Annie may struggle to relate to her non-autistic peers and understand their social cues or communication styles. This lack of mutual understanding can contribute to feelings of isolation or frustration for Annie, as she may struggle to connect with her classmates on a social level.

In Annie's case study, monotropism theory provides insights into her intense interests and focused attention on specific topics, such as maps and directions. Annie's hyperlexia and keen interest in maps and directions align with the characteristics of monotropism. Her early reading abilities and fascination with geographical information suggest a strong preference for specific topics and a tendency to engage in repetitive behaviors related to those interests. Annie's behavior of becoming agitated and anxious when faced with changes in her environment, such as road construction or deviations from planned routes, can be understood through the lens of monotropism. Autistic individuals often find comfort and predictability in routine and familiarity, and disruptions to their preferred activities or environments can evoke strong emotional reactions.

Overall, Annie shows strong interest in areas currently viewed as interfering. However, these interests could be incorporated into classroom routines and help facilitate her participation and engagement in class activities. For example, circle time could use squares where students identify what "country" or "state" they are sitting on and then come up and find it on a globe. Turn taking and listening to others could be facilitated. Providing a map of her day could provide predictability and structure. A "parking lot" for Annie's focused interests could be used to drive the interests over to the parking lot when transitioning to a new activity. Finally, Annie shows incredibly high competence in reading and map skills. How can these competence areas be increased with independent work, pairing with older students in the school, reading clubs, extra library time, etc.? The frustration for children like Annie often arises when teachers and OTPs (1) view these interests as problematic and then (2) subsequently control their use in reward systems only without integrating them into the general education curriculum as a vehicle for learning, regulation, and participation. These are Annie's preferred interests, passions, or meaningful occupations. By shifting to a strength-based frame of reference, an OTP can and should use Annie's strengths to develop an appropriate supportive program.

The minority stress model sheds light on the potential extra stresses and difficulties Annie, an autistic person living in a non-autistic environment, may encounter in her case study. Annie's dependence on outside assistance—such as her computer time behavior plan and her requirement for reminders to finish tasks—may indicate how minority stress affects her capacity for self-control and independent environmental navigation. Annie may encounter obstacles to her complete inclusion and participation in her educational environment if she needs outside assistance to engage in classroom activities. The minority stress model emphasizes how critical it is to identify and solve the extra stress and difficulties that autistic people, such as Annie, have in regular classroom environments. Teachers and OTPs should endeavor to create more inclusive and supportive environments that fit

Annie's specific needs and strengths by understanding the impact of minority stress on her well-being.

OTPs can use a strength-based frame of reference in parallel with other frames of reference that address areas of challenge common in autism. By adopting a strength-based approach focused on fostering independence, enhancing mutual understanding, supporting individual interests, addressing autistic stress beyond typical stressors, and acknowledging the profound influence of the environment on well-being, OTPs can effectively align themselves as allies of the autistic community, a pivotal stakeholder in the therapeutic process. In addition, utilization of strength and interests can help mitigate anxiety (Courchesne et al., 2020; Patten Koenig & Hough Williams, 2017) and generate feelings of well-being, which may ultimately have a positive impact on the quality of life (Pizzi & Richards, 2017; Smerbeck, 2017).

SUPPORTING EVIDENCE

The theoretical base for a strength-based frame of reference for autistic individuals is grounded in the DET, the monotropism theory, and the minority stress model. Adhering to this framework promotes practices that affirm neurodiversity, foster mutual understanding, support individual interests, and address autism-related stressors (Meyer, 2003; Milton, 2012; Murray et al., 2005). Jones et al. (2023) studied how non-autistic adults viewed interactions between autistic and non-autistic individuals. They found that non-autistic participants were more positively perceived when interacting with non-autistic partners, while interactions involving autistic partners were rated less favorably. Mixed interactions were seen as the least successful. Non-autistic adults tended to disclose more to non-autistic partners and rated autistic participants more negatively than the participants themselves did. These results highlight the DET in social interactions involving autistic individuals.

Nowell et al. (2021) conducted a pilot study on the Special Interest Survey with 1,992 autistic children. They found that the most common special interests identified were television, objects, and music. These interests could foster expertise and knowledge acquisition, motivating children to seek information through various channels. Such interests may stem from perceptual neurodevelopmental differences (Mottron, 2017). Additionally, special interests in autistic individuals can offer avenues for social interaction, connection, and well-being (Grove et al., 2018; Klin et al., 2007; Koenig & Williams, 2017). Previous research has shown that special interests facilitate social interactions, generate positive emotions, provide coping strategies, build skills for future employment, and enhance overall well-being (Grove et al., 2018; Jordan & Caldwell-Harris, 2012; Koenig & Williams, 2017; Stratis & LeCavalier, 2013; Teti et al., 2016; Trembath et al., 2012; Winter-Messiers, 2007). A survey of autistic adults revealed that the majority (96.2%) believed special interests should be encouraged in children, citing positive outcomes in their own lives (Koenig & Williams, 2017). Focusing on special interests can increase participation in school and work activities.

Botha and Frost (2020) explored the application of the minority stress model in a study involving 111 autistic adults, focusing on general psychological well-being as the outcome variable. The results showed mixed applicability of the model. While experiences of discrimination and harassment predicted lower levels of psychological well-being as expected, the study revealed that "outness" about one's autism, or publicly identifying as autistic, was also associated with poorer psychological well-being. This finding contrasts somewhat with the minority stress model's expectations, as greater outness would typically be linked with reduced self-stigma and psychological distress. The authors hypothesized that increased outness might lead to heightened perceptions of difference, resulting in increased harassment and discrimination against autistic individuals (Botha & Frost, 2020). Autistic adults have reported that having accepting spaces and communities where they can authentically express themselves reduces burnout and associated psychological distress (Raymaker et al., 2020). Cooper et al. (2017) discovered that autistic social identification served as a protective factor against depression and anxiety, with a positive relationship between autistic social identification and personal self-esteem mediated by collective self-esteem. Another study found that stronger feelings of social identification with other autistic individuals correlated with better mental well-being (Maitland et al., 2021). Therefore, to mitigate minority stress and enhance autistic well-being, adopting the neurodiversity paradigm as the foundation for all therapies and supports is essential.

> I think the benefits of encouraging special interests outweigh their liabilities. To do otherwise is to insist on normalizing an innate behavior pattern that can only cause stress and detract from the originality of the Aspie's life (it's hard to overemphasize the importance of avoiding stress and anxiety). Special interests can be a motivator or a catalyst to learn social, organizational, and communicative skills. ... having finally the ability and the understanding now at age 52 to pursue my special interests – primarily furniture making, luthiery, and motorcycles – I appreciate that following them is when I am most myself. This may sound "autistic," but like writing poetry or playing the violin, they are the expression of my mind's working and are worth doing in themselves.

Source unknown

> "As an autistic individual, I frequently discover that the double empathy theory significantly impacts my social interactions. It's not only that I want to understand non-autistic folks; I want them to understand me. To make matters more difficult, my propensity for intense concentration on certain interests, like baseball stats and history facts, is occasionally misinterpreted, interpreted, or disregarded by others. The stress of being autistic in a non-autistic world can be overwhelming due to the need to fit in and the lack of acceptance. I prefer a world that promotes genuine acceptance and inclusion for everyone; society must acknowledge and address these issues."

Source unknown

REFERENCES

Alkhaldi, R. S., Sheppard, E., & Mitchell, P. (2019). Is there a link between autistic people being perceived unfavorably and having a mind that is difficult to read? *Journal of Autism and Developmental Disorders*, *49*(10), 3973–3982. https://doi.org/10.1007/s10803-019-04101-1

Alkhaldi, R. S., Sheppard, E., Burdett, E., & Mitchell, P. (2021). Do neurotypical people like or dislike autistic people? *Autism in Adulthood: Challenges and Management, 3*(3), 275–279. https://doi.org/10.1089/aut.2020.0059

Barbeau, E. B., Soulières, I., Dawson, M., Zeffiro, T. A., & Mottron, L. (2013). The level and nature of autistic intelligence III: Inspection time. *Journal of Abnormal Psychology*, *122*(1), 295–301. https://doi.org/10.1037/a0029984

Blommaert, J. (2005). *Discourse: A critical introduction*. Cambridge University Press.

Botha, M., & Frost, D. M. (2020). Extending the minority stress model to understand mental health problems experienced by the autistic population. *Society and Mental Health*, *10*(1), 20–34. https://doi.org/10.1177/2156869318804297

Bottema-Beutel, K., Kapp, S. K., Lester, J. N., Sasson, N. J., & Hand, B. N. (2021). Avoiding ableist language: suggestions for autism researchers. *Autism in Adulthood*, *3*(1), 18–29. https://doi.org/10.1089/aut.2020.0014

Bottema-Beutel, K., LaPoint, S. C., Kim, S. Y., Mohiuddin, S., Yu, Q., & McKinnon, R. (2023). An evaluation of intervention research for transition-age autistic youth. *Autism*, *27*(4), 890–904. https://doi.org/10.1177/13623613221128761

Bottema-Beutel, K., Sasson, N. J., McKinnon, R., Braun, C., Guo, R., Hand, B. N., Kapp, S. K., Espinas, D. R., Bailin, A., Lester, J. N., & Yu, B. (2024). Recognizing and resisting ableist language in schools: Suggestions for School-based speech-language pathologists and related professionals. *Language, Speech, and Hearing Services in Schools, 55*(4), 1025–1038. https://doi.org/10.1044/2024_LSHSS-24-00036

Bury, S. M., Jellett, R., Spoor, J. R., & Hedley, D. (2023). "It Defines Who I Am" or "It's Something I Have": What Language Do [Autistic] Australian Adults [on the Autism Spectrum] Prefer? *Journal of Autism and Developmental Disorders*, *53*(53), 677–687. https://doi.org/10.1007/s10803-020-04425-3

Camus, L., Macmillan, K., Rajendran, G., & Stewart, M. W. (2022). "I too, need to belong": Autistic adults' perspectives on misunderstandings and well-being. *PsyArXiv*. https://doi.org/10.31234/osf.io/5mysh

Chapman, R. (2019). Autism as a form of life: Wittgenstein and the psychological coherence of autism. *Metaphilosophy*, *50*(4), 421–440. https://doi.org/10.1111/meta.12366

Chapman, R. (2021). *Negotiating the neurodiversity concept|Psychology today*. https://www.psychologytoday.com/us/blog/neurodiverse-age/202108/negotiating-the-neurodiversity-concept

Chen, Y.-L., Schneider, M., & Patten, K. (2022). Exploring the role of interpersonal contexts in peer relationships among autistic and non-autistic youth in integrated education. *Frontiers in Psychology*, *13*, 946651. https://doi.org/10.3389/fpsyg.2022.946651

Chen, Y.-L., Senande, L. L., Thorsen, M., & Patten, K. (2021). Peer preferences and characteristics of same-group and cross-group social interactions among autistic and non-autistic adolescents. *Autism*, *25*(7), 1885–1900. https://doi.org/10.1177/13623613211005918

Cokley, R. (2020, February 28). Why "special needs" is not helpful. *Medium*. https://rebecca-cokley.medium.com/why-special-needs-is-1959e2a6b0e

Cook, A. (2024). Conceptualisations of neurodiversity and barriers to inclusive pedagogy in schools: A perspective article. *Journal of Research in Special Educational Needs*, *24*(3), 627–636. https://doi.org/10.1111/1471-3802.12656

Cooper, K., Smith, L. G. E., & Russell, A. (2017). Social identity, self-esteem, and mental health in autism. *European Journal of Social Psychology*, *47*(7), 844–854. https://doi.org/10.1002/ejsp.2297

Cosden, M., Koegel, L. K., Koegel, R. L., Greenwell, A., & Klein, E. (2006). Strength-based assessment for children with autism spectrum Disorders. *Research and Practice for Persons with Severe Disabilities*, *31*(2), 134–143. https://doi.org/10.1177/154079690603100206

Courchesne, V., Langlois, V., Gregoire, P., St-Denis, A., Bouvet, L., Ostrolenk, A., & Mottron, L. (2020). Interests and strengths in autism, useful but misunderstood: a pragmatic case-study. *Frontiers in Psychology*, *11*, 569339. https://doi.org/10.3389/fpsyg.2020.569339

Courchesne, V., Meilleur, A.-A. S., Poulin-Lord, M.-P., Dawson, M., & Soulières, I. (2015). Autistic children at risk of being underestimated: school-based pilot study of a strength-informed assessment. *Molecular Autism*, *6*(1), 12. https://doi.org/10.1186/s13229-015-0006-3

Crompton, C. J., Ropar, D., Evans-Williams, C. V., Flynn, E. G., & Fletcher-Watson, S. (2020). Autistic peer-to-peer information transfer is highly effective. *Autism*, *24*(7), 1704–1712. https://doi.org/10.1177/1362361320919286

Dallman, A. R., Williams, K. L., & Villa, L. (2022). Neurodiversity-affirming practices are a moral imperative for occupational therapy. *The Open Journal of Occupational Therapy*, *10*(2), 1–9. https://doi.org/10.15453/2168-6408.1937

Dawson, M., Soulières, I., Gernsbacher, M. A., & Mottron, L. (2007). The level and nature of autistic intelligence. *Psychological Science*, *18*(8), 657–662. https://doi.org/10.1111/j.1467-9280.2007.01954.x

Dunn, D. S., & Andrews, E. E. (2015). Person-first and identity-first language: Developing psychologists' cultural competence using disability language. *American Psychologist*, *70*(3), 255–264. https://doi.org/10.1037/a0038636

Epstein, M. H. (2004). *Behavioral and emotional rating scale: A strength-based approach to assessment* (2nd ed.). PRO-Ed.

Fletcher-Watson, S. (2022). Transdiagnostic research and the neurodiversity paradigm: commentary on the transdiagnostic revolution in neurodevelopmental disorders by Astle et al. *Journal of Child Psychology and Psychiatry*, *63*(4), 418–420. https://doi.org/10.1111/jcpp.13589

Gernsbacher, M. A. (2017). Editorial perspective: the use of person-first language in scholarly writing may accentuate stigma. *Journal of Child Psychology and Psychiatry*, *58*(7), 859–861. https://doi.org/10.1111/jcpp.12706

Grove, R., Hoekstra, R. A., Wierda, M., & Begeer, S. (2018). Special interests and subjective wellbeing in autistic adults. *Autism Research, 11*(5), 766–775. https://doi.org/10.1002/aur.1931

Hatzenbuehler, M. L. (2009). How does sexual minority stigma "get under the skin"? A psychological mediation framework. *Psychological Bulletin, 135*(5), 707–730. https://doi.org/10.1037/a0016441

Jaswal, V. K., Lampi, A. J., & Stockwell, K. M. (2024). Literacy in nonspeaking autistic people. *Autism. 28*(10), 2503–2514. https://doi.org/10.1177/13623613241230709

Jones, D. R., Botha, M., Ackerman, R. A., King, K. M., & Sasson, N. J. (2023). Non-autistic observers both detect and demonstrate the double empathy problem when evaluating interactions between autistic and non-autistic adults. *Autism*, 28(8), 2053–2065. https://doi.org/10.1177/13623613231219743

Jordan, C. J., & Caldwell-Harris, C. L. (2012). Understanding differences in neurotypical and autism spectrum special interests through internet forums. *Intellectual and Developmental Disabilities, 50*(5), 391–402. https://doi.org/10.1352/1934-9556-50.5.391

Karp, S. A., & Konstadt, N. L. (1963). Manual for the children's embedded figures test. In *Manual for the children's embedded figures test.* Consulting Psychologists Press.

Kenny, L., Hattersley, C., Molins, B., Buckley, C., Povey, C., & Pellicano, E. (2016). Which terms should be used to describe autism? Perspectives from the UK autism community. *Autism, 20*(4), 442–462. https://doi.org/10.1177/1362361315588200

Kenworthy, L., Verbalis, A., Bascom, J., daVanport, S., Strang, J. F., Pugliese, C., Freeman, A., Jeppsen, C., Armour, A. C., Jost, G., Hardy, K., & Wallace, G. L. (2022). Adding the missing voice: How self-report of autistic youth self-report on an executive functioning rating scale compares to parent report and that of youth with attention deficit hyperactivity disorder or neurotypical development. *Autism, 26*(2), 422–433. https://doi.org/10.1177/13623613211029117

Klin, A., Danovitch, J. H., Merz, A. B., & Volkmar, F. R. (2007). Circumscribed interests in higher functioning individuals with autism spectrum disorders: an exploratory study. *Research and Practice for Persons with Severe Disabilities, 32*(2), 89–100. https://doi.org/10.2511/rpsd.32.2.89

Koegel, R. L., Fredeen, R., Kim, S., Danial, J., Rubinstein, D., & Koegel, L. (2012). Using perseverative interests to improve interactions between adolescents with autism and their typical peers in school settings. *Journal of Positive Behavior Interventions, 14*(3), 133–141. https://doi.org/10.1177/1098300712437043

Kramer, J., Velden, M. T, Kafkes, A., Basu, S., Federico, J., & Kielhofner, G. (2014). *Child occupational self-assessment* (2.2 ed.). Model of Human Occupation Clearinghouse.

Law, M., Baptiste, S., Carswell, A., McColl, M. A., Polatajko, H., & Pollock, N. (2014). *Canadian occupational performance measure* (5th ed.). CAOT Publications.

Maitland, C. A., Rhodes, S., O'Hare, A., & Stewart, M. E. (2021). Social identities and mental well-being in autistic adults. *Autism, 25*(6), 1771–1783. https://doi.org/10.1177/13623613211004328

Meyer, I. H. (2003). Prejudice, social stress, and mental health in lesbian, gay, and bisexual populations: conceptual issues and research evidence. *Psychological Bulletin, 129*(5), 674–697. https://doi.org/10.1037/0033-2909.129.5.674

Milton, D. E. M. (2012). On the ontological status of autism: the "double empathy problem." *Disability & Society, 27*(6), 883–887. https://doi.org/10.1080/09687599.2012.710008

Milton, D. E. M., Waldock, K. E., & Keates, N. (2023). Autism and the "double empathy problem." In F. Mezzenzana, & D. Peluso (Eds.), *Conversations on empathy: Interdisciplinary perspectives on imagination and radical othering*. Taylor & Francis.

Milton, D., Gurbuz, E., & Lopez, B. (2022). The "double empathy problem": Ten years on. *Autism, 26*(8), 1901–1903. https://doi.org/10.1177/13623613221129123

Mottron, L. (2017). Should we change targets and methods of early intervention in autism, in favor of a strengths-based education? *European Child & Adolescent Psychiatry, 26*(7), 815–825. https://doi.org/10.1007/s00787-017-0955-5

Murray, D., Lesser, M., & Lawson, W. (2005). Attention, monotropism and the diagnostic criteria for autism. *Autism, 9*(2), 139–156. https://doi.org/10.1177/1362361305051398

Murthi, K., Chen, Y.-L., Shore, S., & Patten, K. (2023). Strengths-based practice to enhance mental health for autistic people: a scoping review. *The American Journal of Occupational Therapy*, 77(2), 7702185060. https://doi.org/10.5014/ajot.2023.050074

Murthi, K., & Patten, K. (2023). Improving executive functions using the engineering design process: a peer-mediated problem-solving approach for autistic adolescents. *The American Journal of Occupational Therapy*, 77(2), 7702347010. https://doi.org/10.5014/ajot.2023.050166

Natri, H. M., Chapman, C. R., Heraty, S., Dwyer, P., Walker, N., Kapp, S. K., Dron, H. A., Martínez-Agosto, J. A., Mikkola, L., & Doherty, M. (2023). Ethical challenges in autism genomics: recommendations for researchers. *European Journal of Medical Genetics, 66*(9), 104810–104810. https://doi.org/10.1016/j.ejmg.2023.104810

New York City Public Schools (2024.) *A systems level guide to the language we use when we speak about students with IEPs and the programs and services they receive*. https://pwsblobprd.schools.nyc/prd-pws/docs/default-source/default-document-library/special-education/nycps-iili-glossary.pdf?sfvrsn=59fe3b08_8. Retrieved December 2024.

Nowell, K. P., Bernardin, C. J., Brown, C., & Kanne, S. (2021). Characterization of special interests in autism spectrum disorder: A brief review and pilot study using the special interests survey. *Journal of Autism and Developmental Disorders, 51*(8), 2711–2724. https://doi.org/10.1007/s10803-020-04743-6

Onwumere, D. D., Cruz, Y. M., Harris, L. I., Malfucci, K. A., Seidman, S., Boone, C., & Patten, K. (2021). The impact of an independence curriculum on self-determination and function in middle school autistic students. *Journal of Occupational Therapy, Schools, and Early Intervention, 14*(1), 103–117, https://doi.org/10.1080/19411243.2020.1799904

Parham, D. L., Ecker, C. L., Kuhaneck, H., Henry, D. A., & Glennon, T. J. (2013). *Sensory Processing Measure, Second Edition (SPM-2)*. Western Psychological Services.

Patten Koenig, K., & Hough Williams, L. (2017). Characterization and utilization of preferred interests: A survey of adults on the autism spectrum. *Occupational Therapy in Mental Health, 33*(2), 129–140. https://doi.org/10.1080/0164212x.2016.1248877

Patten Koenig, K., & Shore, S. (2018). Self-determination and a shift to a strengths-based model. In R. Watling & S. Spitzer (Eds.), *Autism: A comprehensive occupational therapy approach* (4th ed.). AOTA Press.

Patten, K. K. (2022). Finding our strengths: Recognizing professional bias and interrogating systems. *The American Journal of Occupational Therapy, 76*(6), 7606150010. https://doi.org/10.5014/ajot.2022.076603

Pizzi, M. A., & Richards, L. G. (2017). Promoting health, well-being, and quality of life in occupational therapy: a commitment to a paradigm shift for the next 100 years. *American Journal of Occupational Therapy, 71*(4), 7104170010p1–7104170010p5. https://doi.org/10.5014/ajot.2017.028456

Rath, T. (2007). *Strengthsfinder 2.0*. Gallup Press.

Raven, J. (1998). Advanced progressive matrices. In J. Raven, J. C. Raven, & J. H. Court (Eds.) *Manual for Raven's progressive matrices and vocabulary scales*. Oxford Psychologists Press Ltd.

Raymaker, D. M., Teo, A. R., Steckler, N. A., Lentz, B., Scharer, M., Delos Santos, A., Kapp, S. K., Hunter, M., Joyce, A., & Nicolaidis, C. (2020). "Having All of Your Internal Resources Exhausted Beyond Measure and Being Left with No Clean-Up Crew": defining autistic burnout. *Autism in Adulthood, 2*(2), 132–143. https://doi.org/10.1089/aut.2019.0079

Saleebey, D. (2001). *The strengths perspective in social work practice* (3rd ed.). Allyn & Bacon.

Sasson, N. J., Faso, D. J., Nugent, J., Lovell, S., Kennedy, D. P., & Grossman, R. B. (2017). Neurotypical peers are less willing to interact with those with autism based on thin slice judgments. *Scientific Reports, 7*(1), 40700. https://doi.org/10.1038/srep40700

Scheerer, N. E., Boucher, T. Q., Sasson, N. J., & Iarocci, G. (2022). Effects of an educational presentation about autism on high school students' perceptions of autistic adults. *Autism in Adulthood, 4*(3), 203–213. https://doi.org/10.1089/aut.2021.0046

Shaw, S. C. K., Doherty, M., McCowan, S., & Eccles, J. A. (2022). Towards a neurodiversity-affirmative approach for an over-represented and under-recognised population: autistic adults in outpatient psychiatry. *Journal of Autism and Developmental Disorders, 52*, 4200–4201. https://doi.org/10.1007/s10803-022-05670-4

Shogren, K. A., & Wehmeyer, M. L. (2017). *Self-determination inventory: Student-Report*. Kansas University Center on Developmental Disabilities.

Shore, S. (2013). *Keeping it real*. www.projectkeepitreal.com; New York University. https://www.projectkeepitreal.com/

Sinclair, J. (1993). *Don't mourn for us. Autism Network International Newsletter: Our Voice, 1*(3). Retrieved February 23, 2025, from https://philosophy.ucsc.edu/SinclairDontMournForUs.pdf

Smerbeck, A. (2017). The survey of favorite interests and activities: assessing and understanding restricted interests in children with autism spectrum disorder. *Autism, 23*(1), 247–259. https://doi.org/10.1177/1362361317742140

Stratis, E. A., & Lecavalier, L. (2013). Restricted and repetitive behaviors and psychiatric symptoms in youth with autism spectrum disorders. *Research in Autism Spectrum Disorders, 7*(6), 757–766. https://doi.org/10.1016/j.rasd.2013.02.017

Taboas, A., Doepke, K., & Zimmerman, C. (2023). Preferences for identity-first versus person-first language in a US sample of autism stakeholders. *Autism, 27*(2), 565–570. https://doi.org/10.1177/13623613221130845

Tan, D. W. (2023). Early-career autism researchers are shifting their research directions: tragedy or opportunity? *Autism in Adulthood, 5*(3). https://doi.org/10.1089/aut.2023.0021

Teti, M., Cheak-Zamora, N., Lolli, B., & Maurer-Batjer, A. (2016). Reframing autism: young adults with autism share their strengths through photo-stories. *Journal of Pediatric Nursing, 31*(6), 619–629. https://doi.org/10.1016/j.pedn.2016.07.002

Trembath, D., Germano, C., Johanson, G., & Dissanayake, C. (2012). The experience of anxiety in young adults with autism spectrum disorders. *Focus on Autism and Other Developmental Disabilities*, *27*(4), 213–224. https://doi.org/10.1177/1088357612454916

Turner-Brown, L. M., Lam, K. S. L., Holtzclaw, T. N., Dichter, G. S., & Bodfish, J. W. (2011). Phenomenology and measurement of circumscribed interests in autism spectrum disorders. *Autism*, *15*(4), 437–456. https://doi.org/10.1177/1362361310386507

Vivanti, G. (2020). Ask the editor: What is the most appropriate way to talk about individuals with a diagnosis of autism? *Journal of Autism and Developmental Disorders*, *50*(2), 691–693. https://doi.org/10.1007/s10803-019-04280-x

Wechsler, D. (2005). *The Wechsler intelligence scales for children: Canadian (WISC-IV)* (4th ed.). Psychological Corporation.

Winter-Messiers, M. A. (2007). From Tarantulas to toilet brushes. Understanding the special interest areas of children and youth with Asperger syndrome. *Remedial and Special Education*, *28*(3), 140–152. https://doi.org/10.1177/07419325070280030301

Wolman, J., Campeau, P., Dubois, P., Mithaug, D., & Stolarski, V. (1994). *AIR self-determination scale and user guide* (pp. 26, 1–47). American Institute for Research.

A Frame of Reference for School-Aged Children With Anxiety and Depression

Susan Cahill ■ Brad Egan ■ Mary "Betsey" Pohl

Mental health refers to the state of psychological well-being. It involves utilizing personal strengths and abilities to foster connection with others, find enjoyment, and effectively navigate everyday life challenges (World Health Organization, 2022). Social and emotional functioning are considered the foundation of mental health (Keyes, 2002), and are supportive of children's learning and participation at school. Children and adolescents with good mental health are goal-oriented, actively participating in their various roles, engaging in positive and meaningful relationships, developing a healthy self-concept, adapting readily to changes, expressing pride in their accomplishments (Keyes, 2002), and making responsible life decisions (Bjørnsen et al., 2023).

Poor mental health may be in response to situational circumstances or organic causes, leading to academic underachievement and reduced participation in meaningful occupations both at home and in school (Cahill & Egan, 2017). Children with symptoms of anxiety and depression often struggle with social and emotional functioning and possess feelings of heightened stress, excessive worry, fear of failure, loneliness, ambivalence, and negativity (Racine et al., 2021). At school, children with symptoms of anxiety and depression may withdraw from opportunities for social participation, avoid academic challenges, and worry more than their peers about their performance on assignments, meeting due dates, and whether they are able to engage in typical daily tasks such as remembering to bring lunch money. In more severe instances of distress, children may experience internalizing behaviors (e.g., depression, anxiety, and somatic complaints) and externalizing behaviors (e.g., aggression, tantrums, clinginess, and running away). School-aged children displaying behaviors of school avoidance or refusal often have an existing diagnosis of anxiety or exhibit clinical levels of anxiety and would likely benefit from further screening and assessment (Heyne & Brouwer-Borhuis, 2022).

The COVID-19 pandemic led to ongoing school disruptions, prolonged social isolation, and a significant increase in student-reported levels of stress, anxiety, and depression (Racine et al., 2021; Waddell et al., 2020). The additional mental health stressors have put an even heavier burden on schools, which by many accounts were already struggling to meet the mental health needs of students before the pandemic (Schaffer et al., 2021) (Figure 16.1). On the other hand, the pandemic has highlighted the importance of mental health, its role in overall health and wellness, and the need to profoundly reorganize and expand school-based mental health services (Sampson et al., 2023).

SAFE
SCHOOL
ZONE
WITHIN 1000 FEET OF A SCHOOL
PENALTIES ARE INCREASED FOR
WEAPONS VIOLATIONS
DRUG VIOLATIONS
GANG RECRUITMENT
REPORT CRIME • DIAL 911
CITY OF CHICAGO
CITY OF CHICAGO

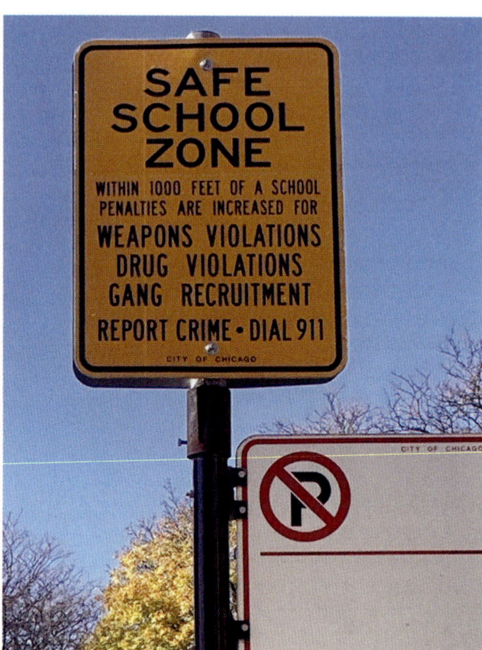

FIGURE 16.1 School safe zone sign.

The frame of reference for school-aged children with anxiety and depression focuses on children in traditional school settings between 6 and 13 years of age. Although children in this age range may experience internalizing behaviors and other symptoms associated with anxiety and depression, the majority of individuals with mental health conditions do not receive diagnoses until they are between the ages of 13 and 25 years (Solmi et al., 2022). Therefore, the focus of this frame of reference is on children experiencing symptoms of anxiety and depression at school, with or without a mental health diagnosis.

THEORETICAL BASE

Occupational therapy (OT) intervention operates on the principle that meaningful participation in occupations and mental health are bidirectional (Parsonage-Harrison et al., 2023). Engagement levels may indicate mental health or mental illness, and an individual's state of mental well-being affects their levels of engagement. Occupational therapists use occupation-based groups to encourage active participation and provide opportunities for children with and at risk for anxiety and depression to enhance their self-efficacy or their beliefs in their abilities to be successful (Olson, 2011). Additionally, they use occupation-based interventions to expose young people to positive childhood experiences (PCEs), which foster resilience (Frederick, 2022) and serve as a buffer from long-term effects of adverse childhood events (ACEs) (Bethell et al., 2019; Rothman & Lynch, 2023).

Academic competence, social participation in the classroom, and adaptive coping skills can be difficult for children with mental health concerns to develop. The centrality of symptoms of anxiety and depression has been highlighted in the growing rates of school refusal and attendance concerns resulting from emotional distress (Heyne & Brouwer-Borhuis, 2022; Leduc et al., 2022). This frame of reference draws on various theories that are related to children's psychological well-being. Constant theoretical information from temperament theories (De Pauw & Mervielde, 2010; Nigg, 2006) and attachment theory (Bowlby, 1988) describe the innate characteristics of children and their support systems. Dynamic concepts explain children's adaptations to the world, and positive psychology and positive education interventions highlight children's psychological and behavioral qualities that promote positive change and support well-being (Coulombe et al., 2020).

Finally, this frame of reference integrates the concept of volition as it is used in the Model of Human Occupation (Taylor et al., 2024) to facilitate children's positive adjustments. This frame of reference addresses the need for cultivating a sense of positive mental health in academic environments for children with symptoms of anxiety or depression using occupation-based interventions.

Developmental Psychopathology

Developmental psychopathology, as defined by Sroufe and Rutter (1984), explores mental health in relation to patterns of adaptation and maladaptation to life circumstances over time. Understanding the mechanisms and causes underlying the development of mental health conditions is critical for designing targeted interventions that can mitigate the impact of these challenges and promote positive mental health. Developmental psychopathology frameworks are essential as they provide a foundation for examining how early adverse experiences, contextual factors, and other influences contribute to the risk of developing mental illnesses or experiencing lifelong mental health challenges (Pollack, 2015). Factors such as temperament, family support, and life experiences are known to play significant roles in shaping mental health development (Pynoos et al., 1999).

Temperament

Temperament and Personality

Temperament is a collection of dispositional traits, thought to be relatively stable after the first two years of life. These traits influence an individual's response systems and can be observed through a patterned set of behaviors (Nigg, 2006; Shiner et al., 2021). Personality, on the other hand, is largely influenced by life experiences and is characterized by gradual changes across the lifespan (Chopik & Kitayama, 2018). Personality traits are commonly classified according to the Big Five model (citations of original theory), which describes behaviors according to extraversion, agreeableness, openness to experience, neuroticism, and conscientiousness (Chopik & Kitayama, 2018; Shiner et al., 2021).

The psychobiological approach views temperament and personality as the result of a combination of hereditary factors and individual differences in self-regulation and reactivity (De Pauw & Mervielde, 2010). Self-regulation is an individual's ability to focus, shift attention, and inhibit behavior when it is appropriate or necessary (De Pauw & Mervielde, 2010). Reactivity is the response of neural systems in relation to the expression of emotions and physical activity such as movement and speech (De Pauw & Mervielde, 2010).

Children experiencing anxiety and depression often display emotional instability (De Pauw & Mervielde, 2010), characterized by heightened withdrawal and negative emotions, particularly fear (Nigg, 2006; Watson, 2005). Children with anxiety have a heightened biologic stress response associated with increased vigilance, alertness, and excitement (De Pauw & Mervielde, 2010). The temperaments and personalities of children with depression typically result in these children having high levels of withdrawal and negative emotions, as well as the presence of anhedonia (i.e., loss of interest) (Nigg, 2006; Watson et al., 2005). Children who are prone to withdrawal and negative affect are considered particularly susceptible to developing anxiety and depression (Nigg, 2006).

Attachment

Early experiences are significant in shaping the child's expectations and connections within the environment (Sroufe et al., 1999). A commonly held belief is that children's mental health development is significantly influenced by the quality of the relationships they have with their first caregivers, typically their parents (Pawl & Milburn, 2006). The experiences infants and young children have with these caregivers, and the predictability of these experiences, are thought to establish a neurobiologic basis for future social relationships and the ability to adapt to challenges (Davis & Glynn, 2024).

Attachment is the bond that forms between infants and their primary caregivers (Bowlby, 1988). This bond develops through the caregiver's responsiveness to the infant's needs. Early attachment forms the basis for trust, feelings of self-worth, and adaptive behaviors (Sroufe et al., 1999). Securely attached children trust their feelings and problem-solving ability in challenging situations (Van der Kolk, 2017). Attachment security also plays a beneficial role in fostering the growth of self-regulation, encouraging the adoption of help-seeking behaviors, and influencing physiologic responses in stressful situations (Whittenburg et al., 2023). Conversely, insecure attachment hampers the development of self-regulation skills (Whittenburg et al., 2023) and is linked to adverse mental and physical health outcomes in children Yaffe, 2021).

One aspect of attachment in early relationships is established by how safe children feel. Starting at birth, children are reliant on caregivers for survival and protection. Children's sense of safety becomes more nuanced as they develop. In the beginning, infants respond to survival threats (e.g., being hungry) and the need for nurturance by crying, social referencing, and trying to elicit care through other nonverbal behaviors (Pynoos et al., 1999). Preschool children may consciously consider their safety as well as the safety of their parents, yet be less aware of threats (e.g., walking into the street to retrieve a ball) and more dependent on adults to initiate protection when encountering potentially harmful circumstances. School-aged children begin to have a more heightened sense of danger and understand the outcomes associated with unsafe physical and emotional situations; however, they may not yet have developed strategies to deal with these situations successfully and independently (Pynoos et al., 1999). During each one of these stages, children compare their perceptions of real or imagined dangerous situations with how their primary caregivers/parents respond (Pynoos et al., 1999). Caregivers/parents' reaction to and framing of events may influence how children interpret them. Overprotective parenting styles, overconcern, uncertainty, overt expressions of fear and anxiety, labeling situations as dangerous or unsolvable, and permitting catastrophic interpretations can intensify children's negative emotions and withdrawal tendencies (Yaffe, 2021).

Life Experiences

There has been a significant body of research that has established the connection between traumatic life experiences and adverse mental health outcomes (Struck et al., 2021). Trauma-informed care practices promote safety and acknowledge the deep impact of generational and personal trauma on a child's present behaviors and future mental health (Shih et al., 2023). The presence of chronic stress and adversity during childhood—such as the death of a parent, abuse, poverty, or displacement from one's home country—has been shown to impact the sympathetic nervous system, immune system, and hypothalamic–pituitary–adrenal axis (Maier et al., 2022).

Adversity is any situation that requires a child to adapt significantly. Over time, persistent stress and adversity weaken the body's ability to adapt to pressures effectively and contribute to poor life adjustment. Life adjustment or adaptation refers to a child's propensity to tolerate or manage ongoing pressures that have the potential to influence psychological and behavioral development (Pynoos et al., 1999). Efficient and effective life adjustment requires children to understand what they have experienced, process their emotions, and plan for the use of protective strategies in future situations (Elrefaay & Elyzal, 2024). The literature suggests that some groups and populations, for example, children and youth who are newcomers to the United States, are expected to make significant life adjustments and that these adjustments may lead to increased stress (Davis et al., 2021). Resilience-building programs that emphasize emotional expression, mental flexibility, problem-solving skills, and coping strategies are effective in helping children adapt to change and manage life stressors (Elrefaay & Elyzal, 2024). Recent research on PCEs, including seven categories of positive interpersonal experiences within home, school, and community contexts, highlights their crucial role in safeguarding individuals against mental health challenges. These protective effects persist even when accounting for the presence of several adverse childhood experiences (Bethell et al., 2019; Breedlove et al., 2020).

Positive Youth Development

The field of positive youth development, rooted in positive psychology, emphasizes children's acquisition of strengths through positive subjective experiences, often in social contexts with peers (Buenconsejo & Datu, 2022). When addressing children's mental health through a positive youth development framework, therapists move from a symptom-oriented or problem-focused approach to prioritizing protective factors and encourage children to develop resilience and master developmental tasks (Elrefaay & Elyzal, 2024). A key feature of positive youth development is enabling children to develop and exercise personal power within structured environments (Buenconsejo & Datu, 2022). Programs offering structured leisure activities and resilience-building initiatives have been shown to promote positive social, emotional, and academic outcomes for children across diverse socioeconomic backgrounds (Buenconsejo & Datu, 2022; Elrefaay & Elyzal, 2024; Breedlove et al., 2020). These outcomes correlated strongly with high levels of psychological well-being among children and youth (Coulombe et al., 2020).

Subjective Well-Being

Subjective well-being is an indicator of life satisfaction and flourishing (Coulombe et al., 2020). It is characterized by recurrent feelings and expressions associated with happiness and the absence of sadness, anger, guilt, shame, fear, and anxiety (Chaves, 2021). Conversely, low subjective well-being is associated with poor life satisfaction, symptoms of mental health disorders, and challenges in academic settings (Chaves, 2021). Recent studies have emphasized the role of the school context in fostering a positive climate that enhances subjective well-being for all students (Moreira et al., 2021). Activities that promote an increased sense of self-efficacy and competence, build on personal strengths, and foster positive relationships with classmates are critical to well-being (Chaves, 2021).

Volition

Another hallmark of the positive youth development movement is the emphasis on cultivating children's volition. Volition is acting autonomously and with a "full sense of choice" (Deci & Ryan, 2008, p. 15). In occupational therapy, volition is described as a multidimensional construct that consists of a person's sense of capacity and self-efficacy (i.e., personal causation), a person's personal convictions and obligations (e.g., values), and a person's preferences and enjoyment associated with occupational performance and participation (e.g., interests) (Basu et al., 2008; Lee & Kielhofner, 2024). Volition is observed through a cycle of "anticipating, choosing, experiencing, and interpreting what one does" (Lee & Kielhofner, 2024, p. 42). Personal circumstances and life histories influence and shape volition (Lee & Kielhofner, 2024). The examination of occupational choices and engagement provides insight into one's sense of volition and their tendency toward taking initiative. Table 16.1 outlines volitional behaviors and their descriptions. These skills and abilities are associated with different levels of volition (i.e., exploration, competency, and achievement) (Lannigan et al., 2024). Volitional development occurs on a continuum, and it is expected

Table 16.1 Descriptions of Volitional Behavior

Volitional Behavior	Description
Initiates actions	Initiates interactions within their environment on their own
Shows preferences	Expresses desire for specific items within the environment
Tries to produce effects	Seeks to cause something to occur because of their actions
Tries new things	Will attempt to do things that they have not done before
Stays engaged	Wants to continue in an activity
Task directed	Tries to complete something or do something until a goal is achieved
Expresses mastery pleasure	Is pleased when a task is completed successfully
Practices skills	Continues to do something until improvement occurs
Tries to solve problems	Attempts to find a way to be successful when engaging in a task or find a way of doing something that leads to success
Pursues activity to completion	Willingness to continue in an activity until the goal is reached
Seeks challenges	Tries to do new and different things
Organizes/modifies environment	Tries to change an aspect of the environment to improve skills and performance
Uses imagination	Engages in imaginary play or creates a pretend environment

that children will first engage in exploration in order to gain confidence in anticipating, choosing, experiencing, and interpreting their own occupational choices and engagement (Lannigan et al., 2024). Children may develop spontaneous volitional behaviors through positive experiences associated with academic competence, engagement in social participation, and effective use of adaptive coping skills.

FUNCTION/DYSFUNCTION CONTINUA

The frame of reference for school-aged children with anxiety and depression has three function–dysfunction continua.

Social Participation in the Classroom

Social participation at school involves engagement in social activities with other people, including peers, teachers, and other adults (e.g., school nurse, parent volunteer) (American Occupational Therapy Association, 2020). Social participation is influenced by feelings of acceptance and power dynamics. It may lead to the expansion of social networks, establishment of new social roles, and cultivating a sense of belonging; or it may lead to unfair social evaluation and exclusion from a group (da Silva & Oliver, 2021). Social participation is influenced by factors internal to the student (e.g., interest, motivation), the social context, the students' actions, and the intended outcomes of participation (Martins et al., 2022). Social participation can be observed in parallel interactions (i.e., working on class assignments or playing side by side), associative interactions (i.e., brief interactions), basic cooperative interactions (i.e., joint implementation of play or working on assignments), supportive cooperative interactions (i.e., joint implementation of play or working on assignments with an emphasis on mutuality), and mature interactions (i.e., engagement in multiple group roles to achieve a joint goal, such as a group project) (Donahue, 2013). Children who function high on this continuum are proficient at interpreting social cues and using social skills; they are friendly, approachable, flexible, and able to easily engage with different people (e.g., teachers, students), and assume a variety of different group roles. In addition, such children demonstrate willingness, and often enthusiasm, to engage in tasks that require interdependence and cooperation (e.g., group work and activities). For example, a child at school might ask to work with a partner or in a small group, rather than work alone. Children who function lower on this continuum may struggle with using social skills, sometimes feel powerless, and present as being avoidant, aloof, withdrawn, and rigid. They may demonstrate a preference for engaging only with certain people, attempt to avoid group situations and prefer to work on assignments independently. Table 16.2 includes indicators of the social participation continuum.

Adaptive Coping Skills

Coping refers to individuals' ability to respond and adapt to stress arising from various circumstances. For children with or susceptible to anxiety and depression, attending school and producing academic tasks can often be stress inducing. Stress and ineffective coping skills can negatively influence a child's competence and desire to participate (Raine et al., 2023; Skinner et al., 2016). Coping styles are strong predictors of academic engagement and success (Raine et al., 2023) and are linked with factors like self-esteem, autonomy, emotional regulation, perspective-taking, and

Table 16.2 Indicators of Function: Social Participation in the Classroom

Function	Dysfunction
Engages in social participation in the classroom	Limited engagement in social participation in the classroom
Indicators of Function	**Indicators of Dysfunction**
Friendly and identifies friends	Aloof, withdrawn, slow to warm; does not identify friends
Attempts to join in play activities with peers and makes an effort to get along well with them, regardless of the group size	Avoids interacting with peers or limits interaction to a small group or specific individuals within a group
Tries different ways to approach a task	Avoids challenging tasks or relies on one way to perform a task and is unwilling to try other ways of doing things
Able to recognize and respond to social cues appropriately	Demonstrates poor social awareness; may misinterpret social cues and events
Communicates well verbally and nonverbally and is able to listen to others	Does not communicate well verbally or nonverbally, has difficulty listening to others
Makes visible efforts to work things out when encountering a challenging situation	Struggles or avoids attempting to work out a difficult situation with peers. May need help to do so, or may have a tantrum
Follows classroom rules and social conventions	Difficulty following some classroom rules (e.g., deadlines for assignments) and social conventions (e.g., attending to student presentations)
Assumes a variety of different roles during a group activity	Difficulty working in groups and assuming different roles

decision making in behavior (Skinner et al., 2016). Research also suggests that using ineffective coping strategies (Table 16.3) is associated with disengagement and poor outcomes related to school transitions (Martins et al., 2022; Raine et al., 2023; Skinner et al., 2016). Children who can effectively cope with and adapt to stressful situations develop resilience and acquire valuable skills that support future success in life.

Academic Competence

Academic competence is children's perception of their ability to perform in the student role and to keep up with peers, make progress, and accomplish goals related to academic work. Children who function high on these continua have a strong sense of self-efficacy and a belief that their efforts will produce positive gains in the classroom and with educational tasks. They may experience minor setbacks related to learning (e.g., struggling initially with learning how to complete long division using a specific strategy). However, they can seek out and utilize supports while maintaining a positive self-concept and demonstrating a high frequency of volitionally related behaviors. Children who function low on this continuum possess negative beliefs about their capacity to produce effects, have a low sense of self-efficacy, and demonstrate few, lower-level volitional behaviors. Such children may also demonstrate a lack of persistence when faced with

Table 16.3 Indicators of Function: Adaptive Coping Skills

Function	Dysfunction
Handles difficult situations effectively	Struggles to deal with difficult situations and has a negative behavioral response
Indicators of Function	**Indicators of Dysfunction**
Feels good about themself as shown by smiles or positive facial expressions	Does not appear to feel good about themself as shown by frowns or negative facial expressions
Emotional reactions are appropriate to the situation	Emotional reactions are not appropriate to the situation
Behaviors are appropriate to the situation	Behaviors are not appropriate to the situation, may act out and have tantrums
Can calm themselves when upset	Requires assistance to calm down when upset and struggles to comprehend their surroundings independently
Shows understanding of how their surroundings can be helpful	Demonstrates a lack of understanding of how things around them can be helpful
Asks for help when needed	Does not realize or avoids asking for help when needed
Seeks help and uses resources appropriately	Does not seek help or does not use resources effectively
Demonstrates awareness of options and appropriate responses to various situations	Unable to recognize choices and lack awareness of how to respond to situation
Recovers and persists after experiencing failures or setbacks	Failures or setbacks result in disengagement and self-blame

academic challenges. Also, they may not seek out assistance or additional support and resources. Table 16.4 includes indicators of function and dysfunction for academic competence.

GUIDE FOR EVALUATION

It is important to note that in some schools, occupational therapists may not be viewed as key team members for screening, assessing, and intervening with students experiencing anxiety and depression. Therefore, it is beneficial for occupational therapists to communicate with and stay informed about screening and assessment tools utilized by other team members, especially social workers and school counselors, who can provide valuable insights to guide further assessment by the occupational therapist. Additionally, advocating for the role of occupational therapy on teams that support students with mental health concerns is crucial for enhancing the impact of the OT profession in school systems.

In some school districts, occupational therapists may be able to provide interventions to students in general education who are at risk for anxiety and/or depression under a multitiered system of support model. Such interventions are designed to support the student's engagement and performance in general education. Before providing interventions to students in general education, occupational therapists should be familiar with their state licensure laws and understand the requirements and limitations associated with providing preventative interventions.

Table 16.4 Indicators of Function: Academic Competence

Function	Dysfunction
Perceives themself as academically competent	Feels inadequate or incompetent academically
Indicators of Function	**Indicators of Dysfunction**
Progress toward academic benchmarks, at or close to the same rate as peers	Lack of progress toward academic benchmarks; achievement discrepancies as compared to peers
Able to ask for and use help	Does not ask for help and does not use it when offered
Demonstrates a future orientation and can set realistic goals	Difficulty seeing the "big picture" and struggles with planning ahead to reach goals; may not be able to set goals; concerned about meeting expectations
Seeks out new academic challenges and shows curiosity and interest in academic tasks	Avoids seeking out new challenges and lacks curiosity or interest in academic tasks.
Demonstrates engagement in academic tasks	Shows disinterest or lack of engagement in academic tasks
Perseveres and remains committed to completing a task	Abandons tasks before completion and lacks persistence
Shows satisfaction through facial expressions upon successful completing a task	Shows indifference or lack of emotional response upon completing a task successfully.

The evaluation for school-aged children with anxiety and depression begins with the occupational profile. The occupational profile includes information about the children's occupational history, performance patterns, and occupational needs (American Occupational Therapy Association, 2021). It is particularly important to develop an occupational profile for children with symptoms of anxiety and depression to understand better when symptoms related to their mental health concerns were first noticed. The occupational profile can also assist the occupational therapist in understanding how the children's environment supports or inhibits occupational performance and participation, and the protective factors associated with positive youth development.

The occupational therapist should first consider the child's occupational performance and determine how it is affected by the child's sense of competence, engagement in social participation, and use of adaptive coping skills. Conducting observations of occupational engagement in different settings and during different periods of the school day will provide an understanding of how initiative, academic functioning, and participation are influenced by the child's underlying mental health concern. Furthermore, such observations will help the therapist frame the child's needs based on the function/dysfunction continua associated with this frame of reference.

Self-report measures provide valuable information about the child's perceptions of competence and subjective well-being. The use of self-report assessment tools for children exhibiting symptoms of anxiety and depression is beneficial. These assessments allow children to reflect on their needs and abilities; providing occupational therapists with firsthand insights from the child's perspective. This personal knowledge is crucial for developing effective and relevant intervention plans that support mental health (Kramer et al., 2012).

In addition to observation-based assessments and self-report rating scales, occupational therapists may collaborate with school teams to screen for specific behaviors associated with mental health conditions. When completed frequently (e.g., once a quarter or semester), team-based rating scales (e.g., the *Student Risk Screening Scale for Internalizing and Externalizing Behaviors* [Lane & Menzies, 2009; Lane et al., 2015; Lane et al., 2023] and the *Social Emotional Distress Scale–Secondary-Brief* [Dowdy et al., 2023]) can be used for school-wide surveillance and to identify changes in a student's behavior that can signal mental health concerns.

Based on the occupational profile and screenings of the child's concerns and strengths, therapists select specific evaluations that provide more in-depth information. Below are some of the alternative assessments a therapist might select.

Observation-Based Assessments

The *Pediatric Volitional Questionnaire* (PVQ) (Basu et al., 2008) (used for children between 2 and 7 years old) and the *Volitional Questionnaire* (VQ) (for children and youth aged 8 and older) (de las Heras et al., 2007) support the therapist's clinical reasoning related to how occupational engagement is impacted by the child's state of mental health. Both the PVQ and the VQ focus on the behavioral indicators of volition and can be used to consider skill development and performance in a variety of domains (Kiraly-Alvarez, 2015). A multitude of school-related occupations, such as playing at recess, completing an independent assignment, eating lunch in the cafeteria, and working on a group project, can be used as the focus for PVQ and VQ observations. Both questionnaires include 14 observable behaviors that can be interpreted to provide insights into where the child is performing on the volitional continuum of exploration, competency, and achievement (Basu et al., 2008; de las Heras et al., 2007).

The *Social Profile* (Donahue, 2013) is a descriptive observation-based assessment tool that provides the occupational therapist with an understanding of how the child participates in group settings. The *children's version* of the *Social Profile* is recommended for early and intermediate elementary school children and examines parallel, associative, and basic cooperative social interactions (Donahue, 2013). The *adult/adolescent version* of the *Social Profile* is for middle school and high school students beginning at age 12 years. This version of the *Social Profile* also examines parallel, associative, basic cooperative, supportive cooperative, and mature types of social participation (Donahue, 2013). The Social Profile can be used as an outcome measure to determine if occupational therapy intervention is successful (Prusnek et al., 2019).

Self-Report Assessment Tools

The *Child Occupational Self-Assessment* (Kramer et al., 2014) is a self-report assessment that is designed to capture a child's perceptions related to competence for daily occupations. The *Child Occupational Self-Assessment* is for a child between the ages of 7 and 17 years. Occupational therapists working with an older child may use the *Occupational Self-Assessment* (Baron et al., 2006). A critical difference between the *Child Occupational Self-Assessment* and the *Occupational Self-Assessment* is the inclusion of a visual rating scale that uses symbols to establish responses. Both the *Child Occupational Self-Assessment* and the *Occupational Self-Assessment* ask a child to rate how well they perform specific occupations and how they value these occupations.

The *Brief Multidimensional Students' Life Satisfaction Scale* measures subjective well-being (Seligson et al., 2003). The *Brief Multidimensional Students' Life Satisfaction Scale* is a five-item self-report that can be administered to a young child or adolescent through 12th grade and examines their sense of subjective well-being. The *Brief Multidimensional Students' Life Satisfaction Scale* provides an opportunity for a child to rate their overall satisfaction with family life, friendships, school experience, the self, and where one lives. Occupational therapists who need more comprehensive information related to subjective well-being may consider using the 40-item *Multidimensional Students' Life Satisfaction Scale* (Huebner, 1994).

Team-Based Rating Scales

The *Student Risk Screening Scale for Internalizing and Externalizing Behaviors* (SRSS-IE, Lane et al., 2015, 2023) is a 12-item questionnaire that asks the team member to rate the level of frequency that an adolescent engages in specific internalizing and externalizing behaviors. Internalizing behaviors are associated with anxiety and depression. Some examples of internalizing behaviors include flat affect, sadness, worry, and loneliness. Occupational therapists working with a younger child may consider using the *Strengths and Difficulties Questionnaire* (Goodman, 1997). The *Strengths and Difficulties Questionnaire* includes 25 items and is appropriate for a child between the ages of 2 and 17 years when information is collected through a caregiver (e.g., parent or teacher) (sdqinfo.org). The *Strengths and Difficulties Questionnaire* provides an opportunity for primary caregivers/parents and educators to rate the child's emotional symptoms, conduct problems, inattention, peer relationship problems, and prosocial behavior (Goodman, 1997). Another option is the *Devereux Student Strengths Assessment Mini* (Naglieri et al., 2011/2014), a universal screener of social–emotional competencies in kindergarten through eighth-grade students. The *Devereux Student Strengths Assessment Mini* includes an eight-item behavior rating scale and allows for progress monitoring and can be completed by a variety of educational team members, parent/guardians, and other professionals who might interact with students outside of the school setting.

Schools or districts may identify their own areas of concern (i.e., "red flags") and develop corresponding screening questions based on local issues, such as homelessness, truancy, gun violence, and those surrounding newcomers such as migrants, refugees, and asylum seekers.

POSTULATES REGARDING CHANGE

Occupational therapists who provide services to a school-aged child with symptoms of anxiety and depression promote mental health and work to improve occupational performance and participation.

General Postulate Regarding Change

Occupational therapy practitioners analyze, adapt, and modify occupations and environments to support occupational engagement and improve mental health. They may provide children with activities where engagement in the occupation serves both as the means and the end, leading to the display of positive mental health behaviors. Additionally, practitioners should approach intervention with sensitivity, considering the child's past life experiences and relationships—both traumatic and affirming—while designing interventions tailored to meet the child's unique mental health needs.

Directional Postulate Regarding Change

The occupational therapy practitioner would generally address the two continua of social participation in the classroom and adaptive coping skills before addressing the continuum of academic competence.

Specific Postulates Regarding Change

This frame of reference presents specific postulates regarding change that focus on aligning the concept of positive youth development and supportive of children's overall functioning at school. Interventions focus on the intentional selection of occupations that highlight the child's strengths, support skill development, and provide the basis to learn strategies. The following are specific postulates regarding change aligned to each of the continuum:

1. Social participation in the classroom

   If the occupational therapist incorporates graded occupations that are satisfying and promote feelings of subjective well-being and accomplishment, while involving peers in authentic environments, the child will demonstrate improved social participation and make meaningful connections to people and places.
2. Adaptive coping skills

   If the therapist promotes the use of various strategies in the context of meaningful occupations with peers, then the child will develop adaptive coping skills with people that will become habitual.
3. Academic competence

   If the therapist provides opportunities where successful engagement in occupations is supported, then the child will develop a more secure occupational identity and improved academic role satisfaction.

APPLICATION TO PRACTICE

Occupational therapy practitioners providing services to school-aged children experiencing symptoms of anxiety and depression work to improve occupational competence, social participation, coping skills, and academic competence. Central to this frame of reference is the use of activities and associated occupations that support the child's feelings of competence and mastery. This intervention encourages the child to use volitional behaviors that promote subjective well-being and coping skills, ultimately reducing symptoms related to anxiety and depression. Interventions take place in familiar school environments such as classrooms, hallways, cafeterias, playgrounds, and after-school programs, ensuring relevance and integration into the child's daily routine.

Given the nature of anxiety and depression, the practitioner develops a unique intervention plan that draws on the child's personal strengths and addresses the most significant areas of difficulty. Thus, intervention plans are very individualized and cannot be specified with a particular protocol. Instead, the challenge is fostering positive change in the school with all its dynamics and the numerous professionals involved in the child's school life. Finally, the intervention plan must address the three continua: social participation, adaptive coping, and academic competence.

Goal Setting

Intervention planning requires an understanding of the child's perceptions of subjective well-being and competence in academic and social situations, as well as the factors that support and inhibit volition. When addressing the mental health concerns of the school-aged child, it is critical to understand their strengths, perspectives, and desires. This understanding facilitates the development of the therapeutic relationship. For a child with anxiety and depression who has experienced trauma or poor attachment to caregivers, this is even more critical.

In addition to gaining the child's perspectives during the evaluation phase of the occupational therapy process, occupational therapists should collaborate with the child to establish goals for intervention. The demands of the school environment are such that occupational therapists should also be aware of others' expectations and negotiate with teachers, administrators, primary caregivers/parents, and other service providers to fully integrate the child into the goal-setting process (O'Connor et al., 2021; Pritchard et al., 2022). The process of goal setting may be overwhelming to the child; therefore, the occupational therapy practitioner should first explain, using language the child can understand, the connection between engaging in occupation and mental health. It is important for the practitioner to clarify how satisfaction in roles relates to competence and volitional behaviors. Empathetic listening should be employed, encouraging the child to use insights obtained from self-assessment tools to explore and identify priority areas (Antoniadou et al., 2024). The child should be invited to propose occupational therapy goals in their own words.

The occupational therapy practitioner may suggest areas for intervention based on information gained from standardized evaluations. However, it is crucial to support the child and allow them to express opinions regarding the course of occupational therapy. Throughout this process, the occupational therapist must demonstrate understanding, respect, and support for the child's values, performance experience, and sense of competency. Whenever possible, a strength-based approach should be used (Patten, 2022).

Use of Activities and Occupation

OT interventions for a school-aged child with anxiety and depression should attend to how symptoms of their mental health conditions affect occupational engagement. Interventions should support the child's competence, social participation, the development of subjective well-being, and coping skills. OT interventions may be provided during typical school occupations and within typical school environments, such as the classroom and the cafeteria. Such interventions focus on developing competence and moving a child along the volitional continuum from exploration to competency, to achievement (Kiraly-Alvarez, 2015; Lee & Kielhofner, 2024; Reilly, 1974).

The exploration, competency, and achievement stages first proposed by Reilly (1974) describe how engagement in an occupation leads to eventual feelings of mastery as the child meets challenges and overcomes them. The first stage, exploration, is derived from an inherent interest in the environment (Reilly, 1974). When a school-aged child experiencing anxiety and depression withdraws from certain environments, it may indicate their effort to self-protect. Before attempting to cultivate interest in activities, occupational therapy practitioners must ensure that the school environments—such as classroom and the treatment space—are supportive. One way that occupational therapists can do this is to employ trauma-informed practices. These practices include understanding how stress affects learning, fostering social connectedness, and building a trusting relationship where students feel safe to take risks (Lynch et al., 2020). Occupational therapy practitioners should offer activities or occupations that provide choices for the child to freely exercise. The complexity of tasks should be adjustable to meet the child's individual needs, facilitating their exploration and engagement in meaningful occupations.

As children progress beyond exploration, they begin attempting to achieve desired outcomes to meet specific demands and receive feedback, while also seeking out small challenges (Reilly, 1974).

This second stage is called competency, where a child actively interacts with the environment. A child experiencing symptoms of anxiety and depression may demonstrate competency behaviors in certain school-related occupations but not in others. The occupational therapy practitioner should observe and take note of which occupations the child engages more readily. They should then identify and analyze the attributes of these occupations, the setting in which they occur, and the social environment surrounding them. This assessment can help therapists determine if these factors can be replicated during other times and in different settings to promote consistent engagement and skill development.

The final stage is based on a child's understanding that they can modify behavior to affect the outcome of the experience. During the achievement stage, a child learns to take calculated risks, experience failure, recover quickly, and try again (Reilly, 1974). Occupational therapy practitioners working with a child with symptoms of anxiety and depression should carefully grade challenges and possibly first present activities that are of high interest but hold low personal significance. Such activities may provide the conditions for a child to take risks while suspending the fear of consequences that may have a lasting impact on their life at school.

Besides ordinary activities and occupations associated with school environments, play addresses motivational factors, encourages social participation, and teaches perspective (Leigers et al., 2016). A focus on leisure for adolescents has been shown to positively influence self-efficacy, self-worth, and competency (Cahill et al., 2020). Occupations associated with caring for others, civic engagement, advocating for justice, and volunteerism are associated with increased engagement, self-confidence, and happiness (Breedlove et al., 2020; Chaves, 2021). These activities can be incorporated throughout the school day during academic and nonacademic periods and in after-school programs.

Group Interventions

Occupation-based group interventions provide opportunities to promote mastery of developmental tasks, enhance social connections, and facilitate the learning of social and adaptive coping skills. Occupational therapy practitioners, particularly those working in school systems, may use group interventions as a targeted Tier 2 intervention in accordance with state and local policies (Egan et al., 2023). Therapeutic groups may follow a psychoeducational approach and emphasize the acquisition of adaptive coping skills. For example, The Zones of Regulation (Kuypers, 2011) is an evidence-informed curriculum that is often presented in groups, teaching children how to manage their emotions and regulate their behaviors for enhanced occupational participation and well-being. Therapeutic groups may also build agency and a sense of belonging by including peers who serve as role models and mentors.

OT group interventions often include familiar and fun activities (e.g., board games, sports, crafts) or provide opportunities to try engagement in new activities. Sometimes, therapists use crafts as they have been found to be supportive for cultivating enjoyment stability, positive routines, problem solving, innovation, socialization, and collaboration (Horghagen et al., 2014; Hansen et al., 2021). Suldo et al. (2014) designed a series of groups to promote subjective well-being. Examples of the group activities associated with promoting subjective well-being and positive youth development included writing in gratitude journals, completing gratitude visits (i.e., telling someone you are grateful for them), and performing random acts of kindness. In the Kia Piki te Hauora (which means "uplifting our health and well-being" in the Māori language) school-based occupational therapy group intervention sessions, students are explicitly taught occupational concepts, engage in a developmentally appropriate occupation, and guided through an occupation-focused reflection that supports their understanding of how occupational choices can impact mental health and well-being (Tokolahi et al., 2018).

In addition to considering the focus of the group intervention, occupational therapists should also consider structuring the activity so that, when possible, all group members experience a positive outcome. One way to ensure that group members experience a positive outcome is to build in routines that promote social participation from all group members (Olson, 2011). Such routines may include ways to greet each other, ways to ask for assistance, ways to offer help, and ways to close the group. Designing groups with signals that follow a predictable flow (i.e., beginning, middle, and end) is also beneficial. Moreover, a design that includes engagement in occupation and directs members to process how the experience relates to their occupational priorities enables an occupation-as-means-and-ends approach. Finally, assuring that a child has enough time to process the group experience and, if necessary, resolve group events is essential (Olson, 2011).

CASE EXAMPLE

Isabela

Isabela is a 12-year-old (sixth-grade) student whose family, including her mother, father, and sister emigrated from Venezuela to the United States 14 months ago. After multiple temporary housing situations, Isabela's family settled into a metropolitan area and are living in a small basement apartment with relatives. Isabela and her younger sister, Mariana (9 years old, third grade) enrolled in their neighborhood school within a large, urban public school district nearly a year ago. Both Isabela and Mariana spoke limited English upon enrollment, and both are receiving English language learning supports.

Isabela's school participates in a district-wide quarterly mental health and wellness screening for all students. Her scores on the internalizing subscale of the Spanish version of the *Student Risk Screening Scale-IE* suggested a moderate risk for behavioral concerns. Additional screening questions based on the four core stressors for refugee and immigrant youth (i.e., trauma, acculturative stress, resettlement stress, and isolation) (Davis et al., 2021) were included for newcomers and their data was tracked over time. Isabela demonstrated concerns for all four core stressors. On the other hand, her younger sister appears to be thriving in all areas, making Isabela's stressors even more noteworthy and concerning.

Isabela is currently being evaluated for special education services focusing on learning and social–emotional skills, with a recommended occupational therapy evaluation. The evaluation team prioritized concerns related to Isabela's mental health due to its potential impact on her academic performance. According to her teacher, Isabela shows increased social withdrawal and disengagement in both academic and nonacademic activities compared to her peers. The teacher noted Isabela's reluctance to participate in small group works, often silent and contributes with head nods and only a few verbal responses, even when encouraged. Her performance is described as "just enough to get by." The school social worker previously suggested several extracurricular options such as drawing club, dance team, and Math Olympiad, but Isabela has not shown interest or signed up for any of these activities. The social worker recommended the occupational therapist assess Isabela's motivation for engaging in school activities and conduct further evaluation of her emotional well-being to identify additional strengths and interests. Isabela's mother provided signed consent for the occupational therapy evaluation.

The occupational therapist, proficient in Spanish, completed an occupational profile (Table 16.5) with Isabela over two consecutive lunch periods using the AOTA Occupational

Table 16.5 Isabela's Occupational Profile Organized by the American Occupational Therapy Association (AOTA) Occupational Profile Template

Student: Isabela	Grade: 6 (Age 12)	
Reason the client is seeking service and concerns related to engagement in occupations	Isabela is a quiet sixth-grade student who historically enjoyed school in her home country, Venezuela. During this academic year, she has become more disengaged and socially withdrawn. She has dismissed attempts by peers to engage in social activities during and after school. Despite encouragement from her teacher and school social worker, Isabela did not sign up for any after-school clubs or activities. She typically goes to the library during her lunch period to avoid socializing with peers and to limit how much English she has to speak	
Occupations in which the client is successful	• Excels at math; this is the one subject area where she appears motivated and consistently engaged • Successfully gets herself and her sister up and ready for school in the morning (includes ensuring they eat breakfast, are well-dressed and groomed, and arrive on time) • Liked to play chess at shelter with older girl	
Personal interests and values	• Values her role as older sister and daughter. She feels it is important for her to make sure her sister is taken care of and her parents do not have to worry about her or her sister • Wants her parents to be proud of her • Interested in anime, pop music, watching TV (cooking shows), YouTube videos, and Facetiming with family in Venezuela	
Occupational history (i.e., life experiences)	Isabela recently moved into a family member's small basement apartment with both her parents and younger sister. Prior to that, her family lived in a variety of shelters and church spaces for migrant families. Both parents work several cash-based day labor jobs, so Isabela is often expected to help take care of her sister and do most of the household chores. She described her life in Venezuela as generally "happy" and filled with good memories spending time with her "big family" and "lots of friends." For reasons she does not fully understand, her family had to flee Venezuela on foot 14 mo ago. She was tearful and described the experience as scary and reported that she was often worried about being kidnapped and separated from her family. She reports that her parents tell her life will get better soon, but she is doubtful and very homesick. Isabela shared that nothing about her life seems "normal" anymore	
Performance patterns (routines, roles, habits, and rituals)	Routines at home are often unpredictable due to the temporary nature of her parents' work assignments and their need to work several jobs to cover household costs. Isabela is often expected to help her younger sister get ready for school, make a simple breakfast, walk her sister and self to school, pick her sister up after school, start dinner, do the dishes, and finish homework. Isabela reports that she skips homework sometimes so that she can video chat with her friends and family members in Venezuela. On days when her parents are home and can watch her sister, she enjoys reading anime comics at the local library branch and listening to music, drawing, and looking at social media	
What aspects of the client's environments or contexts does he or she see as		
	Supports occupational engagement	Barriers to occupational engagement
Physical	Multimedia room (library and computers) ELL teacher's classroom	Describes school as "big and loud"

(*continued*)

Table 16.5 Isabela's Occupational Profile Organized by the American Occupational Therapy Association (AOTA) Occupational Profile Template (Continued)

Social	Classmates have shown interest in being her friend English language learner (ELL) teacher is supportive Several after-school clubs and activities Parents work long hours but are very engaged when they are home.	Does not like speaking English; lacks confidence and is not motivated to improve Minimal involvement with peers outside of school
Cultural	ELL supports available District is expanding services for newcomers Some staff members speak Spanish	Some staff and parents express negative personal feelings about newcomers and resources need to support them Isabela worries that peers make fun of the way she pronounces words
Personal	Handles responsibilities well, cooperative, enjoys being a big sister, values keeping strong relationships with family members	Homesick, worries about losing her heritage and sense of identity, reluctant to learn English because she wants to preserve her culture and heritage, worries she is disappointing her parents, becomes overwhelmed at times by all the responsibilities at home
Temporal	Early adolescence Only been in the United States for 14 mo Had a gap in schooling while traveling from Venezuela and during resettlement	Spends most of her time with her sister and unsupervised by parents because they are working Family schedules are inconsistent Sleep routines vary
Virtual	School provides tablet that can be taken home	Has a smartphone with unlimited data
Client's priorities and desired target outcomes:	Wants to feel comfortable around classmates and make friends Would like to do more fun things	

Template Retrieved from aota-occupational-profile-template.pdf

Profile template (AOTA, 2021). During these sessions, they engaged in assembling a 150-piece jigsaw puzzle. Although the therapist was initially unaware of Isabella's affinity for puzzles, her enthusiasm for the activity became evident through her behavioral responses. Isabela spontaneously started turning over pieces, locating border pieces, and connecting pieces together to begin forming the four corners of the puzzle. Throughout the activity, the therapist observed Isabela staying engaged in the activity, though she would sometimes stop doing the puzzle and put her head on the table when the conversation appeared to cause distress. At times, Isabela responded to questions by saying "no lo entenderías," Spanish for "you wouldn't understand." In these instances, the occupational therapist paused the interview and redirected focus back to the puzzle, inviting Isabela to participate at her own pace. Isabela shared that she would likely feel more confident if she became more proficient in English. Currently, her favorite subject is math because, as she put it, "it's about numbers, not words." This allows her to show her work on the board without having to speak in front of the class. Isabela shared that she would really like to make friends and have more things to do that she enjoys. During the second session of the occupational profile, Isabela continued to work on the puzzle. She spontaneously organized the pieces in new ways to try to find matches, checked the box to see if there were any missing pieces, and stayed a few extra minutes after the interview to complete the puzzle. She smiled upon finishing it and asked if she could take a picture of the completed puzzle with her phone.

In addition to conducting an occupational profile, the occupational therapist observed Isabela during two 20-minute sessions outside of regular classroom instruction to observe her social engagement with peers of her choice. The observations took place in the school library and during gym class. To guide these observations, the occupational therapist used the *Volitional Questionnaire* (de las Heras et al., 2007). Based on findings from the *Volitional Questionnaire*, it was determined that Isabela exhibits passive volitional behaviors in most situations during gym class, whereas she displayed some spontaneous volitional behaviors in the school library.

In the school library, Isabela spontaneously initiated actions, showed preferences, remained focused on tasks, tried to achieve specific outcomes, and engaged in imaginative activities. She selected two anime books and examined them while sitting in a bean bag chair. Isabela sketched some designs but immediately put her drawings away when three peers sat next to her. When they asked to see her drawings, Isabela shook her head "no" and smiled. Instead, she showed them her books, exchanged a few polite words, and then moved to another area of the library to sit alone until her next class.

During gym class, Isabela's class played volleyball. Isabela was hesitant to initiate actions, though she remained task directed. She was hesitant in showing preferences (e.g., did not run or walk quickly to a position on the court when her teacher indicated she could play wherever she liked), or try new things (e.g., appeared reluctant to try to overhand serve). Isabela did not observably express mastery pleasure when she hit the ball over the net, ran for the ball when it was slightly out of arm's reach, or attempted to help a teammate who called to her. Isabela frequently walked away from the ball when it was in her vicinity. After two classmates encouraged her to stand closer to the net, Isabela did so hesitantly but then immediately retreated after the ball was served. Isabela appeared to want to avoid the activity (e.g., frequently left the volleyball activity area to get water, stood near the sidelines, and went to the bleachers several times to "look for something" in her backpack).

In addition to the *Volitional Questionnaire*, the occupational therapist also completed the *Child Occupational Self-Assessment* (Kramer et al., 2014) using the card sort approach to encourage Isabela's engagement. The therapist intentionally took time to discuss Isabela's strengths with her. Isabela categorized several items in the category "I am really good at doing this," such as "keep my body clean," "dress myself," "get my chores done," "take care of my things," "use my hands to work with things," and "following classroom rules." Isabela shared details about her responsibilities related to taking care of her little sister and doing household chores. She expressed pride in being a big sister, helping her parents, and learning how to make simple meals and desserts. Isabela also identified items that she perceived as challenging, such as "having enough time to do things I like," "get enough sleep," "keep my mind on what I am doing," "do things with my friends," "do things with my classmates," "make others understand my ideas," and "ask my teacher questions when I need to." Isabela shared that she would really like to make friends and have more things to do that she enjoys; however, she is worried doing so would leave less time for her to complete all her home responsibilities. Isabela shared stories about the people she met

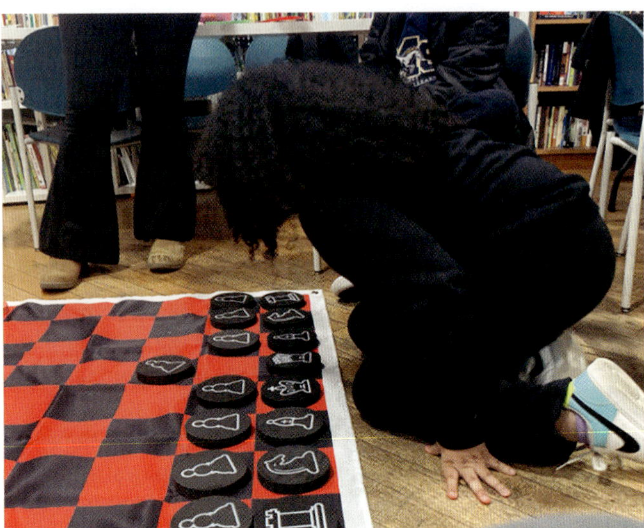

FIGURE 16.2 Isabela learning chess.

on her journey and from her time living in shelters. She told the therapist that she didn't like to think about the children and other people she met whom she believed to still be living there. She also missed her family in Venezuela.

The therapist had permission to evaluate other areas of Isabela's occupational performance. However, before proceeding, Isabela's mother withdrew her consent for evaluation for special education and related services. The occupational therapist shared his initial findings with the evaluation team and Isabela's mother. The occupational therapist recommended that Isabela join the after-school chess club (Figure 16.2) as a way to develop adaptive coping skills and demonstrate spontaneous volitional behaviors. Chess club was selected because of Isabela's previous interest in playing chess. The occupational therapist suggested tasks where Isabela could showcase existing competence, such as setting up the chess board and teaching new players how the chess pieces move. The occupational therapist also suggested that Isabela initially be matched with less skillful players before being introduced to more advanced ones. Additionally, a self-rating form for chess play was proposed, so that the club leader could further support Isabela. The form was to include opportunities to rate statements like, "I had fun today," "I learned something new today," and "I played well today." Engaging in chess strategy and gameplay would enable Isabela to focus on the present moment. Furthermore, participating in chess would introduce Isabela to new peers, learn a game that she could play in different contexts, apply her already well-developed strategic thinking skills, and demonstrate her intelligence to her peers (Figure 16.3).

The occupational therapist suggested to the teacher that she should continue acknowledging Isabela's math skills and consider opportunities for group math activities. This would allow Isabela to interact with her peers during an activity where she feels confident. The therapist also suggested that the classroom teacher incorporate some activities to promote Isabela's subjective well-being and benefit the entire class. Specifically, the occupational therapist recommended teaching the students about random acts of kindness. The therapist selected this activity over other ones that promote subjective well-being (e.g., telling someone you are grateful for them) due to the low language demands. Furthermore, the occupational therapist recommended the teacher to allocate 3 to 5 minutes at the start of each day

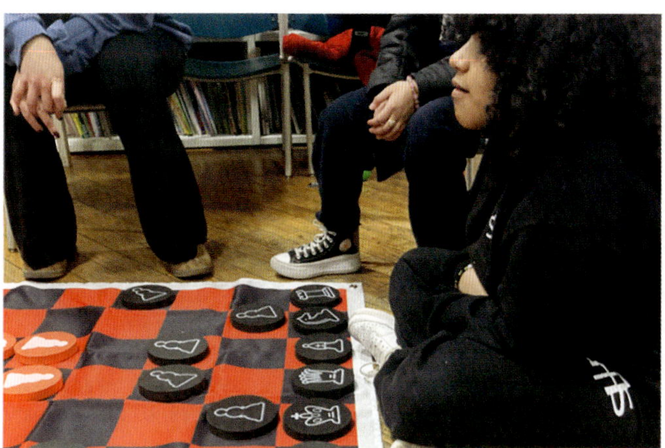

FIGURE 16.3 Isabela demonstrating strong volition while playing chess.

for students to write in a personal gratitude journal. Students would be encouraged to use their preferred language and have the option to draw a picture to represent something they were grateful for. This activity was selected due to its minimal social demands.

The occupational therapist also encouraged Isabela's mom to continue finding time during their busy weeks to engage in activities with Isabela that they both enjoyed doing together. Isabela's mom identified preparing dinner, completing a puzzle, and going to the park on the weekends as things they like to do together.

SUPPORTING EVIDENCE

Cahill et al. (2020) found evidence for the use of occupation and activity-based interventions for children with and at risk for mental health concerns. Group and individual interventions that include the intentional use of occupations can enhance role competence, habitual use of adaptive coping strategies, and meaningful social participation. Occupation-based groups and activities that promote PCEs lead to feelings of subjective well-being and mitigate the effects of adverse childhood experiences (Bethell et al., 2019; Rothman & Lynch, 2023).

Play, crafts, and mindfulness techniques have also been successfully used to meet the needs of children and youth experiencing symptoms of anxiety and depression. Play-based interventions provide children with the opportunity to enhance creativity and volitional development and provide an opportunity to practice using social rules and conventions (Bundy et al., 2017; Cordier, et al., 2009). Crafts have been used to establish positive routines and provide opportunities for problem solving, creativity, and collaboration (Hansen et al., 2021; Horghagen et al., 2014). Mindfulness practices, such as yoga and meditation, have been found to help children and youth cope with everyday stressors and focus attention during times of stress (Rempel, 2012; Zoogman et al., 2014).

Suldo et al. (2014) designed a series of groups to promote subjective well-being. Examples of the group activities associated with promoting subjective well-being and positive youth development included writing in "gratitude journals," completing "gratitude visits" (i.e., telling someone you are grateful for them), and performing random acts of kindness. Students who participated in groups in this study reported greater life satisfaction. Table 16.6 includes an overview of relevant evidence-based literature.

Table 16.6 Overview of Relevant Literature

Concept	Description	Supporting Evidence
Promoting positive childhood experiences (PCEs)	PCEs provide protective advantages and interact in a mitigating capacity with adverse childhood events (ACEs). Children and youth who report greater numbers of PCEs typically exhibit commensurately elevated levels of mental health and well-being and less risk for future mental health challenges, even in the presence of ACEs. Seven PCEs have been identified and included: (1) feeling supported by family during tough times, (2) feels safe and protected by adult(s) at home, (3) feels supported by friends, (4) has two or more nonparent caring adults in their life, (5) able to talk to their family about their feelings, (6) sense of belonging at school, and (7) enjoys participating in their community. Rothman and Lynch (2023) discussed the alignment between PCE items and occupational therapy practice, particularly with respect to the positive impact of protective factors on self-regulation, engaging in school occupations, and social participation at home and school.	Bethell, C., Jones, J., Gombojav, N., Linkenbach, J., & Sege, R. (2019). PCEs and adult mental and relational health in a statewide sample: Associations across adverse childhood experiences levels. *JAMA Pediatrics, 173*(11), 1–10. https://doi.org/10.1001/jamapediatrics.2019.3007 Rothman, E., & Lynch. A. (2023). The state of the science on adverse childhood experiences. *OTJR: Occupational Therapy Journal of Research, 43*(1), 6–13. https://doi.org/10.1177/15394492221120799
Play as a means to increase intrinsic motivation and internal control	Play enables children to take risks in a safe environment, experience success, learn how to control and modify the environment for positive outcomes, and connect with other individuals to learn social rules and conventions.	Cordier, R., Bundy, A., Hocking, C., & Einfeld, S. (2009). A model for play-based intervention for children with ADHD. *Australian Occupational Therapy Journal, 56*(5), 332–340. https://doi.org/10.1111/j.1440-1630.2009.0079 Bundy, A., Engelen, L., Wyver, S., Tranter, P., Ragen, J., Bauman, A., & Naughton, G. (2017). Sydney playground project: a cluster-randomized trial to increase physical activity, play, and social skills. *Journal of School Health, 87*(10), 751–759.
Occupations associated with mindfulness, relaxation, and yoga support positive mental health	Learning how to cope with everyday stressors is an important life skill. Mindfulness practices help to reduce stress and refocus attention.	Rempel, K. D. (2012). Mindfulness for children and youth: A review of the literature with an argument for school-based implementation. *Canadian Journal of Counseling and Psychotherapy, 46*(3), 201–220. Zoogman, S., Goldberg, S. B., Hoyt, W. T., & Miller, L. (2014). Mindfulness interventions with youth: A meta-analysis. *Mindfulness*. https://doi.org/10.1007/s12671-013-0260-4

Table 16.6 Overview of Relevant Literature (Continued)

Concept	Description	Supporting Evidence
Positive youth development (PYD)	The field of PYD is rooted in positive psychology and emphasizes children's proclivity towards thriving and the development of strengths through positive subjective experiences, typically in a social context with other children and youth. Buenconsejo et al. (2023) describe several models of PYD and share indicators of thriving common across models.	Buenconsejo, J. U., & Datu, J. A. (2022). Toward an integrative paradigm of positive youth development: Implications for research, practice, and policy. *Human Development, 66*(6), 381–396. https://doi.org/10.1159/000527122
Use of positive youth development framework in occupational therapy	A review of 11 studies suggests that positive youth development results from the relationship between person, environment, and occupation factors. This relationship suggests an opportunity for occupational therapy to address positive youth development.	Hall, S., McKinstry, C., & Hyett, N. (2015). An occupational perspective of youth positive mental health: A critical review. *British Journal of Occupational Therapy, 78*(5), 276–285.
Cultivation of subjective well-being	Subjective well-being is thought to be an indicator of life satisfaction and children with high subjective well-being tend to be more virtuous, have more meaningful social relationships, engage in more productive pursuits, cope better with stress, and can more easily navigate obstacles. Subjective well-being is often thought of as happiness. Children with higher levels of subjective well-being are less likely to demonstrate internalizing and externalizing behaviors. Interventions that address subjective well-being by focusing on one or more components of positive psychology are effective for children and adolescents.	Chuecas, M. J., Alfaro, J., Benavente, M., & Ditzel, L. (2022). A systematic narrative review of subjective well-being promotion intervention programmes in the school setting. *Review of Education, 10*(1), e3345.
Goal setting with the child	Therapists have an obligation to adjust their approaches to including children in decision making about therapy services based on the child's evolving skills and abilities. When children are more engaged with planning, intervention maybe more successful.	O'Connor, D., Lynch, H., & Boyle, B. (2021). A qualitative study of child participation in decision-making: Exploring rights-based approaches in pediatric occupational therapy. *Plos One, 16*(12), e0260975. Pritchard, L., Phelan, S., McKillop, A., & Andersen, J. (2022). Child, parent, and clinician experiences with a child-driven goal setting approach in paediatric rehabilitation. *Disability and Rehabilitation, 44*(7), 1042–1049.

(*continued*)

Table 16.6 Overview of Relevant Literature (Continued)

Concept	Description	Supporting Evidence
Activity and occupation-based interventions to promote youth mental health.	This systematic review identified outdoor camps, video and computer games, productive occupations and life skills, meditation, animal-assisted interventions, creative arts, play, sports, and yoga. Moderate strength of evidence was found for yoga and sports. Moderate strength of evidence was found for play and creative arts.	Cahill, S. M., Egan, B. E., & Seber, J. (2020). Activity- and occupation-based interventions to support mental health, positive behavior, and social participation for children and youth: A systematic review. *American Journal of Occupational Therapy, 74*, 7402180020. https://doi.org/10.5014/ajot.2020.038687
Occupation-based nonacademic in-school programming	The manualized 8-week school-based occupational therapy group for seventh and eighth graders with subclinical anxiety, Kia Piki te Hauora (Maori for "uplifting our health and well-being"), included weekly instruction on occupational concepts, engagement in developmentally appropriate occupations based on the week's topic, encouraged peer exchanges, and facilitated occupational analysis reflection. Specifically, group members reflected on the relationship between occupational choices, occupational balance, and mental health and well-being. The process highlighted cognitive-behavioral thinking strategies by exploring the reciprocal ways that doing occupation and thinking/feeling can influence each other	Tokolahi, E., Vandal, A. C., Kersten, P., Pearson, J., & Hocking, C. (2018). Cluster-randomised controlled trial of an occupational therapy intervention for children aged 11–13 y, designed to increase participation to prevent symptoms of mental illness. *Child and Adolescent Mental Health, 23*(4), 313–327. https://doi.org/10.1111/camh.12270
Participation in civic engagement and volunteer activities to support mental health and positive youth development	Youth civic engagement, including volunteering and social activism, may affect adolescents' mental health and decrease stress.	Chaves, C. (2021). Wellbeing and flourishing. In M. Kern & M. Wehmeyer (Eds.), *The Palgrave handbook of positive education* (pp. 273–295). Springer International Publishing. Breedlove, M., Choi, J., & Zyromski, B. (2020). Mitigating the effects of adverse childhood experiences: How restorative practices in schools support PCEs and protective factors. *The New Educator, 17*(3), 223–241.
Use of mind-stimulating leisure activities.	Mind-stimulating leisure activities, both solitary and those with a social component, have been found to positively affect mental health outcomes in adults. More research is needed to determine the affects on children and adolescents.	Weziak-Bialowolska, D., Bialowolski, P., & Sacco, P. L. (2023). Mind-stimulating leisure activities: Prospective associations with health, wellbeing, and longevity. *Frontiers in Public Health, 11*, 1117822.

Table 16.6 Overview of Relevant Literature (Continued)

Concept	Description	Supporting Evidence
Use of crafts to support mental health	Crafts have been found to promote creativity and the mind-body connection. Crafts are supportive for cultivating enjoyment, stability, positive routines, problem solving, innovation, socialization, and collaboration in individuals with mental health concerns.	Horghagen, S., Fostvedt, B., & Alsaker, S. (2014). Craft activities in group meeting places: supporting mental health occupations. *Scandinavian Journal of Occupational Therapy, 21*(2), 145–152. https://doi.org/10.3109/11038128.2013.866691 Hansen, B. W., Erlandsson, L. K., & Leufstadius, C. (2021). A concept analysis of creative activities as intervention in occupational therapy. *Scandinavian Journal of Occupational Therapy, 28*(1), 63–77.
Occupations associated with gratitude are associated with increased life satisfaction	Students who participated in groups focused on cultivating gratitude reported greater life satisfaction. Examples of group activities included writing in gratitude journals, completing gratitude visits (i.e., telling someone you are grateful for them), and performing random acts of kindness.	Suldo, S. M., Savage, J. A., & Mercer, S. H. (2014). Increasing middle school students' life satisfaction: Efficacy of a positive psychology group intervention. *Journal of Happiness Studies, 15*(1), 19–42.

Summary

This chapter presents a frame of reference for providing occupational therapy services to school-aged children experiencing symptoms of anxiety and depression. Social participation, adaptive coping skills, and academic competence are central issues to school performance and indicative of positive mental health. This framework includes postulates regarding change, means to assess the need for targeted services, and guidance for intervention. Because engagement in occupation is central to mental health, an emphasis on occupational performance and supporting volitional development through occupation-based interventions is presented.

REFERENCES

American Occupational Therapy Association. (2020). Occupational therapy practice framework: Domain and process (4th ed.). *American Journal of Occupational Therapy*, 74(Suppl 2), 7412410010p1–7412410010p87. https://doi.org/10.5014/ajot.2020.74S2001

American Occupational Therapy Association. (2021). Improve your documentation and quality of care with AOTA's updated Occupational Profile Template. *American Journal of Occupational Therapy*, 75, 7502420010. https://doi.org/10.5014/ajot.2021.752001

Antoniadou, M., Granlund, M., & Andersson, A. K. (2024). Strategies used by professionals in pediatric rehabilitation to engage the child in the intervention process: A scoping review. *Physical & Occupational Therapy in Pediatrics*, 44(4), 461–488. https://doi.org/10.1080/01942638.2023.2290038

Baron, K., Kielhofner, G., Iyenger, A., Goldhammer, V., & Wolenski, J. (2006). *The occupational self-assessment (OSA) (version 2.2)*. Model of Human Occupation Clearinghouse, Department of Occupational Therapy, College of Applied Health Sciences, University of Illinois at Chicago.

Basu, S., Kafkes, A., Schatz, R., Kiraly, A., & Kielhofner, G. (2008). *Pediatric volitional questionnaire (version 2.1)*. Model of Human Occupation Clearinghouse, Department of Occupational Therapy, College of Applied Health Sciences, University of Illinois at Chicago.

Bethell, C., Jones, J., Gombojav, N., Linkenbach, J., & Sege, R. (2019). Positive childhood experiences and adult mental and relational health in a statewide sample: Associations across adverse childhood experiences levels. *JAMA Pediatrics*, *173*(11), e193007. https://doi.org/10.1001/jamapediatrics.2019.3007

Bjørnsen, H. N., Bjørnebekk, G., & Brandmo, C. (2023). Schools as a source of mental health literacy: Adjusting and validating a mental health literacy scale. *Health Promotion Practice*, *24*(2), 391–398. https://doi.org/10.1177/15248399231161090

Bowlby, J. (1988). *A secure base: Parent-child attachment and healthy human development*. Basic Books Inc.

Breedlove, M., Choi, J., & Zyromski, B. (2020). Mitigating the effects of adverse childhood experiences: How restorative practices in schools support positive childhood experiences and protective factors. *The New Educator*, *17*(3), 223–241. https://doi.org/10.1080/1547688X.2020.1807078

Buenconsejo, J. U., & Datu, J. A. D. (2022). Positive youth development: A brief review of literature with implications for school-based psychological interventions. *Journal of Psychologists and Counsellors in Schools*, *32*(2), 275–282. https://doi.org/10.1017/jgc.2021.25

Buenconsejo, J. U. & Datu, J. A. (2023). Toward an integrative paradigm of positive youth development: Implications for research, practice, and policy. *Human Development*, *66*(6), 381–396. https://doi.org/10.1159/000527122

Bundy, A., Engelen, L., Wyver, S., Tranter, P., Ragen, J., Bauman, A., Baur, L., Schiller, W., Simpson, J.M., Niehues, A.N., Perry, G., Jessup, G., & Naughton, G. (2017). Sydney playground project: a cluster-randomized trial to increase physical activity, play, and social skills. *Journal of School Health*, *87*(10), 751–759.

Cahill, S. M., & Egan, B. E. (2017). Identifying youth with mental health conditions at school. *OT Practice, 22*(5), CE-1–CE-8.

Cahill, S. M., Egan, B. E., & Seber, J. (2020). Activity-and occupation-based interventions to support mental health, positive behavior, and social participation for children and youth: A systematic review. *The American Journal of Occupational Therapy*, *74*(2), 7402180020p1–7402180020p28.

Chaves, C. (2021). Wellbeing and flourishing. In: M. L. Kern, M. L. Wehmeyer. (Eds.) *The Palgrave Handbook of Positive Education*. Palgrave Macmillan. https://doi.org/10.1007/978-3-030-64537-3_11

Chopik, W. J., & Kitayama, S. (2018). Personality change across the life span: Insights from a cross-cultural, longitudinal study. *Journal of Personality, 86*(3), 508–521. https://doi.org/10.1111/jopy.12332

Coulombe, S., Hardy, K., & Goldfarb, R. (2020). Promoting wellbeing through positive education: A critical review and proposed social ecological approach. *Theory and Research in Education*, *18*(3), 295–321. https://doi.org/10.1177/1477878520988432

Cordier, R., Bundy, A., Hocking, C., & Einfeld, S. (2009). A model for play-based intervention for children with ADHD. *Australian Occupational Therapy Journal, 56*(5), 332–340. https://doi.org/10.1111/j.1440-1630.2009.00796.x

da Silva, A. C. C., & Oliver, F. C. (2021). Social participation in occupational therapy: Is it possible to establish a consensus? *Australian Occupational Therapy Journal*, *68*(6), 535–545. https://doi.org/10.1111/1440-1630.12763

Deci, E. L., & Ryan, R. M. (2008). Self-determination theory: A macrotheory of human motivation, development, and health. *Canadian Psychology/Psychologie Canadienne*, *49*(3), 182–185. https://doi.org/10.1037/a0012801

de las Heras, C. G., Geist, R., Kielhofner, G., & Li, Y. (2007). *A user's manual for the Volitional Questionnaire (version 4.1)*. Model of Human Occupation Clearinghouse, Department of Occupational Therapy, College of Applied Health Sciences, University of Illinois at Chicago.

DePauw, S. S., & Mervielde, I. (2010). Temperament, personality and developmental psychopathology: A review based on the conceptual dimensions underlying childhood traits. *Child Psychiatry and Human Development*, *41*(3), 313–329. https://doi.org/10.1007/s10578-009-0171-8

Davis, E. P., & Glynn, L. M. (2024). Annual research review: The power of predictability-patterns of signals in early life shape neurodevelopment and mental health trajectories. *Journal of Child Psychology and Psychiatry*, *65*(4), 508–534. https://doi.org/10.1111/jcpp.13958

Davis, S. H., Winer, J. P., Gillespie, S. C., & Mulder, L. A. (2021). The Refugee and Immigrant Core Stressors Toolkit (RICST): Understanding the multifaceted needs of refugee and immigrant youth and families through a four core stressors framework. *Journal of Technology in Behavioral Science*, *6*(4), 620–630.

Donahue, M. (2013). *Social Profile: Assessment of social participation in children, adolescents, and adults*. AOTA Press.

Dowdy, E., Furlong, M. J., Nylund-Gibson, K., Arch, D., Hinton, T., & Carter, D. (2023). Validating a brief student distress measure for schoolwide wellness surveillance. *Assessment for Effective Intervention*, *48*(3), 159–169. https://doi.org/10.1177/15345084221138947

Egan, B. E., Sears, C., & Keener, A. (2023). *Occupational therapy groups for addressing mental health challenges in school-aged populations: A tier 2 resource*. SLACK, Inc.

Elrefaay, S. M. M., & Elyzal, A. S. (2024). Adverse childhood experiences and depression: The mediating role of resilience and emotional regulation. *Journal of Psychosocial Nursing and Mental Health Services*, *62*(1), 45–54. https://doi.org/10.3928/02793695-20230726-06

Frederick, K. (2022). Resilience development in children with adverse childhood experiences: The role of the occupational therapist and the interdisciplinary team. *Student Journal of Occupational Therapy*, *3*(2), 14–29. https://doi.org/10.46409/001.YHFA8315

Goodman, R. (1997). The strengths and difficulties questionnaire: A research note. *Journal of Child Psychology and Psychiatry*, *38*(5), 581–586.

Hansen, B. W., Erlandsson, L. K., & Leufstadius, C. (2021). A concept analysis of creative activities as intervention in occupational therapy. *Scandinavian Journal of Occupational Therapy*, *28*(1), 63–77.

Heyne, D., & Brouwer-Borghuis, M. (2022). Signposts for school refusal interventions, based on the views of stakeholders. *Continuity in Education*, *3*(1), 25–40. https://doi.org/10.53334/cie.42

Horghagen, S., Fostvedt, B., & Alsaker, S. (2014). Craft activities in group meeting places: supporting mental health occupations. *Scandinavian Journal of Occupational Therapy*, *21*(2), 145–152. https://doi.org/10.3109/11038128.2013.866691

Huebner, E. S. (1994). Preliminary development and validation of a multidimensional life satisfaction scale for children, *Psychological Assessment*, *6*(2), 149–158. https://doi.org/10.1037/1040-3590.6.2.149

Keyes, C. L. (2002). The mental health continuum: from languishing to flourishing in life. *Journal of Health and Social Behavior*, *43*(2), 207–222. https://doi.org/10.2307/3090197

Kiraly-Alvarez, A. (2015). Assessing volition in pediatrics: Using the volitional questionnaire and the pediatric volitional questionnaire. *The Open Journal of Occupational Therapy*, *3*(3), 7. https://doi.org/10.15453/2168-6408.1176

Kramer, J., ten Velden, M., Kafkes, A., Basu, S., Federico, J., & Kielhofner, G. (2014). *The child occupational self-assessment (COSA) (version 2.1)*. Model of Human, IL, Occupation Clearinghouse, Department of Occupational Therapy, College of Applied Health Sciences, University of Illinois at Chicago.

Kramer, J., Walker, R., Cohn, E. S., Mermelstein, M., Olsen, S., O'Brien, J., & Bowyer, P. (2012). Striving for shared understandings: therapists' perspectives of the benefits and dilemmas of using a child self-assessment. *OTJR: Occupation, Participation and Health*, *32*(1_Suppl), S48–S58. https://doi.org/10.3928/15394492-20110906-02

Kuypers, L. (2011). *The zones of regulation: A curriculum designed to foster self-regulation and emotional control*. Social Thinking.

Lane, K. L., & Menzies, H. M. (2009). Student Risk Screening Scale for Internalizing and Externalizing (SRSS-IE). Retrieved from http://www.ci3t.org/screening

Lane, K. L., Oakes, W. P., Swogger, E. D., Schatschneider, C., Menzies, H. M., & Sanchez, J. (2015). Student risk screening scale for internalizing and externalizing behaviors: Preliminary cut scores to support data-informed decision making. *Behavioral Disorders*, *40*, 159–170. https://doi.org/10.17988/0198-7429-40.3.159

Lane, K. L., Oakes, W. P., Buckman, M. M., Lane, N. A., Lane, K. S., Fleming, K., Swinburne Romine, R., Sherod, R., Chang, C., & Cantwell, E. D. (2023). Additional evidence of predictive validity of SRSS-IE scores with elementary students. *Behavioral Disorders*, *49*(3), 189–204. https://doi.org/10.1177/0198742923122289

Lannigan, E. G., Raber, C., & Seber, J. (2024). Observational assessments. In R. R. Taylor, P. Bowyer, & G. Fisher (Eds.), *Kielhofner's model of human occupation: Theory and application* (6th ed., pp. 235–255). Wolters Kluwer.

Leduc, K., Tougas, A., Robert, V., & Boulanger, C. (2022). *School refusal in youth: A systematic review of ecological factors*. Child Psychiatry & Human Development.

Lee, S., & Kielhofner, G. (2024). Volition: Pattern of thoughts and feelings about oneself as one anticipates, chooses, experiences, and interprets what one does. In R. Taylor, P. Bowyer, & G. Fisher (Eds.), *Kielhofner's model of human occupation* (6th ed., pp. 41–60). Wolters Kluwer.

Leigers, K., Myers, C., & Schneck, C. (2016). Social participation in schools: a survey of occupational therapy practitioners. *American Journal of Occupational Therapy*, *70*(5), 7005280010p1–7005280010p9. https://doi.org/10.5014/ajot.2016.020768

Lynch, A. K., Ashcraft, R., Mahler, K., Whiting, C. C., Schroeder, K., & Weber, M. (2020). Using a public health model as a foundation for trauma-informed care for occupational therapists in school settings. *Journal of Occupational Therapy, Schools, & Early Intervention*, *13*(3), 219–235. https://doi.org/10.1080/19411243.2020.1732263

Maier, B. C. L., Zillich, L., Streit, F., Wildenberg, K., Rietschel, M., Hammes, H.-P., Witt, S. H., & Deuschle, M. (2022). Adverse childhood experiences and late-life diurnal HPA axis activity: Associations of different childhood adversity types and interaction with timing in a sample of older East Prussian World War II refugees. *Psychoneuroendocrinology*, *139*, 105717. https://doi.org/10.1016/j.psyneuen.2022.105717

Martins, J., Cunha, J., Lopes, S., Moreira, T., & Rosário, P. (2022). School engagement in elementary school: A systematic review of 35 years of research. *Educational psychology review*, *34*(2), 793–849. https://doi.org/10.1007/s10648-021-09642-5

Moreira, A. L., Yunes, M. Â. M., Nascimento, C. R. R., & Bedin, L. M. (2021). Children's subjective well-being, peer relationships and resilience: an integrative literature review. *Child Indicators Research*, *14*(5), 1723–1742. https://doi.org/10.1007/s12187-021-09843-y

Naglieri, J. A., LeBuffe, P. A., & Shapiro, V. B. (2011/2014). The Devereux Student Strengths Assessment – Mini (DESSA-Mini): Assessment, technical manual, and user's guide, Apperson.

Nigg, J. T. (2006). Temperament and developmental psychopathology. *Journal of Child Psychology and Psychiatry*, *47*(3–4), 395–422. https://doi.org/10.1111/j.1469-7610.2006.01612.x

O'Connor, D., Lynch, H., & Boyle, B. (2021). A qualitative study of child participation in decision-making: exploring rights-based approaches in pediatric occupational therapy. *PloS one*, *16*(12), e0260975.

Olson, L. (2011). Development and implementation of groups to foster social participation and mental health. In Bazyk, S. (Ed.), *Mental health promotion, prevention, and intervention with children and youth: A guiding framework for occupational therapy* (pp. 95–115). AOTA Press.

Parsonage-Harrison, J., Birken, M., Harley, D., Dawes, H., & Eklund, M. (2023). A scoping review of interventions using occupation to improve mental health or mental wellbeing in adolescent populations. *British Journal of Occupational Therapy*, *86*(3), 236–250. https://doi.org/10.1177/03080226221110391

Patten, K. K. (2022). Eleanor Clarke Slagle Lecture—Finding our strengths: recognizing professional bias and interrogating systems. *American Journal of Occupational Therapy*, *76*(6), 7606150010. https://doi.org/10.5014/ajot.2022.076603

Pawl, J., & Milburn, L. (2006). Family- and relationship-centered principles. In Foley, G. & Hochman, J. (Eds.), *Mental health in early intervention: Achieving unity in principles and practice* (pp. 191–226). Brookes.

Pollack, S. D. (2015). Developmental psychopathology: Recent advances and future challenges. *World Psychiatry*, *14*(3), 262–269. https://doi.org/10.1002/wps.20237

Pritchard, L., Phelan, S., McKillop, A., & Andersen, J. (2020). Child, parent, and clinician experiences with a child-driven goal setting approach in paediatric rehabilitation. *Disability and Rehabilitation*, *44*(7), 1042–1049. https://doi.org/10.1080/09638288.2020.1788178

Prusnek, L. L., Griffiths, T., & Provident, I. (2019). Implementing the comfortable cafeteria program to foster social participation of students with and without hearing impairments: a look at the outcomes. *Journal of Occupational Therapy, Schools, & Early Intervention*, *12*(2), 239–252. https://doi.org/10.1080/19411243.2019.1592055

Pynoos, R. S., Steinberg, A. M., & Piacentini, J. C. (1999). A developmental psychopathology model of childhood traumatic stress and intersection with anxiety disorders. *Biological Psychiatry*, *46*(11), 1542–1554. https://doi.org/10.1016/S0006-3223(99)00262-0

Raine, K.E., Zimmer-Gemeck, M. J., & Skinner, E. (2023). The role of coping in processes of resilience: the sample case of academic coping during late childhood and early adolescence. *Development and Psychopathology*, *35*(5), 2499–2515. https://doi.org/10.1017/S095457942300072X

Racine, N., McArthur, B. A., Cooke, J. E., Eirich, R., Zhu, J., & Madigan, S. (2021). Global prevalence of depressive and anxiety symptoms in children and adolescents during COVID-19: a meta-analysis. *JAMA Pediatrics*, *175*(11), 1142–1150. https://doi.org/10.1001/jamapediatrics.2021.2482

Reilly, M., (Ed.). (1974). *Play as exploratory learning*. Sage Publications.

Rempel, K. D. (2012). Mindfulness for children and youth: A review of the literature with an argument for school-based implementation. *Canadian Journal of Counseling and Psychotherapy*, *46*(3), 201–220.

Rothman, E., & Lynch. A. (2023). The state of the science on adverse childhood experiences. *OTJR: Occupational Therapy Journal of Research*, *43*(1), 6–13. https://doi.org/10.1177/15394492221120799

Sampson, L., Kubzansky, L. D., & Koenen, K. (2023). The missing piece: A population health perspective to address the U.S. mental health crisis. *Daedalus*, *152*(4), 24–44. https://doi.org/10.1162/daed_a_02030

Schaffer, G. E., Power, E. M., Fisk, A. K., & Trolian, T. L. (2021). Beyond the four walls: the evolution of school psychological services during the COVID-19 outbreak. *Psychology in the Schools*, *58*(7), 1246–1265. https://doi.org/10.1002/pits.22543

Seligson, J. L., Huebner, E. S., & Valois, R. F. (2003). Preliminary validation of the brief multidimensional students' life satisfaction scale (BMSLSS). *Social Indicators Research*, *61*(2), 121–145. https://doi.org/10.1023/A:1021326822957

Shih, E. W., Ahmad, S. I., Bush, N. R., Roubinov, D., Tylavsky, F., Graff, C., Karr, C. J., Sathyanarayana, S., & LeWinn, K. Z. (2023). A path model examination: maternal anxiety and parenting mediate the association between maternal adverse childhood experiences and children's internalizing behaviors. *Psychological Medicine*, *53*(1), 112–122.

Shiner, R. L., Soto, C. J., & De Fruyt, F. (2021). Personality assessment of children and adolescents. *Annual Review of Developmental Psychology*, *3*(1), 113–137. https://doi.org/10.1146/annurev-devpsych-050620-114343

Skinner, E. A., Pitzer, J. R., & Steele, J. S. (2016). Can student engagement serve as a motivational resource for academic coping, persistence, and learning during late elementary and early middle school? *Developmental Psychology, 52*(12), 2099–2117. https://doi.org/10.1037/dev0000232

Solmi, M., Radua, J., Olivola, M., Croce, E., Soardo, L., Salazar de Pablo, G., Il Shin, J., Kirkbride, J. B., Jones, P, Kim, J. H., Kim, J. Y., Carvalho, A. F., Seeman, M. V., Correll, C. U., & Fusar-Poli, P. (2022). Age at onset of mental disorders worldwide: large-scale meta-analysis of 192 epidemiological studies. *Molecular Psychiatry*, *27*(1), 281–295. https://doi.org/10.1038/s41380-021-01161-7

Sroufe, L. A., Carlson, E. A., Levy, A. K., & Egeland, B. (1999). Implications of attachment theory for developmental psychopathology. *Development and Psychopathology, 11*(1), 1–13. https://doi.org/10.1017/S0954579499001923

Sroufe, L. A., & Rutter, M. (1984). The domain of developmental psychopathology. *Child Development, 55*(1), 17–29.

Struck, S., Stewart-Tufescu, A., Asmundson, A. J., Asmundson, G. G., & Afifi, T. O. (2021). Adverse childhood experiences (ACEs) research: A bibliometric analysis of publication trends over the first 20 years. *Child Abuse & Neglect*, *112*, 104895.

Suldo, S. M., Savage, J. A., & Mercer, S. H. (2014). Increasing middle school students' life satisfaction: Efficacy of a positive psychology group intervention. *Journal of Happiness Studies, 15*(1), 19–42. https://doi.org/10.1007/s10902-013-9414-2

Taylor, R., Bowyer, P., & Fisher, G. (Eds.) (2024). *Kielhofner's model of human occupation* (6th ed.). Wolters Kluwer.

Tokolahi, E., Vandal, A. C., Kersten, P., Pearson, J., & Hocking, C. (2018). Cluster-randomised controlled trial of an occupational therapy intervention for children aged 11–13 years, designed to increase participation to prevent symptoms of mental illness. *Child and Adolescent Mental Health*, *23*(4), 313–327. https://doi.org/10.1111/camh.12270

Van der Kolk, B. A. (2017). Developmental trauma disorder: Toward a rational diagnosis for children with complex trauma histories. *Psychiatric Annals, 35*(5), 401–408. https://doi.org/10.3928/00485713-20050501-06

Waddell, C., Schwartz C., Barican J., Yung D., & Gray-Grant D. (2020). *COVID-19 and the impact on children's mental health*. Children's Health Policy Centre, Simon Fraser University.

Watson, D., Gamez, W., & Simms, L. J. (2005). Basic dimensions of temperament and their relation to anxiety and depression: a symptom-based perspective. *Journal of Research in Personality, 39*(1), 46–66. https://doi.org/10.1016/j.jrp.2004.09.006

Whittenburg, P. N., Stern, J. A., Brett, B. E., Straske, M. D., & Cassidy, J. (2023). Maternal depressive symptoms and child behavior problems: attachment security as a protective factor. *Development and Psychopathology, 35*(2), 678–688. https://doi.org/10.1017/S0954579421001802

World Health Organization. (2022). *World mental health report: Transforming mental health for all.* World Health Organization. https://www.who.int/publications/i/item/9789240049338

Yaffe, Y. (2021). A narrative review of the relationship between parenting and anxiety disorders in children and adolescents. *International Journal of Adolescence and Youth*, *26*(1), 449–459.

Zoogman, S., Goldberg, S. B., Hoyt, W. T., & Miller, L. (2014). Mindfulness interventions with youth: A meta-analysis. *Mindfulness, 6,* 290–302. https://doi.org/10.1007/s12671-013-0260-4

Transition From School to Adult Life Frame of Reference

Meira L. Orentlicher

with comments from Samuel J. Hendrickson

Graduating from or aging out of high school is an exciting, yet challenging time for young adults as they prepare for new opportunities and experiences in attending college, starting work, living outside of their parents' home, developing new relationships, and participating in community life. Young adults with intellectual and developmental disabilities (IDD) hold similar aspirations for adulthood, although they face added challenges associated with their disabilities that may require additional supports (Bennet et al., 2018; Carter et al., 2017). Indeed, young adults with IDD lag behind their typical peers in achieving adult outcomes (Griffiths et al., 2024; Hiersteiner et al., 2016; Schutz & Carter, 2022; Wehman et al., 2020).

The Individuals with Disabilities Education Improvement Act of 2004 (IDEA; Pub. L. 108–446) mandates that students who receive special education and related services should be prepared for "further education, employment, and independent living" (§ 1401[d]). This explicit statement clarifies that school personnel, parents, and students must consider adult outcomes as they plan students with IDD's school experiences and individualized education programs (IEPs). To improve adult outcomes for eligible students with disabilities, schools are required to provide transition services beginning no later than age 16 years. IDEA identifies seven areas to focus on when planning and preparing for the transition to adult life: (1) postsecondary education; (2) vocational education; (3) integrated employment (including supported employment); (4) continuing and adult education; (5) adult services; (6) independent living; and (7) community participation. These transition areas are strikingly similar to the *areas of occupation* in the Occupational Therapy Practice Framework (*"Framework,"* 4th edition, American Occupational Therapy Association [AOTA], 2020). The *Framework* introduces successful transition to the next life stage or service as an outcome of occupational therapy services and cites Orentlicher and Gibson's (2015) definition of transition as "movement from one life role or experience to another" which "may require preparation, new knowledge, and time to accommodate to the new situation" (p. 27).

Adolescence is a developmental stage that generally occurs from ages 13 to 19 and is considered the transition between childhood and adulthood. It is a time of major change, and the physical, psychological, and social changes can add additional challenges to the preparation for the transition from school to adult life. This chapter introduces a frame of reference for the transition from school to adult life. It provides the theoretical lens for understanding the transition process, including the major challenges faced by adolescents with IDD and the impact of these challenges on the adolescents' current and future occupational performance. Evaluation and intervention strategies to address these challenges are suggested, as well as the applications to occupational therapy practice. Because transitions are critically important to parents and educators in addition to the student, periodically throughout the chapter, comments from a parent and educator have been included to enhance practitioner's understanding of their perspective.

THEORETICAL BASE

The transition from school to adult life can be understood from a variety of disciplines and theoretical approaches. Anthropologists examine life transitions within the contexts of cultural beliefs and practices (American Anthropology Association, n.d.), while sociologists explore the broader societal trends that reflect changes in populations and subgroups' behavior (Doidge & Saini, 2020). These perspectives help us understand the expectations that young adults and families have about the transition process and outcomes. For example, many young adults view college as a rite of passage. Beyond academics, the college experience is believed to provide preparation for "real" jobs, opportunities to participate in social activities, and growth in independence and self-confidence (Papay & Bambara, 2014; Smith et al., 2018). Psychologists seek to understand individuals' behavior, mental processes, and reactions and responses to transition experiences and other life changes (Gerrig, 2013). During high school, typically developing adolescents explore their identity through experimentation with interests, relationships, images, and behaviors and form self-concept and self-esteem. Evolving identity plays an important role in the young adult's future education, employment, and social relationships. Educators focus on developing and implementing transition programs to support students with IDD during the movement from high school to employment and independence (Wehman, 2013).

Developmental and Natural Transitions

Developmental transitions typically follow a person's lifespan, and most are accepted as natural and reinforced by cultural practices, such as the first day of school, or celebrations marking development stages in adolescence including Sweet 16, Bar or Bat Mitzvah, or Quinceañera (Orentlicher & Gibson, 2015). Other transition markings in adolescence and young adulthood include attending prom, graduating high school, attending college, or getting a first job. These transitions are also referred to as *natural transitions*, which are life transitions that are generally anticipated and prepared for and shared within a cultural context (Orentlicher & Gibson, 2015). The developmental and natural transitions typically encompass shared rules and expectations about the changes pre- and post-transition. For example, young adults are expected to move out of their parents' home and live on their own or with roommates, after college.

Natural transitions usually involve three stages: (1) *Preparation*: time to prepare for the transition and practice the anticipated new roles; (2) *Distinct transition*: the actual time of change; and (3) *Consolidation*: a period of adjustment posttransition (Orentlicher & Gibson, 2015).

Natural transitions, possibly because of their relationship to development and cultural norms, tend to be one directional; once the transition has occurred, there is usually no returning to the pretransition state.

Understanding Adolescence

Adolescence is a time of major change for all individuals. The physical, psychological, and social changes can be challenging for both the adolescents and those around them, such as parents and teachers. As children with IDD move into and through adolescence, they experience many challenges including dealing with the changes of puberty, managing a desire for and expectations of greater independence, developing and maintaining close friendships, preparing for adult roles and skills, and coping with increased academic and vocational demands (Orentlicher & Case, 2018a).

Puberty is the period during which preadolescents and adolescents undergo sexual maturation involving physical changes that end with the young adult achieving fertility. The maturation also results in secondary sex characteristics, which are the physical features associated with adult males and females (Stöppler & Shiel, 2022). In addition to sexual maturation, the adolescent years also include general growth and major changes in height, weight, and body composition. Sexuality and sexual behavior develop and change in response to interactions and social experiences.

Adolescents typically experience *emotional changes* that accompany puberty. Changes can occur in the way teens view themselves and in how they respond to family or friends. Many adolescents experience mood swings, anxiety, confusion, and sensitivity (Memmott-Elison et al., 2020; Stöppler & Shiel, 2022). However, not all emotional changes of puberty are negative. Puberty is also a time in which adolescents learn about their interests and goals and how to relate to others in a more mature way (Stöppler & Shiel, 2022). The typical emotional swings of adolescents also include a desire to separate from parents and achieve independence in activities of daily living, schoolwork, social and recreational participation, and decision making. Typical adolescents provide their parents with "cues" that demonstrate their desire for more independence (Aikins et al., 2009; Ruhl et al., 2015). For example, they push away from their parents and insist on making more independent decisions. From the parents' perspective, when parents of adolescents have high expectations for their children and express strong beliefs in their children's ability to succeed, their children achieve higher levels of success (Xu et al., 2022). Similarly, young adults with IDD whose parents have high expectations about their independence achieve more independence and more successful outcomes as adults (Wehmeyer, 2014).

As adolescents pull away from their parents, *friendships* and peer group acceptance become increasingly more important (Anderson et al., 2016). The development of social connections and friendships is strongly related to an individual's ability to behave in a socially accepted manner. Communication expectations become increasingly complex and social interactions become more abstract (Cresswell et al., 2019). Current technologic developments provide opportunities for adolescents to develop friendships in virtual environments. Friendships developed online, such as in gaming environments, can go beyond superficial connections and develop into meaningful relationships (Gallup et al., 2016).

Adolescence is a time of preparation for lifelong roles. Strong *executive functioning skills* relate to successful adult outcomes (Matthews et al., 2015; Tamm et al., 2022). As adolescents move through high school and transition to postsecondary schooling or vocation, it is expected that they will be able to plan activities, organize materials, plan for time to complete tasks, maintain focus on the task despite other distractions, and problem solve.

Philosophy of Practice

Transition from school to adult life processes is grounded in philosophical underpinnings that guide practice: inclusion, social model of disability, and universal design.

Inclusion

Inclusion means that people with disabilities have the right to full and equitable access to activities, social roles, and relationships alongside typical individuals, with the appropriate supports necessary for successful experiences (AOTA, 2014). Disability is viewed as a natural part of the human experience and it should not diminish the right of individuals to participate in or contribute to society. Individuals who learn, live, work, and receive services in inclusive settings have better outcomes in social interactions and participation in meaningful occupations in their communities (Spence-Cochran et al., 2013). When young adults with IDD transition to new activities, programs, and places, planning and preparation should include consideration of accommodations, systems of support, and activities to allow those individuals access to social, educational, recreational, and vocational opportunities within natural and inclusive settings (Orentlicher & Gibson, 2015).

Social Model of Disability

The social model of disability proposes that people with disabilities have difficulty participating in activities and community settings because of society's failure to provide appropriate accommodations and services (Oliver & Barnes, 1998). Thus, to support young adults with IDD who are transitioning to new environments, programs, and tasks, the focus of intervention should be on changing and accommodating the environment, tools, and tasks, rather than "fixing" the individual (Orentlicher & Gibson, 2015).

Universal Design

Universal design means that to the greatest extent possible, products and environments should be designed in a manner that can be usable by everyone regardless of age, ability, or circumstance (Schoonover, 2019). With roots in architecture, universal design was introduced to create public spaces, buildings, and everyday items that are accessible for people with and without disabilities. Examples of universal design include curb cuts, ramps, levered door handles, braille grids, software operating systems with options such as speech output, captioning of television and films, ergonomic keyboards, voice-activated telephones, or buses with wheelchair lifts.

Best Practices in Transition From School to Adult Life

Research on best practices in transition indicates that they can be ranked from most to least substantiated as follows: paid and unpaid work experiences; employment preparation emphasizing job-searching skills and vocational training; family involvement; inclusion in general education classrooms; social skills and independent living skills training; self-determination; community integration; and interagency collaboration (Mazzotti et al., 2021; Test et al., 2009).

Paid and Unpaid Work Experiences, Employment Preparation Emphasizing Job-Searching Skills and Vocational Training

Employment is a primary pathway to independence and autonomy (Schutz & Carter, 2022). Young adults who participate in vocational training in community employment sites throughout high school and obtain paid or unpaid jobs before graduation, are more successful in obtaining and maintaining paid work in the community as adults (Frentzel et al., 2021; Ogawa et al., 2023; Williams et al., 2019). When young adults with IDD are connected to meaningful work experiences in their communities, achieving their other aspirations becomes much more likely (Wehman et al., 2018). A well-matched job contributes to a sense of accomplishment, self-worth, and independence; it gives the young adults a place to share their strengths in valued ways; and it can help foster new friendships and access to social supports, connections, and community involvement. Meaningful work experience means participating in and contributing to the work environment in some way. For young adults with severe physical and intellectual disabilities, this may mean identifying the one or several tasks that they can do in order to contribute to a work setting in their community (TASH, 2009; Wehman & Brooke, 2013).

The emphasis on integrated employment options in the community is based on the belief that everyone, including those with severe disabilities, can work with the appropriate short- or long-term supports (Dean et al., 2022; Wehman et al., 2018). Successful employment outcomes include self-employment, competitive or supported employment, or customized employment. *Supported employment* means integrated employment in the community, within typical companies, for people with disabilities who traditionally have not had access to the job market (Vigna et al., 2024; Wehman et al., 2014). Supports are provided inside and outside of the workplace and may include a job coach, task and environmental adaptations, assistive technology, and specialized transportation to and from work. The main principle of supported employment is "place then train" (Wehman et al., 2014). The first step in the supported employment process involves securing community-integrated employment for the individual with IDD. Once the employment is secured, the next step includes providing the needed training and support at the job site. This enables individuals with IDD to learn the necessary job skills in real work settings as immediately as possible and without the need to generalize skills between environments. A form of supported employment, *customized employment* is a process in which a new job is created within a business that matches the young adult's abilities and skills (Salon et al., 2019). *Employment preparation programs* are classroom and curriculum-based programs that teach students how to prepare for the workforce and find a job, emphasizing job-search skills and career education (Ogawa et al., 2023; Torres et al., 2022). They also include work–study and internship programs and have been linked to more positive employment outcomes after graduation (Ashworth et al., 2023; Avellone et al., 2023; Mazzotti et al., 2021).

Family Involvement

Family involvement is a key component during transition and is a predictor of postsecondary success for young adults with IDD (Dean et al., 2021; Rispoli et al., 2023). Specifically, young adults with IDD work more hours, earn higher wages, live more independently, and have an overall higher quality of life when their parents are involved in their transition process (Francis et al., 2019). Although formal professional services and supports are critical, the majority of adults with IDD reside with their families, and only 25% are reported to access long-term services and supports through their state (Carter et al., 2017; Larson et al., 2018). Thus, parents, especially mothers, are typically the ones who piece together their children's programs and services and serve as advocates (Orentlicher, 2019). Research also indicates that young adults with IDD often rely on their parents for support when making important decisions or facing problems, they utilize their parents' contacts to secure employment and other community-based opportunities, and they participate in community activities in which their parents engage (Boehm et al., 2015; Carter et al., 2018). The impact of family involvement lasts way beyond high school and into adult life, even when young adults move away from their parents' homes to other residential settings (Gilson et al., 2018; Reynolds et al., 2015; Villaescusa et al., 2021).

Parents of young adults with IDD understand the importance of their involvement in their children's transition planning and expressed concerns about what will happen to their adult son or daughter after the parent's death or when the parent loses the ability to care for their child (Orentlicher, 2018). From a parent's perspective, this is a defining difference between parents of neurotypical children and parents of neurodivergent children. Other challenges were identified by Targett and Wehman (2013) and include: (1) parents devoting much of their time to taking care of their child with disabilities, in addition to being occupied with other important life tasks such as work and household maintenance, which can result in emotional distress; and (2) parents lacking knowledge of available resources. From a parent's perspective, while this may not have been studied in depth in this citation, it appears that parents of children with IDD have marital issues and high incidences of divorce caused by the stress of having a child with a disability. It is important that practitioners understand this when working with these families.

From an educator's perspective, it is important for the team to work with the parents to help them set reasonable expectations for postschool transition and goal setting. When parents accept the classification and limitations that might come with it, the school and the team can implement the most appropriate programs that can lead to more successful transitions. When parents struggle with accepting the needs and realities of their IDD child, it complicates the parent–school/team relationship and can delay positive outcomes.

Inclusion in General Education Classrooms

IDEA 2004 supports the inclusion of students with disabilities in schools and communities, to the maximum extent possible, with the appropriate individualized supports necessary for successful experiences. Researchers have determined that students with IDD who are included in and have access to the general education curriculum have better postschool outcomes (Hadley & Mapondera, 2023; Lund & Cmar, 2020; Morningstar et al., 2017; Rentschler et al., 2023). From an educator's perspective, while the data shows that these students might have better postschool outcomes, one should be careful not to generalize as this is not true of all students. This may be a factor of their specific type of disability and/or classification. Furthermore, receiving a high school diploma and having strong academic skills have been identified as predictors of employment (Getzel & Briel, 2013; Prince et al., 2019). High schools have the potential to foster the growth of students' interests and social relationships beyond the classroom (Asmus et al., 2017; Carter, 2018; Guest, 2018). Some of the extracurricular activities that provide students with opportunities for personal development and social inclusion include sports teams, performing and visual arts groups, special interest clubs, and service projects. By participating in the full range of activities offered in a typical high school, students can develop skills and relationships that are important for active adult life within their communities (Feraco et al., 2022; Lee et al., 2024).

Social Skills and Independent Living Skills Training

Social skills are ways of interacting with others in social and other environments, such as employment settings. They include effective communication, both verbal and nonverbal (Agran et al., 2016; Carter & Hughes, 2013). Social skills are generally comprised of five components: cooperation (i.e., working with others to achieve a task), assertion (i.e., initiating social interactions), self-control (i.e., dealing with emotions constructively), responsibility (i.e., recognizing the impact of actions on others), and empathy (i.e., understanding what others might be feeling) (Gresham et al., 2011).

Having functional daily living skills has been linked to better postschool outcomes, specifically in employment, friendships, social participation, and independent living (Ghanouni & Raphael, 2022; Gray et al., 2013; Gray et al., 2014; Reyes et al., 2022). In addition to ADLs and instrumental activities of daily living (IADLs), evidence shows support for teaching young adults personal responsibility (e.g., habits and patterns such as self-control, ability to save money, punctuality, and the ability to accept criticism) (Wehman, 2013). Independent living skills are viewed as components of self-determination. Independence in living skills increases individuals' sense of dignity, which is vital for self-determination (Lam et al., 2023).

Self-Determination

Self-determination is a predictor of employment, independent living, and community access for students with disabilities (Burke et al., 2020; Jones et al., 2018). As a psychological construct, it refers to volitional actions taken by young adults based on their own will, intention, conscious choice, and decision. In transition preparation, the focus is on the development of cognitive, social, and behavioral skills that are essential for self-determined behavior (Wehmeyer, 2015). Self-determination skills include the ability to make choices and decisions, problem solve, set and attain goals, advocate and be a leader, and self-regulate and control oneself (Biggs & Carter, 2016; Shogren et al., 2015; Wehmeyer, 2015).

Self-determination was identified as the "ultimate goal of education" (Halloran, 1993, p. 213) and the emergence from adolescence to adulthood has been characterized as a quest for self-determination. Self-determination has been linked to increased quality of life, feelings of personal development, and self-fulfillment (Burke et al., 2020; Chou, 2020; Dean et al., 2021; Ghanouni & Raphael, 2022).

Community Integration and Interagency Collaboration

Community integration means the full participation of all people in community life, including living in "ordinary" or "regular" homes, and engaging in employment, education, recreation, and transportation with the necessary supports (Gray et al., 2013; Gray et al., 2014; Lee & Morningstar, 2019).

At its core, community integration also means ensuring that young adults with IDD have opportunities to pursue their interests, desires, and goals; control their own schedules and which activities to pursue; and receive services in integrated settings of their choosing that are appropriate to their needs (Bigby et al., 2018). Community integration allows all people to enjoy the physical surroundings of their neighborhoods and the naturally occurring formal and informal activities. It promotes connection and presence in communal environments (Overmars-Marx et al., 2014).

Interagency collaboration is the coordination between school transition teams and adult agencies who work together to promote students' successful outcomes during transition (Flowers et al., 2018). A seamless transition that includes integrating adult services in school, such as vocational supports from community adult agencies, leads to more successful transition outcomes (Butterworth et al., 2017; Schlegelmilch et al., 2019; Trainor et al., 2012).

FUNCTION/DYSFUNCTION CONTINUA

The following six areas of function/dysfunction continua are identified for this frame of reference:

- Paid and unpaid work experiences, employment preparation emphasizing job-searching skills and vocational training (Table 17.1)
- Family involvement (Table 17.2)
- Inclusion in general education classrooms (Table 17.3)
- Social skills and independent living skills training (Table 17.4)
- Self-determination (Table 17.5)
- Community integration and interagency collaboration (Table 17.6)

Table 17.1 Indicators of Function: Paid and Unpaid Work Experiences, Employment Preparation Emphasizing Job-Searching Skills and Vocational Training

Function	Dysfunction
Participates in and contributes to the work environment in some way in supported employment, customized employment, work–study, or internship.	Does not participate in or contribute to the work environment in some way.
Indicators of Function	**Indicators of Dysfunction**
Participates in vocational training in community employment sites.	Does not participate in vocational training in community employment sites.
Participates in employment preparation program in school.	Does not participate in employment preparation programs in school.
Obtains paid or unpaid job before graduation.	Does not obtain paid or unpaid job before graduation.
Obtains a weekend or a summer job.	Does not obtain a weekend or a summer job.
Identifies and completes tasks that contribute to the work setting.	Does not identify or complete tasks that contribute to the work setting.

Table 17.2 Indicators of Function: Family Involvement

Function	Dysfunction
Parents are involved in the transition process and utilize available state, local, and school-based resources and supports.	Parents are not involved in the transition process and do not utilize available state, local, or school-based resources and supports.
Indicators of Function	**Indicators of Dysfunction**
Parents help child with IDD look for a job, fill out an application, and provide transportation to the job site.	Parents do not help child with IDD look for a job, fill out an application, or provide transportation to the job site.
Parents balance taking care of their child with IDD with other important life tasks such as work and household maintenance.	Parents devote much of their time to taking care of their child with IDD, in addition to being occupied with other important life tasks such as work and household maintenance.
Parents report feelings of well-being.	Parents report being in emotional distress.
Parents understand and utilize available state, local, and school-based resources and supports.	Parents lack knowledge of and do not utilize available state, local, and school-based resources and supports.
Long-term plans for caring for the son or daughter with IDD are developed.	No long-term plans for caring for the son or daughter with IDD.

Table 17.3 Indicators of Function: Inclusion in General Education Classrooms

Function	Dysfunction
Member of an inclusive classroom in high school and participates in the full range of activities offered by the school, including structured and unstructured extracurricular activities.	Member of a segregated classroom in high school and does not participate in the full range of activities offered by the school, including structured and unstructured extracurricular activities.
Indicators of Function	**Indicators of Dysfunction**
Copes with increased academic demands with academic supports and accommodations.	Does not cope with increased academic demands. Not provided with academic supports or accommodations.
Develops and utilizes effective study skills.	Does not develop or utilize effective study skills.
Participates in extracurricular activities, such as sports teams, performing and visual arts groups, special interest clubs, or service projects.	Does not participate in extracurricular activities.
Participates in social activities with typical students.	Does not participate in social activities with typical students.

Table 17.4 Indicators of Function: Social Skills and Independent Living Skills Training

Function	Dysfunction
Effectively interacts and communicates with others in social and other environments. Demonstrates daily living skills including ADLs and IADLs.	Does not effectively interact or communicate with others in social and other environments. Does not demonstrate daily living skills including ADLs or IADLs.
Indicators of Function	**Indicators of Dysfunction**
Communicates with others.	Does not communicate with others.
Understands environmental information, including verbal and nonverbal communication. Interprets body language and responds appropriately.	Does not understand environmental information, including verbal or nonverbal communication. Does not interpret body language or respond appropriately.
Works with others to achieve a task.	Does not work with others to achieve a task.
Initiates and maintains social interactions and close friendships.	Does not initiate or maintain social interactions or close friendships.
Deals with emotions constructively.	Does not deal with emotions constructively.
Recognizes the impact of actions on others.	Does not recognize the impact of actions on others.
Understands what others might be feeling.	Does not understand what others might be feeling.
Healthy and acceptable sexual behavior.	Unhealthy and unacceptable sexual behavior.
Socializes online and through social media.	Does not socialize online or through social media.
Exhibits habits and behaviors indicative of self-control, such as saving money, punctuality, and accepting criticism.	Does not exhibit habits and behaviors indicative of self-control, such as saving money, punctuality, or accepting criticism.
Copes with stress and anxiety.	Does not cope with stress or anxiety.
Independent in ADLs.	Is not independent in ADLs.
Independent in IADLs.	Is not independent in IADLs.
Demonstrates executive functioning skills including planning activities, organizing materials, planning for time to complete tasks, maintaining focus on tasks despite other distractions, and solving problems.	Does not demonstrate executive functioning skills including planning activities, organizing materials, planning for time to complete tasks, maintaining focus on tasks despite other distractions, or solving problems.

Table 17.5 Indicators of Function: Self-Determination

Function	Dysfunction
Takes actions based on own will, intention, conscious choice, and decision.	Does not take actions based on own will, intention, conscious choice, or decision.
Indicators of Function	**Indicators of Dysfunction**
Demonstrates self-determination skills including making choices and decisions, problem solving, setting and attaining goals, advocating and being a leader, self-regulating, and self-control.	Does not demonstrate self-determination skills including making choices and decisions, problem solving, setting or attaining goals, advocating and being a leader, self-regulating, or self-control.
Making daily decisions such as choosing what to do on free time or how to spend personal money.	Does not make daily decisions such as choosing what to do on free time or how to spend personal money.

Table 17.6 Indicators of Function: Community Integration and Interagency Collaboration

Function	Dysfunction
Full participation in community life and engagement in recreation, employment, transportation, and education with the necessary supports. Enjoys the physical surroundings and the naturally occurring formal and informal activities. Has connections and present in communal environments.	Lack of or limited participation in community life and engagement in recreation, employment, transportation, or education. Necessary supports not provided. Does not participate in the physical surroundings or the naturally occurring formal or informal activities. Does not have connections and has no presence in communal environments.
School transition teams and adult agencies coordinate efforts and work together to promote students' transition.	School transition teams and adult agencies do not coordinate efforts and do not work together to promote students' transition.
Indicators of Function	**Indicators of Dysfunction**
Pursues own interests, desires, and goals.	Does not pursue own interests, desires, or goals.
Controls own schedule and chooses which activities to pursue.	Does not control own schedule or choose which activities to pursue.
Participates in chosen activities such as social and structured events in public facilities (e.g., libraries and community centers); religious pursuits in institutions or faith groups; arts and cultural events (e.g., theater, concerts); or volunteer causes.	Does not participate in chosen activities.
Receive services in integrated settings of own choosing that meet needs.	Receive services in segregated settings or settings that do not meet needs.
Lives in "ordinary" or "regular" home.	Lives in segregated home or institution.
Uses public transportation.	Does not use public transportation.
Adult services such as vocational supports are provided in school.	Adult services are not provided in school.

GUIDE FOR EVALUATION

Evaluation of students with IDD's transition readiness and relevant skills should be an ongoing and a dynamic process throughout high school because new self-discoveries and interests, which are a natural part of adolescent development, foster new goals (Orentlicher, 2019). An essential element in high-quality transition evaluation is the integration of the perspectives of individuals who know the student well and are familiar with the current or future environments in which the student will participate, such as parents and teachers (Carter et al., 2014). The Division on Career Development and Transition (DCDT) of the Council for Exceptional Children defines age-appropriate transition assessment as,

> … an ongoing process of collecting information on the youth's needs, strengths, preferences, and interests as they relate to measurable postsecondary goals and the annual goals that will help facilitate attainment of postsecondary goals. This process includes a careful match between the characteristics of the youth and the requirements of secondary environments and postsecondary environments along with recommendations for accommodations, services, supports, and technology to ensure the match (Neubert & Leconte, 2013, p. 74).

The National Secondary Transition Technical Assistance Center (2023) recommends a combination of several types of evaluation including formal and informal tests, student and family interviews, situational assessments, and curriculum-based assessments. *Formal measures* include standardized tools that measure performance skills, client factors, aptitude, interests, adaptive behavior, independent living skills, transition readiness, career abilities, or self-determination (Hughes & Carter, 2002). *Informal measures* are nonstandardized and include interviews or questionnaires, direct observations, anecdotal records, and environmental or situational analyses (Carter et al., 2014). The primary strength of informal measures is their direct relevance to the individual student and the environment in which they plan to learn, work, and live. Informal measures can be developed or modified to focus on specific skills relevant to the particular student and their transition goals and needs rather than generic traits or abilities (Hughes & Carter, 2002). The *Framework* also directs occupational therapists to consider contexts for participation and include observations of task performance in natural environments. From a self-determination perspective, students should be actively involved in their transition evaluation process (Carter et al., 2014). They should participate in decisions regarding which procedures and tools to use, possible modifications, and interpretation and application of the results. By actively choosing and participating in informal evaluations, the students can develop awareness of their own strengths, skills, interests, and preferences relative to opportunities and demands in the environment (Hughes & Carter, 2002). Recommended transition evaluation tools can be found in the Transition Assessment Toolkit of the National Secondary Transition Technical Assistance Center (2013).

The Assess, Plan, Instruct, and Evaluate (APIE) model is a transition assessment framework that incorporates a variety of methods for assessing the student and potential future work, education, or living environments (Sitlington et al., 2007). The APIE model provides therapist with information on how to best match a student with their potential environments and what accommodations or modifications may be required to enhance participation.

- *Step one: Assess:* Assess the student's interests, preferences, and needs related to desired postschool outcomes using formal and informal assessments.
- *Step two: Plan:* Interpret the results from the assessments and incorporate them into the student's IEP.
- *Step three: Instruct:* Teach the student the skills they will need to reach the postschool goals. Recommend accommodations, modifications, and adaptations.
- *Step four: Evaluate:* Evaluate whether progress has been made toward achieving the transition goals and whether the student is better able to engage in desired activities in the potential environments.

Occupational therapists can contribute to the transition evaluation process by completing an occupational profile and analyzing the gap between current and desired occupational performance (Orentlicher, 2019). Once the context or environment is determined, identifying performance needs should be guided by questions such as, will the student need to get to work using public transportation? Will they need to access a bank and use an ATM? Will they live in their own home and need to prepare meals or perform other household chores? Does the student want to adopt a pet? (Orentlicher & Case, 2018b). Once the list of potential activities is complete, an *activity analysis* is used to list the steps necessary to complete each activity, identify the activity demands, and determine the best approaches for training the student to perform the desired activities (Orentlicher, 2019).

The next step is to observe the student performing the activities. Observations in multiple environments help gather information on the environmental elements that provide support for and barriers to participation and the needed adaptations or modifications. For example, individuals with IDD may be more successful purchasing groceries in a small local store that is quieter and has less visual stimulation than in a large supermarket. While observing the student performing the desired activity in a natural environment, the occupational therapists can assess elements such as the type and amount of sensory stimulation and the student's reactions to it, the type and number of people typically present and the interactions among them, and the social skills expected of the student. When the student's occupational performance is analyzed, the following should be considered: sensory and motor skills; cognitive performance; daily living and community living skills; vocational skills; socialization skills; and skills in self-determination and self-advocacy (Orentlicher, 2019).

Another informal method for transition evaluation, which specifically focuses on employment, is *discovery*. Discovery means learning about the student and creating a profile of their interests and strengths, the ideal employment conditions, and available employment opportunities in their community (Wehman & Brooke, 2013). Once the profile is created, the young adult can then pursue internships, competitive or supported employment, or customized employment.

A final stage of the transition evaluation is the creation of a *portfolio* that includes collections of information by and about the student, in order to give a broad view of their abilities, skills, and achievements (Mabry, 1999). The portfolio can include samples of the student's work, narrative descriptions, resume, grades, student self-evaluations, and photographic records, such as pictures of the student performing job tasks (Orentlicher, 2019). The portfolio can then be shared with potential employers or college admissions staff.

POSTULATES REGARDING CHANGE

The general postulate regarding change encompasses best practices in transition and is as follows:

Providing opportunities for students with IDD to identify preferences, make choices, and participate in meaningful activities will result in the student achieving occupational engagement and participation in meaningful activities in natural environments during and after the transition from school to adult life.

The following specific postulates regarding change are organized according to the transition best practices.

1. Providing job sampling opportunities that match students' age, goals, and needs, including short-term exploratory experiences and job shadowing, will prepare students for future employment.
2. Teaching soft skills, such as work completion, task accuracy, punctuality, time management, and appropriate dress will result in long-term engagement in work settings.

   Examples of strategies for teaching *time management* include adding a time component to every task analysis (i.e., specifying the time required to complete each step), setting timers and alarms to motivate targeted behaviors such as transitions between tasks, establishing routines that eliminate wasted time, creating visual schedules and referring to them throughout the day, and attaching a to-do list to the daily schedule and crossing off accomplished tasks.

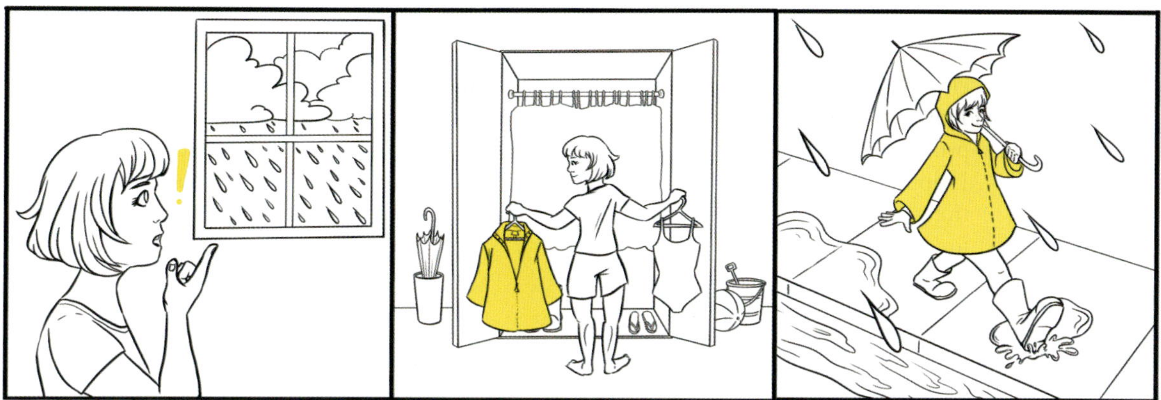

FIGURE 17.1 Person sees visual cue of rain, explores closet for the appropriate clothes, wears appropriate outfit for the weather.

Examples of strategies for teaching *appropriate dress* include visual reminders with pictures of the student wearing appropriate clothing for the weather in each season, or for different occasions such as a job interview, or a company outing (Figure 17.1).

3. Incorporating task and environmental adaptations and modifications will support completion of work tasks.

   Examples of *task and environmental adaptations and modifications* include scheduling optimal shifts/working hours, such as scheduling work around feeding times for a student that is fed by a gastronomy tube; recommending optimal workstation location, such as recommending a workstation close to the accessible bathroom and fire exit for a student who uses a wheelchair; adjusting sensory stimulation, such as light, noise level, or the material of the uniform; or providing assistive devices.

4. Utilizing natural supports and naturally existing cues in the work environment will promote completion of work-related daily tasks.

   Examples of *natural supports* include coworkers, peers, and family members (Nisbet, 1992). These individuals can provide support to the student in naturally occurring events, such as a neighbor who takes the bus to work can assist the student to get on the bus in the morning. Examples of *naturally existing cues* include a clock on the wall that signals break time, or a sign that directs employees to wash hands.

5. Teaching work readiness skills to students in elementary and middle school will assist in the development of work skills in high school and posttransition.

   Work readiness skills can be taught to entire elementary and middle school classrooms or groups of selected students. Examples of work readiness activities include baking and cooking groups, selling school supplies, or developing recycling programs for the school.

6. Teaching executive functioning skills including planning activities, organizing materials, planning for time to complete tasks, and maintaining focus on the task despite other distractions will improve transition outcomes.

Family Involvement

1. Educating families about the disability service system and assisting in navigating the system will increase families' advocacy skills.

2. Helping parents establish daily routines that balance caring for the child with IDD with childcare for siblings, work responsibilities, and household maintenance will enhance parents' availability to participate in transition planning.
3. Supporting parents in identifying and engaging in desired meaningful occupations will promote parents' well-being and self-actualization.
4. Helping parents plan for the long term by identifying relatives, friends, or service organizations that will help support the young adult in the future will ease stresses associated with long-term future planning.

Inclusion in General Education Classrooms

1. Including students with IDD in the full range of activities offered in a typical high school will provide opportunities for identity formation and for developing interpersonal relationships.
2. Providing accommodations, modifications, and assistive technology will broaden students with IDD's opportunities for full inclusion in education and other settings.

   Accommodations are changes made to remove barriers for learning without changing the content of what is being taught or the expectation that students with IDD should meet the performance standards applied to all students (Kochhar-Bryant & Izzo, 2006). *Modifications* are changes to the general education curriculum or other material being taught, which alter the standards or expectations for students with IDD (Kochhar-Bryant & Izzo, 2006). Instruction can be modified so that the material is presented differently and/or the expectations of what the student will master are changed. *Assistive technology* is any device that helps a student with IDD function in a given environment (Schoonover & Orentlicher, 2015). Assistive technology includes both high-tech options as well as simple devices such as laminated pictures for communication, removable highlighter tapes, Velcro, or other low-tech devices.
3. Teaching self-management skills, such as organizational or study skills, will promote participation in educational activities.

   Examples of strategies for teaching *study skills* include breaking large assignments into small steps, using schedules and calendars to establish "mini due dates" for completing the small steps, color coding assignment schedules by subject, using flash cards to summarize major concepts, adapting the sensory characteristics (i.e., noise level, light) of preferred study environments to match the student's needs, and using technology to assist in studying (e.g., PDAs, tablet computers, or assistive technology) (Woods-Groves et al., 2023).

Social Skills and Independent Living Skills Training

1. Utilizing peer-focused strategies will create supportive environments for peer interactions and social skills development.

   Peer-focused strategies include teaching peers and coworkers, and how to interact with the student with IDD (Carter & Hughes, 2013). Further, developing peer mentors can be very helpful for the IDD student. From an educator's perspective, the use of peers and peer mentors can be useful in making the IDD student feel more comfortable and be guided to handle the social situations that frequently arise with young adult population.

2. Teaching social problem solving, perspective taking, and emotional regulation will enhance social competence.

    Social competence is a multidimensional construct that includes sociocognitive skills such as social problem solving and perspective taking (Fraser et al., 2005), as well as skills for emotional regulation (Nigg, 2017; Nuske et al., 2022). It also includes the ability to independently choose friends, network, and initiate social activities. Appropriate expressions of sexuality and participation in recreational activities are also components of social competence.
3. Guiding students with IDD to modulate emotions, use emotions as cues, identify signs of impending emotional stress, read social cues, and interpret the perspectives of others will promote positive interactions in a variety of social situations.
4. Providing social information will reinforce positive social interactions.

    Social information includes providing specific social rules. Strategies for providing social information include rehearsing strategies for social interactions, using peers as models, and providing scripts of what the adolescent should do in particular social situations (Carter & Hughes, 2013).
5. Securing recreational options and leisure activities in integrated settings will promote socialization and making friends.
6. Providing Internet safety training including appropriate online communication with familiar people and strangers, securing personal information, and netiquette, will support young adults with IDD in socializing online and through social media.
7. Teaching financial management skills including saving money, budgeting, and using credit will increase young adults' ability to manage disability benefits.
8. Infusing instructional strategies and intervention approaches including audio cuing, video modeling, behavioral in vivo procedures, and visual cues will improve the functional skills of adolescents with IDD.

    Audio cuing is the use of prerecorded or live audio prompts delivered via earbuds to assist adolescents with IDD to perform tasks (Allen et al., 2012). *Video modeling* involves filming someone (either the adolescent or a peer) correctly performing a selected task. The video is then used to train the adolescent with IDD how to perform the task (Orum Cattik et al., 2024). *Behavioral in vivo procedures* involve observing another person engage in a target behavior (Whittenburg et al., 2022). *Visual cues* are pictures or other visual items used to communicate with adolescents with IDD who have difficulty understanding or using language. Visual cues or supports can be photographs, drawings, objects, written words, or lists (Cannella-Malone et al., 2017; Hong et al., 2017).
9. Encouraging participation in IADLs in children and increasing the expectations for participation as they grow, will promote their maturation into independent adults.

    Strategies for increasing young children's participation in IADLs include engagement in household chores (Orentlicher & Case, 2018b). For example, preschoolers can be expected to pick up and put away their toys. As they grow, they can be expected to help set the table for dinner, feed and clean up after a pet, dust, or rake leaves in the yard (Figures 17.2 and 17.3). Teens can be expected to prepare light meals; budget an allowance; shop for desired items; and help with laundry. When teens attend college, and in the years beyond, they are expected to live independently, manage their own household, participate in community activities, and eventually take care of others (e.g., raise children, care for pets).

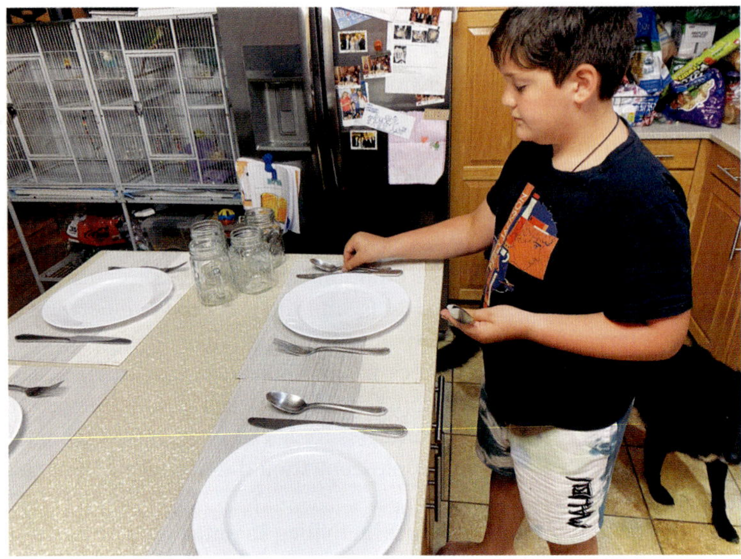

FIGURE 17.2 Child is setting the table independently.

Self-Determination

1. Providing students with IDD with opportunities to make choices, problem solve, set goals, and self-evaluate will result in the development of self-advocacy skills.
2. Mentoring young adults to take control over their own transition plans will increase their self-determination.

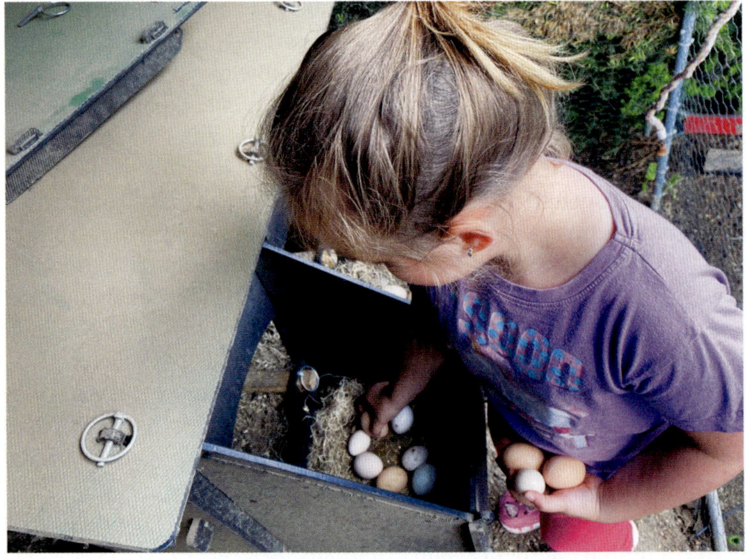

FIGURE 17.3 Child is collecting eggs, which is part of caring for a pet chicken.

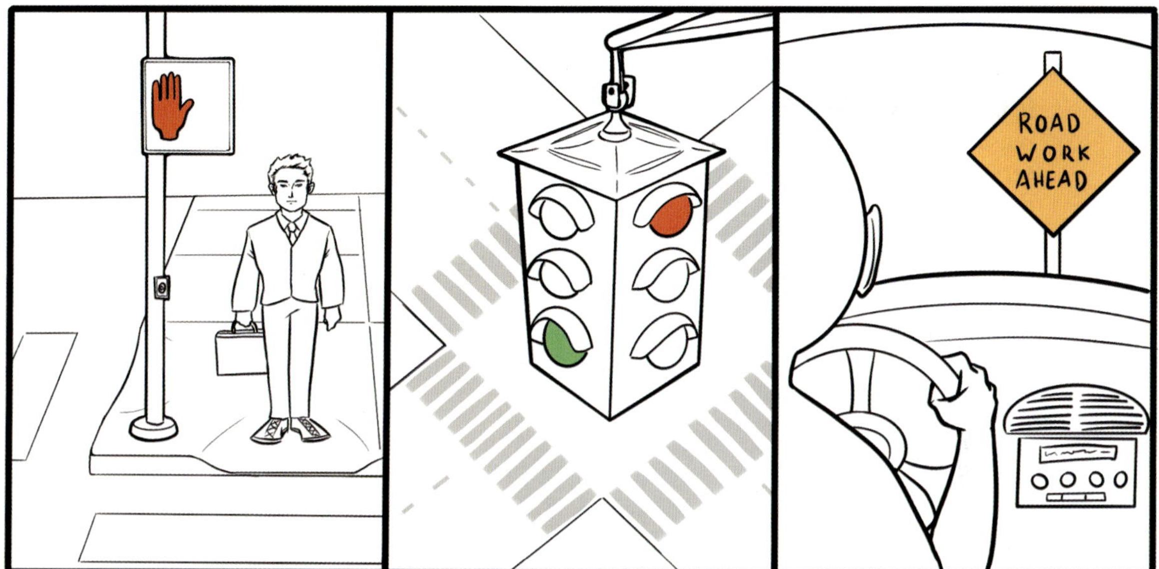

FIGURE 17.4 Person observing several visual signs which will help decide behavior.

Community Integration and Interagency Collaboration

1. Teaching functional skills such as telling time, reading and understanding common signs, counting change, using an ATM, and shopping at a grocery store, will help students with IDD achieve community integration.
2. Providing community-based instruction (CBI) will increase students' skills in performing meaningful activities in natural contexts.

   CBI is typically used to teach skills such as using public transportation, accessing stores and public services, and adjusting to schedules that mirror adult life (White & Weiner, 2004). Providing travel training, including using public transportation, will increase students with IDD's ability to participate in activities within their communities (Figure 17.4).
3. Involving community agencies, including federal, state, and local representatives, as well as local businesses, will create a seamless transition to and important connections within the young adults' communities.
4. Building relationships with community-based agencies, by touring their offices or inviting their representatives to the school, will increase coordination among all transition stakeholders.

APPLICATION TO PRACTICE

Occupational therapy practitioners have a unique expertise in analyzing tasks and determining the needed adaptations and other supports an individual may need in order to engage in meaningful occupations during and after the transition from school to adult life. As a profession, occupational therapy supports nondiscrimination and inclusion (AOTA, 2014). Occupational therapy practitioners believe that "society has an obligation to provide the reasonable accommodations necessary to allow individuals access to social, educational, recreational, and vocational opportunities" (p. S23). Occupational therapy practitioners can utilize their understanding of reasonable accommodations, adaptations, and assistive technology to broaden the focus of their services to influence the students' opportunities for full inclusion in education and other community settings.

Occupational therapy practitioners' focus on occupational performance in natural environments makes them the ideal professionals to provide transition and community-based instruction. Occupational therapy practitioners can utilize task and activity analyses to instruct students to perform meaningful activities in natural environments, including school, home, and the community (Hollenbeck et al., 2015; Orentlicher, 2019). Some strategies to promote successful transition experiences include:

- Providing services in natural environments.
- Promoting accessibility of tasks and environments.
- Modifying tasks and environments to reduce the impact of physical barriers and sensory stimuli.
- Providing activity instructions using visual guides.
- Establishing routines, individualized schedules, and physical organization of materials.

From an educator's perspective, occupational therapy practitioners can be very helpful in working with school personnel to provide social supports and coaching with IDD students so that innocent attempts at social interactions are handled appropriately. Navigating social situations in a way that supports success is critical for these students to develop positive social interactions, where they are accepted and not subjected to a negative experience.

Occupational therapy practitioners should become familiar with the resources within and outside of school, and target community agencies and organizations that can provide support to young adults with IDD who are transitioning to adult life in the community.

CASE EXAMPLE

Ben

Ben is 17 years old and was diagnosed with high-functioning autism when he was 5 years old. He attends a specialized hybrid program at his local high school that combines typical academic classes such as history and science with life skills classes and vocational experiences. Ben enjoys math and science classes and hopes to work in something that will incorporate his strong math skills after high school. It is expected that he will receive a high school diploma from his local district. He is not expected to receive the state's Regents diploma. This means that he will not be eligible to attend a 4-year college.

Although Ben's state requires transition services to begin at age 15, only now, at age 17, Ben and his parents were invited to attend a transition planning meeting at the school. School professionals in attendance included the special education administrator, his homeroom teacher, social worker, psychologist, and Rachel, an occupational therapist. At the meeting, it was decided that once leaving school, Ben will attend a local community college where he can study math and accounting and receive a certificate in bookkeeping.

The community college also offers a specialized life skills program for students with autism. In addition to general vocational and life skills training, students also have opportunities to participate in organized social and recreational activities.

Rachel began the transition evaluation by integrating the perspectives of individuals who know Ben well and are familiar with the current and future environments in which he will participate. She used *formal measures* including the Arc's Self-Determination Scale (Wehmeyer & Kelchner, 1995) to assess Ben's self-determination and the Behavior Rating Inventory of Executive Function (BRIEF; Guy et al., 2004) to assess Ben's executive function. She used *informal measures* including interviews and observations, and reviewed Ben's previous school records to assess his social skills, adaptive behavior, sensory integration, and soft skills related to work.

During an interview, Ben's parents reported that he has been exhibiting many mood swings and behaviors associated with anxiety. They noticed that he has been pulling away from them by refusing to join family activities such as going out for dinner. However, he has not formed any friendships or social connections and instead, spends evenings and weekends alone at home. In conversations with Ben's psychologist, Rachel understood that Ben's mood swings and anxiety are intensified beyond those experienced by typical adolescents because of his autism. Considering the information obtained during interviews, Rachel analyzed the results from the formal and informal assessments and selected five postulates regarding change to guide her intervention this year.

1. *Incorporating task and environmental adaptations and modifications will support completion of work tasks.*

   Taking advantage of Ben's love for and strong understanding of science, Rachel educated Ben about sensory differences and assisted him in identifying and implementing strategies to manage overwhelming sensory inputs. She also taught him to identify when he begins to feel overwhelmed so he can immediately implement strategies to limit the sensory input and regulate his level of alertness. Rachel also guided Ben, his teacher, and his parents on how to modify Ben's environments to lessen sensory sensitivity and increase his ability to register necessary sensory input for occupational participation. She taught them the importance of Ben retreating to a quiet space alone for short periods of time so that he could recover from the stress of social interactions and related sensory experiences. Other recommended environmental adaptations included limiting sounds, keeping wall and floor coverings simple and consistent, and using colored lightbulbs to cut down on color contrast.

   In preparation for college and work, Rachel taught Ben strategies for communicating with others that may put less demand on his ability to analyze multiple sensory inputs. For example, she recommended that whenever possible, Ben should ask his work supervisor or college professors to communicate via e-mail as opposed to face-to-face meetings. She also taught Ben to prepare for face-to-face meetings by writing down major points for the conversation and requesting that, if possible, the meeting should take place in a sensory-limited environment.

2. *Teaching executive functioning skills including planning activities, organizing materials, planning for time to complete tasks, and maintaining focus on the task despite other distractions will improve transition outcomes.*

To address Ben's executive function deficits, Rachel used principles from two occupational therapy frameworks that utilize cognitive-behavioral approaches to intervention, the multicontext approach (Toglia, 2005) and the CO-OP Approach (Polatajko & Mandich, 2004). Both approaches emphasize the importance of metacognitive skills to enhance successful task performance. Metacognitive skills include awareness of personal strengths, one's ability to identify where one is likely to experience challenges in a task, one's ability to predict what strategies may help to overcome these challenges, and one's capacity for monitoring performance.

Rachel assisted Ben in developing awareness of the strategies that he automatically uses to cope with task challenges. She then taught him how to anticipate his needs for strategies and how to go about applying cognitive strategies to improve occupational performance. Other strategies included teaching Ben how to lessen the demands on his executive function capacities. Specifically, she helped him to establish routines using visuals including individualized schedules and physical organization of materials. She taught Ben to use an online calendar to track deadlines, sticky notes to remind him to complete important tasks, and an ongoing list app on his phone to keep up with his to-do list.

3. *Guiding students with IDD to modulate emotions, use emotions as cues, identify signs of impending emotional stress, read social cues, and interpret the perspectives of others will promote positive interactions in a variety of social situations.*

Ben was invited to participate in a psychoeducational group in which the psychologist and Rachel collaborated to teach specific skills, including social skills, emotional self-regulation, sensory regulation strategies, and self-determination. They used strategies such as social stories and comic strip conversations to help Ben and other students generate solutions to social situations they may experience in college and at work.

4. *Providing social information will reinforce positive social interactions.*

Rachel observed that Ben has difficulty reading social cues, which is an ability that is especially important for job interviews. A job interview typically involves many social rules for proper behavior, and Ben will be required to exchange vital information with someone he has not met before and will need to sufficiently impress to secure the job. After becoming employed, Ben will need to maintain work relationships with supervisors and coworkers, and his weak skills in reading the often subtle negative or positive verbal or nonverbal cues can lead to friction, job-related stress, or even the loss of the job.

Rachel reviewed the social rules of job interviews with Ben. She suggested that to avoid the pain of direct eye contact that is caused by Ben's visual hypersensitivity, Ben should learn to look near people's faces rather than right at their eyes and faces. She and Ben rehearsed strategies for social interactions at work and used scripts describing what Ben should do in various social situations that may arise.

5. *Providing students with IDD with opportunities to make choices, problem solve, set goals, and self-evaluate will result in the development of self-advocacy skills.*

At the transition meeting, the team determined that one goal in Ben's IEP should address self-determination, specifically choice making. They hypothesized that giving Ben two or three choices at a time during class time or therapy sessions would decrease his frustration and anxiety. Rachel mentioned that incorporating an emotional check-in with Ben during the choice-making opportunities will help Ben develop emotional awareness and self-regulation skills. Together with Ben, Rachel created an emotional check-in routine with a list of possible coping and regulation techniques.

SUPPORTING EVIDENCE

Transition Outcomes

Approximately 464,000 students with disabilities graduated from or aged-out of high school in 2021 (National Center for Education Statistics, 2024). Compared to typically developing students, young adults with disabilities continue to lag in employment, postsecondary education, and community living skills despite legislation and systematic efforts to improve these outcomes (Cheng & Shaewitz, 2020). In fact, data indicates that in 2018, 20.2% of young adults with disabilities were neither in school nor in the labor force, compared to 5.7% of their typical peers. These young adults report living with their parents and doing nothing specific during the day.

Cheng and Shaewitz (2020) explain that the reasons for the continued gaps between young people with and without disabilities could be the result of inequities in the education and workforce systems. For example, in 2017, the National Center for Learning Disabilities (NCLD) reported that only 17% of general education teachers felt highly prepared to teach children with learning disabilities, even though more than 63% of students with disabilities were in general education classrooms more than 80% of the time (Horowitz et al., 2017). Similarly, colleges and universities are often unprepared to help students with disabilities to succeed, and the disability stigma among employers continues to deter young adults with disabilities from obtaining jobs (Cheng & Shaewitz, 2020).

Predictors

Transition outcomes vary greatly by individual, familial, and contextual factors. Students with IDD are more likely to be members of racial, ethnic, and disadvantaged socioeconomic groups and have fewer familial resources, both social and financial (Cheatham & Randolph, 2022).

Individual factors include race, gender, and disability. According to the secondary analysis of the Second National Longitudinal Transition Study (SNLTS; Wagner et al., 2003), 67% of young adults with IDD who had paid work were White. Similar findings were reported more recently (Cheatham & Randolph, 2022; Lindsay et al., 2022). Students with disabilities from ethnic minorities, and especially students who are Black, had poorer transition outcomes and had significantly decreased odds of productive participation in postschool activities.

Erickson et al. (2013) documented that 31.1% of women with disabilities between the ages of 21 and 64 years were employed, compared with 35.9% of men. Women with disabilities who are employed are more likely to work fewer hours, hold lower-status occupations, and have significantly lower starting wages compared to men with disabilities. Furthermore, in comparison to men, women with disabilities face additional challenges including lowered family expectations and social supports, gendered role assumptions, and limited vocational training (Lindsay et al., 2018; Sung et al., 2015).

Students with cognitive disabilities are 44% less likely to graduate from high school as compared to their typical peers and 55% less likely to graduate from high school than their peers with physical disabilities (Cheatham & Randolph, 2022). Postschool outcomes indicate that individuals with severe disabilities are 73% less likely, and individuals with low-severity disabilities are 45% less likely than their typical peers to report engagement in postschool activities such as education or employment (Cheatham & Randolph, 2022). More specifically, young adults with emotional disturbances (Wagner et al., 2017), autism spectrum disorder (Alverson & Yamamoto, 2017), and mild intellectual disabilities (Bouck, 2017) have the poorest transition outcomes.

Employment

In 2023, young adults with IDD, ages 20 to 24, were 20.7% less likely to be part of the labor force (51.8%) than their typical peers (72.5%). The unemployment rate for young adults with IDD was 11.8% in comparison to 6.4% for those without disabilities (Office of Disability Employment Policy, 2024). Young adults with IDD are also 10% more likely to live in poverty (Cheng & Shaewitz, 2020).

Evidence indicates that most young adults with IDD and their families prefer competitive integrated employment to segregated employment or day services (Gilson et al., 2018; Siperstein et al., 2014). Supported employment was found to be both cost-effective and a predictor of positive employment outcomes (Schutz & Carter, 2022; Vigna et al., 2024). However, in 2015, only 19% of young adults with IDD were working in paid jobs in the community (Hiersteiner et al., 2018). The poor employment outcomes for young adults with IDD are attributed to limited emphasis on integrated employment and limited vocational experiences while in school (Butterworth et al., 2017; Carter et al., 2011), insufficient family engagement in transition planning and inadequate collaboration between schools and adult agencies (Hirano et al., 2018; Plotner & Marshall, 2015), and schools inconsistently implementing evidence-based practices that support positive postschool outcomes (Mazzotti et al., 2021). The substantiated evidence-based practices guide the postulates regarding change and recommended OT transition interventions in this frame of reference.

Transition Services

One key factor that influences postschool outcomes is transition services and supports (Benson et al., 2021; Carlson et al., 2019; Lee & Carter, 2012). Describing the benefits of services and supports offered through high school, family members, teachers, rehabilitation counselors and young adults with IDD emphasized that having a transition specialist at school helped young adults in the transition process by providing assistance such as helping with resumes, interviews, job opportunities, and postsecondary education (Lindstrom et al., 2011). When comparing the transition outcomes between students who began the transition process at age 14 and those who began at age 16, Cimera et al. (2013) found that students who began transition services at age 14 had higher rates of employment and higher salaries, indicating the need for earlier transition services in high school.

REFERENCES

Agran, M., Hughes, C., Thoma, C. A., & Scott, L. A. (2016). Employment social skills: What skills are really valued? *Career Development and Transition for Exceptional Individuals*, *39*(2), 111–120. https://doi.org/10.1177/2165143414546741

Aikins, J. W., Howes, C., & Hamilton, C. (2009). Attachment stability and the emergence of unresolved representations during adolescence. *Attachment & Human Development*, *11*(5), 491–512. https://doi.org/10.1080/14616730903017019

Allen, K. D., Burke, R. V., Howard, M. R., Wallace, D. P., & Bowen, S. L. (2012). Use of audio cuing to expand employment opportunities for adolescents with autism spectrum disorders and intellectual disabilities. *Journal of Autism and Developmental Disorders*, *42*(11), 2410–2419. https://doi.org/10.1007/s10803-012-1519-7

Alverson, C. Y., & Yamamoto, S. H. (2017). Employment outcomes of vocational rehabilitation of clients with autism spectrum disorders. *Career Development and Transition for Exceptional Individuals*, *40*(3), 144–155. https://doi.org/10.1177/2165143416629366

American Anthropology Association. (n.d.). *What is anthropology?* https://americananthro.org/learn-teach/what-is-anthropology/

American Occupational Therapy Association (AOTA). (2014). Occupational therapy's commitment to nondiscrimination and inclusion. *American Journal of Occupational Therapy*, *68*(Supplement_3), S23–S24. https://doi.org/10.5014/ajot.2014.686s05

American Occupational Therapy Association (AOTA). (2020). Occupational therapy practice framework: domain and process—fourth edition. *American Journal of Occupational Therapy*, *74*(Supplement 2), 7412410010p1–7412410010p87. https://doi.org/10.5014/ajot.2020.74s2001

Anderson, K. A., McDonald, T. A., Edsall, D., Smith, L. E., & Taylor, J. L. (2016). Postsecondary expectations of high-school students with autism spectrum disorders. *Focus on Autism and Other Developmental Disabilities*, *31*(1), 16–26. https://doi.org/10.1177/1088357615610107

Ashworth, M., Heasman, B., Crane, L., & Remington, A. (2023). Evaluating a new supported employment internship programme for autistic young adults without intellectual disability. *Autism*, *28*(8), 1934–1946. https://doi.org/10.1177/13623613231214834

Asmus, J. M., Carter, E. W., Moss, C. K., Biggs, E. E., Bolt, D. M., Born, T. L., Bottema-Beutel, K., Brock, M. E., Cattey, G. N., Cooney, M., Fesperman, E. S., Hochman, J. M., Huber, H. B., Lequia, J. L., Lyons, G. L., Vincent, L. B., & Weir, K. (2017). Efficacy and social validity of peer network interventions for high school students with severe disabilities. *American Journal on Intellectual and Developmental Disabilities*, *122*(2), 118–137. https://doi.org/10.1352/1944-7558-122.2.118

Avellone, L., Taylor, J., Ham, W., Schall, C., Wehman, P., Brooke, V., & Strauser, D. (2023). A scoping review on internship programs and employment outcomes for youth and young adults with intellectual and developmental disabilities. *Rehabilitation Counselors and Educators Journal*, *12*(1). https://doi.org/10.52017/001c.38785

Bennet, M., Webster, A. A., Goodall, E., & Rowland, S. (2018). *Life on the autism spectrum. Translating myths and misconceptions into positive futures*. Springer. https://doi.org/10.1007/978-981-13-3359-0

Benson, J. D., Tokarski, R., Blaskowitz, M. G., & Geubtner, A. (2021). Phenomenological study of the transition process for adolescents with intellectual and developmental disabilities. *American Journal of Occupational Therapy*, *75*(3), 7503180040. https://doi.org/10.5014/ajot.2021.044289

Bigby, C., Anderson, S., & Cameron, N. (2018). Identifying conceptualizations and theories of change embedded in interventions to facilitate community participation for people with intellectual disability: A scoping review. *Journal of Applied Research in Intellectual Disabilities*, *31*(2), 165–180. https://doi.org/10.1111/jar.12390

Biggs, E. E., & Carter, E. W. (2016). Quality of life for transition-age youth with autism or intellectual disability. *Journal of Autism and Developmental Disorders*, *46*(1), 190–204. https://doi.org/10.1007/s10803-015-2563-x

Boehm, T. L., Carter, E. W., & Taylor, J. L. (2015). Family quality of life during the transition to adulthood for individuals with intellectual disability and/or autism spectrum disorders. *American Journal on Intellectual and Developmental Disabilities*, *120*(5), 395–411. https://doi.org/10.1352/1944-7558-120.5.395

Bouck, E. C. (2017). Educational outcomes for secondary students with mild intellectual disability. *Education and Training in Autism and Developmental Disabilities*, *52*(4), 369–382.

Burke, K. M., Raley, S. K., Shogren, K. A., Hagiwara, M., Mumbardó-Adam, C., Uyanik, H., & Behrens, S. (2020). A meta-analysis of interventions to promote self-determination for students with disabilities. *Remedial and Special Education*, *41*(3), 176–188.

Butterworth, J., Christensen, J., & Flippo, K. (2017). Partnerships in employment: building strong coalitions to facilitate systems change for youth and young adults. *Journal of Vocational Rehabilitation*, *47*(3), 265–276. https://doi.org/10.3233/jvr-170901

Cannella-Malone, H. I., Chan, J. M., & Jimenez, E. D. (2017). Comparing self-directed video prompting to least-to-most prompting in post-secondary students with moderate intellectual disabilities. *International Journal of Developmental Disabilities*, *63*(4), 211–220.

Carlson, S. R., Munandar, V. D., Wehmeyer, M. L., & Thompson, J. R. (2019). Special education transition services for students with extensive support needs. In *Special education transition services for students with disabilities* (Vol. 35, pp. 117–136). Emerald Publishing Limited. https://doi.org/10.1108/S0270-401320190000035015

Carter, E. W. (2018). Supporting the social lives of secondary students with severe disabilities: considerations for effective intervention. *Journal of Emotional and Behavioral Disorders*, *26*(1), 52–61. https://doi.org/10.1177/1063426617739253

Carter, E. W., Bendeston, S., & Guiden, C. H. (2018). Family perspectives on the appeals of and alternatives to sheltered employment for individuals with severe disabilities. *Research and Practice for Persons with Severe Disabilities*, *43*(3), 145–164. https://doi.org/10.1177/1540796918778293

Carter, E. W., Brock, M. E., & Trainor, A. A. (2014). Transition assessment and planning for youth with severe intellectual and developmental disabilities. *The Journal of Special Education*, *47*(4), 245–255. https://doi.org/10.1177/0022466912456241

Carter, E. W., & Hughes, C. (2013). Teaching social skills and promoting supportive relationships. In P. Wehman (Ed.), *Life beyond the classroom: Transition strategies for young people with disabilities* (5th ed., pp. 261–281). Paul H. Brookes.

Carter, E. W., McMillan, E., & Willis, W. (2017). The TennesseeWorks Partnership: Elevating employment outcomes for people with intellectual and developmental disabilities. *Journal of Vocational Rehabilitation*, *47*(3), 365–378. https://doi.org/10.3233/jvr-170909

Carter, E. W., Trainor, A. A., Ditchman, N., Swedeen, B., & Owens, L. (2011). Community-based work experiences of adolescents with high-incidence disabilities. *Journal of Special Education*, *45*(2), 89–103. https://doi.org/10.1177/0022466909353204

Cheatham, L. P., & Randolph, K. (2022). Education and employment transitions among young adults with disabilities: Comparisons by disability status, type and severity. *International Journal of Disability, Development and Education*, *69*(2), 467–490. https://doi.org/10.1080/1034912x.2020.1722073

Cheng, L., & Shaewitz, D. (2020). *The 2020 youth transition report: Outcomes for youth and young adults with disabilities*. Institute for Educational Leadership.

Cimera, R. E., Burgess, S., & Wiley, A. (2013). Does providing transition services early enable students with ASD to achieve better vocational outcomes as adults? *Research and Practice for Persons with Severe Disabilities*, *38*(2), 88–93. https://journals.sagepub.com/doi/abs/10.2511/027494813807714474

Chou, Y. C. (2020). Navigation of social engagement (NOSE) project: Using a self-directed problem solving model to enhance social problem-solving and self-determination in youth with autism spectrum disorders. *Education and Training in Autism and Developmental Disabilities*, *55*(1), 101–114. https://www.jstor.org/stable/26898717

Cresswell, L., Hinch, R., & Cage, E. (2019). The experiences of peer relationships amongst autistic adolescents: a systematic review of the qualitative evidence. *Research in Autism Spectrum Disorders*, *61*, 45–60. https://doi.org/10.1016/j.rasd.2019.01.003

Dean, E. E., Hagiwara, M., Shogren, K. A., Wehmeyer, M. L., & Shrum, J. (2022). Promoting career design in youth and young adults with ASD: A feasibility study. *Journal of Autism and Developmental Disorders*, *52*(6), 2689–2700. https://doi.org/10.1007/s10803-021-05146-x

Dean, E. E., Kirby, A. V., Hagiwara, M., Shogren, K. A., Ersan, D. T., & Brown, S. (2021). Family role in the development of self-determination for youth with intellectual and developmental disabilities: a scoping review. *Intellectual and Developmental Disabilities*, *59*(4), 315–334. https://doi.org/10.1352/1934-9556-59.4.315

Doidge, M., & Saini, R. (2020). *The short guide to sociology*. Policy Press.

Erickson, W., Lee, C., & von Schrader, S. (2013). *Disability statistics from the 2011 American Community Survey (ACS)*. Cornell University Employment and Disability Institute.

Feraco, T., Resnati, D., Fregonese, D., Spoto, A., & Meneghetti, C. (2022). Soft skills and extracurricular activities sustain motivation and self-regulated learning at school. *Journal of Experimental Education*, *90*(3), 550–569. https://doi.org/10.1080/00220973.2021.1873090

Flowers, C., Test, D. W., Povenmire-Kirk, T. C., Diegelmann, K. M., Bunch-Crump, K. R., Kemp-Inman, A., & Goodnight, C. I. (2018). A demonstration model of interagency collaboration for students with disabilities: a multilevel approach. *The Journal of Special Education*, *51*(4), 211–221. https://doi.org/10.1177/0022466917720764

Francis, G. L., Regester, A., & Reed, A. S. (2019). Barriers and supports to parent involvement and collaboration during transition to adulthood. *Career Development and Transition for Exceptional Individuals*, *42*(4), 235–245. https://doi.org/10.1177/2165143418813912

Fraser, M. W., Galinsky, M. J., Smokowski, P. R., Day, S. H., Terzian, M. A., Rose, R. A., & Guo, S. (2005). Social information-processing skills training to promote social competence and prevent aggressive behavior in the third grade. *Journal of Consulting and Clinical Psychology*, *73*(6), 1045–1055.

Frentzel, E., Geyman, Z., Rasmussen, J., Nye, C., & Murphy, K. M. (2021). Pre-employment transition services for students with disabilities: A scoping review. *Journal of Vocational Rehabilitation*, *54*(2), 103–116. https://doi.org/10.3233/jvr-201123

Gallup, J., Duff, C., Serianni, B., & Gallup, A. (2016). An exploration of friendships and socialization for adolescents with autism engaged in massively multiplayer online role-playing games (MMORPG). *Education and Training in Autism and Developmental Disabilities*, *51*(3), 223–237.

Gerrig, R. J. (2013). *Psychology and life: Pearson new international edition* (20 ed.). Pearson.

Getzel, E. E., & Briel, L. W. (2013). Pursuing postsecondary education opportunities for individuals with disabilities. In P. Wehman (Ed.), *Life beyond the classroom: Transition strategies for young people with disabilities* (5th ed., pp. 363–376). Paul H. Brookes.

Ghanouni, P., & Raphael, R. (2022). Transition to adulthood in individuals with ASD: What does the employment look like? *Journal of Education and Work*, *35*(3), 307–325. https://doi.org/10.1080/13639080.2022.2048253

Gilson, C. B., Carter, E. W., Bumble, J. L., & McMillan, E. D. (2018). Family perspectives on integrated employment for adults with intellectual and developmental disabilities. *Research and Practice for Persons with Severe Disabilities*, *43*(1), 20–37. https://doi.org/10.1177/1540796917751134

Gray, K. M., Keating, C. M., Taffe, J. R., Brereton, A. V., Einfeld, S. L., Reardon, T. C., & Tonge, B. J. (2014). Adult outcomes in autism: community inclusion and living skills. *Journal of Autism and Developmental Disorders*, *44*(12), 3006–3015. https://doi.org/10.1007/s10803-014-2159-x

Gray, K. M., Piccinin, A., Keating, C. M., Taffe, J., Parmenter, T. R., Hofer, S., Einfeld, S. L., & Tonge, B. J. (2013). Outcomes in young adulthood: are we achieving community participation and inclusion? *Journal of Intellectual Disability Research*, *58*(8), 734–745. https://doi.org/10.1111/jir.12069

Gresham, F. M., Elliott, S. N., Vance, M. J., & Cook, C. R. (2011). Comparability of the social skills rating system to the social skills improvement system: content and psychometric comparisons across elementary and secondary age levels. *School Psychology Quarterly*, *26*(1), 27–44. https://doi.org/10.1037/a0022662

Griffiths, A. J., Torres, R., Delgado, R., Hurley-Hanson, A. E., Giannantonio, C. M., Walrod, W., Maupin, Z., & Brady, J. (2024). Understanding unique employability skill sets of autistic individuals: a systematic review. *Journal of Employment Counseling*, *6*(2), 74–104. https://doi.org/10.1002/joec.12223

Guest, A. M. (2018). The social organization of extracurricular activities: Interpreting developmental meanings in contrasting high schools. *Qualitative Psychology*, *5*(1), 41–58. https://doi.org/10.1037/qup0000069

Guy, S. C., Isquith, P. K., & Gioia, G. A. (2004). *Behavior raging inventory of executive function-self-report version (BRIEF-SR)*. Psychological Assessment Resources.

Hadley, W., & Mapondera, A. (2023). Students with autism transitioning into higher education: a systematic review of literature. *Review Journal of Autism and Developmental Disorders*. https://doi.org/10.1007/s40489-023-00413-2

Halloran, W. D. (1993). Transition services requirement: Issues, implications, challenge. In R. C. Eaves & P. J. McLaughlin (Eds.), *Recent advances in special education and rehabilitation* (pp. 210–224). Andover Medical.

Hiersteiner, D., Bershadsky, J., Bonardi, A., & Butterworth, J. (2016). *Working in the community: The status and outcomes of people with intellectual and developmental disabilities in integrated employment-Update 2 (NCI data brief)*. Human Services Research Institute.

Hiersteiner, D., Butterworth, J., Bershadsky, J., & Bonardi, A. (2018). *Working in the community: The status and outcomes of people with intellectual and developmental disabilities in integrated employment: Update 3*. Human Services Research Institute.

Hirano, K. A., Rowe, D., Lindstrom, L., & Chan, P. (2018). Systemic barriers to family involvement in transition planning for youth with disabilities: a qualitative metasynthesis. *Journal of Child and Family Studies*, *27*(11), 3440–3456. https://doi.org/10.1007/s10826-018-1189-y

Hollenbeck, J., Orentlicher, M. L., & Handley-More, D. (2015). Expanding roles, expanding impact: supporting work readiness in middle school. *Early Intervention & School Special Interest Section Quarterly*, *22*(3), 1–4.

Hong, E. R., Ganz, J. B., Morin, K., Davis, J. L., Ninci, J., Neely, L., & Boles, M. B. (2017). Functional living skills and adolescents and adults with autism spectrum disorder: A meta-analysis. *Education and Training in Autism and Developmental Disabilities*, *52*(3), 268–279.

Horowitz, S. H., Rawe, J., & Whittaker, M. C. (2017). *The state of learning disabilities: Understanding the 1 in 5*. National Center for Learning Disabilities.

Hughes, C., & Carter, E. W. (2002). Informal assessment procedures. In C. L. Sax & C. A. Thoma (Eds.), *Transition assessment: Wide practices for quality lives* (pp. 51–69). Paul H. Brookes.

Individuals with Disabilities Education Improvement Act of 2004. P.L. 108–446, 20 U.S.C. § 1400 *et. seq.*

Jones, J. L., Shogren, K. A., Grandfield, E. M., Vierling, K. L., Gallus, K. L., & Shaw, L. A. (2018). Examining predictors of self-determination in adults with intellectual and developmental disabilities. *Journal of Developmental and Physical Disabilities*, *30*(5), 601–614. https://doi.org/10.1007/s10882-018-9607-z

Kochhar-Bryant, C. A., & Izzo, M. V. (2006). Access to post-high school services: Transition assessment and the summary of performance. *Career Development for Exceptional Individuals*, *29*, 70–89.

Lam, G. Y. H., Timmons, J., & Zalewska, A. (2023). Program logic model and impacts perceived by stakeholders in a post-school transition program for autistic young adults. *Research in Autism Spectrum Disorders*, *107*, 102220. https://doi.org/10.1016/j.rasd.2023.102220

Larson, S., Eschenbacher, H., Anderson, L., Pettingell, S., & Hewitt, A. (2018). *In-home and residential long-term supports and services for persons with intellectual or developmental disabilities: Status and trends through 2016*. Institute on Community Integration, University of Minnesota. https://ici.umn.edu/products/view/1005

Lee, G. K., & Carter, E. W. (2012). Preparing transition-age students with high-functioning autism spectrum disorders for meaningful work. *Psychology in the School*, *49*(10), 988–1000. https://doi.org/10.1002/pits.21651

Lee, H., & Morningstar, M. E. (2019). Exploring predictors of community participation among young adults with severe disabilities. *Research and Practice for Persons with Severe Disabilities*, *44*(3), 186–199. https://doi.org/10.1177/1540796919863650

Lee, N. R., McQuaid, G. A., Grosman, H. E., Jayaram, S., & Wallace, G. L. (2024). Vocational outcomes in ASD: An examination of work readiness skills as well as barriers and facilitators to employment identified by autistic adults. *Journal of Autism and Developmental Disorders*, *54*(2), 477–490. https://doi.org/10.1007/s10803-022-05804-8

Lindsay, S., Cagliostro, E., Albarico, M., Srikanthan, D., & Mortaji, N. (2018). A systematic review of the role of gender in securing and maintaining employment among youth and young adults with disabilities. *Journal of Occupational Rehabilitation*, *28*(2), 232–251.

Lindsay, S., Varahra, A., Ahmed, H., Abrahamson, S., Pulver, S., Primucci, M., & Wong, K. (2022). Exploring the relationships between race, ethnicity, and school and work outcomes among youth and young adults with disabilities: a scoping review. *Disability and Rehabilitation*, *44*(25), 8110. https://doi.org/10.1080/09638288.2021.2001056

Lindstrom, L., Doren, B., & Miesch, J. (2011). Waging a living: Career development and long-term employment outcomes for young adults with disabilities. *Exceptional Children*, *77*(4), 423–434.

Lund, E. M., & Cmar, J. L. (2020). A systematic review of factors related to employment in transition-age youth with visual impairments. *Rehabilitation Psychology*, *65*(2), 122–136. https://doi.org/10.1037/rep0000303

Mabry, L. (1999). *Portfolios plus: A critical guide to alternative assessment*. Corwin Press.

Matthews, N. L., Smith, C. J., Pollard, E., Ober-Reynolds, S., Kirwan, J., & Malligo, A. (2015). Adaptive functioning in autism spectrum disorder during the transition to adulthood. *Journal of Autism and Developmental Disorders*, *45*(8), 2349–2360. https://doi.org/10.1007/s10803-015-2400-2

Mazzotti, V. L., Rowe, D. A., Kwiatek, S., Voggt, A., Chang, W.-H., Fowler, C. H., Poppen, M., Sinclair, J., & Test, D. W. (2021). Secondary transition predictors of postschool success: An update to the research base. *Career Development and Transition for Exceptional Individuals*, *44*(1), 47–64. https://doi.org/10.1177/2165143420959793

Memmott-Elison, M. K., Moilanen, K. L., & Padilla-Walker, L. M. (2020). Latent growth in self-regulatory subdimensions in relation to adjustment outcomes in youth aged 12–19 [Article]. *Journal of Research on Adolescence*, *30*(3), 651–668. https://doi.org/10.1111/jora.12550

Morningstar, M. E., Kurth, J. A., & Johnson, P. E. (2017). Examining national trends in educational placements for students with significant disabilities. *Remedial and Special Education*, *38*(1), 3–12. https://doi.org/10.1177/0741932516678327

National Center for Education Statistics. (2024). *Students with disabilities: Condition of education*. U.S. Department of Education, Institute of Education Sciences. https://nces.ed.gov/programs/coe/indicator/cgg

National Secondary Transition Technical Assistance Center. (2023). *Age appropriate transition assessment toolkit*. University of North Carolina at Charlotte. https://transitionta.org/wp-content/uploads/docs/TransitionAssessmentToolkit_Updated_2023b.pdf

Neubert, D. A., & Leconte, P. J. (2013). Age-appropriate transition assessment: the position of the division on career development and transition. *Career Development for Exceptional Individuals*, *36*(2), 72–83. https://doi.org/10.1177/2165143413487768

Nigg, J. T. (2017). Annual research review: On the relations among self-regulation, self-control, executive functioning, effortful control, cognitive control, impulsivity, risk-taking, and inhibition for developmental psychopathology. *Journal of Child Psychology and Psychiatry*, *58*(4), 361–383. https://doi.org/10.1111/jcpp.12675

Nisbet, J. (Ed.). (1992). *Natural supports at home, work, and in the community for people with severe disabilities*. Paul H. Brookes.

Nuske, H. J., Shih, W. I., Sparapani, N., Baczewski, L., Dimachkie Nunnally, A., Hochheimer, S., Garcia, C., Castellon, F., Levato, L., Fischer, E., Atkinson-Diaz, Z. L., Li, J., Mandell, D. S., & Kasari, C. (2022). Self-regulation predicts companionship in children with autism. *International Journal of Developmental Disabilities*, *68*(6), 889–899. https://doi.org/10.1080/20473869.2021.1917109

Office of Disability Employment Policy. (2024). *Disability employment statistics*. U.S. Department of Labor. https://www.dol.gov/agencies/odep/research-evaluation/statistics

Ogawa, Y., Itani, O., Jike, M., & Watanabe, N. (2023). Psychosocial interventions for employment of individuals with autism spectrum disorder: a systematic review and meta-analysis of randomized clinical trials. *Review Journal of Autism and Developmental Disorders*, *10*(1), 38–50. https://doi.org/10.1007/s40489-021-00285-4

Oliver, M., & Barnes, C. (1998). *Disabled people and social policy: From exclusion and inclusion*. Addison Wesley Longman.

Orentlicher, M. L. (2018). Participatory action research on the experiences and perceptions of people who receive disability funding through consumer-directed funding models. *Manuscript submitted for publication*.

Orentlicher, M. L. (2019). Best practices in transition planning for independent living and workplace readiness. In G. Frolek Clark, J. E. Rioux, & B. Chandler (Eds.), *Best practices for occupational therapy in schools* (2nd ed., pp. 193–199). AOTA Press.

Orentlicher, M. L., & Case, D. (2018a). Adolescence and ASD. In R. Watling & S. L. Spitzer (Eds.), *Autism across the lifespan: A comprehensive occupational therapy approach* (4th ed., pp. 243–253). AOTA Press.

Orentlicher, M. L., & Case, D. (2018b). Intervention for participation in IADLs and independent living for individuals with ASD. In R. Watling & S. L. Spitzer (Eds.), *Autism across the lifespan: A comprehensive occupational therapy approach* (4th ed., pp. 287–303). AOTA Press.

Orentlicher, M. L., & Gibson, R. W. (2015). Foundations of transition. In M. L. Orentlicher, S. Schefkind, & R. W. Gibson (Eds.), *Transitions across the lifespan: An occupational therapy approach* (pp. 21–30). AOTA Press.

Orum Cattik, E., Dogan Aslan, S., & Ergenekon, Y. (2024). The effectiveness of video model with Bug-in-Ear coaching in the instruction of employment skills to adolescents with autism spectrum disorder. *International Journal of Developmental Disabilities*, 1–14. https://doi.org/10.1080/20473869.2024.2331809

Overmars-Marx, T., Thomése, F., Verdonschot, M., & Meininger, H. (2014). Advancing social inclusion in the neighbourhood for people with an intellectual disability: an exploration of the literature. *Disability & Society*, *29*(2), 255–274.

Papay, C. K., & Bambara, L. M. (2014). Best practices in transition to adult life for youth with intellectual disability. *Career Development and Transition for Exceptional Individuals*, *37*(3), 136–148. https://doi.org/10.1177/2165143413486693

Plotner, A. J., & Marshall, K. J. (2015). Postsecondary education programs for students with an intellectual disability: Facilitators and barriers to implementation. *Intellectual and Developmental Disabilities*, *53*(1), 58–69. https://doi.org/10.1352/1934-9556-53.1.58

Polatajko, H. J., & Mandich, A. (2004). *Enabling occupation in children: The Cognitive Orientation to daily Occupational Performance (CO-OP) Approach*. CAOT Publications ACE.

Prince, A. M. T., Plotner, A. J., & Bridges, W. C. (2019). Postschool engagement predictors for youth with intellectual disability: Results from South Carolina. *Exceptionality*, *27*(4), 247–261. https://doi.org/10.1080/09362835.2018.1480946

Rentschler, L. F., Hume, K. A., & Steinbrenner, J. R. (2023). Building inclusive high school communities for autistic students. *Teaching Exceptional Children*, *56*(2), 98–106.

Reyes, C., Perzynski, A., Kralovic, S., Gerry, T. H., Wexberg, S., Zhu, S., Frazier, T. W., & Roizen, N. (2022). Factors associated with transition planning in autism and other developmental disabilities. *Journal of Developmental and Physical Disabilities*, *34*(1), 43–56. https://doi.org/10.1007/s10882-020-09785-3

Reynolds, M. C., Gotto, G. S., Arnold, C., Boehm, T. L., Magana, S., & Shaffert, R. (2015). National goals for supporting families across the life course. *Inclusion*, *3*(4), 260–268.

Rispoli, K. M., Lee, G. K., Okyere, C., Nelson, S. R., & Norman, M. Z. (2023). Parent expectations for postsecondary transition among youth with ASD: Exploring the role of family mental health. *Contemporary School Psychology*, *28*, 524–536. https://doi.org/10.1007/s40688-023-00466-4

Ruhl, H., Dolan, E. A., & Buhrmester, D. (2015). Adolescent attachment trajectories with mothers and fathers: The importance of parent-child relationship experiences and gender. *Journal of Research on Adolescence*, *25*(3), 427–442. https://doi.org/10.1111/jora.12144

Salon, R. S., Boutot, N., Ozols, K., Keeton, B., & Steveley, J. (2019). New approaches to customized employment: Enhancing cross-system partnerships. *Journal of Vocational Rehabilitation*, *50*(3), 317–323. https://doi.org/10.3233/jvr-191013

Schlegelmilch, A., Roskowski, M., Anderson, C., Hartman, E., & Decker-Maurer, H. (2019). The impact of work incentives benefits counseling on employment outcomes of transition-age youth receiving Supplemental Security Income (SSI) benefits. *Journal of Vocational Rehabilitation*, *51*(2), 127–136. https://doi.org/10.3233/jvr-191032

Schoonover, J. (2019). Best practices in Universal Design for Learning. In G. Frolek Clark, J. E. Rioux, & B. E. Chandler (Eds.), *Best practices for occupational therapy in schools* (2nd ed., pp. 161–176). AOTA Press.

Schoonover, J. W., & Orentlicher, M. L. (2015). Supportive environments for transition. In M. L. Orentlicher, S. Schefkind, & R. W. Gibson (Eds.), *Transitions across the lifespan: An occupational therapy approach* (pp. 213–236). AOTA Press.

Schutz, M. A., & Carter, E. W. (2022). Elevating the employment outcomes of transition-age youth with disabilities: Four decades of intervention research. *Journal of Vocational Rehabilitation*, *57*(1), 1–21. https://doi.org/10.3233/jvr-221194

Shogren, K., Wehmeyer, M., Palmer, S., Rifenbark, G., & Little, T. (2015). Relationships between self-determination and postschool outcomes for youth with disabilities. *Journal of Special Education*, *48*(4), 256–267.

Siperstein, G. N., Heyman, M., & Stokes, J. E. (2014). Pathways to employment: A national survey of adults with intellectual disabilities. *Journal of Vocational Rehabilitation*, *41*(3), 165–178. https://doi.org/10.3233/JVR-140711

Sitlington, P. L., Neubert, D. A., Begun, W. H., Lombard, R. C., & Lecconte, P. J. (2007). *Assess for success: A practitioner's handbook on transition assessment* (2nd ed.). Corwin Press.

Smith, F., Grigal, M., & Shepard, J. (2018). Postsecondary education and employment outcomes for youth with intellectual disability served by vocational rehabilitation. *Think College Fast Facts*, (18), 1–2.

Spence-Cochran, K., Pearl, C. E., & Walker, Z. (2013). Full inclusion into schools: Strategies for collaborative instruction. In P. Wehman (Ed.), *Life beyond the classroom: Transition strategies for young people with disabilities* (5th ed., pp. 175–195). Paul H. Brookes.

Stöppler, M. C., & Shiel, W. C. (2022). Puberty. *MedicineNet*. https://www.medicinenet.com/puberty/article.htm

Sung, C., Sánchez, J., Kuo, H.-J., Wang, C.-C., & Leahy, M. J. (2015). Gender differences in vocational rehabilitation service predictors of successful competitive employment for transition-aged individuals with autism. *Journal of Autism and Developmental Disorders*, *45*(10), 3204–3218. https://doi.org/10.1007/s10803-015-2480-z

Tamm, L., Day, H. A., & Duncan, A. (2022). Comparison of adaptive functioning measures in adolescents with autism spectrum disorder without intellectual disability. *Journal of Autism and Developmental Disorders*, *52*(3), 1247–1256. https://doi.org/10.1007/s10803-021-05013-9

Targett, P., & Wehman, P. (2013). Families and young people with disabilities: Listening to their voices. In P. Wehman (Ed.), *Life beyond the classroom: Transition strategies for young people with disabilities* (5th ed., pp. 69–94). Paul H. Brookes.

TASH. (2009). *TASH resolution on integrated employment*. http://tash.org/advocacy-issues/employment/

Test, D. W., Fowler, C. H., Richter, S. M., White, J., Mazzotti, V., Walker, A. R., Kohler, P., & Kortering, L. (2009). Evidence-based practices in secondary transition. *Career Development for Exceptional Individuals*, *32*, 115–128.

Toglia, J. P. (2005). A dynamic interactional approach to cognitive rehabilitation. In N. Katz (Ed.), *Cognition and occupation across the lifespan: Models for intervention in occupational therapy* (2nd ed., pp. 29–72). American Occupational Therapy Association.

Torres, A., Kearney, K. B., Berlingo, L., & Brady, M. P. (2022). "What ELSE about this job?" Teaching job decision-making to college students with intellectual and developmental disabilities. *Journal of Developmental and Physical Disabilities*, *34*(4), 673–692. https://doi.org/10.1007/s10882-021-09820-x

Trainor, A. A., Carter, E. W., Swedeen, B., & Pickett, K. (2012). Community conversations: An approach for expanding and connecting opportunities for employment for adolescents with disabilities. *Career Development for Exceptional Individuals*, *35*, 50–60. https://doi.org/10.1177/0885728811419166

Vigna, E., Meek, A., & Beyer, S. (2024). Supported employment, quality of jobs and employment typicalness: the experience of the Engage to Change project. *Journal of Applied Research in Intellectual Disabilities*, *37*(3), e13226. https://doi.org/10.1111/jar.13226

Villaescusa, M., Martínez-Rueda, N., & Fernández, A. (2021). Support for families of youths and adults with intellectual disabilities: contributions of a program from families' and specialists' perspectives. *Education Sciences*, *11*(2), 88. https://doi.org/10.3390/educsci11020088

Wagner, M., Cameto, R., & Newman, L. (2003). *Youth with disabilities: A changing population*. SRI International.

Wagner, M., Newman, L. A., & Javitz, H. S. (2017). Vocational education course taking and post-high school employment of youth with emotional disturbances. *Career Development and Transition for Exceptional Individuals*, *40*(2), 132–143. https://doi.org/10.1177/2165143415626399

Wehman, P. (2013). Transition: New horizons and challenges. In P. Wehman (Ed.), *Life beyond the classroom: Transition strategies for young people with disabilities* (5th ed., pp. 3–39). Paul H. Brookes.

Wehman, P., & Brooke, V. (2013). Securing meaningful work in the community. In P. Wehman (Ed.), *Life beyond the classroom: Transition strategies for young people with disabilities* (5th ed., pp. 309–337). Paul H. Brookes.

Wehman, P., Chan, F., Ditchman, N., & Kang, H. J. (2014). Effect of supported employment on vocational rehabilitation outcomes of transition-age youth with intellectual and developmental disabilities: A case control study. *Intellectual and Developmental Disabilities*, *52*(4), 296–310.

Wehman, P., Schall, C., McDonough, J., Sima, A., Brooke, A., Ham, W., Whittenburg, H., Brooke, V., Avellone, L., & Riehle, E. (2020). Competitive employment for transition-aged youth with significant impact from autism: A multi-site randomized clinical trial. *Journal of Autism and Developmental Disorders*, *50*(6), 1882–1897. https://doi.org/10.1007/s10803-019-03940-2

Wehman, P., Taylor, J., Brooke, V., Avellone, L., Whittenburg, H., Ham, W., Brooke, A. M., & Carr, S. (2018). Toward competitive employment for persons with intellectual and developmental disabilities: What progress have we made and where do we need to go. *Research and Practice for Persons with Severe Disabilities*, *43*(3), 131–144. https://doi.org/10.1177/1540796918777730

Wehmeyer, M. (2015). Framing the future: Self-determination. *Remedial and Special Education*, *36*, 20–23.

Wehmeyer, M. L. (2014). Self-determination: a family affair. *Family Relations*, *63*(1), 178–184. http://www.jstor.org/stable/43695339

Wehmeyer, M., & Kelchner, K. (1995). *The Arc's Self-Determination Scale: Adolescent version* http://www.thearc.org/document.doc?id=3670

White, J., & Weiner, J. S. (2004). Influence of least restrictive environment and community based training on integrated employment outcomes for transitioning students with severe disabilities. *Journal of Vocational Rehabilitation*, *21*(3), 149–156.

Whittenburg, H. N., Xu, Y., Thoma, C. A., Schall, C., & Ham, W. (2022). Effects of behavioral skills training with video modeling and In Situ training on workplace conversational skills of students with autism. *Focus on Autism and Other Developmental Disabilities*, *38*(3), 188–198. https://doi.org/10.1177/10883576221127971

Williams, B., Lo, W. J., Hill, J., Ezike, N., & Huddleston, J. (2019). Employment supports in early work experiences for transition-age youth with disabilities who receive Supplemental Security Income (SSI). *Journal of Vocational Rehabilitation*, *51*(2), 159–166. https://doi.org/10.3233/jvr-191035

Woods-Groves, S., Balint-Langel, K., Rodgers, D. B., Song, H., & Hendrickson, J. M. (2023). College students with intellectual and developmental disabilities use assistive technology in living, learning, and working tasks: A 20-year systematic review and meta-analysis. *Education and Training in Autism and Developmental Disabilities*, *58*(4), 375–395.

Xu, L., Ma, L., & Duan, P. (2022). Relationship between perceived parental academic expectations and students' self-regulated learning ability: A cross-sectional study. *Frontiers in Psychology*, *13*. https://doi.org/10.3389/fpsyg.2022.786298

Index

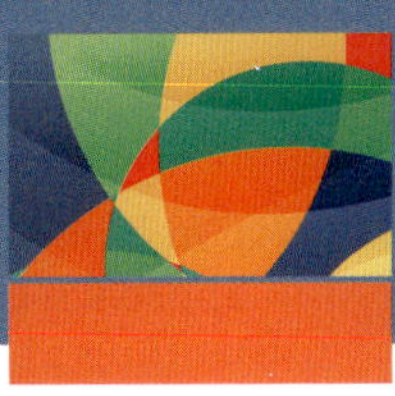

Note: Page numbers followed by "f" indicate figures and "t" indicate tables.

B

P

T

V

Z